Healing Passage

A Midwife's Guide to the Care and Repair of the Tissues Involved in Birth

Sixth Edition

Anne Frye, CPM

BA, Holistic Midwifery

Illustrated by Rhonda Baker

Labrys Press
a division of
Matrix Midwifery Enterprises, Ltd.
Portland, Oregon

Sixth edition, 5000 copies
Printed in the United States of America on acid-free paper by Sheridan Books, Inc., Chelsea, MI

ISBN: 978-1-891145-58-2

Library of Congress Control Number: 2007907324

Previous editions:
1st ed (1982); 2nd ed (1982); 3rd ed (1985) SUTURING FOR MIDWIVES
4th ed (1991) HEALING PASSAGE: A SUTURING MANUAL FOR MIDWIVES
5th ed (1995) HEALING PASSAGE: A MIDWIFE'S GUIDE TO THE CARE AND REPAIR OF THE TISSUES INVOLVED IN BIRTH

Other publications by Anne Frye and Labrys Press:
UNDERSTANDING DIAGNOSTIC TESTS IN THE CHILDBEARING YEAR: A HOLISTIC GUIDE
HOLISTIC MIDWIFERY, A COMPREHENSIVE TEXTBOOK FOR MIDWIVES IN HOMEBIRTH PRACTICE:
Volume I: Care during Pregnancy
Volume II: Care during Labor and Birth
SUTURING TECHNIQUES FOR MIDWIVES (DVD)
FEMALE PELVIC ANATOMY (DVD)

For more information or customer service, please contact:
Labrys Press, 7528 NE Oregon St., Portland, OR 97213 USA
(503) 255-3378 FAX (503) 255-1474
I have three web addresses all of which take you to the same home page:
http://www.midwiferybooks.com
http//www.LabrysPress.com
http://www.AnneFrye.com E-mail me at: info@midwiferybooks.com

Call or visit the web site regarding current editions and pricing. Please report any defects in materials or workmanship as soon as they are noted. A mechanism can be found on the web site for posting errors you may discover in the text. Additions to the texts as well as noted errors along with corrections are posted there as well. Go to the home page of the title you want to check out and you will find a link to any changes that have been posted.

ACKNOWLEDGMENTS

Thanks to the following individuals whose input and support made this book possible:

·To Rhonda Baker for her beautiful artwork, as always, an invaluable contribution to the text.

·To Randy Baker, a graphics wizard, who not only used the computer to label most of the drawings that required it, but taught me how to do it as well.

·To Eiris Baldwin and K Hindall for their editing expertise.

·To John DeLancey, who was kind enough to answer several e-mails early in the process of my research into pelvic anatomy. I am grateful to him for not only pointing me in the right direction for my research but also being such a prolific writer on a variety of topics: his work is heavily referenced in this text.

·To Bev Standish for working on the animation for the anatomy DVD, which helped me understand the 3-dimensional relationships of the parts much more clearly.

·To Jennifer Warnock, a rising star in the midwifery community, who was a student at Birthingway College of Midwifery. She pointed me toward the information that led to my complete rewrite of the chapter covering pelvic floor preparation. Her untimely death in February, 2010 saddened the entire local birth community and represents a real loss to both midwives and mothers.

·To the several others who have helped with suggestions for topics to include or editing or both, including Holly Scholles, Rhonda Baker, Kerri-Anne Gifford, Holly Scholles and Karen Strange.

·To Sara Wickham for responding to a desperate e-mail question in the middle of her night on the eve of my finishing the book.

·To all of you, my readers, whose positive energy and enthusiasm for my work is more helpful than you know.

PREFACE

This book, now in its sixth edition, is required reading in most of the midwifery schools in North America. This new edition includes such sweeping changes that it renders all previous editions obsolete. Rhonda and I have worked diligently to create accurate visual representations of the anatomy, many of them new, and the anatomy section includes much exciting new information. The knot tying chapter as well as those on repairing the external and internal anal sphincters have also undergone intense revisions, as have many other parts of the book. As a result, the book has almost doubled in size.

While material still builds on itself throughout the text, sections have been rearranged a bit to provide a better flow of information, while maintaining the flow from theoretical and background material to clinical application as much as possible. A great deal of detail has been added to all instructional and clinically intense chapters to enhance learning and understanding for students.

As usual, just as I was ready to go to press, I was presented with new information that needed to be addressed. This entailed an extra week or so of research to understand more about prion diseases and how they are being addressed as far as decontamination and sterility is concerned both here and abroad.

So, I present to you the 6th edition of HEALING PASSAGE. I trust it will continue to serve as a significant learning tool for all those who care for women in childbirth.

Sincerely,

Anne Frye
Portland, OR

June 25, 2010

About the Title

Birth is a healing rite of passage for mothers, their newborns and families, and frequently for their midwives as well. As such, it has the powerful potential to transform the lives of women and all those whom birth touches.

So, it is with recognition of the multifaceted healing that birth represents that I have named this book "Healing Passage." Even though it focuses largely on the physical aspects of protecting and caring for the passages of birth, we must never forget that the physical is but a very small part of a process larger than ourselves: the means by which life renews itself.

Table of Contents

How to Use This Manual

This textbook is intended as a complete midwifery-level guide to the care and repair of the perineum and related tissues. Read it through once to familiarize yourself with the entire content. If you have access to the companion suturing techniques DVD (the first edition of which was sold as a video tape), review the lessons you will find on the PDF "DVD manual" file on the DVD as you study the book.

The book is written in a progressive fashion, with information building on previous topics. Complete information about a given subject may not be repeated in every section. Details that are most critical are reiterated where appropriate. Notes are inserted to inform you when it may be important to go back and review another section before you begin the one that follows; in that way, comprehension will be enhanced and no vital information overlooked.

Terminology and phonetic spelling

I have tried to define all terms directly related to suturing that may be new to students. However, the text assumes a basic knowledge of maternal and fetal structures. If some terms are unfamiliar, I recommend TABER'S CYCLOPEDIC MEDICAL DICTIONARY as an excellent reference. Directional terms used in the anatomy descriptions are covered in my HOLISTIC MIDWIFERY, VOL. I. A few vocabulary changes have been incorporated into the language of this text because I feel they are more accurate than those currently in use. These are as follows:

Surgical delivery or surgical birth: To emphasize that a Cesarean is major surgery, I shall refer to Cesarean section as a "surgical delivery" or "surgical birth."

Clitorotomy: The clitoris (not the yoni) is the focal point of the more superficial parts of the female pelvic structures and is a far more complex organ than is generally understood. Acknowledging this changes the emphasis of how we think of the pelvic region. It also changes the understanding of what we do when we cut a woman's perineal body. When the female genitals are cut, circulatory tissues and nerves linked to the clitoris are cut as well. The yoni is surrounded by clitoral tissues, making it a clitoral orifice. To help dispel the rather cavalier attitude regarding this form of genital mutilation, which takes place frequently in the United States and other Western countries, this text will refer to the procedure commonly known as an "episiotomy" by the name "clitorotomy," which means "to cut the clitoris." As you read the chapters in the part entitled "Pertinent Anatomy," you will understand why.

Yoni: Matteo Realdo (a.k.a. Renaldus) Colombo (1559) was the first medical figure to name the birth passage the "vagina." Most midwives I have talked to have been as appalled as I was to learn that the Latin word "vagina" means "scabbard," that is, a sheath for a sword. Given this meaning, it is likely that this was also a slang term for "woman" used by Latin-speaking men in earlier centuries. When I asked Sheila Kitzinger (who has done extensive research into word origins used in obstetrics) if there wasn't a friendlier word in some other language, she said that most words from other languages meant something even worse. I guess the patriarchy doesn't think much of women's genitals other than how they can serve men. The obvious lack of respect, sadism and overt misogyny implied in this word have led me to conclude that midwives should launch a campaign for the adoption of a more enlightened term.

After discussing this with many other midwives and brainstorming for possible words to use instead of "vagina," most liked "yoni" as an alternative. "Yoni" is a Sanskrit word that is used in various contexts, including referral to the vulva, genitalia or vagina. The yoni is a primary object of Tantric worship, representing the Great Mother. It's original meaning is "source or origin of life." It later acquired a secondary meaning: "divine passage." It thus seems a respectful and fitting substitute for the name of the birth canal. Because of these meanings, even though the translation is not precise, this book will replace the word "vagina" with the word "yoni." For the sake of continuity with other texts, terms that incorporate the word "vagina" (such as pubovaginal) will remain unchanged. Although I do not expect that the term "yoni" will formally replace "vagina" in the literature, I think it is important for at least one source to raise consciousness on this issue.

YBAC: Now that I've decided to change the term "vagina" to "yoni," what about the phrase "vaginal birth after Cesarean"?" I have decided to call it "yoni birth after Cesarean": YBAC.

Phonetics: I have included a phonetic spelling for most anatomical words because they may not frequently be spoken aloud or are confusing to pronounce. Most of them appear in the chapters in the part entitled "Pertinent Anatomy," where the word is introduced for the first time.

Vocabulary used on the audiovisual aid: I have decided not to incorporate any vocabulary changes into the audio track when I revise the video into a DVD. This is primarily because this production is used in a wide variety of domestic and international settings. I wanted to avoid unnecessary confusion for viewers that may result from hearing unfamiliar words as there was not adequate time on the DVD itself to explain the reasoning behind changes in terminology.

To students of suturing

This book assumes you know basically nothing about suturing and related topics. It begins with lessons on anatomy and moves on to the primary skills you will need when you begin to attend births so you can protect the perineum from tearing. Then it covers the basic manual skills needed to use the instruments. Finally, it covers how to perform repairs when tears do occur.

By writing this guide and providing the suturing techniques DVD, I do not mean to imply that supervised hands-on training is not important. If you are a student, ideally you will read the book cover to cover and work with the DVD until you are proficient with basic techniques. This will minimize feeling overwhelmed when you begin hands-on clinical training. After you have at least begun to feel proficient with basic techniques, I hope you will avail yourself of training with the midwife or educational program of your choice.

The tissues of the yoni, as one doctor told me, are very forgiving. Therefore, you can get away with simple repairs without much experience; healing will usually turn out fine. Even so, there is no excuse for poor technique. Although it is possible to do basic suturing without training (and, yes, that is how I started), it is also essential not to assume that you can proceed in all situations with no prior supervision. Don't be arrogant about what you can and cannot do without supervision or, at the very least, some experience followed by clinical instruction (i.e., watching and discussing more complicated repairs). If you are in a situation where unsupervised learning is your only option, scrupulously monitor the healing of all repairs so that mistakes in technique can be corrected. Furthermore, you must always explain to your clients the limits of your training, skills and experience.

On the other hand, repairs of the cervix, anterior yoni wall or anal regions need to be done right the first time. These areas are not forgiving, and mistakes can cause serious, long-term problems. As a rule of thumb, unless you have absolutely no alternative, you should not perform repairs in these areas without first having plenty of experience with simple repairs that heal well, followed by clinical observation, instruction and, preferably, supervision of your skills with more complex repairs. Even though I have extensive knowledge and experience in repairing a variety of tears, I have only repaired two third- or fourth-degree tears and have never repaired a cervix or the upper wall of the yoni. (The one woman I have seen with a nasty upper yoni vault tear, I transported.)

I do, however, recognize that midwives are working all over the world in a wide variety of settings and many simply have no alternative but to perform complex repairs themselves. I also know that there may be times when midwives working in more resource-rich environments cannot transport for some reason. Therefore, because I feel it is important for you to understand what is entailed, every variety of repair is explained in this text. If you do get stuck with no other choice but to proceed yourself, far better for you to have detailed information about what is indicated than not.

Locating subject matter

Although the book is laid out in a logical order, not everything is in sequence. Information that is needed only rarely is not included in the main sequence format. Here is a master list of topics covered, incorporating all the possible procedures in the appropriate order. This order may vary slightly depending upon the individual situation. Exceptions are discussed in the appropriate chapters. The bold items are the techniques and procedures you'll be using most frequently:

1. **Allow time for mother-infant interaction immediately after birth (p. 464).**
2. **Make sure the placenta is born and the mother and baby are stable (p. 464).**
3. Position the mother for examination (p. 467).
4. **Wash your hands (p. 438) and don sterile gloves (p. 443).**
5. **Examine the perineum for damage (p. 466).**
6. **Assess the degree of damage (if any) and the need for repair (p. 484).**
7. Staunch bleeding from lacerated blood vessel(s) (p. 571).
8. Catheterize to assess upper yoni wall damage (p. 566).
9. **If needed, prepare the mother for repair (p. 492).**

10. Set up equipment (p. 492).
11. Administer anesthetic (p. 429).
12. If the tear is extensive, insert a retractor (p. 421).
13. Repair the cervix (p. 562).
14. Remove skin tags at the introitus that may interfere with yoni repair (p. 554).
15. Repair the anterior yoni wall (p. 566).
16. Insert a tampon (p. 495).
17. Repair the rectal mucosa (p. 528).
18. Check rectally and remove misplaced sutures (pp. 530, 532).
19. Repair the internal anal sphincter (p. 536).
20. Check rectally and remove misplaced sutures (pp. 530, 532).
21. Repair the external anal sphincter (p. 534).
22. Check rectally and remove misplaced sutures (pp. 530, 532).
23. Remove inclusion cysts (p. 569).
24. Repair the posterior yoni wall (p. 504).
25. Place a deep layer of stitches in the posterior yoni wall, if necessary (p. 511, 512).
26. Check rectally and remove misplaced sutures (pp. 530, 532).
27. Remove the retractor, if in place (p. 421).
28. Repair the subcutaneous tissue of the perineum (p. 517).
29. Repair the subcuticular tissue of the perineum (p. 519).
30. Remove or repair skin tags at the introitus (p. 555).
31. Repair the periurethral and labia area (p.550).
32. Remove the tampon (p. 522).
33. Remove debris from the area (p. 522).
34. Account for all needles, pieces of gauze and other materials used so as not to leave them in the repair or the bedclothes (p. 522).
35. Clean and sterilize equipment (p. 334).

The part entitled "Pertinent Anatomy"

Even if you have already studied pelvic anatomy extensively, you *still* need to study this section because it includes loads of updated information on such structures as the urethral musculature, the clitoris and the levator ani muscles. Understanding female pelvic anatomy is fundamental to grasping much of the information that follows. Study it thoroughly before proceeding to the rest of the text. I know some of you who have been practicing a while are thinking maybe you can just tiptoe by that chapter and I won't notice. After all, you've gotten this far without any more than the vaguest understanding of the perineal muscles. You figure, why torture yourself again trying to learn them when it has always been so fruitless? I have felt the same way, and we are not alone.

Clarity is especially elusive when trying to understand the levator ani muscles. Kearney and colleagues (2004) did a thorough literature review and found that, although the origin–insertion pairs quoted for these muscles were relatively consistent among authors, the terminology used to name the muscles was not. They found 16 terms used for the five primary components of this muscle complex. This overabundant terminology compounds the difficulty in understanding the shape and function of these, the most difficult to understand of all the clinically important muscles. In addition, the tendency to refer to male anatomy as the default with sometimes peripheral or no mention of corresponding female anatomy (or no clarification of the differences between the two anatomies), renders writings on the pelvic floor confusing even for seasoned researchers and leaves little wonder why students have such a hard time understanding it.

Please, give it one more shot. This section has consistently been daunting to research and difficult to write. Through great effort on my part, much that was wrong in the previous editions has been corrected. I really think that now you will "get it" if you go through the chapter carefully and then explore it in three dimensions by constructing the model described in the APPENDICES. If nothing else, doesn't the thought of making a pelvic model of the soft tissues excite you? And coloring by number? If so, read on.

Illustrations

Many of the illustrations in the part entitled "Pertinent Anatomy" are an attempt to marry tissue relationships based on living MRI images with the detail that can only be obtained during dissections. This must be kept in mind during your studies as there is nothing precise about these illustrations. Even though every effort has been made to be as accurate as possible, there are very few reference drawings to work from as we attempt to depict the anatomy as accurately as possible. In the remaining text, drawings emphasize certain anatomical features or the path and direction of the suture. Therefore, most of those showing repairs are not embellished with hands, needles, etc. Needle entry and exit points are indicated by small arrows. All sequences of drawings proceed from left to right. To simplify and focus the illustrations, some anatomical features may be left out. Likewise, even though an attempt has been made to be anatomically correct, it is difficult to demonstrate the actual depth of tissue layers (particularly muscle layers) in a flat illustration. Therefore, the drawings demonstrating stitches are to give you a general idea of the anatomy and a specific idea of the techniques. If in doubt, refer to the text for accurate anatomical relationships.

Measurements

Because virtually all references address anatomical measurements in metric terms, measurements are given in centimeters. All inch equivalents below are correct within a thirty-second of an inch.

0.64 cm = 0.25 inch	1.95 cm = 0.75 inch	5.0 cm = 2 inches
1.00 cm = = ⅜ inch	2.54 cm = 1.0 inch	7.0 cm = 2.75 inches
1.27 cm. = 0.5 inch	2.70 cm = 1⅛ inch	7.5 cm = 3 inches
1.60 cm. = ⅝ inch	3.50 cm = 1⅜ inch	10 cm = 4 inches
1.70 cm. = ⅔ inch	4.0 cm = 1⅝ inch	14 cm = 5.5 inches

If you are left-hand dominant

All of the written descriptions can be followed by persons with either hand dominant. The drawings and most of the suturing DVD presentations are demonstrated for right-hand–dominant techniques. The illustrations in the chapter entitled "Tying Surgical Knots" have been printed for right-hand–dominant students as well. If you are left-handed and are having trouble visualizing other maneuvers from your point of view, prop the book in front of a mirror so you can see the reverse images as you practice. When you have time, visit my website at (www.LabrysPress.com), go to the home page for HEALING PASSAGE and find the link for left-hand–dominant readers. There, you will find a PDF file with the left-hand dominant version of the knot-tying chapter that you can print out.

References

Each introductory chapter ends with its own list of references. Titled sections each end with lists of references that were used for the preceding chapters. Those references used for more than one chapter are grouped together at the beginning of each bibliographical chapter under a separate header. The chapters at the beginning of the text each have their own reference list (as below) when relevant.

Index listings

Index listings that include the word "about" indicate that more details are included about the topic, beginning on the page listed, at that location. The "about" listings often start on the page noted and extend for one or more of the pages that follow.

REFERENCES AND FURTHER READING

Colombo MR. DE RE ANATOMICA. LIBRI XV. Venetiis, ex. Typog. N. Beuilacquose, 1559. Quoted by Krantz KE. "The gross and microscopic anatomy of the human vagina," ANN NY ACAD SCI, 83(2):89-104, Nov 18, 1959.

Haubrich W. MEDICAL MEANINGS: A GLOSSARY OF WORD ORIGINS. Harcourt Brace Jovanovich, San Diego CA, 1984.

Kearney R, et al. "Levator ani muscle anatomy evaluated by origin-insertion pairs," OBSTET GYNECOL, 104(1):168-173, Jul, 2004.

Ethical Considerations

The practice of midwifery: An ethic of risk

For the past 800 years or so, a concerted effort has been put forth to wipe out midwifery. Erasing midwifery was attempted in a literal fashion during the burning times, a grizzly holocaust that persisted for hundreds of years throughout Europe. Together, the church and state tried to subdue the general population by killing their healers and midwives, who were often accused of consorting with the devil and branded as witches; some estimate, based on records dated after 1486, that as many as nine million women were murdered (Starhawk, 1982), although this high figure has been disputed by other scholars. No one knows how many unrecorded deaths took place prior to 1486. It is known that, in some cases, entire villages were left without a single living woman. Today most history books either leave out this holocaust altogether or gloss over it, to the point that it seems like only a very few women actually met their death. Likewise, most texts never mention the special persecution of midwives. A third instance of historical revision occurs when researchers and historians claim that the dawn of obstetrics was also the dawn of midwifery and men are named exclusively as the fathers of midwifery. (This revision effectively erases women's central role in the work of birth for thousands of years beforehand and helped to transfer the work of birth into the hands of men.)

Even today, the struggle continues. Right now, independent midwives are legally restricted from practice for daring to stand for the higher ethics of personal freedom of practice and upholding the right of individuals to choose their health care. Midwives are arrested for practicing in states that won't legally recognize them. Should a baby die at home, the midwife is frequently held responsible automatically; this assumption can occur even in states where she is practicing legally and is almost inevitable if she is practicing where she is not legally recognized.

Nurse-midwifery, by its very nature, attempts to stay within the dotted lines of what our patriarchal culture accepts. Even so, nurse-midwives frequently find that the more noninterventively they practice, the more they stand up for the rights of the woman and not the policies of the institutions in which they work, the more flack and the less support they receive. It was nurse-midwives who coined the term "burn-out."

Like our sisters before us, we are so busy doing what obviously and desperately needs to be done that self-protection is usually not our primary concern. Once we step out of the arena of seeking the approval of the fathers (patriarchy) and into the woman's wilderness of taking responsibility and helping other women do the same, we are taking risks. As is true whenever women stand up for themselves against the status quo, for whatever reason, everything we do can be seen in this light. When we see babies born at home and not taken from their mothers, when we see women have a healing birth experience rather than coming home from the hospital battered and abused, the ethical choices we have made to practice (even without the sanction of the medical or legal community) are so clear. When a nurse-midwife literally holds her foot against the door to keep the doctors at bay so a woman can have her baby in the position she chooses without being cut, she also takes a risk. Therefore, we must learn to view our actions with this ethic of risk in mind. The ultimate price today, most likely, would be our freedom. In the past, the ultimate price has been our lives. In the midst of this risk-taking, the decision to include suturing in your practice still stands out as a controversial issue. I shall attempt to explore some of those issues here.

Should you learn to suture?

In the United States, professional independent midwifery once again came into its own with the advent of the Certified Professional Midwife (CPM) credential in the 1990s. This nationally standardized avenue to credentialing is what I think of as a "gateway" process because one can become a CPM via a variety of educational routes. This is not true of nurse-midwives, who must complete a university-based educational program in order to become credentialed. The CPM process includes a psychometrically sound written examination. This exam has been offered to state governments, to allow them to bypass the cumbersome process of formulating and overseeing their own test. As of October 2008, 24 states have accepted the examination as part of their state licensure process and the CPM credential itself as an avenue to licensure. With this process came a more explicit understanding of what constitutes midwifery-model care. In particular, most midwives agreed that suturing and urinary catheterization should be included in the scope of practice of all CPMs.

Even so, controversy still exists among some independent midwives about whether suturing is an appropriate midwifery skill. For licensed midwives, the advantage is obvious. Nonetheless, many still point to the medical and technical nature of these skills. Some feel that while suturing is important, it should take place in a hospital, that the need for stitches places the situation outside the realm of "normal" and beyond our domain. Many CPMs note that they have few tears and get good results without suturing the ones they see. Therefore, although they must have some training in suturing to qualify for their CPM, they do not feel the need to apply suturing in their practice and, due to a lack of regular use of the skills involved, may not feel confident about suturing when it is needed. Finally, many midwives who still practice in settings where formal education is out of reach hesitate to suture, quite reasonably, because they have had no clinical training. All of these considerations have ethical overtones. Part of your decision to suture will be based, no doubt, on practicalities. If you live and work rurally, far from hospital care, suturing may be a necessity. On the other hand, if good backup is down the street, you may feel it is not worth the bother of learning.

There may also be feelings that suturing is a form of violence. It is daunting to contemplate inserting a needle into living tissue, and it is certainly violent in that sense yet sometimes a small violence (such as pruning a hedge, weeding a garden or suturing a tear) yields the healthiest result. Plus, knowing how to suture avoids taking women to the hospital, where they may be subjected to separation from their infant and, depending on the hospital, negative ideas about homebirth, which has been known to adversely impact the care they receive.

If you question whether to learn suturing or not, I suggest talking to different midwives and examining what else you are willing or unwilling to do in your practice. In this way you will gain clarity about where you are drawing lines and why. This will aid your decision-making process. At the same time you should keep in mind that knowing how to suture is one more powerful tool you can use to insulate women from the mainstream medical system.

Practicing medicine without a license: If you are a nurse-midwife, this may not be a big issue for you (although it may be if you are forbidden to practice at home or in the way you choose). If you are an RN practicing as an independent midwife, however, state nursing regulations may leave you more restricted than your licensed or unlicensed independent midwife sisters.

In states where independent midwifery is still illegal, just about everything we do as competent practicing midwives constitutes practicing medicine without a license. In some places, practice may constitute a misdemeanor with a fine of a few hundred dollars, while in others it may be classified as a felony with a penalty of years in jail or a massive fine. Many states define the practice of medicine in economic terms (i.e., those who get paid for rendering medical assistance); others, in terms of what is actually done. In general, diagnosing, prescribing and surgery to treat any physical condition are the principle things considered to be within the jurisdiction of physicians. Exceptions are made, however, for nurse-midwives and, in some states, licensed independent midwives, who are legally permitted to cut and repair clitorotomies and to prescribe certain pharmaceutical agents in specific situations (e.g., oxytocin to stop a hemorrhage).

In regions where there is no independent midwifery regulation or where minimal laws exist, independent midwifery practice is legal by technicality only. Diagnosing and treating common discomforts of pregnancy, performing surgery (e.g., cutting clitorotomies, if necessary, and sewing tears), administering prescription or herbal agents for hemorrhage, administering oxygen for fetal distress, as well as performing internal exams, may all be within the domain of practicing medicine, depending upon where you live. If the state wanted to prosecute a midwife on these points, it could be done with the greatest of ease.

Therefore, if you are avoiding suturing because you don't want to break the law, but you still do any of these other things, you are already breaking the law. Alternatively, almost everything mentioned above can remain between yourself and your clients. Sutures, once placed, cannot be removed. If a problem arises postpartum that necessitates hospital care or doctor consultation, there is a good possibility that your stitches will be discovered. This is the source of a real dilemma: if you do suture and further postpartum problems arise, you may be tempted to postpone transport or consultation. If your midwife or doctor backup is supportive, the discovery of your repair may not be an issue, but taking a woman to a strange doctor or not-too-supportive hospital may create an unwanted uproar about your practice.

Choosing not to suture also presents legal and ethical challenges. On the one hand, transporting for repair places some midwives in a compromised legal position if they are in an illegal jurisdiction. On the other hand, not transporting may leave a tear unsutured that clearly needs repair. If you don't suture a tear that really needs it, you will be practicing negligently.

If you practice in a gray legal situation or your practice is frankly illegal, think through your options and about reactions should you suture and then need medical assistance for your client. You may decide, despite the hassle, it is simplest and safest to transport your clients for repairs. Another possibility is to wait a couple of hours after the birth to suture. Those first few hours hold the highest risk for a critical emergency, so you reduce the chances of raising a furor over your work if you wait to see if transport will be necessary.

Other considerations include how you feel about practicing illegally in general, and how you will explain possession of suture materials and other regulated accoutrements (anesthetic, syringes, etc.).

Whatever you decide, it is important that you feel clear about what you are doing. To be harboring paranoia about getting caught will only draw you into unpleasant situations. Be aware and be careful, but be proud of what you do and know you have a right to do it. It does not do you, your clients or the midwifery community any good for you to practice in fear.

When clients refuse sutures

Parents who have strong feelings regarding ways of dealing with complications usually make this known during the consultation visit. If a woman does not want to be sutured, she will usually tell you then. That may be one reason she is seeking a homebirth or independent midwifery care in the first place. You need to ask further questions to clarify what she means. No sutures under any circumstances? What about a torn anal sphincter or extensive upper vault damage? Does she understand the consequences of her decision, such as possible incontinence? Be sure you are clear with her about your professional limits. Can you, in good conscience, agree to forego suturing or transport to the hospital in a situation that may leave her permanently rectally incontinent as a result? Does she really understand what this means? Discuss why she feels this way. You may uncover feelings about previous traumatic experiences or inaccurate beliefs about suturing that you can clarify or correct.

Leaving minimal to moderate second–degree tears unsutured and caring for the area with herbs and reduced activity is a controversial practice that has been widely used in the US and UK. While minimal damage can heal well with proper care, there are no good, long-term studies to confirm what the lasting impact of not suturing will be on a wide range of important outcome variables. Tears should be left to heal on their own only when a woman has minimal damage and clearly refuses suturing. How to tell which tears these are and why leaving tears unsutured may not be advisable will be explored at appropriate points throughout the book.

If you agree to help a woman who does not want to be sutured and she does have a bad tear, decide in advance what will you do. One solution would be to write out a statement describing the extent of the tear, your recommended course of action and the possible consequences of not suturing, and have both parents sign it. You should explain this waiver process (or any other creative means of dealing with the situation to your mutual satisfaction) at your initial visit. This kind of waiver does not cover you legally, but it should make them think twice and, in my opinion, covers you ethically.

Alternatively, as a responsible midwife, it is perfectly legitimate to refuse to participate. The parents have rights, but so do you. If you feel uncomfortable practicing within the parameters of what parents are requesting, you have every right to say so. You should make this clear at the consultation visit and not after you have taken them on as clients. If you are the only midwifery care provider available to them and they want to have an attendant at their birth, then you need to make some arrangement that feels comfortable to everyone concerned.

This is an unlikely scenario; in fact, most parents are relieved to hear that suturing is among your repertoire of skills because it means one less thing that could require hospital transport. It does happen that women refuse suturing, though, and your reaction is worth pondering.

Knowing your own limits

After the birth of the placenta, the next order of midwifery business is a thorough yoni inspection. Don't be tempted to part the labia quickly and declare "No tears." (That kind of exam would have completely missed the severed anal sphincter I once found behind an intact perineal body.)

Honesty with your clients is of foremost importance. If you know what is damaged and feel you can do the job, explain the parameters of your experience and offer the choice of staying home and having you perform the repair. If the tear is of a type you've never seen or repaired before, tell the mother. Be sure to include the consequences of an inadequate repair and what can and cannot be done to correct it later (when suboptimal results are more likely).

At other times, a tear may be just plain horrible, but the upper vault and rectal area are intact. You can see clearly what is damaged, but your skills may or may not be up to the task at hand; in this case, it is a toss-up. You could transport to the hospital, but will that practitioner have much experience repairing funny-looking tears? Maybe not, since they are probably much more used to sewing straight incisions. Explain to the mother that it is a very bad tear and what your feelings are about transport. If she wants you to go ahead, tell her you'll do the best you can.

If you know you do not have the proper skills, materials or equipment to do a repair, explain this to the parents and insist on transport. Don't put yourself in the position of having a client with an incontinent anal sphincter or a fistula on your conscience just because you told yourself you could make do with what you had on hand. It just isn't worth the risk.

Never be afraid to admit that you are unsure of something, regardless of your experience level. Your clients are depending on your skills, and an important one is knowing and admitting when you don't know!

Animal rights and the use of gut suture material

Surgical gut is not made from the intestines of deceased surgeons who have donated their guts to science. You may be relieved to know that it is not made from those of cats either. However, raw material is derived as a by-product from sheep and cattle who are killed to harvest their body parts. Use of gut materials definitely promotes the enslavement and exploitation of animals for human benefit. If you avoid wearing leather, don't eat meat, or you or your client has an ethical objection to using other animal products out of compassion, you or she may or may not feel comfortable using natural gut suture materials. (Again, you must examine how much you adhere to this ethic. For example, if you use dairy products or eggs, factory-style production is abusive to the animals.) Some of your clients may prefer that you use synthetic suture if given the choice. It's just another thing to consider.

REFERENCES AND FURTHER READING

Barstow A. WITCHCRAZE: A NEW HISTORY OF THE EUROPEAN WITCH HUNTS. HarperCollins, San Francisco CA, 1995.

Daly M. GYN/ECOLOGY: THE METAETHICS OF RADICAL FEMINISM. Beacon Press, Boston MA, 1978.

Starhawk. DREAMING THE DARK: MAGIC, SEX, AND POLITICS. Beacon Press, Boston MA, 1982.

NOTES:

PERTINENT ANATOMY

NOTE: Read about changes in terminology on page 1 before studying this part, and read and understand this part of the book before proceeding to the rest of the text.

Understanding Female Pelvic Anatomy: An Introduction

The chapters in this part of the book offer a foundation for understanding basic pelvic and genital anatomy. Female anatomy is presented unless otherwise noted, with a focus on tissues that can be seen and repaired at a birth and that pertain to performing a basic screening evaluation of pelvic floor health. Some parts or landmarks are mentioned only to provide context for discussing another part that is more relevant to midwifery practice. Most structures that are mentioned, however, are explained in more detail or at least defined somewhere in this part of the book.

Problems Inherent in the Study of Female Pelvic Anatomy

The study of pelvic anatomy in general is a daunting undertaking. As far as female anatomy goes, this difficulty has been compounded by the traditional tendency to discuss female parts as counterparts to the male, rather than presenting them as unique in and of themselves, even though significant gender differences exist. As a result, there are profound deficiencies in most descriptions of female pelvic anatomy. These shortages, in combination with the lack of standardized terminology for describing the parts and the exuberant proliferation of unexplained synonyms in the literature have made it nearly impossible to compare the findings from different studies (Van Houten, 2006).

To start with, dissection of the female pelvic soft tissues is challenging because so many small, complex, multilayered, interdependent and comingled structures are packed into such a difficult-to-access space. Removing small, delicate and interrelated structures to reveal underlying ones disrupts surrounding tissues and alters anatomical relationships. A variety of factors, such as the length of time a cadaver has been an object of study, have a huge bearing on the condition of the tissues. Age- and childbirth-related changes alter the muscles and connective tissues, sometimes dramatically. As a woman ages, distinct pelvic muscle bundles are gradually infiltrated with more fibrous and elastic connective tissue. These changes obscure the precise anatomy and are especially problematic when the only cadavers available are those of elderly women.

DeLancey (1996) pointed out that much of this confusion can be traced to the supine position in which the pelvic soft tissues are normally examined in life and prepared and dissected after death. The pelvic tissues are designed to provide support when a woman is standing. Thus, misunderstandings are inevitable when studying the tissues out of their normal orientation. Moreover, the behavior of these tissues in living subjects is altered quite a bit upon death, and anyone performing dissections must keep this in mind. Authors often neglect to detail or take into account how specimens were prepared when explaining their findings. Apart from positioning, cadaver preparation itself can dramatically alter the shape of the soft tissues, but this is frequently not considered, especially in older studies. While there are processes that can be used to retain more life-like tissue relationships, they require forethought and access to fresh specimens so they can be properly prepared. Finally, significant anatomical variations exist among normal individuals, limiting the value of studies that include only a few specimens, which has frequently occurred when female specimens were examined as an adjunct to studies that focused primarily on male anatomy.

Contemporary anatomists are striving to better understand and more accurately depict the female pelvic soft tissues. However, since normal tissue relationships only exist in life and detailed tissue examination is only possible after death, this presents a challenging dichotomy for the best medical illustrator. Moreover, the complex, three-dimensional nature of this anatomy makes it difficult to accurately represent the different planes of the muscles and connective tissues, and how they interact, in a drawing. Throughout this chapter, when relevant, the way the drawings were developed (with reference to MRI images or cadaver-derived illustrations or both) will be given so you know better what you are looking at. Many publishers have not invested the time or money to include truly good drawings that provide accurate depictions in three dimensions. Another factor that makes clinical application difficult is that most perineal muscle layers are demarcated by microscopic tissue differences instead of the well-defined and easy-to-see structures that characterize many other muscle groups (Kolder, 1990). (See the chapter entitled "How to Use This Manual.")

Because the current literature on this topic is still so inconsistent, this chapter includes many details of pelvic anatomy in more depth than the average midwife will ever require. The material is too complex and, presented any other way, too confusing. When necessary, I have included points of controversy so that you can more intelligently evaluate what might or might not be correct when you study other sources.

I have chosen to discuss the pelvic muscles most involved in the birth process as well as a few others to which these are attached. Although other muscles could be damaged during birth, they probably won't be unless the tissue is very unhealthy or an operative or traumatic delivery occurs (specifically clitorotomy, use of forceps, vacuum extraction or unusually severe perineal trauma due to a difficult spontaneous birth).

Connective tissues can also be damaged during birth, but this type of damage is generally invisible to the midwife on gross examination just after the birth. While the connective tissues directly involved in a visible tear will be brought together with the other tissues as they are sutured, internal damage can occur that is not obvious in a visible tear, but that can still result in eventual weakening of the pelvic soft tissue support system. Any damage that does not heal completely may eventually lead to changes that can be identified after the postpartum period and that may require surgical repair. Because the midwife will not be working directly with these deeper tissues, however, I have chosen to review these complex connective tissue supports, as well as nerve, blood vessel and lymph supplies, in less detail.

As you go through this section, please take one step at a time. Write down terms you do not know and check them off as they are explained. I suggest that you have a medical dictionary and a general anatomy textbook, such as GRAY'S ANATOMY FOR STUDENTS, on hand as you study. The anatomy textbook is to look up information on other areas of the body. Do not rely on it to double-check what you find in this section on female pelvic soft tissue anatomy as there is no single text that has the pelvic anatomy completely correct, and this is true of this edition of HEALING PASSAGE as well. This is the case because the understanding of the female pelvic region is currently in a state of constant flux.

Due to the complexity of the material, plan on reading it through several times to gain the best understanding. That this material is broken up into separate chapters should help you find specific information more easily. Each chapter in this section builds on the next, however, so initially they should be studied in sequence. As you read, I also recommend referring to the various full-page drawings included at the end of this section. (More about how to use them can be found just before the pages of drawings.)

As hard as I have tried to explain these structures with words and pictures, I realize that, for some, it just won't be adequate. When you have studied this chapter thoroughly, I suggest that you obtain my audiovisual presentation that covers pelvic anatomy, which should help. In addition, the pelvic floor model in the back of the book has been updated to match the new information in this section. I have done a ton of homework to make this easier for you. I hope you will find my observations helpful.

If you require additional information, refer to any new edition of a urogynecology text or a gynecologic-surgery text that includes a comprehensive chapter on pelvic anatomy that is authored by John DeLancey. He is one of the foremost urogynecologists in the US and has made a huge effort to clarify many points of female anatomy. He is referenced frequently throughout this part of the book. Also check (www.PubMed.gov) for articles on the topics of interest as this is where the newest peer-reviewed medical research is first published.

Orientation of the Woman's Body

As each part is discussed, assume that the woman is standing unless the text says otherwise. Although the natural orientation for these structures is an upright position, some parts, such as the external genitals, can only be seen if you are looking between a woman's open legs. When a supine position is noted, assume that the woman is lying on her back with her legs open. Anatomical terms are used to describe the parts in relationship to each other and to the body in general. These terms, including "right" and "left" and "superior" and "inferior," are applicable regardless of a person's position because they always locate parts from the point of view of the "anatomical" position, which is standing face forward, with the arms to the sides and palms forward. These terms are discussed in Vol. I of HOLISTIC MIDWIFERY, and in nearly all anatomy textbooks. Whenever nonanatomical directional terms are used, such as "up" or "down," "above" or "below," at least one anatomical term will also be included as well to avoid any confusion about what is meant.

THE EXTERNAL GENITALIA

This chapter reviews the external female genitalia, which consist of the structures of the surface anatomy that lie between the inguinal-gluteal folds and that extend from the exterior surface of the hymen outward. The region reaches from the mons pubis to the anus. As you read this chapter, refer to the illustration below and keep in mind that the appearance of the genitalia varies considerably among individuals. Assume that the woman is lying on her back with her legs relaxed and apart.

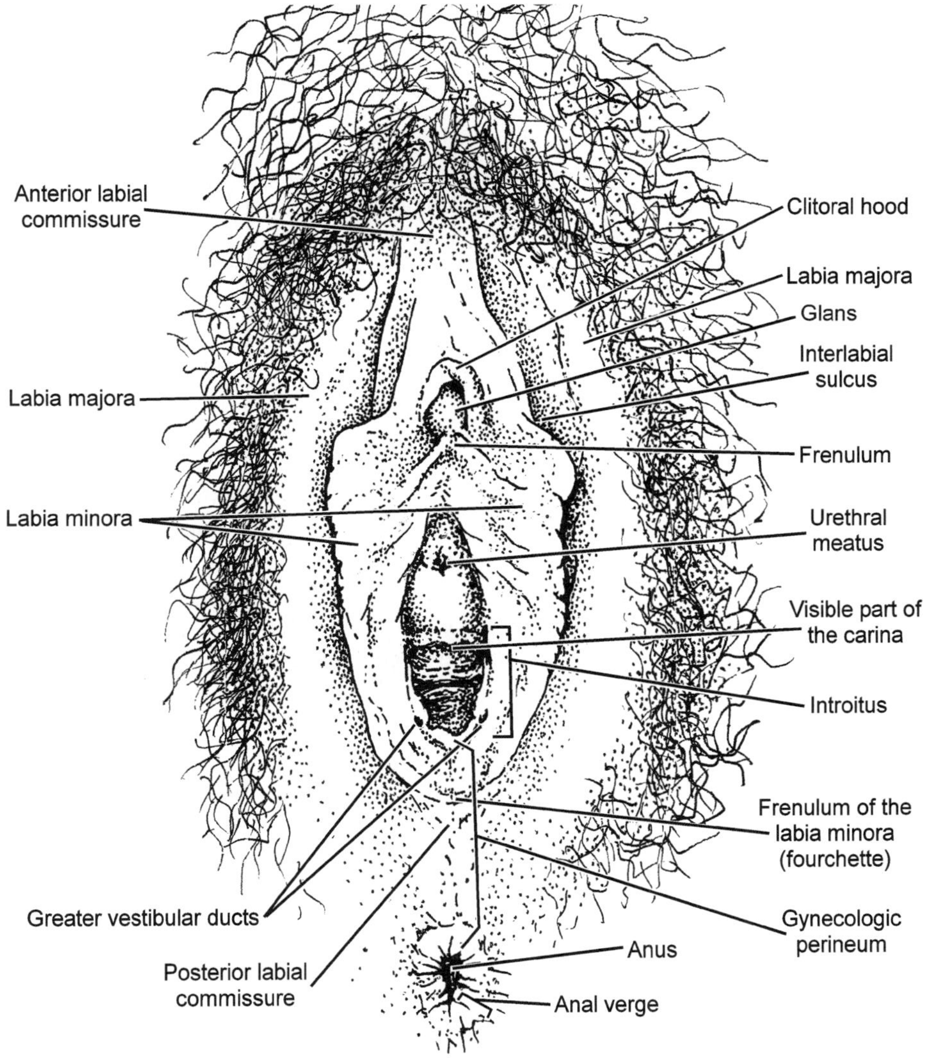

The external female genitalia with labia majora and minora parted to reveal the vulval vestibule.

Vulva (VUHL-va)/pudenda (pew-DEN-dah)

The "vulva" refers to the urogenital or pudendal cleft or space (rima) located between the thighs. This region encompasses the mons pubis, labia majora, labia minora, clitoral glans, vestibule, hymen, and the orifices of the urethra and yoni; a few authors also include the gynecologic perineum and the anus. In most writings, however, the anterior and posterior vulval boundaries extend from the mons pubis to the posterior commissure of the labia majora. Laterally the vulval boundaries are marked by the **genitocrural folds** (creases of the thighs). Some authors also include internal structures such as the female prostate (or Skene) glands and the vestibular (or Bartholin) glands as well as the clitoral (vestibular) bulbs as parts of the vulva (Deliveliotou & Creatsas, 2006); these are covered in another chapter.

Layered divisions of the vulva

Some sources divide the entire vulva into layered superficial and deep compartments, using the sheet-like superficial (Colles) fascia as the boundary between them. Structures in the superficial vulval compartment lie superficial to this sheet and include the skin, skin appendages (hair follicles, glands, etc.) and subcutaneous fat. The deep vulval compartment lies above this sheet of fascia (and is, at times, confusingly referred to as the "superficial perineal pouch"). It includes the clitoral body and glans, which are embedded in the fatty tissue of the anterior labial commissure; the distal urethra and yoni canals; the clitoral bulbs; the vestibular glands; the bulbocavernosus, ischiocavernosus and superficial transverse perineal muscles; and the perineal body. The superior (deepest) internal boundary of the vulva is the inferior surface of the perineal membrane complex (Dennerstein et al., 2005).

Vulval skin

Most vulval skin consists of keratinized squamous epithelium studded with hair follicles, sebaceous (oil-secreting) glands and typical coiled eccrine sweat glands. It also contains specialized **apocrine sweat glands** that are only found in the axillary and genital regions and are usually associated with hair follicles. They secrete a viscous, fat-rich sweat that reacts with skin bacteria to produce odor. Genital skin contains a large number of melanocytes per square millimeter of skin surface, resulting in its typically darker appearance in comparison with other skin regions. The vulval skin is discussed in more detail, beginning on page 27 and in the excellent article by Erickson and Montagna (1972).

Vulval nerve, blood and lymph supplies

The vulva's primary blood supply comes from the femoral artery via the external and internal pudendal arteries. Venous drainage occurs via the internal pudendal veins. Lym-phatic drainage occurs primarily via the superficial and deep inguinal nodes and along the dorsal vein of the clitoris, directly into the iliac nodes.

Branches of several nerves supply the vulva, including the ilioinguinal nerve, the genital branch of the genitofemoral nerve, the perineal branch of the lateral femoral cutaneous nerve of the thigh, and the perineal branch of the pudendal nerve (Deliveliotou & Creatsas, 2006). More about the nerve endings in the vulval skin and the yoni can be found on page 29.

Mons pubis (PEW-bis) (mons veneris [mons vee-NEER-us])

The broad anterior border of the vulva is formed by the mons pubis. The mons consists of a rounded, fat-filled pad of tissue that overlies the pubic symphysis. Under this superficial fat lies the fan-shaped superficial suspensory ligament of the clitoris, which converges in the midline and extends down to attach to the clitoral body and glans. Inferolaterally, this fan-shaped layer extends into the labia majora and attaches to the clitoral crura and the clitoral bulbs, where it forms the large, superficial part of the suspensory ligament of the clitoris, which stabilizes these parts of the clitoris as well as the labia majora (Rees et al., 2000).

At the onset of puberty, the mons gradually becomes covered with "terminal" hair that is usually coarser than other body hair. The pattern of hair growth is sometimes referred to as the **escutcheon (es-CUT-chin)**. In most women, the pubic hair forms a more or less horizontal upper margin where it meets the abdominal wall and appears as a downwardly pointed triangle when they are standing. In 25% of women, hair growth extends up the midline toward their navel, creating a diamond shape. In Asian and Native American women, pubic hair is more sparse than in Caucasian women, and may only grow down the center of the mons and along the medial edges of the labia majora (Farage et al., 2006).

Labia majora (LAY-bee-ah ma-JOR-ah)

The labia majora, or "great lips," form the lateral boundaries of the urogenital cleft. These prominent, fleshy, fibroadipose lips extend on either side from the mons pubis, passing posteriorly between the legs on either side and joining just below the inferior border of the yoni introitus. These lips are 7 to 8 cm long, 2 to 3 cm wide, and 1 to 1.5 cm thick. Their size is directly related to their fat content.

The labia majora are thicker anteriorly where they join in the midline between the posterior border of the mons pubis and anterior part of the clitoral body. This joining point is called the **anterior (labial) commissure**. It forms a protective pad above and to either side of the external clitoral structures, which project into it. Posteriorly, the fleshy lips taper as they approach the midline, wrap below the introitus and merge, forming a small transverse ridge that lies just posterior to the yoni orifice; this joining point is called the **posterior (labial) commissure** and is usually said to demarcate the lowermost boundary of the vulva (sometimes referred to as the **posterior boundary of the pudendum**). The **labiocrural fold** is where the lateral borders of the labia majora meet the most medial skin of the inner thighs. The **labial fold** or **interlabial sulcus** is the longitudinal depression between the medial borders of the labia majora and the lateral borders of the labial minora on either side.

In nulliparas the excitement phase of sexual response results in the labia majora becoming thinner and flatter and retracting slightly in an upward and outward direction. In multiparas the labia tend to become markedly distended with venous blood, especially in the presence of varicosities. No further changes occur until after orgasm, when the tissues return rapidly to a resting state (Masters & Johnson, 1966).

Skin: The labia majora have two skin regions with differing characteristics. The outer, hair-covered surface of each labia may be slightly rugose (wrinkled) in the unaroused state and is covered with ordinary, darkly pigmented skin (compared to most of the skin). It is studded with apocrine, eccrine and sebaceous glands. Blood flow is brisk; twice that of the forearm skin. Skin permeability to hydrocortisone is 2.8 to 7 times greater than that of the forearm, although permeability varies greatly among different agents (Farage & Maibach, 2006).

The inner surfaces of the labia majora have moist, smooth, shiny, more delicately pink skin containing many large sebaceous, apocrine and eccrine glands, but no hair follicles. Superficial sebaceous glands present as tiny yellowish bumps called **Fordyce spots**. Vulval apocrine glands resemble those of the breast and axillary areas.

Internal structure: The subcutaneous labial tissues consist of fat interlaced with connective tissue septa that have no well-defined layering and unattached borders, although regional variations in the quantity of fat and connective tissues do exist. This tissue is an extension of the fatty layer known as **Camper fascia** (the fatty, subcutaneous layer of tissue overlying the abdomen) (DeLancey, 2003b). The fibrous and fatty tissues of the labia are mixed with smooth muscle; as well as nerves, glands and many blood vessels, derived mostly from the external pudendal vessels. The round ligaments of the uterus terminate in the lateral borders of the labia majora to either side of the clitoral glans. During pregnancy, traction on these ligaments can cause discomfort as the uterus enlarges.

Birth-related trauma: The labia majora very rarely sustain birth-related tears. However, they may harbor varicose veins that are subject to trauma from pressure, to rupture and to hematoma formation, if they are damaged during birth.

Labia minora (LAY-bee-ah meh-NOR-ah) (nymphae)

The labia minora, or "little lips," are the two thinner skin folds that form soft, moist, inner flaps located medial to and parallel with the labia majora.

Originating at the clitoral glans, these lips extend vertically downward on either side of the urethral and yoni openings. They average 4 cm in length, but their size may be unequal and their appearance varies widely. The labia minora may be enclosed by the labia majora, in which case the large lips must be parted to reveal the labia minora. Often, however, the labia minora project beyond the labial majora, sometimes as much as five inches (12.5 cm). This is particularly common among certain ethnic groups of color. Some women have an extra fold of tissue known as a **labium tertium** on one or both sides between the labia minora and majora (Göttlicher, 1994).

Posteriorly, the labia minora taper and then join in the midline, between the introitus and the posterior labial commissure, to form the **fourchette** or **frenulum of the labia minora**.

Anteriorly, the labia minora merge in the midline, forming two layers or folds of skin that protect and support the clitoral glans from above and below.

Clitoral hood (prepuce [PREH-pus]/clitoral foreskin/preputium clitoridis): The top layer forms a lateral, crescent-shaped fold that overlies the clitoral body, forming an awning over the glans known as the "clitoral hood." The sides of the hood pass down to merge with the larger folds of the labia minora on either side (O'Connell & Sanjeevan, 2006).

Frenulum (FREN-you-lum) of the clitoris: The frenulum is a discrete fold of skin at the posterior border of the clitoral glans. It marks the transition between the labial skin and the skin that overlies the anterior vestibule (O'Connell et al., 2004). It is created by the anterior (upper) ends of the labia minora as they taper, converge to a point, join in the midline and merge on the underside of the glans. In many women, the edges of the labia minora are slightly ruffled just below (posterior to) this attachment (Dickinson, 1949).

With the exception of the clitoris, the labia minora undergo the most definitive changes of all the genital tissues during sexual response. During a well-established excitement phase, they expand markedly in diameter. By the plateau phase they have enlarged by two to three times, adding at least 1 cm to the clinical length of the yoni. Once enlarged, they undergo dramatic color changes ranging from pink to bright red in nulliparas and bright red to deep wine in multiparas. The degree of color change correlates with the intensity of sexual excitement and reliably precedes orgasm. These changes resolve within 10 to 15 seconds after orgasm (Masters & Johnson 1966).

Skin: The thin, supple, elastic skin of the labia minora is similar to mucous membrane in color and texture, with numerous sebaceous follicles (Fordyce spots), but no hair follicles, sweat glands or fat.

It overlies a matrix of elastic fibers and erectile tissue as well as dense but loosely woven connective tissue that allows movement during sexual activity and birth.

Birth-related trauma: The labia minora may sustain skin splits and tears during birth.

Vestibule (VES-ti-beuwl) of the vulva

The vulval vestibule is the teardrop-shaped region. Its anterior border is formed by the clitoral hood and its posterior border consists of the fourchette of the labia minora. Its interior boundary is the hymen, and its lateral boundaries are the medial borders of the labia minora. Several structures and landmarks are located within this area. (The term "vestibule" is also used to refer to the region just inside the yoni introitus to the depth of the hymen. It is discussed on page 52.)

Skin: The vulval vestibule is demarcated by a dermatological boundary known as the Hart line. Within this boundary, the skin is not keratinized (i.e., lacks a stratum corneum layer) and has loosely packed cells, a less-structured fat layer and a thinner epithelial layer than regular skin. This renders it roughly ten times more permeable to water than keratinized tissue (a statement based on studies of buccal and yoni membranes, to which it is similar) (Farage & Maibach, 2006). The clitoral glans and the openings of the yoni, the urethra, the vestibular glands, and numerous small mucinous glands are situated within the vestibule. Some women have tiny soft projections called **vestibular papillae** randomly scattered around their vestibule.

Within the vulval vestibule, the following structures and landmarks are identified:

Clitoral glans: The clitoris is a complex, mostly internal organ. Its only exposed part, the glans, forms a small, inverted-acorn–shaped terminus on the end of the internal clitoral body. The glans is covered by a thin, hairless, stratified epithelium that is studded with a few minor vestibular glands (Stilwell, 1976) and an underlying dermis that is densely vascular (O'Connell et al., 2004). The glans projects forward at an angle from under the clitoral hood, which covers it to a variable extent. Above the glans the clitoral body and its suspensory ligament, though covered by the clitoral hood, can be easily palpated as a firm, longitudinally oriented column overlying the anterior surface of the pubic symphysis. The internal anatomy of the glans is explained in more detail on page 63.

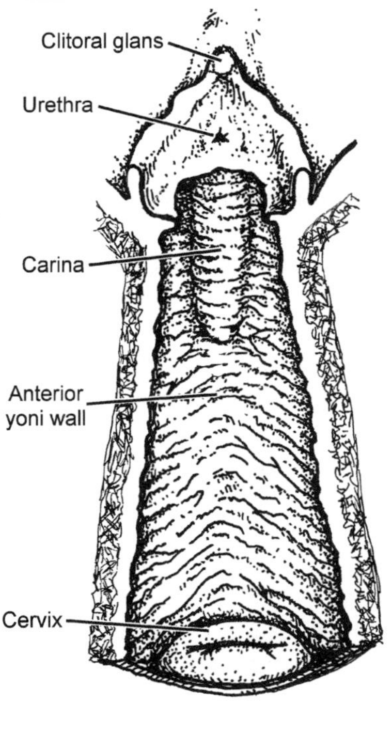

View of the entire anterior yoni wall showing the carina

Urethral meatus (you-REE-thrall mee-AY- tuss): This orifice lies below the junction of the labia minora, 1.25 to 3.5 cm below the clitoral glans (Narjani, 1924). Its appearance varies: presenting a tiny vertical slit, a crescent- or star-shaped opening or a round opening that may appear as a small bulge or a dimple with slightly everted edges (O'Connell & Sanjeevan, 2006).

Carina (ca-REEN-ah) of the urethra or yoni (carina

urethralis vaginae/urethral ridge/carina vaginae): The carina is the longitudinal bulge that runs along the midline, distal third of the anterior yoni wall that is created by the urethral canal. This bulge is visible in the distal rugose yoni wall immediately beneath the urethral meatus at and just inside the introitus. At times, the term "carina" appears to be used to refer to this visible part specifically, which is why it is included here. The carina is often more obvious in parous women.

Introitus: The introitus is the yoni opening. It presents as a vertical slit with irregular edges and is located below (posterior to) the urethral meatus. The hymen forms the deepest boundary of the introitus and is discussed on page 52. Because the anterior third of the yoni is surrounded by clitoral structures, the introitus is a clitoral orifice (O'Connell & Sanjeevan, 2006).

Vestibular ducts: Each vestibular gland has a 2 cm long duct that opens 3 to 4 mm into the groove between the hymen and the labia minora (the vestibule of the yoni), at about 4 and 8 o'clock. The vestibular glands are discussed in detail on page 64.

Fourchette (foor-SHET): The fourchette is the posterior border of the vestibule of the vulva. It consists of the delicate, semicircular, membranous bridge formed by the posterior frenulum of the labia minora.

Perineum (per-i-NEE-um)

The **anatomic perineum** includes the entire region between the thighs that is shaped like an elongated diamond. It is bounded on either side by the ischial tuberosities. Its longitudi-nal dimension extends from the mons pubis to the coccyx. The levator ani muscles form its superior boundary (or ceiling), and its inferior boundary is the skin.

Clinically, however, the term "perineum" most often refers exclusively to the **gynecologic** or **obstetric perineum**, which extends from the inferior border of the introitus to the superior border of the anal opening (Joseph, 1982; van der Putte, 2005), especially in the midline. The surface anatomy is called the **pudenda** in a few sources. The gynecologic perineum is also referred to as the **perineal body,** especially when discussing the three-dimensional musculofibrous anatomy that fills the space between the yoni wall and the anal canal. A detailed discussion of this internal anatomy starts on page 70. Beyond the anatomy section, the term "perineum" refers to the gynecologic perineum, except as otherwise noted.

Skin: Although the gynecologic perineum is the focus of the most frequently performed surgical procedure (clitorotomy), there is relatively little specific information about the skin in this area. The perineal body is covered with ordinary squamous epithelium, bearing both sebaceous and sweat glands. Hair follicles are also present, except along a variably wide, hairless region that spans the longitudinal midline between the introitus and the anus.

Length: The length of the perineum between the introitus and the anus varies among women, generally ranging between 3 to 6 cm and averaging 4 cm. A short perineum is under 3 cm in length; a long perineum is over 6 cm in length (Kalis et al., 2005). Length influences whether and to what extent the tissues tear during birth (see page 169 for more details).

Little is known regarding ethnic variations in perineal length. A study of 1000 women (25% Asian and 75% Caucasian), found no real differences overall, except that more Caucasian women had long perineums than would be expected. There was no correlation between perineal length and height, weight or body mass index (BMI) (Dua et al., 2008).

Perineal raphe (RAY-fee): A very small, longitudinal ridge extends along the midline of the perineum from the introitus to the anus (also see page 38). The perineal raphe is much more prominent in men.

Perianal region and anus

The **perianal region** surrounds the anal orifice. This skin contains mammary-like glands (see page 25) as well as eccrine sweat glands and many apocrine sweat glands, although most of the apocrine glands are nonfunctional. A variable number of sebaceous glands are also found in the perianal region, some of these open into a hair follicle and others are individual, or "free," glands not associated with a hair follicle and are found along the anal verge. (More about the perianal glands can be found on page 103.) The **anal verge** is the external region immediately surrounding of the anus; it represents the transition zone between the perianal skin and the moist, hairless, modified skin of the distal anal canal.

The **anus** is the opening of the anal canal, through which feces pass. It faces downward and posteriorly and lies in the midline about 4 cm below and anterior to the tip of the coccyx. It is not considered a part of the "genitalia" per se because it looks the same in both sexes. The skin of the anal orifice is uniformly puckered in a purse-string fashion (the corrugator cutis ani), an important feature when examining for anal sphincter damage. Uneven or absent puckering indicates underlying damage to the external anal sphincter (Ellis & Dussek, 1999).

Postperineum

"Postperineum" is a rarely used term that refers to the midline region between the posterior border of the anus and the tip of the coccyx.

External genital skin

The gynecologic perineum and the labia minora are the primary sites of skin trauma or deeper tearing during birth. Because the skin overlying these areas is sparsely discussed in most texts, it is reviewed here in some depth.

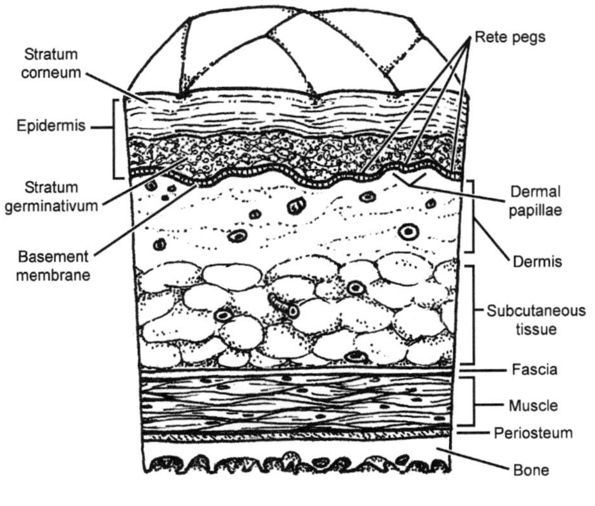

Layers of the skin and deeper structures

Review of skin anatomy: First, lets briefly review basic skin, or integument, anatomy with a focus on features relevant to surgical repair. Although the skin and fascia involve a complex system of organs and anatomic structures, it is the way the skin is layered that is most relevant to wound repair and healing. These layers include the epidermis, dermis, superficial fascia and deep fascia. After this overview, there are more details on the vulval skin.

Epidermis: The skin has two primary layers, the epidermis and the dermis. The epidermis, is the epithelial, or surface layer, of the integument. It protects against bacterial invasion and toxic substances and regulates the loss of water and electrolytes. It consists entirely of squamous epithelial cells and contains no organs, nerve endings or blood vessels. Nourishment diffuses into this layer from capillaries in the underlying dermis. The epidermis is thin, averaging about 0.12 mm and ranging between 75 to 150 μm (another source says 0.06 to 0.6 mm) in thickness.

The epidermis is composed of five thin layers, or strata, of epithelial cells at different stages of differentiation, from the most superficial to the deepest layer, these are as follows:

1. **Stratum corneum:** The outermost layer consists of varying layers of flat, closely packed, dead cells that are constantly being lost due to abrasion.
2. **Stratum lucidum:** The second layer forms a band of clear, closely packed cells with indistinct outer boundaries. It is most prominent in regions where the skin is thick and is absent in some locations.
3. **Stratum granulosum:** The third layer consists of flat cells arranged in about three layers. These cells contain granules that grow in size as their nucleus disintegrates and dies; the outermost cells of this layer are dead.
4. **Stratum spinosum:** The fourth layer also tends to become somewhat flattened and appears to have extensions connected to other cells.
5. **Stratum germinativum:** Finally the bottom layer, where new cells are born, sits directly on top of the dermis. Melanin is formed here to protect against ultraviolet radiation.

The number and thickness of these epithelial layers vary depending upon the location of the skin (Spence, 1990).

Two epidermal layers are of particular importance in the healing of surface wounds. The first is the **stratum germinativum**, or **basal layer**, where new skin cells are formed during healing. Also of special interest is the **stratum corneum**, the outermost visible layer that functions as a barrier and gives the skin its final cosmetic appearance. This protective layer is deeper in thick skin than in thin skin. Cells are constantly being lost and replaced by new cells that move up from underlying strata. Turnover takes 28 to 40 days. As epidermal cells approach the stratum corneum, they become flat and horny (i.e., dead) as their cytoplasm is replaced by large amounts of a protein called **keratin (KER-ah-tin)**. Keratin is not found in mucous membrane, which heals by a process of regeneration, where injured tissues are replaced by the same kind of tissue that was destroyed. Otherwise, scar tissue is formed during healing, as is true in skin and muscle.

Rete ridges (epidermal ridges) are found in the deepest part of the epidermis. These avascular ridges project down into the vascularized dermis below, where they interdigitate with dermal papillae that help nourish the epidermis. The **dermal papillae** are superficial projections of the papillary dermis (papillary corium) that contain vascular loops and specialized nerve endings, and are arranged in raised lines most prominent in the hand and foot.

The **basement membrane** is sandwiched between the epidermis and the dermis. It supports the epidermis and filters substances moving between the dermis and epidermis.

Dermis (subcuticular [SUB-cue-TICK-you-lar] tissue/subepidermal): The **dermal** layer is immediately below the basement membrane. In most regions it ranges from 0.5 to 2.5 mm in thickness. The dermis is deeper on the palms and as thick as 4 mm on the soles of the feet. Technically, this is the true **subcuticular layer** (Carter, 1992; Skandalakis et al., 2009), although the superficial fascial layer appears to be referred to as "subcuticular" in some descriptions of surgical repairs because it is also below the epidermis.

The dermis has two layers of cells, although they are less defined than those of the epidermis. The thin, superficial **papillary dermis** consists of loosely woven elastic connective fibers that are embedded in a gelatinous matrix, or ground substance, that is well supplied with blood vessels and nerves. It contributes to the elasticity and tear resistance of the skin.

Below the papillary dermis lies the main fibrous bed of the dermis, the **reticular dermis**, which consists of dense, irregular connective tissue. It houses most of the accessory structures of the skin, including sweat glands, sebaceous glands and hair follicles; these structures may penetrate into the subcutaneous layer that underlies the skin. This layer is the most important contributor to the skin's overall strength and elasticity.

In most areas of the body, sebaceous glands open into hair follicles. In hairless regions of the vulva, such as the labia minora and the medial aspect of the labia majora, however, the sebaceous glands are more superficially placed and open directly onto the skin surface. They are usually visible as small, yellow-tinted bumps (Fordyce spots) and are typically less than 2 mm in diameter (Dennerstein et al., 2005).

Mammary like glands are a type of skin appendage unique to the anogenital region. In women, they are most abundant in the interlabial sulci. They are also found, to a lesser extent, in the perineal and perianal skin. Anogenital mammary like glands have some features of both apocrine and eccrine glands. They resemble typical lactiferous ducts and glands of the breast in some respects; they have diverticula, branches and lobules as well as estrogen and progesterone receptors but have a simpler structure. They are not considered supernumerary and are not derived from mammary ridges (van der Putte, 1994). Genital conditions such as hidradenoma papilliferum (a benign epithelial cystic tumor that most commonly occurs in the labia majora) and mammary conditions of the vulva such as ectopic breast or breast tissue, fibroadenoma, phyllodes tumor and primary breast like adeno-carcinoma appear to be derived from these mammary like glands (Scurry & Melville, 2007).

The dermis is the most important skin layer in relation to proper repair of surface wounds. Although the epidermis is a separate layer, it is too thin to be distinguished with the naked eye. Thus, closure of the epidermis is accomplished by reapproximating the dermis, which provides an anchoring site for both percutaneous and deep sutures. Placing stitches in these shallow tissues is more painful because of the nerve endings in this layer. The dermis heals by forming scar tissue, therefore only skin tags that are too damaged to repair or to heal well on their own should be trimmed away before repair.

Subcutaneous (SUB-cue-TAY-nee-us) tissue: Subcutaneous means "below the skin." The irregular subcutaneous layer lies between the dermis and the deep muscular fascia. It is also called the **hypodermis** or **superficial fascia** and may be what is meant when the term "subcuticular" is used by certain authors (Trott, 2005). While the term "subcutaneous" refers to this specific layer of fascia from an anatomical point of view, surgeons sometimes seem to use the term when referring to any tissue that lies beneath the dermal layer.

This tissue is penetrated by and gains support from skin ligaments linking the dermis to the underlying fasciae. It is composed of loose connective tissue and varying amounts of fat as well as sweat glands, superficial blood vessels, lymphatic vessels and cutaneous nerves that send terminal branches to the skin. It is recognized by a yellowish cast to the tissue. In some areas it may also contain a muscle layer, a fibrous layer or both. In other areas it consists of a thin membranous layer that is nearly devoid of fat, as is true in the labia minora.

Sensory nerve branches traverse the superficial fascia just below the dermis. When local anesthetic is injected along the plane between the dermis and the superficial fasciae, it spreads easily underneath the dermis and quickly abolishes sensation in the overlying skin.

HISTOLOGICAL FEATURES OF THE SKIN OF THE PERINEUM

Region	Epithelium Type	Hair Follicles	Eccrine Sweat Glands	Apocrine Sweat Glands	Sebaceous Glands	Mammary-like Glands
Mons pubis	Keratinized	+	+	–	+	–
Clitoral hood	Thinly keratinized	–	–	–	–	–
Clitoral glans¤	Thinly keratinized (?)	–	–	–	–	–
Labia majora (lateral surface)	Keratinized	+	+	+	+	–
Labia majora (medial surface)	Thinly keratinized	–	–	–	+	–
Labia minora (lateral surface)	Thinly keratinized	–	+/–	–	+	–
Labia minora (medial surface)	Nonkeratinized in 62% of women	–	–	–	–	–
Interlabial sulcus	Thinly keratinized	–	–	–	–	+
Vestibule¤ (inside Hart line)	Nonkeratinized	–	–	–	Rare	–
Vestibule (outside Hart line)	Keratinized	–	–	–	+	–
Gynecologic perineum (midline)*	Keratinized	–	+	+ (?)	+	+ (?)
Perianal skin	Keratinized	+	+	+	+	+

+: present –: absent (?): I think this is right, but the literature was not entirely clear on this point

¤Lesser vestibular glands are also present on the glans, but originate beneath the skin layer.

*Information on the specific epidermal histology of the gynecologic perineum is almost nonexistent. To the best of my ability this area is described correctly (adapted from Berg & Davis, 2006).

The superficial layer of vulval connective tissue is called **Colles fascia**. This layer is continuous with **Scarpa fascia** (the membranous layer of the subcutaneous tissue of the abdomen that underlies Camper fascia). Thus Colles fascia is the membranous layer of the subcutaneous tissue of the perineum, which has less fat and more interlaced connective tissue septa than does Camper fascia (see page 20). It is also distinguished by its subcutaneous septa that are attached to the ischiopubic rami laterally and that are fused posteriorly to the posterior border of the perineal membrane. The anterior border of this layer is unattached, permitting communication behind this layer of fascia and the abdominal wall. The attached parts limit the expansion of hematomas and infections into the deep anterior compartment, but this anterior opening allows them to spread into the abdomen (DeLancey, 2003b). No fat underlies the midline skin of the gynecologic perineum (Woodman & Graney, 2002).

Below the subcutaneous layer lies a relatively thick, dense and discrete fibrous layer of **deep parietal fascia** (Gallaudet fascia) that acts as a basement layer for the superficial fasciae. This tissue forms an off-white sheath that overlies the muscles. Lacerations of the parietal fascia require closure to restore the protective and supportive functions of this layer. These layers are also discussed on page 32.

Vulval skin: The lower urogenital tract is the only part of the female anatomy that is derived from all three embryonic cell layers. The keratinized cutaneous epithelium of the mons pubis, labia majora, clitoral body and glans, part of the labia minora and the gynecologic perineum derive from the ectoderm. Most of the bladder and the skin overlying the vestibule derive from the endoderm. The skin of the hymen, posterior urethral wall and bladder trigone derive from the mesoderm (Farage & Maibach, 2006; Humphrey, 2008).

The skin of the mons pubis, labia majora and gynecologic perineum is similar to that found elsewhere, consisting of keratinized, stratified, squamous epithelium with sweat glands, sebaceous glands and pigment storage sites (Farage & Maibach, 2006). Hair follicles are present, except in the vestibule and the variably wide midline region of the perineum.

The epidermis overlying the gynecologic perineum averages about 20 cells in thickness. The stratum corneum varies between 5 to 15 cells thick and the stratum granulosum is only 2 to 3 cells thick (Sargeant et al., 1996).

The skin overlying the labia minora is among the thinnest anywhere on the body and is generally lacking in secondary skin structures. The lateral aspects may have a few sweat glands, sebaceous glands and hair follicles. Along the inner third of the medial aspect of the labia minora (inside the Hart line, see below), the skin transitions into nonkeratinized epithelium, which lacks secondary skin structures and has a flat papillary basal layer; however, like keratinized skin, it does support continuous cell regeneration.

The vulval epidermis overlies a sturdy layer of papillary dermis that protects it against tangential forces. The thickness of the stratum corneum layer and the degree of keratinization are relatively high across the mons pubis and labia majora, decreasing over the anterior portions of the clitoris and declining progressively from the outer surface to the inner surface of the labia minora.

Vestibular epithelium varies from 20 to 25 cell layers thick and resembles that of the yoni and the oral mucosa (Sargeant et al., 1996). The teardrop-shaped **Hart line** marks the boundary between the nonkeratinized skin of the vulvar vestibule and the thinly keratinized skin of the labia minora. It begins beneath the glans and follows the inner third of the medial labia minora laterally and the medial edge of the frenulum of the labia minora inferiorly.

Vulval skin has high concentrations of androgen and estrogen receptors. The thickness of the layers of keratin and epithelium in the labial tissues varies throughout life as estrogen levels rise and fall. Thin in newborns, it becomes thicker after menarche and reaches a maximum thickness during the reproductive years, when vulval epithelium has a more or less constant thickness that is not influenced by the phase of the menstrual cycle. After menopause, these layers gradually thin again.

The vulva and the yoni wall display hormone-dependent changes during the menstrual cycle. The surface cells are predominantly orthokeratotic (lacking nuclei) at the beginning and end of the cycle and increasingly parakeratotic (bearing degenerated nuclei) at midcycle.

Jones (1983) examined genital skin specimens obtained from 52 subjects in order to establish reference values for the thickness of the keratin layer, the epithelium and the dermis at various ages. Labial biopsies were taken from adults. Juvenile specimens were obtained from cadavers. The next table shows the mean tissue depth for various age groups.

AGE	MEAN DEPTH OF LAYERS OF LABIAL SKIN (µM=MICROMETER)		
	KERATIN	EPITHELIUM	DERMIS
< 12 months	36.6 µm*	70.5 µm	1187.0 µm
1-14 years	16.2 µm	50.9 µm	1193.4 µm
15-50 years	20.9 µm	75.1 µm	2058.0 µm
51-60 years	15.9 µm	60.8 µm	1849.3 µm
61-86 years	14.6 µm	60.4 µm	1610.8 µm

*µm–micromillimeters

Biopsies were taken from four locations labeled A, B, C and D. The table below shows the mean depth of layers according to the location of each measurement. At the 6 and 12 o'clock positions (the fourchette and the clitoral hood), where there were no labial lips, specimens were divided equally into four levels that approximated the locations of the other specimens. Specifics about the findings at 6 and 12 o'clock were not given in the article. The findings below indicate the mean combined depth at each location.

LOCATION OF SAMPLE	MEAN DEPTH OF SKIN LAYERS		
	KERATIN	EPITHELIUM	DERMIS
A. Center of medial labia minora, fourchette or clitoral hood	9.9 µm	85.6 µm	2040.6 µm
B. Center of lateral labia minora, fourchette or clitoral hood	23.2 µm	63.3 µm	1631.4 µm
C. Center of medial labia majora, fourchette or clitoral hood	19.6 µm	55.2 µm	1395.8 µm
D. Center of lateral labia majora, fourchette or clitoral hood	23.2 µm	50.7 µm	1589.5 µm

The relationship between a woman's age and the relative thickness of tissue at each location was fairly consistent throughout the lifespan (for example, the medial vulval skin typically had a thicker layer of keratin than did the lateral vulval skin, independent of age after menarche). This thicker layer of keratin is protective, raising the threshold for stimulation of nerve endings, making the skin more tolerant of friction (Jones, 1983).

Compared to exposed skin, vulval skin is more hydrated and resists water loss better. It is also generally more permeable than elsewhere, with the skin of the vestibule and the lining of the yoni being the most permeable of all. Even so, skin permeability is a complex phenomenon that is difficult to predict for a given substance (Farage & Maibach, 2006).

Nerve endings in the skin of the vulva and the yoni: The skin of the mons and labia majora possess all types of nerve endings that are all defined in the second table below. These tables are derived from Krantz's study (1958) of the microscopic innervation of the female genitals. The pluses (+) indicate the relative number of endings in that location.

QUANTITATIVE DISTRIBUTION OF FREE NERVE ENDINGS IN THE FEMALE GENITALIA							
Anatomical part or region	Tactile Discrimination (Touch)			Vibration	Pain	Stretch	Pressure
	Meissner corpuscles	Merkel tactile discs	Peritrichial endings	Pacinian corpuscles	Free nerve endings	Ruffini corpuscles	Dogiel-Krause corpuscles
Mons pubis	++++	++++	++++	+++	+++	++++	++
Labia majora	+++	++++	+++	+++	+++	+++	++
Labia minora	++	++	None	++	++	++	+++
Clitoral glans	+	+	None	++++	+++	+++	+++
Hymenal ring	None	+	None	None	+++	None	None
Yoni wall	None	None	None	None	Few	None	None

Nerve Ending Type	Sensations Conveyed	Location
Meissner (tactile)* corpuscle	Vibration, most sensitive in 20-40 Hz range	Dermis of hairless (glabrous) skin
Merkel tactile discs (Tactile meniscus)	Variant of Meissner corpuscle	
Peritrichial nerve ending (hair receptor)	Hair displacement	Surrounding all hair follicles
Pacinian (laminated) corpuscle	Vibration, most sensitive in 150-300 Hz range.	Deep dermis of hairy and hairless skin
Free nerve endings (terminationes)	Different types respond to pressure, temperature and pain	Various types found throughout the skin
Ruffini corpuscles (endings)	Pressure	Dermis of hairy and hairless skin
Dogiel-Krause corpuscles (corpuscula bulboidea)		Lips, tongue and genitals

*Alternate terms in parentheses.

The skin and stratum germinativum of the gynecologic perineum and other genitalia are rich in free nerve endings for sensing pressure, temperature and pain. These nerves are especially dense in the clitoral hood and the dorsal surface of the clitoral glans. There are very few tactile receptors in the deeper tissues of the vestibule and clitoral body (Hoyt, 2006).

Pacinian corpuscles are located in the subcutaneous tissues of the mons and labia majora, but are more common in the skin of the glans, hood and upper labia minora. The labia majora also have a variable number of Meissner corpuscles. Merkel tactile disks are found in the labia minora and clitoral hood. Ruffini and Dogiel-Krause corpuscles are found in variably large numbers in the deep subcutaneous connective tissues of the glans, hood and the labia minora (Krantz, 1958). The skin overlying the clitoral glans, hood, labia minora and vestibule also has specialized nerves that do not appear to be sensorial (Hoyt, 2006).

The Pelvic Support System and Soft Tissues: An Overview

This chapter lays a foundation for understanding pelvic soft and bony internal structures. It discusses a variety of schemes used to divide the pelvic soft tissues into three-dimensional regions or compartments. Some general introductory information is also included regarding the pelvic floor, pelvic connective tissues and muscle fibers. Page numbers in parentheses—(p. #)—indicate where more information about the part can be found in this text.

The Bony Pelvis

Pelvic support begins with the pelvic bones. In adults, the pelvis consists of a ring of three large, complexly shaped bones (the two ilia and the sacrum) and one small bone (the coccyx). These bones, the tissues that join them and the ligaments that overlie and reinforce their joints create a rigid framework with flexible joints to which the muscles, connective tissues and pelvic organs are attached, either directly or by connection to tissues that are themselves so attached. The importance of these attachments is illustrated when the organs and other soft tissues are dissected away from the pelvic bones, causing these soft tissues to lose their shape and lie in a lumpy puddle. Illustrations of the pelvis appear on the next page.

When a woman is standing, the anterior, superior iliac spine and the pubic tubercle are vertically aligned; the anterior surface of the pubic bone is angled downward; the pelvic brim is tilted at about a 120° angle when measured from her left (or about 60° when measured from her right); and the yoni and urethral orifices are directed toward the ground (the introitus points more or less straight down and the anus points in a postero-oblique direction). These relationships direct intra-abdominal pressure and much of the weight of the pelvic contents toward the bones of the pubic arch and pubic rami (lateral borders of the pubic bone) instead of directly down on the muscle and connective tissue attachments within the pelvic cavity. This arrangement takes some pressure off the pelvic muscles and connective tissues, relieving them of some of the constant strain they are subjected to as a result of an upright posture (Barber, 2005).

Variations in the shape of the pelvis and spine have been associated with a higher incidence of pelvic organ prolapse (Barber, 2005). See page 92 for more details.

The drawing to the right and those on the next page review landmarks of the bony pelvis. For more complete anatomical details of the bony pelvic anatomy, refer to HOLISTIC MIDWIFERY, VOLS. I and II.

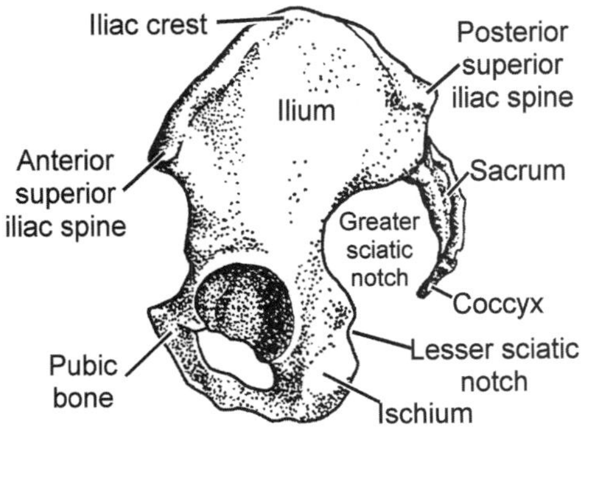

Pelvis: lateral view, standing position

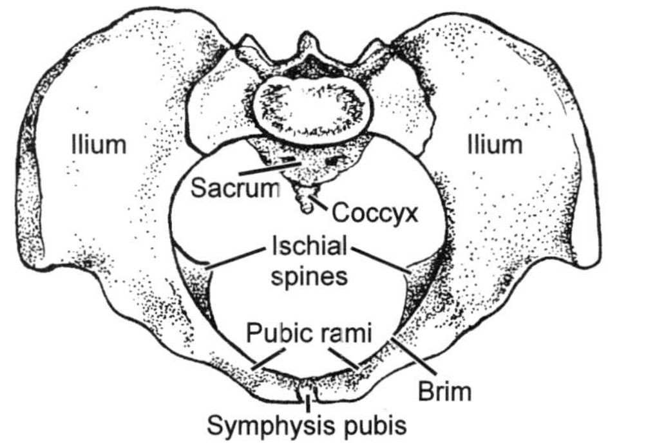

Pelvis: superior view, looking straight down

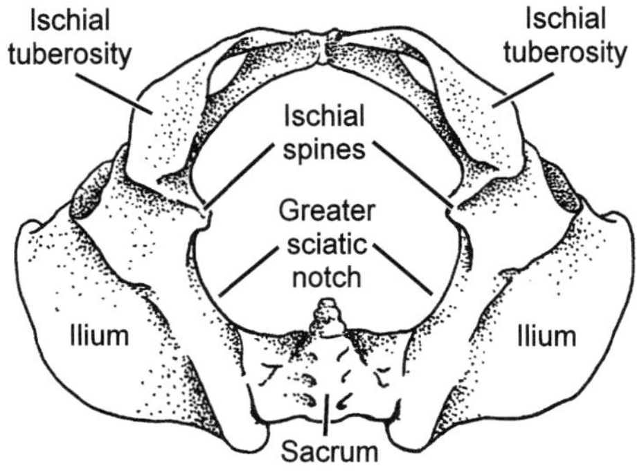

Pelvis: inferior view, looking straight up

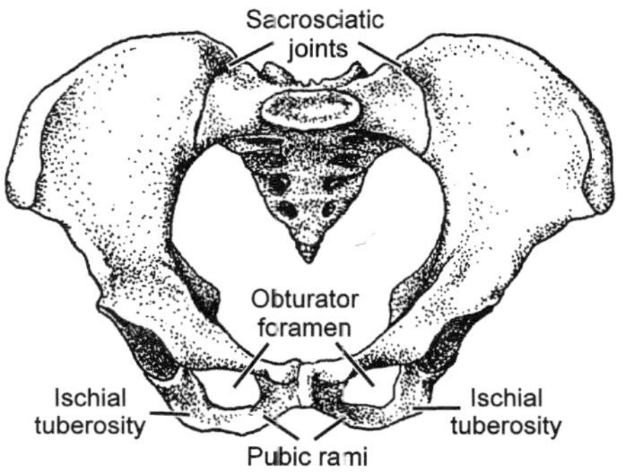

Pelvis: anterior view, standing position

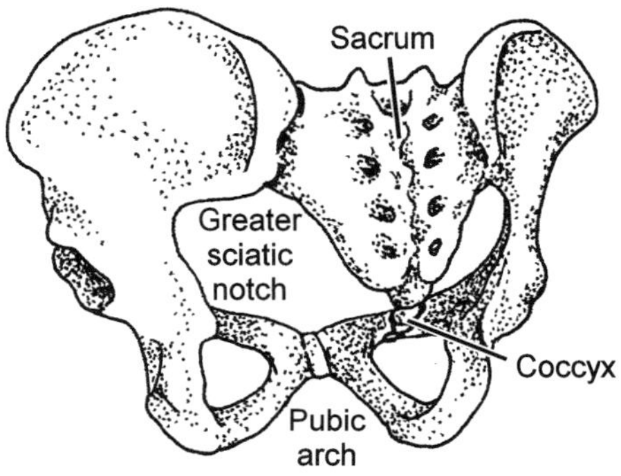

Pelvis: postero-oblique view, standing position

Regional Divisions of the Pelvic Soft Tissues

There are several different ways that the pelvic cavity is layered and otherwise divided by anatomists and surgeons. These schemes often overlap and have similar or identical names, making it hard to determine what is meant when terms are used but left undefined.

Tissue layers of the anatomic perineum

The perineal tissue layers are as follows:

1) The several layers of the skin
2) A layer of subcutaneous fat of variable thickness depending on its location
3) A layer of superficial fascia, which, depending upon its location, consists of either one or two layers, as is true elsewhere in the body
   - -The lower abdominal wall has two layers of superficial fascia. The superficial layer is called Camper fascia. The deeper layer is called Scarpa fascia; it is composed mostly of yellow elastic fibers with little fat.
   - -The anatomical perineum is usually considered to have one superficial fascial layer that is an extension of Scarpa fascia. This perineal layer is variously called the superficial perineal fascia, Colles fascia or the membranous layer

of the superficial fascia.

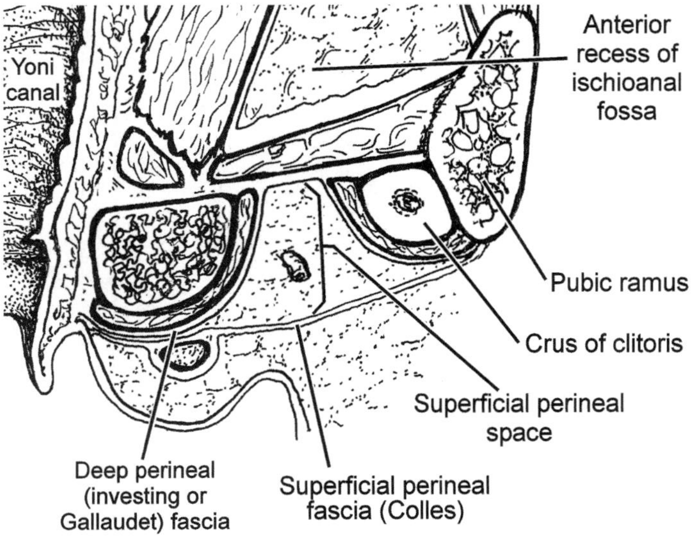

Coronal section (woman's left side from divided midline) showing tissue layers and spaces of the anatomical perineum

4) The deep perineal fascia is an extension of the layer on the abdominal wall called the deep abdominal fascia. This is the parietal fascia covering the surfaces of the external oblique and internal oblique abdominal muscles (it is not the same as the transversalis fascia). Where this deep fascia extends onto or into the perineum it has been referred to as the deep perineal fascia, investing fascia or fascia of Gallaudet; this layer appears to serve as the parietal fascia for the bulbocavernosus and ischiocavernosus muscles. Elsewhere it appears to really be part of the superficial fibers of the perineal membrane. (Note: Some texts consider the superficial perineal fascia [3] and the deep perineal fascia [4] to be fused into one layer. This combined layer is called Colles fascia and refers to the same layer described here as Colles fascia in [3]). Other texts consider 3 and 4 to be two separate layers. Whether superficial and deep perineal fascia are separate or fused is not that important for a midwifery-level understanding of anatomy–it is mentioned here to avoid confusion if you find reference to it in other sources.)

6) Perineal membrane, which demarcates the boundary between the superficial and deep perineal pouch/compartment. (Anatomy helpers, 2009)

Triangular divisions of the pelvic outlet

The pelvic outlet is often divided into two triangular regions. The base of each triangle is formed by a line that runs between the ischial tuberosities. These triangular regions are used when discussing the corresponding external anatomy as well as internal pelvic anatomy that lies between the skin and the inferior surface of the levator ani muscle complex.

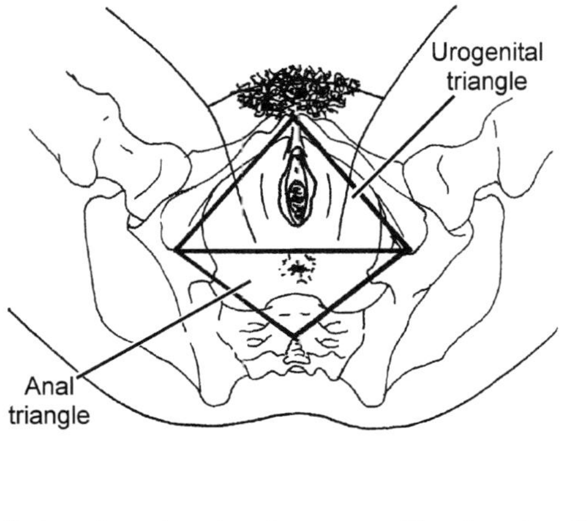

Inferior view showing the external landmarks of the urogenital and anal triangles when a woman is lying supine

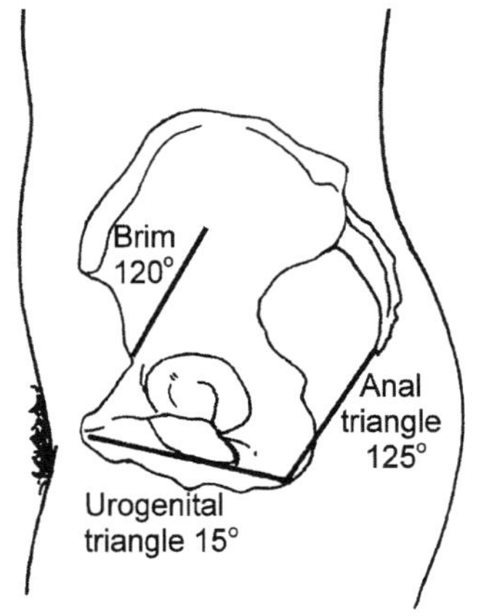

The planes of these triangular regions when a woman is standing (left lateral view)

Urogenital (you-row-GEN-ah-tal)/anterior triangle: The uppermost division is referred to as the **urogenital** or **anterior triangle**. This triangle is somewhat larger than the anal triangle. Its base spans the area between the ischial tuberosities. Its apex extends to the symphysis pubis above, and the sides are formed by the descending pubic rami. The pubic rami are directed toward the floor at about a 10 to 30° angle when a woman is standing (measured from her left; if measured from the right, the angle is 170 to 150°). This angle is derived from a horizontal line drawn level with the tip of the coccyx to the upper inside border of the pubic bone. This angle varies among individuals and is influenced by such things as ethnicity and pelvic type.

Depending on the source, the urogenital triangle is divided into either three regions or layers or into deep and superficial compartments. DeLancey (2003b) noted three layers similar to those found in the abdominal wall. The **deep perineal space, layer** or **compartment** lies superior to (above) the anterior surface of the perineal membrane. It includes the three dimensional connective tissues of the perineal membrane complex in which the following structures are either embedded or to which they attach: the urogenital sphincter muscles and the portions of the urethra and the yoni that they surround. The **middle layer** or **superficial perineal compartment** or **space** lies inferior or superficial to (below) the surface of the perineal membrane complex and the perineal deep investing fascia and superior to Colles fascia. It includes the most distal parts of the urethral and yoni canals; the clitoral body, glans and crura; neurological and vascular structures of the clitoris, including the clitoral bulbs; the vestibular glands; and the ischiocavernosus, bulbocavernosus and superficial transverse perineal muscles. The **skin** comprises the **third layer**, which includes the external vulval structures and Camper and Colles fasciae. The perineal body fills the space between the introitus and the anterior border of the anal canal and is also included in the urogenital triangle.

Anal/posterior triangle: The lowermost region of the external perineum forms the shorter, broad-based, downwardly pointed **anal** or **posterior triangle**. The anatomical apex of the triangle is formed by the tip of the coccyx (as opposed to the obstetrical apex, which is located at the sacrococcygeal junction). The lateral boundaries extend from the coccyx on either side up to the ischial tuberosities; at this level the base meets that of the urogenital triangle. The anal triangle faces posteriorly at about a 125° angle when measured from the left (or 55° when measured from the right) when a woman is standing (this angle is derived from a horizontal line drawn level with the tip of the ischial tuberosity in a side view).

The anal triangle includes the anal canal, anal sphincters, anus, ischioanal fossae (the pelvic spaces filled with fat and loose connective tissue to either side of the anal canal that lie inferior to [below] the levator ani muscle complex) and, according to some sources, the puborectalis muscle. It is not divided into deep and superficial compartments.

Pelvic compartments demarcated by the pelvic organs

The deep pelvic cavity is also divided into two or sometimes three compartments that are defined by the organs that each contains. The floor of the deep pelvic cavity is formed by the superior surface of the levator ani muscle complex. The **anterior pelvic compartment** includes the bladder, the urethra and associated tissues. The yoni, which is connected on either side to the pelvic sidewalls by connective tissues, divides the deep pelvic cavity into anterior and posterior compartments. Some authors have formally designated the yoni canal as the **middle pelvic compartment**. The **posterior pelvic compartment** includes the rectosigmoid colon, the posterior cul-de-sac and associated tissues (Kurtz et al., 1979).

The anatomy of each pelvic region is presented in separate chapters in the following order: the urogenital triangle and associated structures, the levator ani muscles and associated structures, and the anal triangle and associated structures.

Supportive Soft Tissues of the Pelvis

Pelvic floor is a term applied generically to both the muscles and the connective tissues of the pelvis, as well as to the levator ani muscles specifically. In the generic sense, the pelvic floor consists of complex layers of soft tissues that close the pelvic cavity and support the organs within it. These tissues can be roughly divided into three supportive layers:

1. The superficial layer consists of the bulbocavernosus muscle and the tissue immediately superior to it, namely the anterior portion of the **perineal membrane connective tissue complex** (for brevity, hereafter usually referred to as the perineal membrane complex [p. 57]). The superficial layer also includes the perineal body (p. 70), the external anal sphincter (p. 97) and the anococcygeal ligament (p. 89). Fibers from all these parts link together, forming a midline bridge between the pubic bone and the coccyx that resists downward forces.
2. The middle layer consists of the levator ani muscles (p. 75), which provide most of the soft tissue support for the pelvic organs. Other pelvic muscles line the pelvic sidewalls, which overlie openings between the pelvic bones or ligaments or both. The muscles of the levator ani complex work together with these other

muscles to support the pelvic contents, maintain urinary continence and close the pelvic cavity in the midline. Interspersed between the organs and the muscles are loosely arranged connective tissues that act like packing material.

3. The deepest supportive layer consists of endopelvic connective tissues (pp. 36 and 114) that suspend the pelvic organs and extend to the pelvic sidewalls (DeLancey, 2002a).

Levator ani muscle complex

The levator ani muscle complex includes the pubovisceral (pubococcygeus) and its various parts, the iliococcygeus muscles and puborectalis muscle as well as parts of the anococcygeal ligament. Some authors also include the coccygeus (ischiococcygeus) muscles in this group. Parts of these muscles underlie the urogenital or anal triangle or both, depending upon the muscle in question.

Different Types of Pelvic Soft Tissues

Pelvic connective tissues

"Fascia" (FASH-ah) is a catch-all term that has been applied to a wide variety of different types of dissectible connective tissue aggregations. These range from membranous sheets that, when dissected from the surface of muscles, are similar in appearance to a placental membrane, to loosely woven collagenous fibers with no apparent strength (think of pink cotton candy and the way it is spun into long strips or sheets). While these *are* types of fascia in the broadest sense, the use of the same term to describe them all suggests that they are anatomically and functionally similar, which is not the case.

The use of the term "fascia" to describe the intrapelvic connective tissues has resulted in considerable confusion, leading Weber and Walters (1997), among others, to call for a change of terminology. Instead of referring to the loose tissues that serve as coverings for the pelvic organs as "fasciae," they propose the term **adventitiae** (ad-ven-TISH-ee) (singular, adventitia) with the location specified.

"Adventitia" is a somewhat generic term that describes subperitoneal, perivascular and areolar tissue ("areolar" refers to loose, irregularly arranged connective tissue) found in the pelvis and some other parts of the body that consists of elastin, fat, collagen and some nonvascular smooth muscle fibers in which blood vessels and nerve bundles are embedded. The protein elastin allows the tissues to stretch and return to their original shape. The protein collagen contributes strength (O'Dell & Morse, 2008). In most regions of the body, adventitia is primarily associated with blood vessels and does not have a distinct orientation, as does parietal fascia.

Thinking of the loose pelvic tissues as "fasciae" has been so misleading that surgeons have based corrective pelvic surgery techniques on this understanding. Such repairs tend to fail because adventitiae do not have sufficient strength to suspend or stabilize organs by themselves (Otcenasek et al., 2008).

With these distinctions in mind, it is helpful to distinguish the different types of fascia in the pelvic region as follows:

- **Subcutaneous fat (superficial fascia/hypodermis):** A layer of loose connective tissue underlies most of the dermis of the urogenital region. It consists of a web of collagen fibers interspersed with many fat cells. Anteriorly this fat extends a short distance above (anterosuperior to) the perineal membrane complex, where it forms the bulk of the mons pubis and labia majora. Posteriorly this fatty layer expands to fill the ischioanal fossa ("fossa" refers to a space or depression), which fills the large space superior to the banded portion of the perineal membrane, a space bounded by the inferior surface of the muscles of the pelvic floor, the pelvic walls, the anorectum and the skin (except the skin underlying the midline of the gynecologic perineum, which is free of fat) (van Houten, 2006).
- **Parietal fascia:** This tissue consists of a variably thin, tough layer that overlies all the muscles and some vital organs. It is usually what comes to mind when the term "fascia" is used. The parietal fascia is continuous with the deep investing fasciae surrounding the bones and the striated muscles elsewhere in the body. ("Investment" refers to the ensheathing or intimate enclosure of a specific group of muscles.) This dense parietal fascia is fused with the epimysium (the fibrous connective tissue layer that surrounds each muscle like a skin). The parietal fascia divides to cover groups of muscles, spans gaps between muscles and fuses with the periosteal fasciae that cover the bones. Parietal fascia envelopes each muscle and forms a continuous layer linking the muscles together, although this understanding is obscured by naming regions of fascia after each muscle with which it is directly associated, such as the "obturator internus fascia." These names designate localized regions of parietal fascia, not separate structures (van Houten, 2006).
- **Endopelvic fascia:** The endopelvic pelvic fascia forms a continuous three-dimensional mass of variably dense connective tissue in which the pelvic organs are embedded. It acts as a loose packing material that drapes over the organs in sheets (again, think of cotton candy), that is penetrated by nerves, blood and lymph vessels. This adventitia protects and stabilizes organs, while allowing them to change shape (Ercoli et al., 2005).

  Another term sometimes used with respect to the pelvic structures is **visceral pelvic fascia**. Although in the TERMINOLOGIA ANATOMICA the term "endopelvic fascia" is listed as a synonym for "pelvic investing fascia," in the clinical literature the term "endopelvic fascia" is generally used as a synonym for "visceral pelvic fascia" (van Houten, 2006). "Viscera" is another word for organs and, while some organs do have a distinct layer of fascia that encloses them, the pelvic organs do not.

More about the pelvic connective tissues can be found on page 114.

Pertinent anatomy related to muscles

Muscle fibers: There are two types of muscle fibers. **Skeletal** or **voluntary muscles** have striations that result from the overlapping of thick and thin muscular fibers. **Smooth muscle fibers** lack striations and are involuntary; that is, they cannot be consciously controlled.

Some muscles contain a mixture of both types of fibers. **Detrusor muscle** is composed of smooth fibers that act by expelling a substance; the wall of the urinary bladder is composed mostly of these types of fibers.

Skeletal muscle consists of bundles of individual fibers called **myocytes**. Each myocyte contains many **myofibrils**, which are strands of proteins (actin and myosin) that grab hold of each other and pull, shortening or contracting the fibers. The nature of these contractions is governed by two types of striated fibers: slow twitch (Type I) and fast twitch (Type II).

Human striated muscles contain a genetically determined mix of both slow- and fast-twitch fibers. In most voluntary muscles, there are an equal number of both types of fibers. Slow-twitch fibers use oxygen more efficiently and respond more slowly than do fast-twitch fibers. They produce continuous, low-intensity, repetitive muscle contractions and can remain stimulated for a long time before they tire. Therefore, slow-twitch fibers help maintain more or less constant muscle tone.

In contrast, fast-twitch fiber activity occurs by a process of anaerobic metabolism. These fibers generally produce the same amount of force per contraction as do slow-twitch fibers, but they are able to do so much more rapidly, providing short bursts of high-intensity contraction. They also fatigue much more quickly, so an intense contraction cannot be sustained for long. Fast-twitch fibers are an asset in the pelvic area when continence must be maintained or restored under pressure (Bodyandfitness.com, 2008; Quinn, 2008). There is some evidence that, with training, skeletal muscle fiber types can be converted from fast to slow or vice versa.

Connections between muscles and between muscles and other structures: The following terms will be used to discuss ways that muscles connect to themselves and other structures:

Decussate (DEE-coo-sate): "Decussation" refers to the interweaving of fibers from two different parts of the same muscle (as in a pair of muscle parts) or of fibers from completely different muscles. At their meeting point, the fibers cross over each other, forming an "X". There may be one or more crisscrossings of fibers.

Digastric (DIE-gastric): Digastric muscles have two fleshy, usually symmetrical parts that are connected by a tendinous region. Muscle fibers may decussate before entering a tendinous region as well as within it.

Origin and insertion: These terms describe the attachment points at either end of a muscle part. The **origin** of a muscle denotes the proximal, less mobile point of attachment, i.e., the part attached to the more fixed part of the skeleton or (in some cases) soft tissue. The **insertion** of a muscle refers to the other, more distal end that is connected to a more mobile part of the skeleton or soft tissue.

Raphe (RAY-fee): A raphe is the union of two contiguous, bilaterally symmetrical parts. A tendinous region uniting muscle fibers may also be referred to as a raphe.

Tendinous (TEN-dun-us): True tendons are part of a muscle or muscle complex. Tendons consist of nondistensible fibrous bands of variable length that connect the fleshy part of a muscle to a bone or another structure. Pure tendons consist of bundles of densely arranged, almost parallel collagenous fibers; rows of elongated connective tissue cells; and a minimal amount of ground substance. A tendon may unite with the end of the fleshy part of a muscle, or it may run parallel with or extend from the center of the fleshy part of a muscle for a longer or shorter distance, receiving muscle fibers along its path. When determining the length of a muscle, the tendinous and fleshy parts are measured together. Certain attachments of the pelvic muscles are referred to as "tendinous," which means that they are anatomically similar to tendons and function in similar ways, but that their tissue construction is not identical in every respect (Stedman's, 2007).

The Urogenital Triangle and Related Structures

This chapter begins with an explanation of the major clinical landmarks related to the urogenital triangle: the bladder, urethra, and yoni and some related structures. Then, adjacent structures within the urogenital triangle are discussed, including the urethrovaginal sphincter muscle complex, the perineal membrane connective tissue complex, the clitoral complex and the perineal body.

Bladder

The urinary bladder is a hollow, globular organ that is collapsed when completely empty. Its anteroinferior (lower front) wall rests upon the connective tissues overlying the inner surface of the pubic bone. The posteroinferior (lower back) wall rests upon the upper yoni wall and the posterosuperior (upper back) wall abuts the anterior uterine wall.

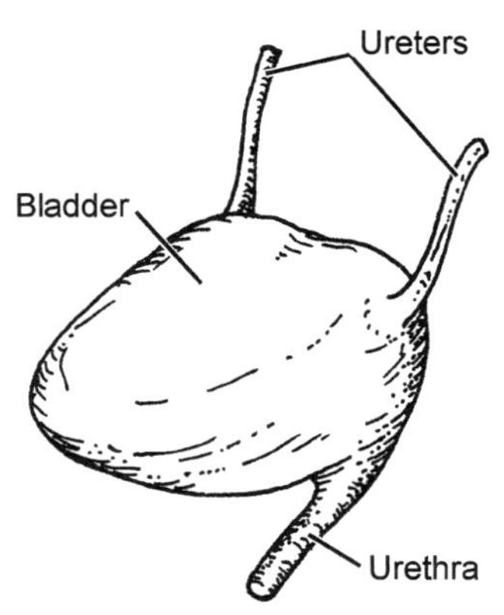

Bladder (antero-oblique view)

The bladder is lined with mucosa that overlies a loose submucosa. Its walls are made up of coarse bundles of smooth muscle fibers.

The wall of the upper part, or dome, is thin and distensible. It consists of poorly defined layers of detrusor muscle fibers that run in various directions. At the level of the vesical neck (the part of the urethra that passes through the bladder wall), the muscle layers of the bladder wall become more distinct. The bladder base consists of the wall that lies below the level of the internal ureteral orifices (of the tubes that extend from each kidney) and is the least distensible.

The internal urethral orifice is surrounded by two U-shaped muscular bands that overlap in opposite directions. These bands may provide a sphincteric action around the urethra as it passes through the bladder wall. Proper autonomic innervation would allow these muscles to work together: when the dome contracts to expel urine, the muscles surrounding the visceral neck would relax; when the dome relaxes to accommodate urine, the muscles adjacent to the visceral neck would contract to maintain a watertight seal.

Subtle tonic responses from type 1 (slow-twitch) muscle fibers occur during bladder filling as part of the **guarding reflex**, a primitive sacrospinal reflex involving nerve impulses triggered by bladder distension that lead to stimulation of the pelvic floor and the external urethral sphincter. These responses increase the continence threshold as the bladder fills and are dependent upon a neurologically responsive pelvic floor (Lukban & Whitmore, 2002).

The **trigone** is a slightly elevated triangular area of smooth muscle at the internal base of the bladder. The lower point of the trigone meets the internal urethral orifice. The ureteral orifices mark its upper two points, which in the undistended bladder are spaced about 3 cm apart (Stepp & Walters, 2007). At the level of the ureteral orifices, the trigone widens into a ring. The trigone is thought to serve as an internal urethral sphincter that assists in the involuntary closure of the proximal urethra (DeLancey, 2003a). The bladder gradually fills during sexual excitement (Schultz et al, 1999), perhaps nature's way of ensuring that the urethra will be flushed out shortly after sexual activity to protect against infection.

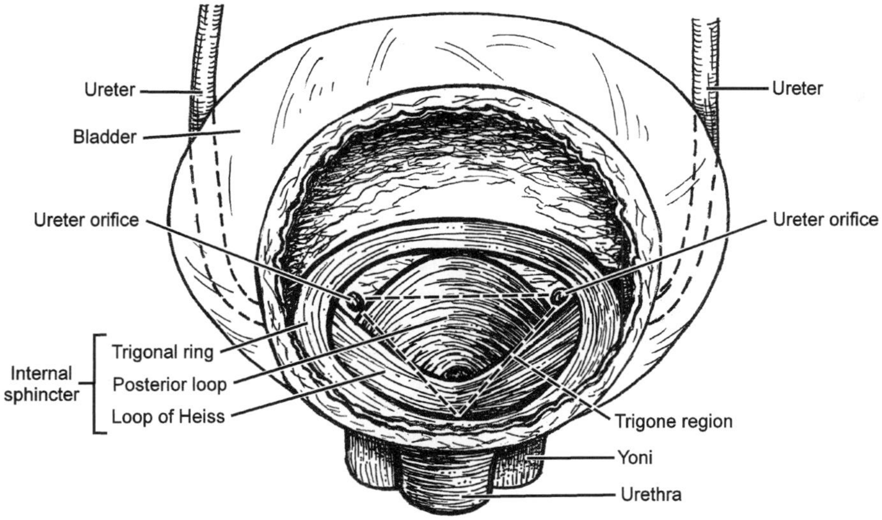

Landmarks inside the bladder: frontal view with anterior bladder wall partially cut away

Birth-related trauma: The bladder does not usually sustain damage during normal childbirth, but when it does, it needs to be repaired in a hospital whenever possible.

Pubovesical muscles

The smooth fibers of the pubovesical muscles are an extension of the detrusor muscle of the bladder wall. In the midline they decussate with detrusor fibers of the external, superior urethral wall as it exits the bladder. The pubovesical muscles lie within connective tissue; when the muscles and connective tissues are considered together, they are known as the "pubovesical 'ligaments'" (although they are not true ligaments). The pubovesical muscles reach from the bladder wall to the **tendinous arch of the pelvic fasciae** (see page 118).

Detrusor muscle fibers can withstand a great deal of stretching, and thus these pubovesical attachments are unsuited to provide support under stress. Indeed, they are located superior to the vesical neck, not under it, so they cannot do so. The pubovesical muscles may help to open the vesical neck at the onset of urination by contracting to pull the anterior wall of the vesical neck forward (DeLancey, 2002a). There are other anterior urethral support structures that are not detailed here. This muscle is included because it is immediately superior to the pubovaginal region of the pubovisceral complex and because it is mentioned later in this text in the context of tissue changes that occur during fetal descent (see page 163).

Urethra (you-REE-thrah)

The urethra is the centrally located, flexible, slightly concavely curved, collapsed muscular tube through which urine leaves the body. Clitoral structures surround the distal urethra to a variable degree, usually with the only gap being where the urethra is embedded in the distal yoni wall. Thus, the urethra can be regarded as a clitoral orifice (O'Connell et al., 2008). The urethra ranges in length from 3 to 5 cm and is inclined in a slightly posterior direction. Its posterior wall exits the bladder at an angle of nearly 90° (the posterior urethrovesical angle). This sharp angle helps maintain continence; it relaxes during voiding. This angle is usually not depicted in illustrations because it is relaxed in dissected tissues. From the point that the urethra exits the bladder, its floor is embedded in a trough like indentation (the carina) in the ceiling of the lower third of the anterior yoni wall.

The lining of the urethral lumen (**lumen** refers to the space within any tube-shaped structure) has numerous longitudinal folds, allowing the urethra to expand. At rest, the lumen forms a horizontal slit about 6 mm in diameter, but it can dilate to a diameter of over 1 cm. The urethra elongates on standing, during late pregnancy and during labor.

Within the bladder, the internal urethral orifice lies about 1.25 cm below the horizontal plane that passes through the upper border of the **pubic symphysis** (sim-FAH-sis). Below that, the intramural part or visceral neck (both terms refer to the portion of the urethra that passes through the bladder wall) is less than 1 cm long and accounts for the first 15 to 20% of its total length (assuming that the internal orifice is 0 and the external orifice is 100%). The midurethra (20 to 60% of its total length) is covered by the striated urethral sphincter muscle. The next 60 to 80% of the urethral canal passes through the deeper connective tissues of the perineal membrane complex. This part is covered by the compressor urethrae muscle and by the urethrovaginal sphincter. The most distal portion (80 to 100% of its length) courses beyond the inferior border of the perineal membrane complex and through the arch formed by the bulbocavernosus muscles before opening into the upper vestibule, about 2.5 cm below the clitoral glans (Sevely, 1987). (These adjacent parts are discussed later in this chapter.)

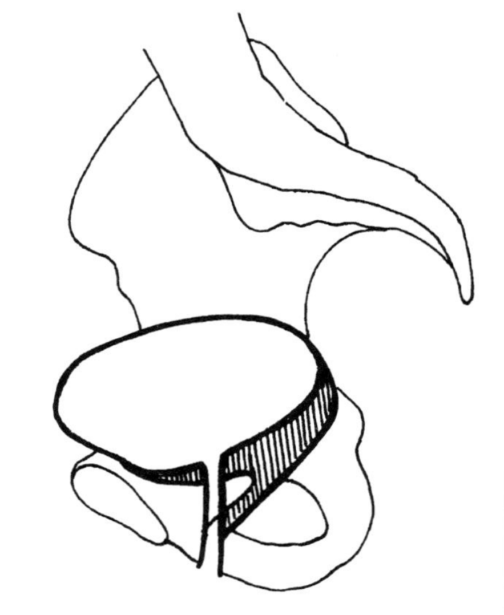

Sagittal view: bladder and urethra in the pelvis (white: at rest; shaded: voiding)

Attachments: The urethra is supported along its length by various connections between the yoni and the periurethral tissues to the muscles and fasciae of the pelvic wall. The primary layer of tissue that supports the urethra has two lateral attachments: an adventitial attachment and a muscular one.

The primary adventitial attachment connects the periurethral tissues and anterior yoni wall to the arcus tendineus fasciae pelvis. Contraction of the pubovisceral complex is believed to assist in stabilizing these tissues and may relieve strain on the arcus tendineus fasciae pelvis to some extent (DeLancey, 1994; Stein & DeLancey, 2008).

The primary muscular support for the urethra consists of the vaginolevator attachments, which span between the anterosuperior "corner" of the yoni wall and the medial surface of the puboanalis muscle. These attachments, augmented by the endopelvic adventitiae attachments on either side, form a hammock that supports the midthird of the urethra. During an exam, the vaginolevator attachments can be identified by the distinct superolateral sulcus grooves of the lateral yoni walls.

In addition, as it nears the meatus, the urethra is increasingly embedded in dense connective tissues that are primarily part of the perineal membrane complex and are continuous with the suspensory ligament of the clitoris and the fascial sheaths of the external genital muscles. This fibrous tissue has been called the "pubourethral ligament," although these tissues do not form a true ligament (DeLancey, 1986) and are better thought of as pubourethral supports, a term that refers to a group of related structures with a common function (DeLancey, 1988).

These muscular and connective tissue attachments determine the position of the urethra. When at rest, the visceral neck is held high within the pelvis, about 3 cm above the lower border of the pubic bone, a position maintained by the constant muscular tone of the pubovisceral complex (a part of the levator ani muscle complex).

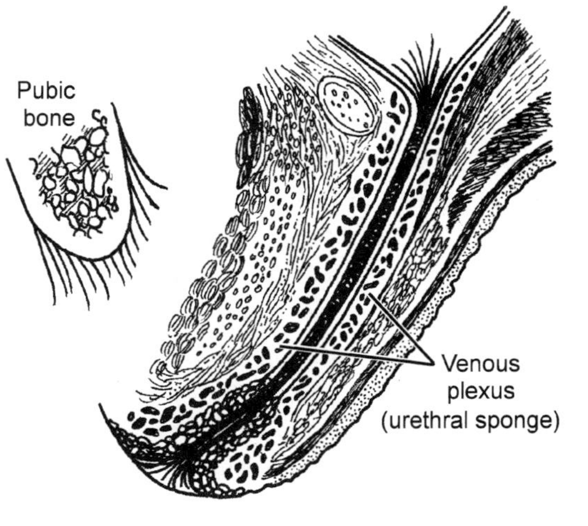

Urethral sponge (sagittal view)

<u>**The urethral sponge:**</u> As is typical of other tubular structures, the wall of the urethra, from the outside in, consists of adventitial, muscular and submucosal (sub-mew-KOH-sal) layers with a layer of mucous membrane lining the lumen. Embedded within the submucosa (DeLancey, 2003b) is a spongy encasement of clitoral circulatory tissue that encloses the top and sides of the length of the urethra all the way up to the bladder neck. This has been called the **urethral sponge** by feminist writers (Downer et al., 1991). The urethral sponge is 1 to 1.5 mm thick throughout most of its length, thinning somewhat near the meatus and widening slightly as it approaches the upper end of the urethra, near the bladder. It underlies the urethral smooth muscle layers and surrounds the female prostate glands (discussed shortly). Although this tissue is vascular and the urethra is surrounded by the clitoral bulbs, there does not appear to be any separate erectile tissue in the urethral wall itself (O'Connell et al., 2008). Engorgement of the urethral sponge may assist in creating a watertight seal in the urethral lumen and contributes to the pelvic engorgement referred to as the "orgasmic platform," a term coined by Masters and Johnson (1966) to describe the vasocongestion that occurs during the plateau phase of sexual arousal.

<u>**Urethral glands (female prostate/paraurethral [pair-ah-you-REE-thral] Skene glands):**</u>
The female prostate glands were first noted by Reinier De Graaf way back in 1672, but,

like so many things female, this knowledge got pushed aside for many centuries (Jocelyn & Setchell, 1972).

It is now recognized that female prostate glands are embedded in the submucosa of the urethral wall. Though these glands are still often referred to as paraurethral glands ("para" meaning "near or alongside"), the most precise way to describe them reflects their true histology: female prostate or urethral glands. The use of other terms (Skene or paraurethral glands) is now considered inaccurate (Zaviacic et al., 2002). For some time these glands were considered insignificant (vestigal) in females; this attitude is giving way as they become better understood.

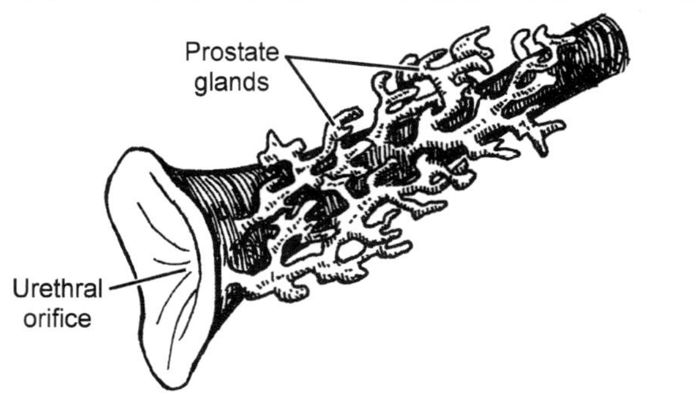

Female prostate glands

These glands consist of widespread branching ductal channels that open into the urethral lumen and less numerous glands that together resemble the stunted branches of a tree, the trunk of which is the urethral canal. The glands are richly supplied with smooth muscle fibers.

The number and distribution of these glands varies widely among women and is probably influenced by such factors as childbearing, hormonal balance and age. The ducts and glands surround the female urethra on all sides and are scattered most abundantly laterally in 70% of women, but may extend the full length of the urethra and, in some cases, encircle it on all sides. Ten percent of women have glands along the floor of the outer third to half of their urethra, where they may create a slight bulge in the ceiling of the yoni. Glandular weight ranges between 2.6 to 5.2 g. The glands average 3.3 cm in length, 1.9 cm in width, and 1 cm in height. Women also have folds and tiny pit-like recesses called **lacunae,** or tiny pockets, that open into the lumen of the urethra, nearer the bladder end, which may be smaller versions of these glands.

Near the external urethral orifice, several urethral glands often merge and open into larger ducts. When present, these ducts are embedded in the submucosal tissue of the urethral canal. In some cases, they merge into a single duct that exits along the posterior wall of the urethra. Other women have a pair of larger ducts that end in small internal openings on either side of the distal urethral canal or along the lateral margin of the external urethral orifice, matching the classic description of the orifices of the paraurethral glands. These orifices are usually more obvious in multiparas in whom their location may be revealed due to flattening and eversion of the urethral meatus as a consequence of the pressure from fetal descent. In nulliparas, the urethral meatus is usually well defined and not everted; the internal openings, when present, are not often visible unless the meatus is parted to expose its most distal lining (Huffman, 1948). In some cases, the orifices noted are actually the mouths of minor vestibular glands.

Prostate gland secretions are emitted from the urethra and are biochemically similar to male prostate fluid (as compared to urine). Female prostatic fluids consist primarily of female prostate-specific antigen (PSA), prostate-specific acid phosphatase (PSAP), glucose and creatinine. The fluid may also contain blood urea nitrogen (BUN), potassium, sodium and chloride (Wimpissinger et al., 2007).

These prostatic secretions contribute to female ejaculate, which some women report during orgasm. Monique Wittig (1935-2003), a French lesbian feminist theorist, noting the lack of specific terminology to refer to female sexual fluids, coined the term **cyprine** (see-preen) to describe the combined secretions produced during female arousal and orgasm (the homologue of semen) (Shaktini, 2005). The quantity of cyprine varies widely, from a few drops to as much as two cups; because of this wide variation in quantity, many more women may ejaculate than are aware of it (The-Clitoris.com, 2008).

The female prostate appears to be far less susceptible to serious disease than its male counterpart, with benign enlargement, inflammation and cancer the main problems that arise, although the actual incidence of such disease in women is not known (Zaviacic et al., 2002).

Functioning: The upper two-thirds of the urethra is mobile and under voluntary control. At the onset of urination, the levator ani muscles relax, allowing the urethra to descend, which straightens the posterior urethrovesical angle and allows the urine to flow. After urination, the normal resting tone of the muscles returns, and the urethrovesical angle is restored (DeLancey, 2002b).

Birth-related trauma: It is uncommon for the urethra to be damaged during childbirth. When it is, however, it is best repaired in hospital, as repair can be difficult and damage may be more extensive than is obvious.

Yoni (YO-nee) (birth canal/vagina [vah-JI-nah])

The yoni is a centrally located, hollow, collapsed, distensible, fibromuscular tube with distinct anatomical regions. The lower third of the yoni is unique because the urethra is embedded in its anterior wall and because its most distal region is intimately related to the clitoris. Clitoral circulatory structures are embedded in its anterolateral walls (the clitoral bulbs) and in the perineal body (the perineal sponge) inferiorly. Because of this, the yoni can be regarded as a clitoral orifice. The remaining two-thirds of the yoni canal appears to be nearly devoid of sexually responsive structures (Jannini et al., 2006).

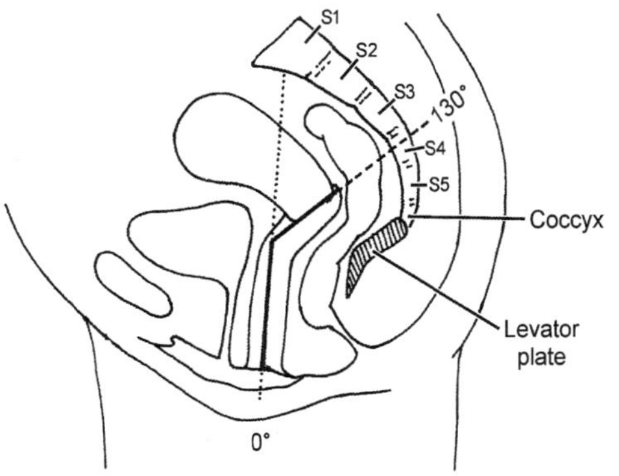

Axis of yoni canal (sagittal view)

Yoni axis: According to Funt and colleagues (1978), when a woman is standing, the distal two-thirds of the yoni canal rises up from the introitus toward the center of S1 (the first sacral vertebra). The upper 3 to 4 cm of the canal then bends, achieving an angle of, on average, 130° or so in the direction of the sacrum (this angle is derived from a line drawn through the center of the yoni canal to the center of S1 and measured from the posterior side of the yoni canal at the level of the bend). In most women, this bend causes the upper third of the canal to point toward S3 or S4 (ranging between S2 and S5). This bend reflects normal muscular support. It exists because the upper third of the yoni rests on the rectum, which itself rests on the supportive shelf formed by the **levator plate** (explained on page 89).

This normal bend is obliterated in routinely prepared cadavers because all the muscles are completely relaxed and thus the support from the levator plate and the pubovisceral complex is withdrawn. This is why most illustrations depict the yoni as straighter than it actually is in living women whose levator plate is well toned.

Dimensions: Overall the yoni ranges between 7 and 10 cm in length. The posterior yoni wall is always longer than the anterior wall by 1.5 to 2 cm (Krantz, 1959). The posterior wall averages 7.5 cm in length among nulliparas; it tends to lengthen more with childbirth, after which it averages 8.7 cm. The anterior wall averages 7 cm from the introitus to the external cervical os; it is somewhat shorter than the posterior wall because the lower end of the cervix occupies the anterior yoni vault. At the deepest end, where the cervix projects into the tube, the anterior vault (the area in front of the cervix) averages 3.5 cm deep and the posterior vault (the area behind the cervix) averages 1.75 cm deep (Hirst, 1903). The yoni canal becomes progressively wider as it nears the cervix. Its midportion is 2.5 cm wide. The width at the deepest end is about 5 cm.

Tissue layers: Although the overall thickness of the yoni wall is only 0.35 cm, it is, as is true for all tubular structures, made up of several layers. Starting with the outer wall, these are:

- **Adventitial or outer coat:** The outermost or adventitial layer consists of a thin matrix of dense connective tissue that is an extension of adjacent endopelvic adventitiae. It is composed of areolar tissue with variable amounts of collagen, elastin and fat. Blood vessels, lymphatics and nerves are embedded within it. This soft layer surrounds the yoni and adjacent pelvic organs, allowing them to expand and contract independently. The adventitial coat links with the superolateral ligaments (cardinal or transverse) and portions of the pubocervical (pubourethral) ligament. These connections help anchor the yoni canal to the pelvis along the sides and from above. Along the posterior outer yoni wall, the adventitial coat is sparse, with only a few fibers reaching completely under the tube, leaving little, if any, adventitial tissue from the yoni wall to lie between the adventitial covering of the rectal wall and the yoni's fibromuscular layer (DeLancey, 1999).
- **Fibromuscular coat:** Next is a thin coat of well-developed smooth muscle consisting of interdigitating circular and longitudinal fibers. The more abundant longitudinal fibers are found primarily along the sides of the yoni, especially near the distal end of the canal, where they are joined by striated fibers from the puboanalis muscle and the anal sphincter. The circular fibers surround the entire

tube (Wendell-Smith & Wilson, 1991). The muscle fibers in this layer are connected by obliquely oriented decussating fibers of connective tissue (Jannini et al., 2006).

- **Submucosa:** Underlying the fibromuscular coat is a loose, indefinite submucosa that attaches the muscular layer to the lamina propria (Krantz, 1959).
- **Lamina propria mucosae:** The lamina propria ("mucosae" is usually left off in modern usage but is more accurate) is the deep component of a mucosal wall. The lamina propria of the yoni wall consists of a relatively thick layer of moderately dense, highly elastic, papillated connective tissue that is heavily laced with lymphocytes and blood vessels and may contain some lymph follicles, but lacks glands. It underlies the epithelium. The term "mucosa" or "mucous membrane" always refers to both the epithelium and the lamina propria (Burkitt et al., 1993; Wendell-Smith & Wilson, 1991).
- **Mucosal epithelial stratum:** The thick epithelial lining of the yoni is 0.15 to 0.2 mm deep. It is made up of loosely arranged, nonkeratinized, stratified squamous epithelium. This layer is relatively tough, and its structure is very close to that of ordinary skin except that it lacks secondary skin structures (hair follicles, sebaceous glands and sweat glands), a feature that prevents microorganisms from entering the yoni wall (Wendell-Smith & Wilson, 1991). It has a flat papillary base layer. Its cells are continuously regenerating at a rate two to four times faster than that of ordinary skin (where cell turnover takes about a week). Hormonally mediated changes become apparent in the yoni mucosa in one to two days; similar changes take twice as long to appear in vulval skin.

The muscular layer and highly elastic lamina propria account for the remarkable distention that the yoni wall can sustain. After coitus, the wall involuntarily contracts, which helps maintain a pool of semen in the region of the cervix (Burkitt et al., 1993).

Trauma may cause the yoni wall's mucosal layer to separate from its muscular layer, resulting in a tear that has two visible layers of tissue, one overlying the other. This can happen from the level of the introitus all the way back to the internal apex of the tear. When it occurs, both layers can be gathered into each stitch as the repair proceeds. A tear of sufficient length may also reveal the rectovaginal space (explained further on page 48).

Blood and nerve supply: The lamina propria contains an extensive network of large, almost cavernous, interconnected, thin-walled venous spaces that are most abundant along the lateral yoni walls. These venous plexuses can be over 1 cm in diameter in young women, but their diameter may reduce to less than 0.5 cm in older women due to hormonal changes (O'Connell & Sanjeevan, 2006). This vascular bed can convert the walls of the yoni into erectile tissue. When engorged during sexual arousal, these vessels secrete fluid through the walls of the yoni into the lumen of the canal (DeLancey, 2003b; Wendell-Smith & Wilson, 1991).

The upper two-thirds of the yoni is supplied by branches of the superior and inferior vesical arteries, which join with branches of the uterine artery. The urethra and the lower third of the yoni are supplied by branches of the bulbar artery (which stem from the perineal division of the internal pudendal artery). The dorsal clitoral arteries also supply the distal yoni where it is attached to the urethra and clitoral bulbs (O'Connell & Sanjeevan, 2006). For more details about the yoni blood supply, see the work of Krantz (1959).

Autonomic nerves form a dense plexus that extends from the rectum and runs along the sides of the upper two-thirds of the yoni. This plexus also supplies the cavernosal nerves of the clitoral body at the level of the upper urethra (O'Connell & Sanjeevan, 2006).

Functions: The yoni is the passageway for the menstrual flow, sexual penetration, fertilization, and childbirth. The yoni allows indirect stimulation of sensitive vascular and nerve tissues of the clitoris and of the female prostate glands during sexual activity.

Contacts with surrounding structures: The most distal part of the yoni is fused anteriorly with the urethra; is flanked laterally by the clitoral bulbs and, behind them, the bands of the perineal membrane; and is fused posteriorly with the perineal body. The upper part of the most distal third is bounded anteriorly by the upper part of the urethra, posteriorly by the rectal wall and laterally by the vaginolevator links to the medial edges of the puboanalis muscle. The midthird of the yoni is adjacent to the visceral neck and bladder anteriorly, is suspended from the cardinal ligaments from above and is bounded by the ureters and the uterine arteries on either side; its posterior wall meets the peritoneal lining of the rectouterine pouch. This pouch is the part of the peritoneum that covers the posterior yoni fornix and, in some women, also covers the upper third of the yoni wall (DeLancey, 2003b; Kuhn & Hollyhock, 1982). The uppermost apex of the yoni is normally level with the ischial spines.

The rectovaginal space: The pelvic "spaces," are really cleavage planes; that is, potential spaces filled or loosely covered with connective tissue that lie between structures. A surgeon can easily separate adjacent structures by peeling apart the loose connective tissue that lies between the parts, thus creating "spaces."

The rectovaginal space is the one that midwives are most likely to encounter during suturing. It begins at the internal apex of the perineal body, 2 to 3 cm above the level of the hymenal ring, and extends posteriorly to the rectouterine pouch and laterally around the sides of the rectum to where the rectovaginal adventitia meets the endopelvic adventitia. At the level of the cervix, some fibers of the **cardinal-uterosacral ligaments** extend down behind the yoni, attaching it to the lateral rectal walls and then to the sacrum. These "rectal pillars" separate the midline rectovaginal space from the "pararectal spaces" to either side of the rectum.

A birth-related yoni tear often leaves all involved layers of the yoni wall attached, resulting in a V-shaped laceration that passes straight down through the perineal body. If the tear extends posteriorly to the part of the yoni floor that overlies the rectal wall, the connective tissue layers sometimes come apart, separating the yoni floor from the underlying loose mesh of adventitiae. When this happens, the torn edges of the yoni floor hang suspended above the (usually) intact rectal wall. This opens an area in the rectovaginal space, creating a gap beneath a portion of or along the entire length of the tear in the part of yoni floor that overlies the rectal wall that looks like this [_] in cross-section. (The top "edges" represent the torn edges of the yoni floor; the space below, the rectovaginal space;

and the solid line below that, the intact rectal wall.) More distally, where the yoni overlies the perineal body, separation of the mucosal layer of the floor of the yoni wall from its muscular layer can present a similar appearance. (For a review of other pelvic "spaces," see page 48.)

Connective tissue surrounding the yoni and bladder: Some organs, such as the heart, lungs and digestive tract, have distinct bursal coverings consisting of closed, double-layered, membranous envelopes, with an epimysial layer—the visceral, skin-like covering that is fused to the surface of the organs—and a parietal layer that contacts other body parts (Moore & Dalley, 2006). The yoni, however, is separated from the bladder anteriorly only by a continuation of the loose areolar tissue that merges with the yoni adventitia. At the level of the urethra, this adventitial tissue is even less distinct and the muscular layers of the yoni and urethra are fused. Neither the yoni, the bladder, nor the uterus have a distinct bursal covering.

The looser covering that is present allows these organs to expand and contract independently. The covering and the surrounding mesh of loose connective tissue provides a framework that stabilizes and anchors the yoni canal. Yoni support is also provided by various muscles, especially those of the levator ani and urethrovaginal sphincter muscle complexes.

The layer of "fascia" widely described as lying between the anterior yoni and the urethra is a surgical artifact created by splitting the yoni epithelium away from the muscular coat of the urethra or by dividing the yoni's anterior muscular coat into two layers (Weber & Walters, 1997).

The rectovaginal septum: The presence of a layer of fascia sandwiched between approximately the midthird of the posterior yoni wall and the anterior rectal wall has been a matter of debate for well over one hundred years. Despite numerous reports claiming to have found such a layer and the persistence of descriptions in much of the medical literature, the growing consensus, based on careful histological studies, is that a distinct fascial layer does not exist (Goff, 1931; Kleeman et al., 2005; Ricci et al., 1947). The distal ends of the posterior yoni wall and the anterior rectal wall are attached to dense connective tissue overlying the superior surface of the perineal body, but with no plane of cleavage. The midthird or so of the posterior yoni wall is superior to the posterior apex of the perineal body and directly overlies the rectal wall. Here, the connective tissue between the anterior outer muscular wall of the rectum and the posterior fibromuscular wall of the yoni consists of a mesh of fatty tissue mixed with discontinuous bundles of fibrous tissue, blood vessels and many elastic fibers. Superior to the midthird of the yoni wall, the tissue between the walls of the yoni and the rectum consists primarily of fatty tissue.

None of these interspersed tissues can rightly be called a discrete layer of fascia. The "fascia" that has been widely described is actually an artifact produced when the adventitial and fibromuscular layers of the yoni are separated from the lamina propria of the yoni wall during surgery. The terms "fascia," "Denonvilliers fascia" and "rectovaginal septum" should not be used to describe this tissue because they are inaccurate and misleading, oversimplifying a complex arrangement of connective tissue and muscle fibers that support the anterior rectal wall (Kleeman et al., 2005).

The loose mesh of connective tissue that is present merges with the cardinal uterosacral ligamentous complex posteriorly. Laterally, it extends from the sidewalls of the yoni and merges with the true fascial layer of the levator ani muscle complex. Anteriorly, it merges with the perineal body. These extensions consist of a mixture of collagen, smooth muscle and very dense elastin fibers and are a part of the endopelvic adventitiae. These tissues help to support the perineal body and to prevent the rectal wall from bulging into the yoni (Richardson, 1993).

Shape of the yoni canal: The yoni is narrowest at the introitus and becomes progressively wider as it approaches the cervix. On coronal section, the shape of the passage also varies along its length. The orifice is a vertical slit. The shape of the lumen is irregular at the level of the hymen. Superior to the hymen, the anterior and posterior walls touch, forming an H shape in cross section, a configuration that creates four walls: two lateral walls, a posterior wall (floor) and an anterior wall (ceiling). The shape of the yoni walls vary according to the adjacent external connective tissue attachments throughout their length. The H of the first third of the yoni above the hymen is formed by the adventitial connections at the four "corners" of the anterior end and is most obvious after a woman has just given birth. The H shape is asymmetric or absent in some women (Fielding et al., 2000), which may reflect connective tissue weakness. The midthird of the posterior yoni wall is shaped like a "W" because in this area the depression created by the urethra is no longer present in the anterior yoni wall, while the rectal canal, below the yoni, creates a bulge in the posterior wall. The posterior wall of the upper third of the yoni is shaped like a "U" where the cervix dips down to fill the anterosuperior region. Longitudinally, the yoni canal has a slightly convex curve throughout its lower two-thirds, a shape created by pressure from the rectal canal that is immediately posterior to it.

Characteristics of the yoni lumen (LOO-men): Behind the hymenal ring, the lumen of the yoni is primarily oriented transversely, that is, a horizontal slit. The walls of the lumen are in contact except at the upper end, where they are held apart by the cervix.

The anterior and posterior walls form two softly rounded, longitudinally oriented ridges, called "columns," (column rugarum). In the area of the urethra this ridge becomes more prominent and is called the "urethral carina." These columns are covered with numerous transverse wrinkles, called **rugae** (RUE-gay), that are interspersed with furrows of varying depth. The rugae are most numerous near the introitus, especially in women who have never given birth. The rugae are a product of both the irregular surface of the yoni epithelium, due to variations in its thickness, and the intact connective tissue that underlies the yoni wall. The rugae allow the yoni walls to distend rapidly and enormously to accommodate sexual penetration and childbirth.

In the region of the vesical neck, a deep lateral fold and groove are present. The anterior fold, in conjunction with a similar, less prominent fold in the posterior yoni wall at the upper level of the levator ani complex has been called the "fold of Shaw" (Krantz, 1959).

Structures within the yoni lumen: The following structures are found within the lumen of the yoni, starting with the deepest first and working outward.

Cervix (SER-viks): The cervix is the constricted, tube-shaped neck of the uterus. The internal os (orifice) opens into the uterus, and the external os opens into the yoni. The lower end of the cervix is called the **exocervix** or **ectocervix**. It protrudes into the upper vault of the yoni. In nulliparous women, the entire cervix is 2 to 4 cm long, with the exocervix comprising one-third of its length. The cervical diameter is about 2.5 cm with a tight, round opening, called the **os**. In parous women, the cervix is a little larger in diameter with a horizontally oriented, slit-shaped os.

The closed cervix protects the uterine cavity from microorganisms, allows for the flow of menstrual blood; admits semen for fertilization; produces, after conception, a protective mucus plug that acts as a uterine barrier; and dilates during birth to allow passage of the baby.

The cervix sometimes sustains birth-related damage needing repair. The sides of the cervix are less fibrous and less muscular than the anterior and posterior lips; thus, when tears occur, they are most often found at 3 or 9 o'clock. Cervical tears are tricky to repair and are best handled in a hospital if transport is an option.

Vault: The vault is the enlarged upper end of the yoni into which the exocervix projects.

Fornices (FOR-nih-sees): The protrusion of the exocervix into the vault of the yoni and adjacent connective tissue arrangements external to the yoni combine to create a circumferential recessed area between the exocervix and the yoni walls. This recessed area is divided into four regions called "fornices." Even though the fornices have no physical divisions, regional names have been assigned. The lateral fornices flank the sides of the cervix. The ureters and uterine arteries are adjacent to the lateral fornices on either side. The posterior fornix borders the retrouterine pouch and is the deepest of all. The anterior fornix borders the base of the bladder and the uterus and is formed by the fusion of the fibromuscular layer of the anterior yoni wall to the pericervical ring. The thin walls of the fornices allow palpation of nearby pelvic structures.

Sulcus (SUL-kuss) grooves: There are four sulcus grooves that are formed by the two uprights of the "H" in the H-shaped portion of the yoni where the sidewalls meet the anterior and posterior columns. The two upper (anterior) and two lower (posterior) grooves on either side contribute to the shape of the canal. Tears can occur along these grooves.

Gräfenberg spot: Most of the yoni wall is considered quite insensitive to touch. The one exception is the Gräfenberg spot, which is relatively sensitive to electrical stimulation. It is variably located somewhere along the midline of the anterior yoni wall, about halfway between the pubic bone and the cervix. Ultrasound studies have correlated the site of greatest sensitivity with the location of the external urethral sphincter muscle. It has been named the "Gräfenberg spot" (G-spot), for the doctor who first described this area in 1950.

Stimulation of the G-spot produces a variety of initial sensations, ranging from discomfort, to a sensation of urination, to pleasure. With additional stimulation, the area starts to swell, and in some women this alone produces an intense orgasm. It is theorized that this sensitivity is linked to the erectile tissue (the urethral sponge) that surrounds the top and sides of the urethra. Some women report that stimulation leading to orgasm also results in the discharge of thin, clear fluids, or cyprine, that differs from urine and can be copious. A portion of this fluid is produced by the female prostate glands.

There is much skepticism about the presence of an anatomically distinct entity in this area. Part of the reason is that, although over 250 articles have been published on this topic, most have not appeared in peer-reviewed journals. In addition, not all women can identify this area, and when it is present, its location appears to vary widely among women (Jannini et al., 2006; O'Connell & Sanjeevan, 2006). Nevertheless, many women report significant sexual sensitivity in this area, and that seems to me to be the best confirmation of all.

***Hymen (HI-men)*:** The hymen is a thin, circular or crescent-shaped fold of mucous membrane located just inside the introitus at a depth that varies between 0.5 to 2 cm. The hymen is absent in some women. Hymenal tissue consists of stratified squamous epithelium, fibrous tissue, and a few small blood vessels. It is richly supplied with free nerve endings (Krantz, 1958). The hymen is the interior boundary of the yoni vestibule.

The intact hymen presents as a band of varying thickness, shape and size with an opening in its center. Most commonly it forms a ring that is widest posteriorly or a crescent with its open margin directed toward the pubes. Other variations include a fringed band, a perforated membrane or a membranous septum so substantial that it may partially block the introitus. The medial edges of the hymenal band may touch. Sometimes the hymen is imperforate; if so, this is discovered at puberty when the menstrual blood begins to back up and create pressure.

Historically, the hymen has received more detailed description than any other part of the female genitalia, emphasizing its sociolegal importance to patriarchal cultures. The presence of an undamaged hymen has long been considered proof that a woman has not had heterosexual intercourse; that is, that she is a virgin. In reality, the hymen can be altered by normal activities, such as self-pleasuring or even horseback riding, so that it appears as though intercourse has occurred. Some women are born with a ruffled hymen that may give the appearance of having been damaged by heterosexual intercourse; in others, the hymen remains virginal in appearance regardless of sexual activity. In multiparas and in nulliparous women with damaged hymens, it consists of tags of firm, fibrous scar tissue on either side. These remnants are known as **caruncúlae myrtiformes (car-RUNK-kew-lah MUR-tee-form-es)** or **hymenales** but are most commonly referred to as **hymenal tags**. Hymenal tags are important landmarks during suturing and can also be used to help locate the inner edges of the puboanalis muscle during a digital exam.

***Introitus (in-TROY-tus)*:** The external opening of the yoni is called the "introitus." Because it is surrounded by clitoral circulatory tissue, it may be considered a clitoral orifice. The appearance of the introitus varies considerably with age. It is highly elastic and is able to stretch to accommodate the fetal parts during birth and yet return to a relatively small resting size of 3 to 4 cm (O'Connell et al., 2008).

***Vestibule of the yoni (fossa navicularis)*:** This is the entryway of the yoni. It consists of a shallow depression that lies between the anterior border of the hymen and the frenulum of the labia minora (the fourchette).

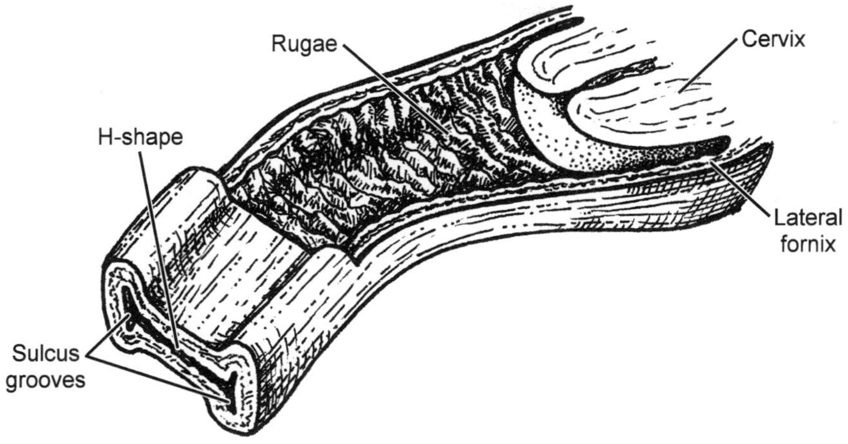

Upper two-thirds of the yoni canal (above the urethra)

Deep perineal (or urogenital) compartment (space, pouch or capsule)

The deep perineal compartment is an open-topped, three-dimensional, irregularly shaped region (here, the term "perineal" is used in the anatomical sense). Its inferior boundary is formed by the pubic bones and the inferior surface of the perineal membrane connective tissue complex (discussed on page 57). Its lateral boundaries are formed by the parietal fascia covering the medial surfaces of the obturator internus muscles and its posterior boundary is formed by the superior surface of the perineal body. Above the inferior surface of the perineal membrane complex, the deep perineal compartment is continuous with the pelvic cavity; its only superior boundary being the inferior fascia of the pubovisceral complex and the connective tissue that passes down around the edges and through the urogenital hiatus to intermingle with the connective tissue mass of the perineal membrane complex that lies to either side of the urethra (Stein & DeLancey, 2008).

Imagine the woman lying on her back with her legs spread. The deep perineal compartment can be divided into a ventral (anterior or upper) part that lies to either side of the urethra and a dorsal (posterior or lower) part that lies to either side of the yoni. The structures within the deep perineal compartment contribute to the pelvic floor (in its generic sense) and lend support to parts of the urogenital organs. The structures of the ventral portion include the urethral canal, the parts of the urethral sphincter muscle that are superior to the surface of the perineal membrane complex, and a mass of connective tissues intermingled with smooth muscle (discussed on page 56). The dorsal neurovasculature of the clitoral glans, body and crura also occupy this area. The structures included in the dorsal region of the compartment are the anterior third of the yoni canal and the anterior portions of the ischioanal fossa.

Urethrovaginal sphincter (sFINCK-ter) muscle complex: Now that we have some understanding of the placement and structure of the urethra and yoni, we will study the urethral sphincter muscles within the anterior compartment. These muscles have been poorly understood for many decades for a couple of reasons. Although they start out as fairly distinct striated muscles in early life, these small, difficult-to-identify striated fibers (30% smaller than most others) become increasingly and variably infiltrated with connective tissue and smooth muscle fibers as a woman ages, obscuring the anatomy considerably.

For many years, the understanding of these tissues was based primarily on the findings of Henle (1873), who described a sheet of muscle sandwiched between two layers of fasciae, giving rise to the concept of a "urogenital diaphragm." This teaching prevailed and was largely left unchallenged for well over a century.

In 1983, Oelrich observed that no researchers after Henle had confirmed the presence of a urogenital diaphragm, yet "all subsequent textbook writers had reiterated this concept with unerring accuracy" (including myself in previous editions). He undertook a comprehensive study of female specimens of varying ages and found that the widely repeated description of a "urogenital diaphragm" and "deep transverse muscle" were not anatomically accurate.

Oelrich described the striated urogenital sphincter as consisting primarily of three complexly innervated muscles that work together to contribute to urinary continence.

1) A urethral sphincter that surrounds the midthird of the urethra, just below the visceral neck.
2) Next, a compressor muscle that forms an arch over the anterior wall of the urethra.
3) A urethrovaginal sphincter that surrounds the distal urethra and yoni canal together.

The following description of these structures in adults is quite detailed. I feel it is important to explain this anatomy in depth because it is either poorly explained in or entirely missing from most other texts. For even greater detail, I refer you to Oelrich's original article. We begin with the deepest structures first.

Urethral sphincter (rhabdosphincter): The deepest of these muscles is the urethral sphincter, which forms the outermost muscular coat overlying the midthird of the urethra (thus Oelrich called it the "external urethral sphincter"). It consists of a nearly circumferential crescent of muscle that begins at the bladder neck and extends along the urethra for about 1.5 cm. (Oelrich [1983] described this muscle as covering the midthird of the urethra because the proximal end of the urethra extends up through the wall of the bladder and the urethral sphincter begins at the neck of the bladder [i.e., where the urethra exits the bladder wall].) The deepest section of the urethral sphincter is in the pelvic cavity, the midportion is level with the urogenital hiatus of the puboanalis muscle, and the most superficial portion traverses the superficial part of the perineal body.

In adults, the sphincter's striated fibers vary in their density and the degree to which they encircle the urethra. The underside of the urethral sphincter is relatively thick with a midline raphe made up primarily of smooth muscle fibers of the urethra, into which the sphincter fibers attach. The muscle becomes thinner as the fibers circle around to meet along the anterior urethra in the midline. Yucel and Baskin (2004) described the muscle as "horseshoe-shaped." At the base of the bladder, the sphincter's fibers intermingle with those of the bladder's circular smooth muscle coat. Between the base of the bladder and a point about 1.3 to 1.6 cm proximal to the external urethral meatus, the fibers of the bladder's smooth muscle coat are gradually replaced by those of the urethral sphincter. The urethral sphincter muscle overlies the area of highest urethral closure pressure and is probably involved in a sustained response to control the passage of urine.

Compressor urethra muscles (transverse urethral muscle): Distal to and directly continuous with the lower border of the urethral sphincter lies the next most shallow pair of muscles, the compressor urethra. Each half originates near the anterior border of the ischial tuberosities (or in some women at a variable distance from this point), as small tendons about 2 mm in diameter. These fibers extend two thin, flat bands from either side that rise toward the anterior wall of the urethra, paralleling the ischiopubic rami, forming an angle of about 130° with the urethra. As they do, they widen into muscular bands about 6 mm wide. As each band approaches the midline, it rises up and over the urethra. In the center, the two bands meet, forming an arch that lies between the urethral sphincter (posteriorly) and the urethrovaginalis sphincter (anteriorly). A few fibers attach to the side-walls of the urethra. The fibers of the compressor urethra merge with those of the urethral sphincter, which lies above it, and with the urethrovaginalis sphincter, which lies below (in front of or anterior to) it. The compressor urethra muscles serve as secondary urethral sphincters, drawing the anterior portion of the urethra downward and backward or stabilizing it when the bladder neck is lifted, thus elongating the urethra and assisting in continence.

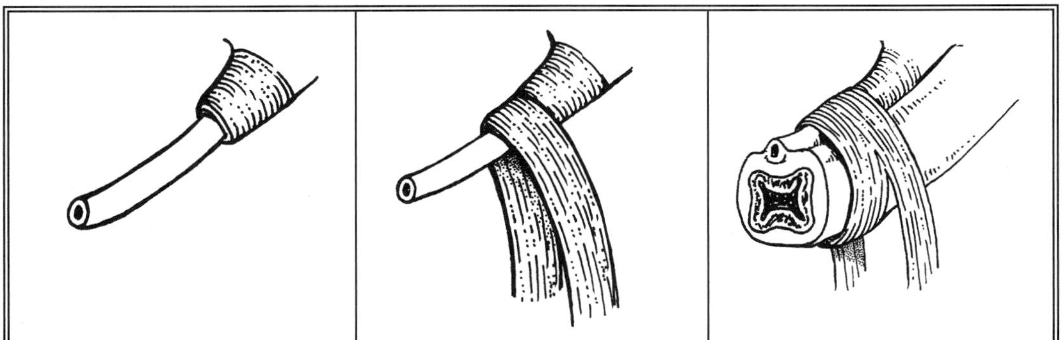

Urethral sphincter and urethra | Compressor urethra | Urethrovaginal sphincter with yoni included

Urethrovaginal sphincter muscle (vaginal sphincter/vestibular sphincter/constrictor cunni profundus/sphincter urethrovaginalis): Lying edge to edge with the compressor urethra is the most superficial (perineal) pair of these muscles. Each half consists of a thin, flat, 5 mm-wide muscle that originates at the posterior midline of the yoni canal (an attachment that is extremely difficult to identify in multiparous women). From the ventral side of the urethra just behind the upper border of the clitoral bulbs, each half passes down from the urethra along the sides of the yoni to the posterior midline, where they interdigitate with the fibers from the other side, forming a single ring that encompasses both the yoni and urethral canals. It is separated from the clitoral bulbs by a very thin layer of membrane.

The urethrovaginal sphincter muscles are primarily composed of slow-twitch, tonic fibers that help close the yoni and urethral canals. Contraction of this sphincter constricts the lumen of the upper urethra and compresses its lower end. These actions assist in the maintenance of continence, via compression retraction and elongation of the urethra, especially when the bladder is full and urination must be delayed, a situation that also prompts the woman to actively contract her pelvic floor (DeLancey, 2003b; Oelrich, 1983).

Transverse yoni muscles: From the medial edges of the two arms of the compressor urethra, striated muscle fibers radiate toward the midline from either side, attaching to the anterior portion of the lateral yoni wall just behind the urethrovaginal sphincter. These stabilizing transverse muscle fibers typically form a thin, fan-shaped attachment that usually does not reach all the way to the posterior yoni wall and therefore does not communicate with the perineal body in most cases. The transverse yoni and compressor urethra muscle fibers form a continuous muscle, but have different courses, thicknesses, and attachments. For this reason, Oelrich (1983) decided to assign individual names to each of these parts.

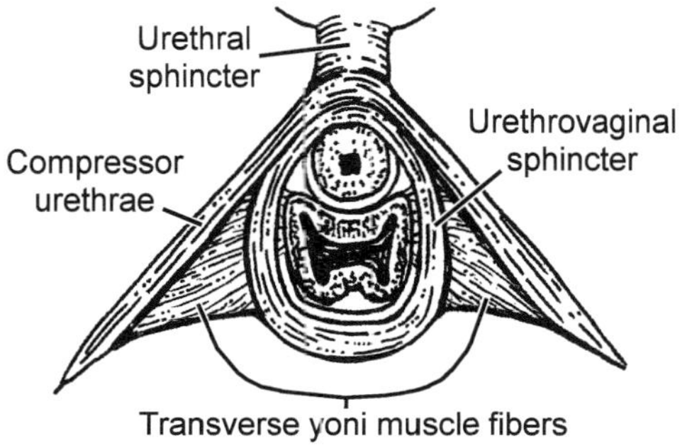

Transverse yoni muscle fibers (inferior view)

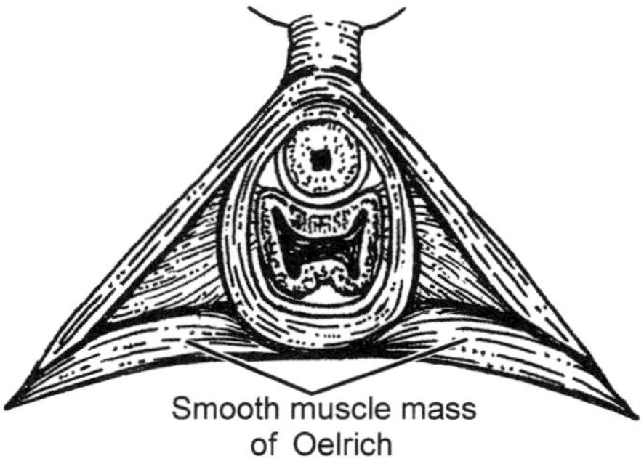

Banded portion of the perineal membrane complex (smooth muscle mass)

Smooth muscle mass: Oelrich found the deep perineal compartment of adult women to contain an extensive fibromuscular mass, consisting of smooth muscle fibers that were difficult to separate from the intermingled connective tissue. This muscle mass infiltrates the region from the ischiopubic rami to the portions of the lateral walls of the urethra and yoni that lie between the surface of the perineal membrane complex and the uppermost connective tissues of the urethrovaginal compartment. This tissue is apparently represented by the bands he simply labels as "smooth muscle" in the illustration in his article. These bands border the transverse yoni muscle fibers, and some authors label them as the "deep transverse perineal muscle," although Oelrich was clear that they were not. These fibers add definition to the lower border of the perineal membrane complex. In the first 15 years of life, most of this tissue consists of striated fibers that are gradually replaced, to a varying extent, with smooth muscle fibers as a woman ages. The striated muscle is not covered with a distinct layer of fascia, and this makes dissecting it from the smooth muscle extremely difficult. This tissue has been designated by Stein and DeLancey (2008) as the perineal membrane connective tissue complex.

What about the deep transverse perineal muscle? Luschka (1864) was the first to describe urethral sphincter muscles that most closely matched Oelrich's findings. He also found a "deep transverse" muscle that extended from the ischium to the perineal body. Later, Henle (1873) described two sheets of fascia sandwiching a deep transverse perineal muscle. This muscle was said to surround the urethra in both sexes and span the space between the pubic rami above and reach to each ischial tuberosity at its posterior border forming, more or less, a triangle shape. Since that time, authors that mention it at all have often described the urethral sphincter as a part of a deep transverse perineal muscle that is encased within two sheets of fascia and called this the "urogenital diaphragm," with only a few more contemporary authors questioning the validity of this concept (Dorschner et al., 1999; Mirilas & Shandalakis, 2004; Oelrich, 1983).

Oelrich (1983) could not locate a true deep transverse perineal muscle or a superior layer of fascia in any of the 29 female specimens he dissected. MRI studies undertaken by Dorschner and colleagues (1999) found no such muscle among 50 live male subjects. In 2007, Guo and Li studied a total of 152 live subjects in a mixed-sex population and found a muscle matching the classical description in only one female.

Oelrich postulated that misidentification of tissue might occur during dissections because of variations in the anatomy of the lower border of the perineal membrane tissue complex, which itself is easily recognized by the arteries, veins and nerves passing through it. In many specimens, the lower border of the perineal membrane complex reaches halfway down around the sides of the rectal wall and contains fibers from the superficial transverse perineal muscle that may also be misidentified as being part of a deep transverse perineal muscle.

In summary, the presence of a true deep transverse muscle is an exceedingly rare exception rather than the rule. Today, the classical description of a deep transverse perineal muscle persists in many textbooks, even though some acknowledge that it is not always present in females (Wendell-Smith & Wilson, 1991).

Perineal membrane connective tissue complex

The true anatomy of the connective tissue of the urogenital triangle has been obscured by the long-standing belief that it consists of two thin sheets of fascia that sandwich the deep transverse muscle. When Oelrich found this to be incorrect, he renamed the superficial component of the urogenital diaphragm (the only part he confirmed) the perineal membrane (1983). Oelrich himself described the region to either side of and posterior to the urethra as consisting of a commingled mass of muscle fibers and connective tissues, with the connective tissues continuing superiorly through the urogenital hiatus (the part of the hiatus anterosuperior to the yoni).

Stein and DeLancey (2008) described the perineal membrane as a complex, three-dimensional mass of tissue that is intimately connected to a variety of adjacent structures and is only one part of a larger assembly of supportive tissues. Thus, although the term "perineal membrane" has been formally adopted, the term "membrane" is, unfortunately, very misleading. It is the term we are stuck with for the present, however, since it is the one currently accepted in the TERMINOLOGIA ANATOMICA (Whitmore, 1998). It is much more accurate to think of it as the **perineal membrane connective tissue complex**, a designation that reminds us of its' three-dimensional nature.

Parts of the complex: This complex can be divided into two distinct regions. A ventral or anterior part (or upper part if the woman is lying on her back and you are looking between her legs) that consists of a three-dimensional mass of tissue adjacent to the urethra that is continuous with the other paraurethral and paravaginal connective tissues in this region. The other part of the complex is the posterior (dorsal or lower) portion that consists of bilateral transverse bands that extend from the lateral yoni walls and the perineal body to attach to the ischiopubic rami on either side.

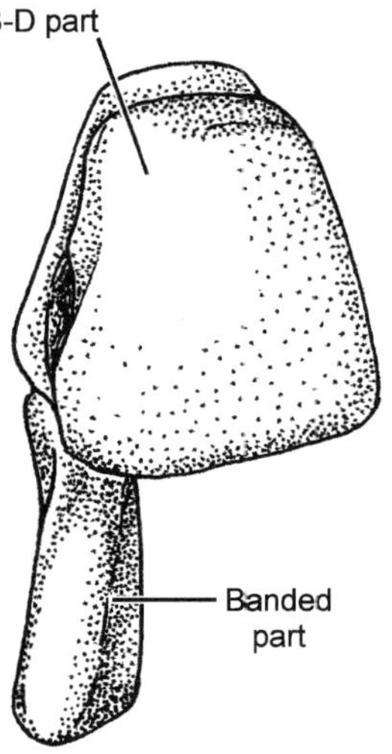

Lateral schematic of upper and lower parts of perineal membrane, showing the differences in thickness of the two parts.

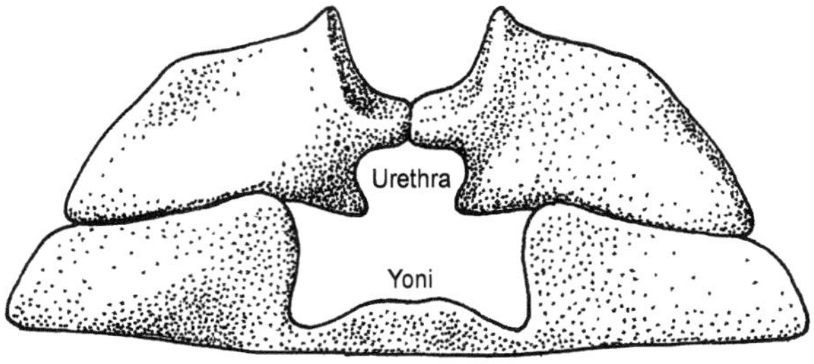

Anterior schematic of perineal membrane

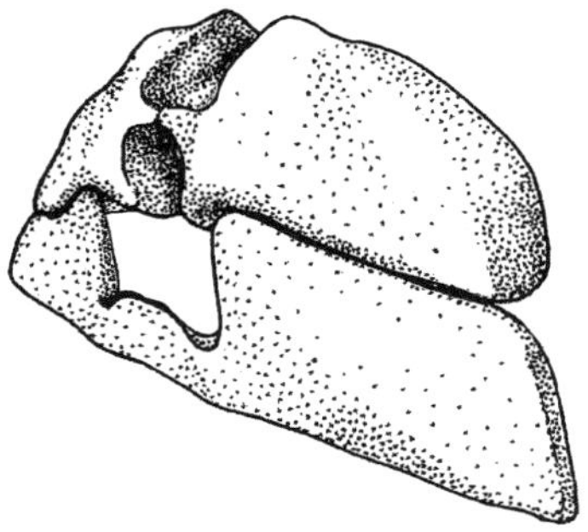

Three-quarter view of perineal membrane

(These schematic images are our best guesses, based on available information.)

Anterior 3-D part: The anterior (ventral) portion of the perineal membrane complex lies superior to the yoni and lateral to the urethra. It forms a three-dimensional mass of connective tissue that fills the space adjacent to either side of the symphysis and extends along the sides of the yoni and urethra, where it is continuous with the other connective tissues that flank these canals. Imagine pink cotton candy packed in among the structures that occupy this part of the pelvic cavity.

In the midline, the tissues of the perineal membrane are thin and interdigitate with or attach to the compressor urethra and the urethrovaginal sphincter (Kato, et al., 2008). More laterally, the compressor urethra and urethrovaginal sphincter muscles of the distal urethra are embedded within it (but the urethral sphincter is not). The most anterior margin of the tissue blends into the tendinous arch of the pelvic fasciae at the point where the arch inserts into the pubic bone. The parietal fascia of the levator ani muscles is attached to the superior surface of the perineal membrane complex and the clitoral bulbs and clitoral crura are fused to its inferior surface. The pudendal neurovascular bundle is embedded in the lateral part of this mass, near the periosteum overlying the pubic bone.

The tissues of the 3-D part of the perineal membrane complex intermingle with others in the area: the superior fascia of the levator ani muscles merges with the bony insertion of the tendinous arch of the pelvic fasciae, which is continuous with the connective tissue supports to either side of the urethra, which are continuous with the ventral portion of the perineal membrane complex. Superiorly, as the space between the anterior midline structures and the pubic bone widens, the tissues of the perineal membrane complex widen to fill the resulting space.

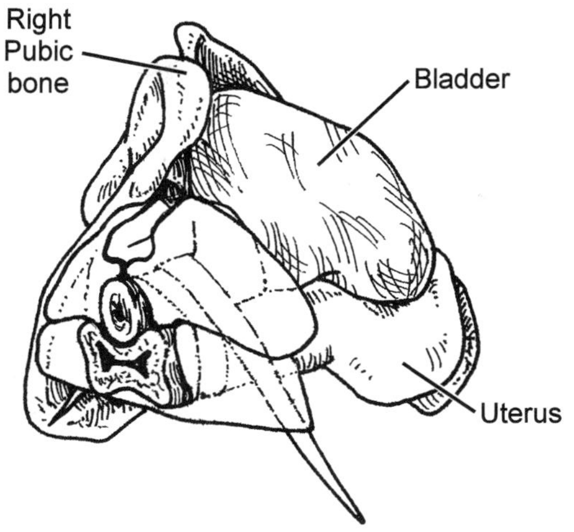

Perineal membrane complex with left half of bones removed to reveal relationship of the membrane to the embedded and adjacent parts

Posterior banded part: The posterior (dorsal or lower) portion of the perineal membrane complex consists of two wide, transversely oriented, fibrous bands that lack striated fibers. They are connected to the perineal body inferiorly, to the lateral walls of the yoni in the midline and to the ischiopubic rami on either side (Stein & DeLancey, 2008).

The bands are sandwiched between the fatty tissues of the ischiorectal fossa superiorly (i.e., from behind or above, if the woman is standing) and the lower ends of the clitoral bulbs, as well as the lower parts of the clitoral crura and bulbocavernosus and ischiocavernosus muscles that overlie the bands inferiorly. Although pubovisceral and puborectalis muscle fibers insert directly into the posterior surfaces of the bands, the bands are nevertheless distinct structures. They are less interconnected with surrounding structures than the ventral portion of the complex and create a true "deep space" behind (or superior to) them that is filled with the fatty connective tissue of the ischioanal fossa.

The superficial transverse perineal muscle overlies the surface of the lower edges of the bands on either side. The lower edge of the bands connects the perineal body to the ischia, which helps it to stabilize the position of the anorectum.

The lower border of the bands also contains the transverse perineal artery and a venous plexus. When an extension of the transverse perineal artery gives rise to the most anterior of the inferior rectal arteries, the lower border of the banded part of the perineal membrane complex may curve backward (Wendell-Smith & Wilson, 1991), extending two narrow, obliquely oriented tails that form a V shape in the midline below the yoni canal, connecting the lower border of the membrane complex to the anorectal canal and to the perineal body. In other women, the lower border of the membrane's bands curve forward rather than backward (Wendell-Smith & Wilson, 1991). DeLancey (1999) also stated that the connection between the posterior edges of the perineal membrane complex has a tapered tail that extends posteriorly about 2 to 3 cm beyond the level of the hymenal ring. The tail's distal end is thick and dense, becoming progressively thinner as it approaches its proximal tip. Stein and DeLancey did not mention this tail in their more recent article (2008).

Functions of the perineal membrane: The perineal membrane may play a dynamic role in the function of the levator ani muscles. The 3-D part's association with the dense connective tissues around the symphysis may serve to stabilize the action of the pubovisceral complex in the midline. By virtue of its attachment to the pubic rami, the banded portion of the perineal membrane complex supports the perineal body and the lateral yoni walls. As feces distend the anal canal and as the baby distends the yoni during labor, these attachments help hold the yoni walls and perineal body in place as pressure builds. In women with normal pelvic support, the perineal body descends significantly during straining. Therefore, it is likely that the levator ani muscles support the perineal body during normal activities. When the levator ani muscles relax, however, it is likely that the attachment between the perineal membrane complex and the perineal body limits the downward motion of the perineal body (Brandon et al., 2009; Stein & DeLancey, 2008).

Birth-related trauma: That the perineal membrane complex is connected to several other structures, including the inferior surface of the pubovisceral complex, means that midline separation of the membrane complex's dorsal bands, which can occur when the perineal body is torn or cut, causes the attached structures to move apart. A tear can thus widen the urogenital hiatus, even when the pubovisceral complex or the puborectalis muscle is not damaged. Repair of the midline separation in the perineal body brings the perineal membrane complex back together as well, realigning and restoring the normal anatomy of the two sides of the pubovisceral complex as well as other attached structures.

The part of the perineal membrane complex most likely to be injured during a spontaneous birth without a clitorotomy is the center of the lower border. Although a small midline tear into the gynecologic perineum might not damage this attachment, a large median incision will cut through it, and a mediolateral incision will cut through a much wider part of the banded portion on one side, which may compromise its function as an anchor for that side of the levator ani muscles as well as the external anal sphincter (Hudson et al., 2002).

Clitoral complex

Superficial to the perineal membrane complex, we find the next layer of tissues in the urogenital triangle, most of which are parts of or intimately associated with the clitoris.

For decades, textbooks have fostered the notion that all there is to the clitoris is a tiny knob of nerves at the junction of the labia minora, if they bothered to mention the clitoris at all. Although texts go on at length explaining penile anatomy, only in the last decade or so of the twentieth century have authors started to try and explain female anatomy in equal depth, although most still have a way to go to achieve this goal. The first modern textbook that researched clitoral anatomy from an entirely feminist perspective was entitled A NEW VIEW OF A WOMAN'S BODY (Federation of Feminist Women's Health Centers, 1981), although this work did not include any new dissection studies. Beginning in about 1997, ongoing research, much of which has been done by Helen O'Connell, has confirmed the complexity of clitoral anatomy. In fact, almost every structure of the female genitalia is either an extension of clitoral tissue or involved in its support, protection or function.

Across all species, the clitoris is the only organ apparently designed purely for pleasure. In humans, it consists of a three-dimensional complex of several interrelated parts that include the distal yoni and urethra. All these parts share circulatory and neurological supplies and all respond together, although in different ways, during sexual stimulation.

We start our discussion with a description of the core parts of the clitoris: the body, glans, crura and root. The body and crura form a wishbone shape. The wishbone's arms are formed by the crura, and its joint is formed by the body, which terminates in the glans. Imagine that the woman is lying, legs spread, and you are looking between her legs.

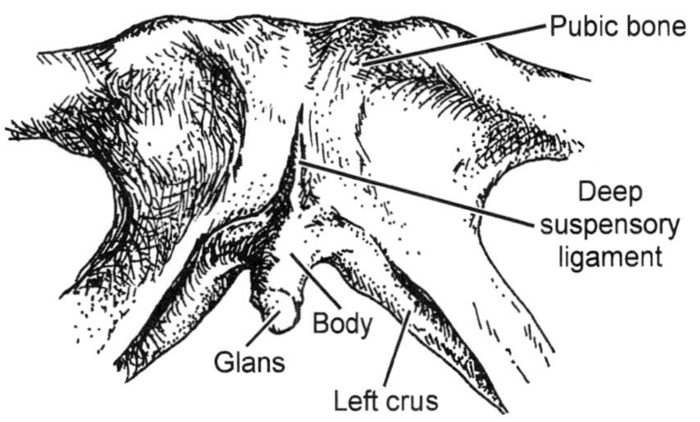

Dissection of clitoral glans, body and crura down to the tunica albuginea, showing how the deep suspensory ligament attaches the body to the pubic bone

Clitoral body (corpora [CORE-poor-ah])/shaft/corpora cavernosa clitoridis): The "clitoral body" refers to a pair of longitudinally oriented columns of erectile tissue that are attached to the surface of the pubic symphysis. At rest, the clitoral body (not including the glans) ranges from 0.5 to 2.0 cm wide, 1 to 2 cm deep and 2 to 4 cm long. When viewed from the side (sagittal section), the body may be either concavely or convexly curved (O'Connell & DeLancey, 2005; O'Connell et al., 2004) as it projects outward from the pubic bone and terminates in an exposed tip: the glans.

The body consists of two thin-walled, parallel columns or corpora are highly vascular and contain cavernous, erectile sinuses. The walls of these sinuses are endothelial with no smooth muscle and few elastic fibers (van Turnhout et al., 1995). These sinuses are surrounded by plexuses of **trabeculae** made up of smooth muscle fibers (Danesino & Martella, 1976; O'Connell, et al. 2004). (Trabeculae [sing., trabecula] are fibromuscular bands or cords that provide 3-D support within a structure.) The cavernous spaces are largest centrally and gradually become smaller toward the periphery of each corpus (van Turnhout et al., 1995). Histological analysis of a series of specimens of the body, crura, glans and bulbs from women of varying ages show significant changes in size and tissue composition with increasing age. Specimens from elderly women, especially those with fatal cardio-vascular disease, display significant fibrosis (O'Connell et al., 2004).

The corpora are surrounded by a thick capsule of connective tissue called the **tunica albuginea**. From the ventral or underside, an incomplete fibrous septum extends up between the corpora and runs along most of their length (Stilwell, 1976). This septum has numerous slits that are crossed by vessels that connect the two corpora (Danesino & Martella, 1976). Continuing in the midline, the septum extends halfway into the glans at the 6 o'clock point

(Baskin et al., 1999).

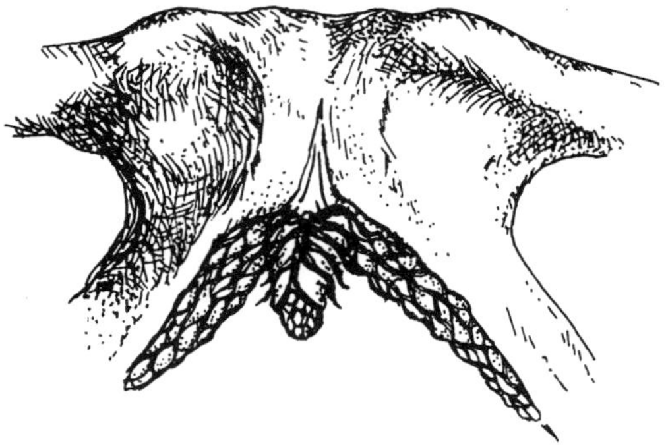
Dorsal vein and venous plexus of crura, body and glans

Nerve and blood supply: The clitoral body and glans as well as the gynecologic perineum are innervated by paired branches of the pudendal neurovascular bundles that arise at the pelvic sidewalls. The clitoral bundles ascend along the periosteum of the ischiopubic ramus on either side to meet the neurovascular bundle from the other side close to the midline. At the joining point of the crura, the clitoral neurovascular bundles pass to the superior surface of the clitoral body to either side of the 12 o'clock point. After some minimal branching, the anteriorly located "dorsal" nerve of the clitoris passes mostly intact into the clitoral glans. This nerve, which is 2 mm in diameter, and is quite large, even in infants. While branches of the cavernous nerve join the dorsal nerve in the midline of the clitoral body, the cavernous nerve originates from the nerves that supply the yoni. The perineal neurovascular bundle passes under the pubic arch on either side to supply the urethra and clitoral bulbs.

The tunica albuginea is embraced by the ventral clitoral neurovascular bundles, which branch along the length of the body as they approach the glans. The bulk of this nerve trunk enters the glans intact.

Pacinian corpuscles are found in association with the nerve trunks of the body and the glans. These sensory receptors are typically found in the dermis and are characterized by rapidly adapting receptors that are sensitive to vibration. In female genitals, they are more prevalent in clitoral structures (part not specified) than in the surrounding skin (Krantz, 1958) and may play a role in generating clitoral sensation during clitoral engorgement. Studies show that the Pacinian corpuscles of the clitoris are midway in sensitivity between the skin of the fingers and feet in response to vibratory stimulation (Helstrom & Lundberg, 1992).

Large arteries and veins follow the course of the nerve trunks along the length of the clitoral body. The cavernous tissue within the body is highly vascular, composed of vascular sinuses surrounded by smooth muscle trabeculae and connective tissue. These sinuses have an endothelium but no obvious smooth muscle in their walls. A moderately large cavernosal artery runs down the midline of each corpora, close to the septum.

Suspensory ligaments of the clitoris: The deep and superficial suspensory ligaments of the clitoris provide a broad-based external support for the clitoral body and glans. The deep suspensory ligament of the clitoris is a relatively rigid, fibrous attachment. It originates from a narrow longitudinal point on the symphysis pubis, attaches to the superior and lateral borders of the clitoral body and then continues deeply and posteriorly to attach to the clitoral bulbs. The ligament may be up to 1 cm wide at its clitoral attachment on the tunica albuginea at the base of the body and the most medial parts of the crura (Stilwell, 1976).

The superficial suspensory ligament of the clitoris arises as a thick, fan-shaped, variably fibrofatty structure from a 7 to 8 cm wide horizontal line of origin within the deep fascia of the mons pubis. These fibers converge as they attach along the body of the clitoris, all the way to the glans. From the undersurface of the superficial ligament, two 8 to 9 cm sheet-like extensions pass posteriorly into the medial tissues of the labia majora, helping to stabilize all these parts (O'Connell & Sanjeevan, 2006; Rees et al. 2000). The clitoral body is also supported by the urethra and yoni and their attachments to the puboanalis muscle and bony pelvis.

The clitoral ligaments anchor the clitoral body to the lower third of the pubic bone and create the bend at its upper end. They allow a range of motion up and down, from about midpubis to around an inch (2.5 cm) below the pubic arch (Stilwell, 1976). The body can become erect during sexual arousal, but its forward movement is significantly restricted by the attached ligaments (O'Connell et al., 2008).

Glans: The clitoral body terminates in an exposed tip, the glans, that lies immediately beneath or projects slightly beyond the lip of the clitoral hood. Its tip is located 1.25 to 3.5 cm above the urethral orifice (Narjani, 1924). "Glans" is Latin for "acorn," and it forms a small, rimmed, stocking-cap shape that fits over the end of the body. It has a discrete skinfold (the frenulum of the clitoris) where its posterior rim merges with the upper tips of the labia minora. The glans is attached to the upper ends of the clitoral bulbs by two extensions of erectile tissue that pass from the root, along the underside (the side against the pubic bone) of the clitoral body and partway into the underside of the glans.

The glans is typically smaller than a pencil eraser. Its average width is 3.4 mm (0.13") with a range of 2.4 to 4.4 mm (0.09 to 0.17"). The length averages 5.1 mm (0.20"), with a range of 3.7 to 6.5 mm (0.15 to 0.26"). The length of the glans and body together averages 16 mm (0.63") with a range of 11.7 mm to 20.3 mm (0.46 to 0.80"), although Masters and Johnson (1966) point out that measuring any part of the clitoris is exceedingly imprecise, that there is a wide normal variation in size and that size is altered dramatically during sexual stimulation. There appears to be no correlation between age, height, weight or use of oral contraceptives and the size of the body and glans, although women who have given birth tend to have significantly larger clitoral structures (Verkauf et al., 1992).

The skin of the glans consists of a thin, hairless squamous mucosa without glands, rete ridges or papillae (Wilkinson & Hardt, 2007) that overlies a densely vascular dermis. Next comes a layer of loose connective tissue that supports the nerves in this area. Below that, the tunica albuginea and enclosed cavernous tissue of the body extend into the upper end of the glans, but the cavernous tissue does not reach the tip (O'Connell et al., 2004). The midline tunica septum continues into the proximal end of the glans at the 6 o'clock point.

The glans is generally considered a noncavernous structure. Whether the glans has erectile properties of its own is confirmed by some authors and denied by others, although most consider it at least partly erectile and that it is directly continuous with the erectile tissues to which it is attached.

Within the tip of the glans, Kobelt found the tiny beginnings of the most anterior branches of the dorsal veins of the clitoris. Larger venous branches pass from the depth of the glans to emerge under its posterior border. The glans has two dorsal arteries, which supply it almost exclusively (Kobelt [1844] 1978).

The glans is also rich in nerves endings, especially Pacini corpuscles, which provide deep sensation and sense vibration. Pacini corpuscles are also closely related to the neurovascular bundles and their branches that surround the body. From the body, most of the dorsal nerve continues intact into the glans (O'Connell et al., 2005). Kobelt notes that, in most women, each nerve divides into three thick branches that pass to the rim of the glans. Within the glans, the nerves fibers disperse into a complex, interlacing plexus among the blood vessels; some of these nerves enter the clitoral hood as arch-shaped loops (Kobelt [1844] 1978). There is a lack of nerves at 12 o'clock position, the lowest nerve density being in the region adjacent to the septum (Baskin, 1999).

Root of the clitoris (pars intermedia/corpus spongiosum): The glans encloses a mesh of very fine veins that arises out of the pars intermedia or root of the clitoris, which connects it to the clitoral bulbs. The root is discussed in more detail on page 66.

Crura (CREW-rah) (singular: crus): The crura are bilateral extensions of the corpora. Starting at a variable point above the clitoral glans, the paired clitoral corpora diverge and narrow into two 5 to 9 cm long tapered extensions, the crura, that form an inverted V of typical cavernous erectile tissue that is fused to the anteroinferior surface of the pubic rami and that extend toward the ischial tuberosities on either side. The superior surfaces of the crura are fused to the perineal membrane complex. They are each partially covered by the tunica albuginea, which is absent where they attach to the bone and where the ischiocavernosus muscles overlie their anterior surfaces. The crura are adjacent to the dorsal clitoral neurovascular bundle, although neither large nerves nor vascular trunks appear within them (O'Connell & Sanjeevan, 2006).

Erectile characteristics of the clitoral body and crura: That the clitoral body and crura are composed of erectile tissue that is surrounded by a dense fibrous capsule results in a type of erection when these parts are engorged with blood. The term "erection" connotes a firm, unyielding rigidity that can cause a structure to rise up. Thus, the term "erectile" can describe clitoral structures, even though it more precisely applies to the more mobile penis than the curved and relatively fixed clitoral crura and body (O'Connell et al., 2004).

Birth-related trauma: The location of the clitoral body, crura, glans and bulbs on the outside of the pubic arch means that they can spread apart, be displaced forward and out of the way, avoiding being crushed between the baby's head and the bones as the baby dilates the vulval tissues. This anatomy protects these tissues to a great extent, although occasionally a blood vessel from these parts is ruptured during birth or a nerve that supplies the clitoris is injured due to periurethral tearing (Kobelt [1844] 1978).

Greater vestibular (VEST-TIB- you-ler) (Bartholin) glands: The two lobulated greater vestibular glands are about 1 cm in diameter. They are located at a depth of 2 cm on either side, between the yoni wall and the clitoral bulbs or just below them at about the level of the posterior end of the labia minora. They are nestled in fat and are sandwiched between the bulbocavernosus muscles and the inferior surface of the banded part of the perineal membrane complex, to which they are fused. Each gland has a 2 cm long duct that opens 3 to 4 mm to either side of the hymen into the groove between the hymen and the labia minora (the vestibule of the yoni), at about 4 and 8 o'clock. These tubuloacinar secretory glands are the primary mucinous glands of the vulva. They contribute a small quantity of lubricating fluids to the other cyprine secretions during sexual arousal (Masters & Johnson, 1966; O'Connell & Sanjeevan, 2006).

A widely variable number of **lesser vestibular glands**, ranging from 1 to 100, open into the mucous membrane of the vestibule. These small, branched tubular, mucous glands are arranged in a circle or in parallel lines beginning at the orifices of the ducts of the greater vestibular glands and extending anteriorly to the level of the urethra.

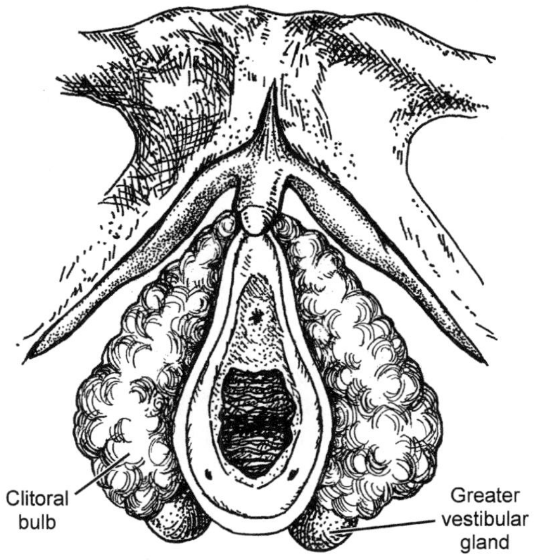

Clitoral bulbs with greater vestibular glands behind the tips on either side

Bulbs of clitoris (clitoral bulbs/ clitoral sponge/ bulbs of the vestibule/ vestibular bulbs): These two dense matrixes of circulatory tissue are shaped more or less like an inflated wishbone that is straddled by the crura and lies dorsal to the clitoral body. The upper ends of each bulb are joined by the **root of the clitoris (pars intermedia)**, which consists of a vascular plexus that projects from the underside of the body, between the clitoral glans and the urethral meatus, superficial to the crura. From this midline connection, two crescentic or triangular arms extend downward on either side, filling the space between the clitoral crura and the body. They lie ventral (superficial to) the urethra, always extending far enough to flank the lateral walls of the distal urethra and usually as far as the distal yoni. In younger women the bulbs often extend as far as the perineal body. Each arm ranges from 3 to 7 cm long, 1 to 2 cm wide, and 0.5 to 1 cm thick. The bulbs underlie the vestibular skin (they do not fill the labia minora, as some texts describe) and lie in a plane superficial to the ischiopubic rami (DeLancey, 2003b). The position of the bulbs relates consistently to that of the clitoral body, crura and glans, rather than the vestibule; because of this they are most appropriately named "clitoral," rather than "vestibular," bulbs. Each is fused to the caudal surface of the perineal membrane complex (Stein & DeLancey, 2008).

The bulbs consist of cavernous erectile tissue that differs from that of the clitoral body and crura. Their vascular spaces are larger and their trabeculae thicker than in other cavernous clitoral tissues. They also lack vascular and neural channels (O'Connell et al., 2004).

The bulbs are surrounded by a delicate membrane that is more translucent than the thick tunica. This allows more of their true color to show through, causing them to appear blue-purple, rather than pink-red, on dissection. When the bulbs are engorged during sexual activity or, to a lesser extent, during pregnancy, this thin enclosing capsule is likely to allow them to expand and become swollen rather than erect (O'Connell & Sanjeevan, 2006; O'Connell et al., 2004).

Root of the clitoris (pars intermedia/corpus spongiosum): In the space between the frenulum and the urethral orifice lies "the root of the clitoris," a term coined by O'Connell and colleagues (2008) to refer to this area where all the clitoral erectile tissues come together.

Van Turnhout and associates (1995) named this part the "corpus spongiosum" and as of this writing, their work offers the most complete contemporary research on this tissue. They described a network of erectile tissue that directly underlies the vestibular skin. Concentrations of spongeous tissue lie on both sides of the midline with no clear septum between them. It consists of irregular spaces, or lacunae, lined with endothelium. These lacunae are separated by fat-free trabeculae consisting of collagen as well as elastic and smooth muscle fibers. These tissues converge underneath the point clitoral frenulum and are continuous with the bilateral clitoral bulbs. Upon joining in the midline, they pass along the underside of the clitoral body to terminate within the glans. The number of vascular spaces diminish as the spongy tissues enter the glans.

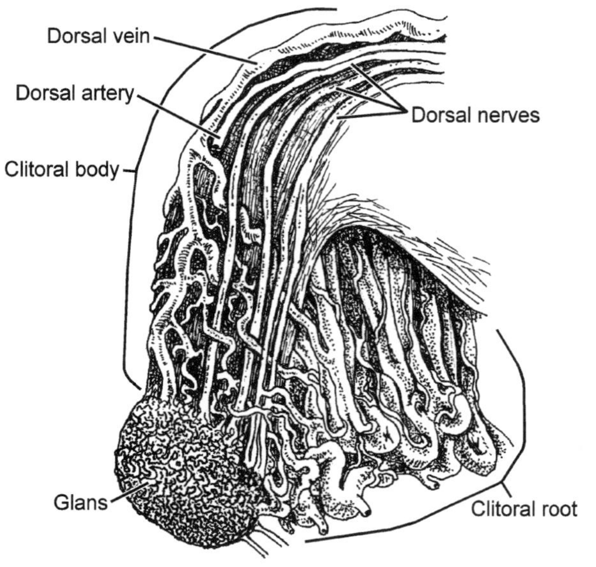

Detail of the part of the clitoral root that underlies the clitoral body and glans; the part best seen on dissection (after Kobelt [1844] 1978)

In 1844, the renowned German anatomist George Ludwig Kobelt published detailed descriptions, unmatched to this day, of a vascular bridge connecting the body and glans of the clitoris to the clitoral bulbs. He reported that injecting either the arteries or veins of one of the bulbs caused both sides to fill, thus confirming a communicating link. O'Connell and colleagues (2005) identified a double row of veins surrounding the distal urethra adjacent to the bulbs. Suh and associates (2003) studied 21 women, performing MRI studies that revealed the bulbs convening anteriorly at the level of the commissure, close to the clitoral body and glans. In many subjects, there appeared to be a point of communication where the bulbs met the clitoral body. This part of the root is most readily identified during dissections and was the only part I could find illustrated anywhere, as shown on the preceding page.

Kobelt found a longitudinal convolution of capillaries and veinous branches of various sizes underlying both columns of the clitoral body. Blood flows through this network from front to back. The veins of the clitoral glans pass posteroinferiorly to the root, linking the vascular network of the clitoral glans and body. The posterior vessels of the root extend inferolaterally to join those of the clitoral bulbs, which hug either side of the introitus.

According to Kobelt, the veins of this root have no valves and make several connections. From the root, lateral branches of the dorsal veins of the clitoris pass in an upward direction, wrapping themselves around the side and surface of the clitoral body. From these branches arise two more or less regularly arranged rows of connecting veins that lie close together against the surface of the clitoral body and penetrate into the body via two rows of openings on either side of the septum. From below, the clitoral root receives several more veins. The anterior veins stem from the frenulum and labia minora, and the more posterior veins come from the labia majora.

Kobelt described the arteries of the central section of the root as encased in a network of capillaries that send separate veins in all directions and that ascend, with the connecting veins, into the interior of the clitoral body. Filaments from the nerves supplying the labia majora pass through the network of vessels within the root.

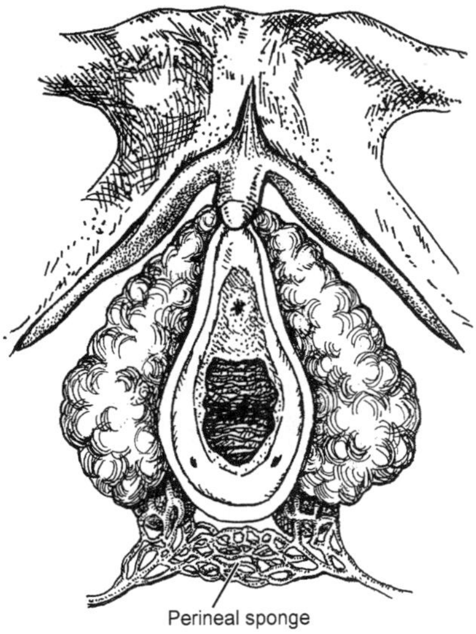

Clitoral bulbs with vestibular glands and perineal sponge below

Perineal sponge: The "perineal sponge" is the name coined by Downer and colleagues (1991) for the extensive vascular network that is interwoven among the musculofascial fibers that traverse the perineal body. The perineal sponge becomes engorged during sexual arousal. Gage, the artist for Downer and colleagues (1991), showed it connected to the clitoral bulbs. Although I could find no confirmation of this from anatomical studies, that there are many branches that extend from the vessels in this region is not in dispute. The perineal sponge is not referred to in standard anatomy textbooks.

Since the introitus and the urethra are surrounded by clitoral tissue, this makes them clitoral orifices and places a *routine* episiotomy, more precisely named a **clitorotomy**, in the dual category of both genital and clitoral mutilation.

Superficial muscles of the urogenital triangle

The next most superficial urogenital structures overlie the clitoral structures just described, completing the internal parts of the urogenital triangle.

Ischiocavernosus (IS-keh-oh-ca-ver-NOH-sus) muscles: These two muscles encase the crura of the clitoris on either side. Each muscle originates at the ischial tuberosity and from the unattached surfaces of the crus, extends toward the pubic symphysis for a variable distance and then inserts into the unattached surfaces of the crus on either side. Most commonly, these muscles terminate about four-fifths of the way up as they approach the midline, although they extend all the way to the clitoral body in some women (Thorek, 1985). (See drawing I. "Coronal section," at the end of the chapter.) These muscles contract the crura during sexual arousal, moving blood toward the clitoral body and glans. They are rarely damaged during childbirth.

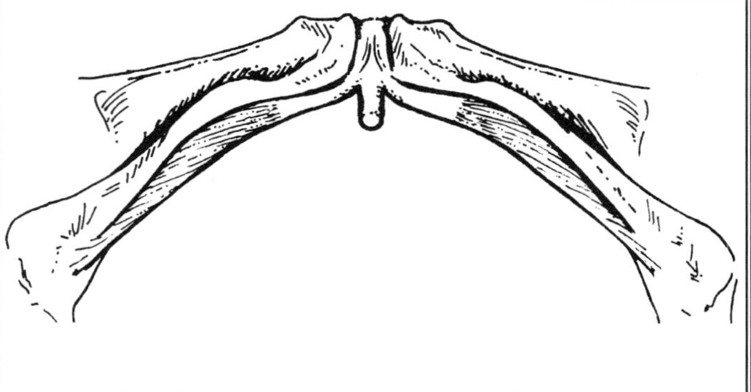

Ischiocavernosus muscles overlying crura

Superficial transverse perineal muscle: This muscle originates from each ischial tuberosity, extending as two narrow bands, often composed of only a few wispy muscle fibers, that run along the lower border of the bands of the perineal membrane complex, attaching just above or adjacent to the ischial tuberosities on either side. These bands usually underlie the fibers that connect the bulbocavernosus muscle to the subcuticular anal sphincter that also traverse the perineal body. The most posterior fibers of the superficial transverse muscle and the most anterior fibers of the main part of the external anal sphincter often overlap (Rociu et al., 2000; Shafik et al., 2007a).

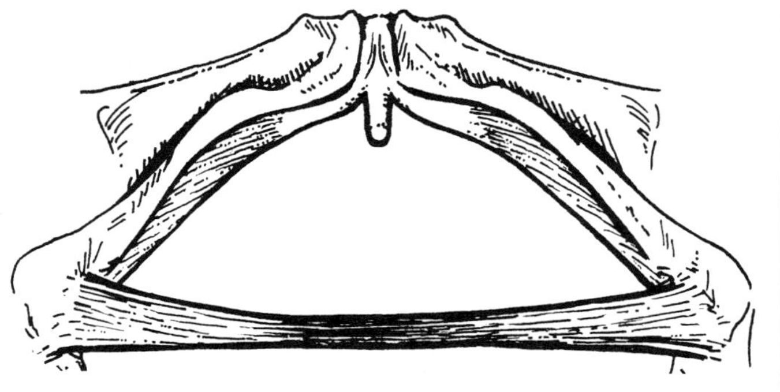

Superficial transverse perineal muscle

Fine tendinous fibers reach out from either side toward the midline where they decussate with those from the opposite side, remaining continuous as they cross the midline. The region of decussation to which they contribute extends from the anal orifice to the posterior commissure and is classically and incorrectly referred to as the **anogenital raphe**. It is not a true raphe because most of the fibers pass uninterruptedly across the midline, where they form the most superficial layer of muscle fibers in the perineal body (blended fibers of the bulbocavernosus and subcutaneous anal sphincter pass over this muscle to either side of the midline). The superficial transverse perineal muscle helps to anchor the perineal body.

The superficial transverse muscle is absent in some women. When present, it completes the bottom (inferior) border of the urogenital triangle (Shafik et al., 2007a).

Bulbocavernosus (bulbospongiosus) (bul-bow-CAV-er- NO-sus/bul-bow-SPONGE-e-OH-sus) muscles: The paired bulbocavernosus muscles are the most superficial muscles that are adjacent to the lateral yoni walls. Some authors characterize these muscles as a sphincter, and while they do assist in closing the introitus, they do not insert in the midline beneath the introitus, as has been classically described.

Some of the uppermost fibers of the bulbocavernosus muscles join as they arch over the clitoral body. Other fibers pass anterolaterally to blend with those of the ischio-cavernosus muscles to either side of the body (only when the ischiocavernosus muscles reach all the way to the midline?—not sure about this, no source was specific on this point) (Drake et al., 2005). Downward pressure on the perineal body does not put tension on the bulbo-cavernosus muscles because of the muscles' sole insertion into soft clitoral structures, which move down with it (DeLancey 1999). A few fibers form a sling below the clitoral glans and its dorsal vein; these fibers may compress these parts of the clitoris during sexual arousal (Wendell-Smith & Wilson, 1991).

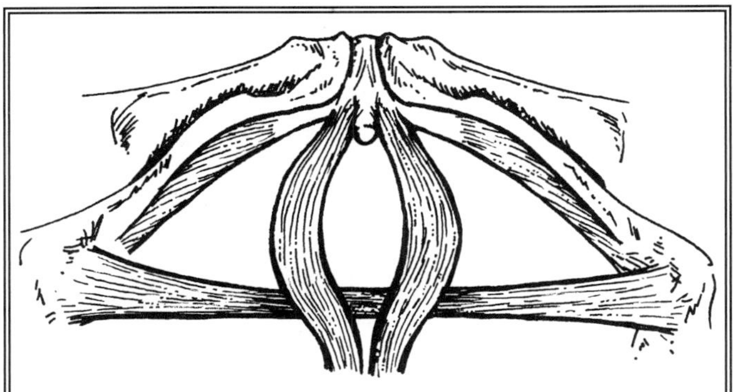

Bulbocavernosus muscles

From these midline attachments, the bulbocavernosus muscles extend as two bands down past the urethra, covering the clitoral bulbs on either side. The inner edges of the bulbocavernosus muscles lie about 0.5 cm deep to the lateral yoni lumen. The posterolateral edge of each muscle band is fused to the surface of the perineal membrane complex and the superior surface of each bulbocavernosus muscle is attached to the inferior surface of the thin membrane overlying the clitoral bulbs. Many illustrations depict the medial edges of the bulbocavernosus muscles as not completely covering the medial edges of the clitoral bulbs, but I did not find this discussed in any source. The lower ends of the bulbocavernosus muscles overlie whatever portion of the greater vestibular glands that is not covered by the clitoral bulbs. At the level of the lower sulcus grooves of the yoni wall, the two arms of the bulbocavernosus muscles pass straight down into the perineal body on either side of the midline (DeLancey, 1999), superficial to those of the superficial transverse perineal muscle (Shafik et al., 2005).

Shafik and colleagues (2007b) confirmed that bulbocavernosus muscle fibers intermix with fibers that pass up through the perineal body from the subcutaneous part of the external anal sphincter. At the level of the fourchette, these sphincter fibers diverge laterally into two groups. Each group of fibers continues up to blend with the bulbocavernosus muscle on the either side, all the way to the anterior midline attachment of the bulbocavernosus (see also the discussion that begins on page 97). Most fibers are longitudinally oriented as they pass through the perineal body, meaning that a midline tear would part, but not sever, them. In a small number of women, a few superficial sphincter fibers crisscross in the midline and join the contralateral bulbocavernosus fibers. This arrangement seems to enhance their constrictive action on the clitoral bulbs, but crossing fibers appear to be the exception, rather than the rule. This means that, in most women, a midline perineal tear will tend to divide, rather than tear through, these longitudinal fibers.

Electrical stimulation of the nerves that supply either the anal sphincter or the bulbocavernosus causes both muscles to contract simultaneously, thus Shafik's group concluded that the two muscles are functionally one. This connection may help close the anus, reducing the risk of flatal or fecal leakage. The bulbocavernosus muscles also appear to work in concert with those of the external anal sphincter to compress the top and sides of the clitoral bulbs during orgasm. For more details about the connection between the bulbocavernosus and the external anal sphincter muscles, see page 100.

Perineal body

The perineal body is, on average, a 4 cm three-dimensional mass of fibromuscular and vascular tissue located between the posterior fourchette and the anus. In a short gynecologic perineum, the perineal body is much more compact, bringing the openings of the yoni and anus closer together.

The perineal body is shaped like a modified pyramid because the base is slightly elongated in its transverse dimension. Between the lower ends of the canals of the yoni and anus, the pyramid's four sidewalls extend superiorly and taper to a point, forming the tip of the pyramid. The pyramid's base (inferior surface) is formed by the skin surface of the gynecologic perineum and is slightly concave when the pelvic muscles are well toned. The gynecologic perineum and the anal opening both lie in the plane just superior to the level of the ischial tuberosities (in the standing position). The posterior surface of the pyramid is fused to the anterior wall of the anal canal and the external sphincter. Its anterior surface is fused to the distal third of the posterior yoni wall.

Classically, the perineal body is simply described as a pyramid, but a pyramid's square base is inadequate to describe the lateral extensions that reach out toward the ischial spines on either side (Soga et al., 2007). The size of these lateral extensions varies and tends to be larger in older, multiparous women. The sides of the base are bounded by the bulbocavernosus muscles on either side, by the lower ends of the clitoral bulbs in some women, by the main part of the external anal sphincter and by the puborectalis muscle. The upper, distal border of the perineal body attaches to the lower part of the perineal membrane complex. Superficially, the sides of the perineal body also receive fibers from the superficial transverse perineal muscles. Deeper inside the perineal body, fibers of the puboperinealis muscle pass through it.

The internal apex (superior tip) of the pyramid is about 2 to 3 cm posterior to the hymenal ring (DeLancey, 2003b); superior to this tip, the posterior midthird of the yoni wall and the anterior rectal wall are gently attached to each other by loose connective tissue. The tip of the pyramid also marks the plane of the rectoanal junction.

The **central point of the perineum** is in the midline, where fibers from various tissues overlap and, in some cases, crisscross. Although this region has classically been referred to as the central perineal tendon, this is not anatomically correct, as most of the muscle fibers it contains actually cross the midline, rather than insert into it (Shafik et al., 2007b). The benefits of this arrangement are explained below.

The complex intermingling of tissues within the perineal body makes dissection difficult. Thus there is very little in the literature about the specific anatomy of this region and even less in relation to female anatomy. I have cobbled together a description based on the best research I could find, which wasn't a lot. Shafik and colleagues (2007b) offered one of the most distinct descriptions. I have combined their findings with DeLancey's. Shafik's team found muscle fibers arranged in three primary layers that do not insert into the perineal body, as is widely described. Rather, most of these fibers either pass straight through the perineal body or decussate with fibers of their opposite half as they pass, uninterrupted, through the perineal body to the contralateral side.

Immediately beneath the posterior distal yoni wall, the sides of the perineal body receive fibers from the puboperinealis portion of the pubovisceral complex that cross the midline (DeLancey, 2003b). Also underlying the yoni wall superior to these fibers are a few from the urethrovaginal sphincter muscle (Oelrich, 1983).

From deepest to most superficial layers, Shafik and associates (2007b) described deep fibers from muscle tissue that they referred to as the "deep transverse perineal muscle," fibers that they stated originate from the ischial rami. These fibers are probably from the superficial transverse perineal muscle or smooth muscle fibers from the perineal membrane complex. Similar fibers were found in both sexes.

In the posterior midline they found tendinous fibers that, though interwoven, did not cross the midline. (Oelrich said that the posterior fibers of the urethrovaginal sphincter interdigitate in the midline. "Interdigitation" describes fibers that meet and interlock but do not cross to the other side.) Next, the dorsal portion of the perineal membrane complex attaches to the perineal body, connecting it to the pubic rami and to the ischial tuberosities.

The next most superficial layer includes decussated fibers of the superficial transverse perineal muscle (Shafik et al., 2007b). Rociu and colleagues (2000) found that, in most women, the superficial transverse muscle is positioned anterosuperior to the anal sphincter, although it is unclear whether this refers to the main part of the sphincter or some other.

The most superficial muscle layer of all included longitudinally oriented fibers of both the bulbocavernosus muscles and the subcutaneous part of the external anal sphincter; in fact, a significant portion of the perineal body is contributed by the main and subcutaneous parts of the external anal sphincter. It was difficult to tell where one ended and the other began.

DeLancey (1999) noted that most of the fibers from the bulbocavernosus muscles pass down through the perineal body on either side, with very few actually crossing in the midline. Shafik and colleagues (2007a) also found superficial external anal sphincter fibers passing straight up through the perineal body, diverging at the level of the fourchette and continuing up either side of the midline where they blend with bulbocavernosus fibers to the level of the clitoral bulbs. The joining of anal sphincter fibers with those of the bulbocavernosus links the perineal body to the coccyx. Together, these layers form the primary bulk of the perineal body. In combination, these connections hold the perineal body in position (DeLancey, 2003b). The perineal body also contains circulatory tissue of the clitoris (the perineal sponge), connective tissue, fatty tissue to either side of the midline, and nerve endings.

Shafik and colleagues (2005) mentioned no puboperinealis, puborectalis or urethrovaginal sphincter muscle fibers in the perineal body in their article, although other authors have found fibers from all these muscles there. (When present, puborectalis fibers would be from those few that wrap around the anterior wall of the rectal canal.) From the numerous and differing findings of published anatomical studies, it appears that the fibers that contribute to the perineal body may vary among individuals.

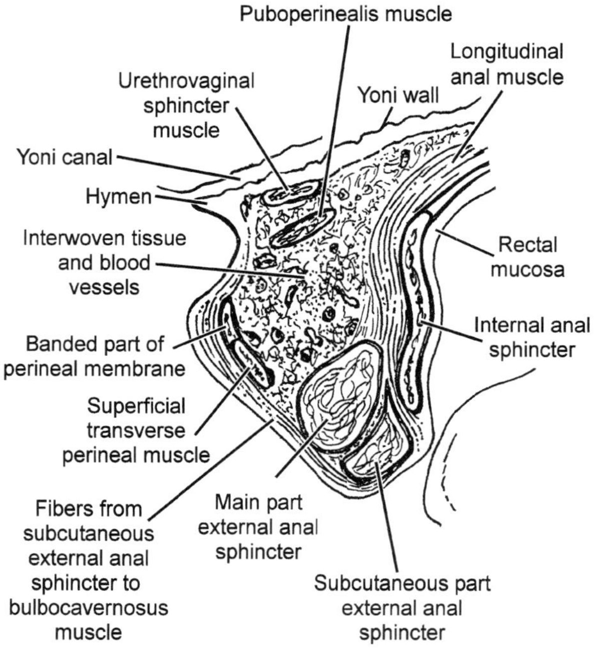

The perineal body

The central point of the perineum: The center of the perineum lies within the midline region of the perineal body, where various musculofascial fibers traverse the tissue. The tissues that meet in the center are (listed from the most superficial structure back):

- Mostly longitudinal fibers of the bulbocavernosus muscle/subcutaneous part of the external sphincter
- The superficial transverse perineal muscle from either side
- The lower edge of the banded portion of the perineal membrane tissue complex from above, which passes laterally
- The anterior parts of the superficial and main external anal sphincter, which pass across the midline, contributing to the bulk of the muscle fibers found here
- The urethrovaginalis sphincter muscle from above
- In the rare case when it is present, the deep transverse perineal muscle, with fibers that pass from side to side
- The U-shaped puboperinealis portion of the pubovisceral complex, which also passes side to side across the midline.
- In addition, the perineal body is interlaced throughout with the vascular network of the perineal sponge.

The central point of the perineum is located between the upper border of the anus and the lower border of the introitus, beginning at an average depth of 0.5 cm posterior to the perineal skin surface and is of variable thickness depending upon the length of the perineal body (everything is more bunched together when the perineum is short). Its topmost border begins approximately 0.35 cm below the surface of the yoni floor, just inside the introitus.

In a short gynecologic perineum, the perineal body is smaller, causing these structures to be more bunched up as they traverse the midline. This may place the superficial transverse muscle level with the sphincter, rather than slightly above it as is usually the case.

The benefits of decussation: Decussation of the muscle fibers within the perineal body occurs when fibers of one muscle overlap crossways in relation to the fibers of another or when fibers within the same muscle cross. Either configuration allows the tissue to stretch up and down and from side to side, in much the same way as a piece of fishnet stocking will do when pulled in either direction. Interwoven fibers of two muscle parts allow each part to contract simultaneously, causing them to shorten or widen, yet function together as one.

Within the perineal body, this creates a highly flexible yet firm arrangement of tissues that can adjust continuously, responding quickly and easily in coordination with respiration, intra-abdominal pressure changes, distension, straining and childbirth (Shafik et al., 2007b). This ability, however, may be exceeded when the tissue is maximally stressed, which can occur when the laboring mother is forced to push lying flat on her back or when the fetal presenting part is unusually large (Sutton, 2001). The perineum is much more likely to remain intact when the mother pushes in an upright position with her pelvic brim tilted forward, a position that, to the extent possible, relieves direct pressure on the perineal body by guiding the descending weight of the fetus directly toward the introitus.

Functions of the perineal body: The perineal body serves many important functions. The attachment of the external sphincter within the well-toned, intact perineal body anchors the lower anorectum and helps maintain fecal continence. The perineal body acts as a spacer between the rectum and yoni, protecting the yoni from contamination during defecation and helping to protect the rectum from damage during childbirth. It also means that anal sphincter dysfunction may accompany damage to the perineal body. When the perineal body is short, it forms only a thin pad of tissue, leaving the sphincter more vulnerable to damage during birth (Woodman & Graney, 2002).

The interweaving of muscle fibers and connective tissue from the superficial and deep perineal compartments within the perineal body helps to anchor these tissues in the midline and keep the yoni closed. While these attachments limit downward motion of the perineal body when the levator ani muscles are relaxed, normal levator ani muscle tone is the most significant factor in maintaining the position of the perineal body over the long term because even extensive damage to the perineal body does not usually result in significant organ prolapse by itself (Stein & DeLancey, 2008). Liu (Miller, 2008) pointed out that, in women with normal pelvic tone, the perineal body can descend up to 2.5 cm during voluntary straining, and thus he felt it cannot provide primary support for the genital outlet. That the perineal body can also be displaced inward 3 to 4 cm toward the sacrum when a weighted speculum is placed in the posterior yoni likewise suggests that the position of the perineal body at rest is primarily determined by the condition of the levator ani muscles.

The perineal body also plays a vital role in maintaining normal sexual function. The perineal sponge contained within it is an integral component of the orgasmic platform. The sponge is part of the extensive vascular complex of the clitoris that surrounds the entire lower third of the yoni and the urethra. When the perineal body is damaged, the function of the perineal sponge may be impaired as well (Woodman & Graney, 2002).

Damage to the muscles of the pelvic floor or its nerve supply may also contribute to weakening or loss of function in the urethrovaginal sphincter muscle because these structures are all connected (Oelrich, 1983). Nerve endings of some of the perineal and inferior rectal branches of the pudendal nerve are embedded within the perineal body. When women are forced to push on their back, when they are encouraged to push on command rather than when they feel the urge, or when the tissues are highly resistant to fetal descent, excessive stretching of the perineal body and the nerves that pass through it may occur. This can result in nerve damage and thus disrupt function in the tissues that the nerves supply.

Finally, the perineal body is the meeting point for the two halves of the inferior border of the banded part of the perineal membrane connective tissue complex. That the lower third of the yoni wall is fused with the perineal membrane complex as well as the medial edges of the puboanalis and puborectalis muscles and the superior surface of the perineal body means that the intact perineal body maintains all these tissues in their normal positions and allows them to work together to assist in tightening and narrowing the genital hiatus, which is, on average, a 5.4 cm^2 oval (the range is 3.69 to 7.1cm^2). The importance of these attachments increases when intrapelvic pressure rises. (The cubic cm figure is derived from two external measurements: the anteroposterior length extending from the symphysis pubis to the dense connective tissue palpable within the perineal body and the widest distance between the palpable inner borders of the puboanalis muscle as they pass up toward the pubic symphysis on either side of the yoni [DeLancey & Hurd, 1998].) Disruption of these connections within the perineal body, whether from a tear or an incision, results in a loss of perineal body support and laterally displaces the perineal membrane, as well as all the tissues that are attached to it, thus widening the urogenital hiatus. Suturing the sides of the perineal body back together pulls all the attached tissues back into alignment, restoring their normal relationships.

THE LEVATOR ANI MUSCLE COMPLEX AND RELATED STRUCTURES

This chapter covers the levator ani muscle complex, the obturator internus muscles, the urogenital hiatus, the anococcygeal ligament, including the concept of the levator plate, and the ischiorectal fossa.

An Overview of the Levator Ani Musculature

Difficulties in understanding the primary muscles of the pelvic floor begin with their name: the levator ani ("lifter of the anus"). Unlike any other muscle group in the body, the pelvic floor muscles are often referred to simply as the "levator ani muscle" as though they were a single muscle, when there are actually at least three different muscles involved. This imprecision frequently results in general references to the "levator ani muscle" in texts and drawings, which is confusing because it obscures what part is being discussed and distracts from the function of each individual muscle. It is more accurate, therefore, to think of them as the levator ani muscle complex.

I shall explain the levator ani musculature starting with the most central part and working outward, toward the pelvic sidewalls. First I will present a simplified explanation of how this muscle group is shaped and how it behaves. Try to grasp this first before moving on to the more detailed descriptions that follow. It may help to draw the shapes yourself as you are reading. Try not to anticipate where other structures may be located. Since the relationship of these muscles is very complex, it will help to take it one step at a time.

The levator ani muscles are often referred to as the "pelvic floor" or "pelvic diaphragm." These muscles form the ceiling for the superficial urogenital structures and a floor under the pelvic organs that actively supports them by closing the pelvic cavity. When the muscles are normally toned, they completely support the pelvic organs (the bladder, urethra, uterus, yoni and anorectal canal), allowing them to rest on the muscles without tension.

The levator ani muscles function collectively and assume a complex and varying shape. To begin to get a general idea of how they look, start by imagining all the muscles together as though they were one. Think of a round sheet of muscle that is attached around its outer edges and slightly baggy in the center, like a trampoline that is a little too big for its frame.

In life, these muscles normally assume a bowl shape only when a person is actively bearing down and when the baby's presenting part fills the pelvis. (References to concavity or convexity of a part assume that you are looking down on it through the pelvic brim.) Unless specimens are specially prepared to better approximate normal tissue relationships, this concave bowl shape becomes permanent in cadavers because the muscles are fully and permanently relaxed.

To better understand why this is so, a comparison with the muscular diaphragm that lies between the lungs and the abdominal organs is helpful. Both are alike in being attached around most of their circumferences and in being free of bony attachments elsewhere; thus both can flex up and down. But, unlike the thoracic diaphragm, there are no organs underneath the pelvic muscles and other soft tissues to help hold them in a particular shape after death. This means the levator ani muscles are more mobile, allowing their position to vary widely with activity and rest. It also means that these unsupported muscles collapse into a very unlifelike shape with damage or after death. As the pelvic muscles move, the organs and other tissues to which they are attached move along with them. Thus, the orientation of connective tissue supports and organ positions all become grossly distorted after death.

During the preservation process, these distortions are exaggerated when embalming fluid is injected into the abdomen. Fluid pressure balloons the relaxed tissues downward even more. This is why virtually all illustrations of the levator ani muscles depict them as shaped like a bowl or basin, leading to the erroneous impression that the pelvic floor is always shaped like this. Nevertheless, the bowl shape is the most uniform and therefore easiest to visualize of all the shapes that the levator ani complex can assume. Therefore, we will begin our understanding there.

When fully relaxed the levator ani muscles descend, forming a teardrop-shaped bowl with its pointed end toward the symphysis pubis. The rim of each side of the bowl attaches along a thickened ridge in the parietal fascia that overlies the obturator internus muscles that line the pelvic sidewalls.

Imagine removing a V-shaped area from the central edge of the rounded posterior end of the bowl. Now, cut off the first inch of the pointed end. Then cut out a U-shaped piece from the pointed end, with the bend in the U directed toward the posterior end of the bowl. The lower sacrum and coccyx project into the V-shaped area. The U-shaped space is called the **urogenital hiatus**. The bend in the U wraps behind the rectal canal. The edges of the U attach to the pubic bone in front and the edges of the bowl attach to the pelvic sidewalls. The deepest part of the rounded part of the bowl has a base that is formed by the anal sphincter. This gives you a general idea of the bowl shape of the pelvic floor in a cadaver.

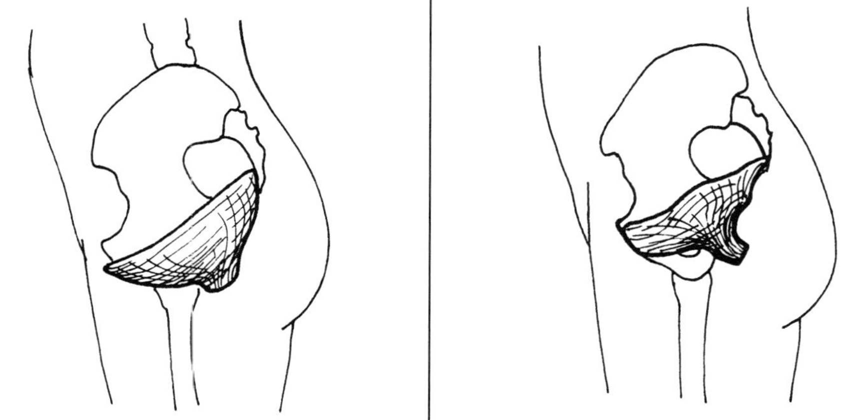

Lateral view: the classic idea of the pelvic floor as a flaccid bowl as is true in cadavers

Lateral view: the new understanding of the living pelvic floor lifted when at rest

Remember, that, in life, the at-rest pelvic floor is not normally shaped like a bowl. The muscles of the levator ani complex and anal sphincter are among the few skeletal muscles in the body that, when not producing movement, remain toned when at rest. They can respond continuously to physical activity. This tone is relaxed during voiding, during defecation, during the Valsalva maneuver (holding the breath and bearing down) and during labor when the baby is filling the pelvis. Some tone remains even when a person is asleep, under anesthesia or upside down (Wilson, 1973).

To get a better idea of how these muscles normally look at rest, imagine a breeze passing up between the legs and through the pelvis, lifting the walls of the muscular bowl from below upward except along the attached edges. In the midline, the medial edges of the U-shaped opening are attached to the midline pelvic organs and the V-shaped area is attached to the coccyx. Laterally, the edges are still attached to the tendinous arch of the levator ani. As the breeze lifts (or your fingers push) the muscles upward to either side of the hiatus, a wall of muscle rises up, hugging the midline organs and billowing the walls of the bowl on either side of the U-shaped space upward, like a parachute filling with air; converting the bowl into a double dome shape because the attached lower edges of the U-shaped area create a depression in the midline. The other image that may be helpful is an unbuttoned, standing collar with flared sides that curve down around the outer edges toward the shoulders. The neck of the collar is the urogenital hiatus. If none of those images are useful, try imagining a U-shaped funnel with flared, convexly cupped sides.

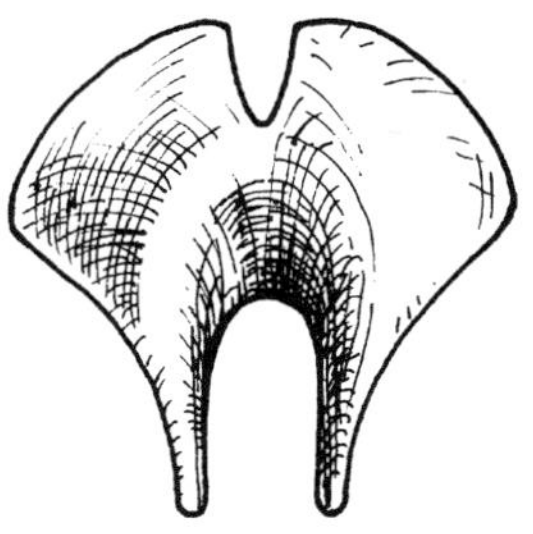

Superior view of living pelvic floor at rest

Hjartardóttir and colleagues (1997) did MRI studies of healthy women to gain insight into how the levator ani muscles normally behave. At rest in supine women, they found that the walls of the posterior half of the bowl (the region of the iliococcygeus muscles) invert, curving upward. During muscle contraction, the iliococcygeus muscle rises upward as it shortens, straightens (i.e., flattens) and becomes more horizontal. Upon bearing down, the iliococcygeus muscle descends from its double dome shape anywhere from 4 to 26 mm in nulliparas and 16 to 35 mm in multiparas. That the inner edges of the U-shaped part of the levator ani complex are tethered to the yoni and rectal canals and to the iliococcygeus muscle via the iliococcygeal ligament causes the organs to rise or descend along with the muscles as they change position.

Guo and Li (2007) did even more extensive MRI studies on subjects of both sexes. They found that when a woman's pelvic floor is at rest it is basin shaped around the bladder neck, funnel shaped adjacent to the yoni, and dome shaped in the anal and postanal regions.

While illuminating, there are problems inherent in MRI studies that must be taken into account. Distinct images are not possible, and the tissues can only be viewed in slices, which can lead to misinterpretation of the anatomy. The other big problem is that these studies were done with MRI machines that require the subject to be supine in order to obtain the images. Lying supine puts pressure against the buttocks, forcing the ischiorectal fat upward, which likely results in some distortion of the posterior levator ani and anal sphincter muscles; the effects of gravity may also alter the positioning of the connective tissues to an extent (DeLancey, 1996). In addition, it causes the soft tissues to settle toward the sacrum, thus likely distorting organ positioning somewhat. As of this writing, standing MRI machines are available, but no studies have yet been done to see what differences there may be in standing anatomy. Because of these limitations, existing MRI studies may not be showing us exactly what the pelvic floor looks like when a woman is upright. Because these muscles retain tone when at rest, however, these images are likely to offer a more accurate understanding of the complex shapes the muscles assume when a woman is standing than do drawings from dissections.

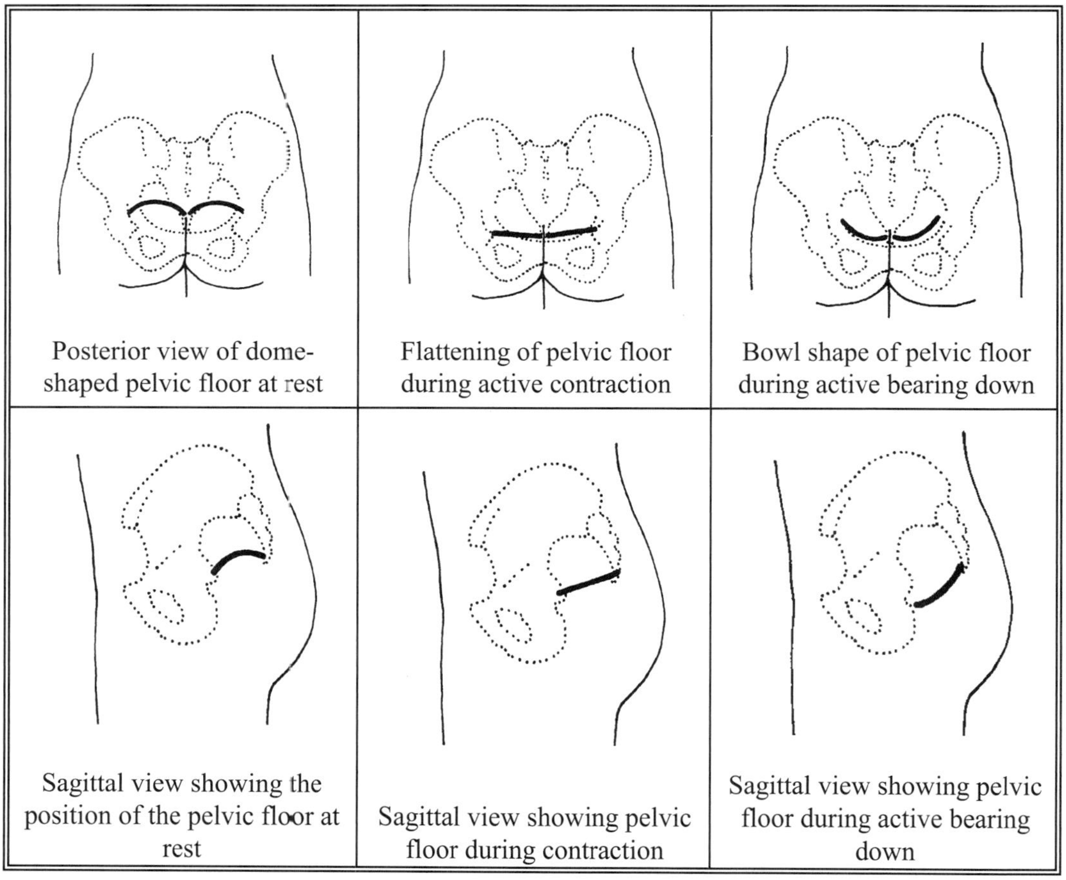

Posterior view of dome-shaped pelvic floor at rest

Flattening of pelvic floor during active contraction

Bowl shape of pelvic floor during active bearing down

Sagittal view showing the position of the pelvic floor at rest

Sagittal view showing pelvic floor during contraction

Sagittal view showing pelvic floor during active bearing down

A Closer Look at the Pelvic Floor

The following is a detailed description of the component muscles that make up the "loose trampoline" we have just discussed, plus a few others. Finding an image to use as a prototype for the way this muscle complex looks during life was challenging. After looking a numerous illustrations and MRI images, I chose to use the three-dimensional reconstruction of the pelvic floor presented on page S5 (Figure 3) in the article by Barber (2005). It made the most sense to me and offered four different views. Using it as a baseline, I referred to various descriptions, MRI studies and drawings from dissections to arrive at a detailed image and anatomy.

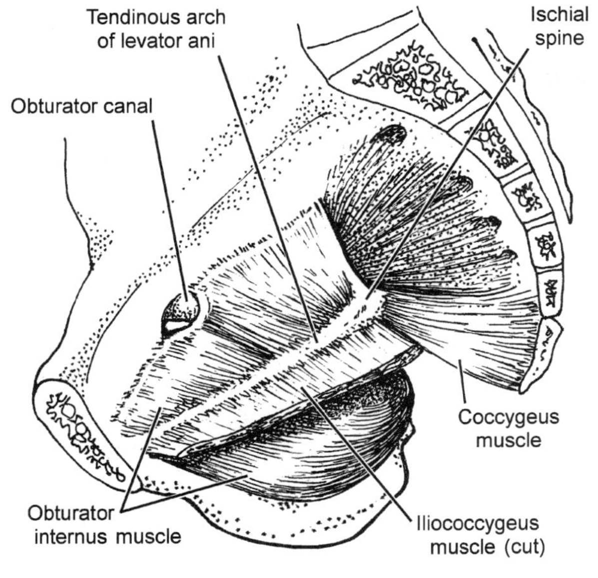

The right obturator internus muscle with superior parietal fascia, showing the location of the tendinous arch of the levator ani

Obturator internus (OB- tuh-RAY-tor in-TERN-us) muscles

The obturator internus muscles are important to our discussion because they are where the iliococcygeal muscles originate. The main body of each of the two obturator internus muscles is shaped roughly like a butterfly wing. The muscles line either side of the inner anterolateral pelvis, where they cover the obturator foramina (the openings created by the pubic rami). They also attach to the inner surface of the obturator (arcuate) tendon on either side. The urethropelvic ligament and periurethral adventitiae that support the bladder and urethra attach to the obturator tendon as well.

Each obturator internus muscle has a tail that makes a 120° turn as it passes through the lessor sciatic notch below the ischial spine to the posterior aspect of the greater trochanter of the femur. The obturator internus muscle works to rotate and abduct the thighs. Muscle contraction has a pulley action that also lifts the bladder and the urethra (Hulme, 2002).

A ridge of dense connective tissue arises from the fascia covering the inner surface of the obturator internus muscle on either side. It follows a curved path that runs along the pelvic sidewall from the ischial spine to the area lateral to the symphysis pubis. It is called the **tendinous arch of the levator ani** and is where the iliococcygeus muscles and, in some women, the lateral edges of the puboanalis portion of the pubovisceral complex originate.

The **obturator canal** is an opening through the obturator foramen in the superior part of the obturator membrane through which the obturator nerve and vessels pass from the pelvic cavity into the thigh.

Levator ani (leh-VAY-tore A-nigh) muscle complex

The levator ani complex makes up most of the muscles of the pelvic floor. In concert with the anterior part of the bony pelvis (the pubic symphysis and adjacent pubic rami), this dynamic muscular diaphragm helps prevent the abdominal and pelvic organs from falling through the hollow bony ring of the pelvis. It assists with sphincteric control of the urethra, yoni and anus, and it stimulates the clitoris and yoni by contracting during orgasm. The levator ani muscle complex is made up of three (some say four) primary muscles with several subdivisions that all work together to accomplish these tasks.

While the names for the major muscles of the levator ani are pretty consistent among sources, there is real confusion regarding the labeling and anatomy of the various muscle subdivisions and other soft-tissue parts. When reading any work on this topic, be aware that authors often have assigned their own terms to parts with no correlation to terms assigned by other writers. It may be impossible to determine what is meant by the numerous terms employed. As one attempts to gain clarity by studying a variety of sources, the confusion only mounts. When I first encountered this problem in the literature, I was left completely confused and thought it was just me. Now, this problem is widely acknowledged by contemporary researchers.

Muscle names refer to the origin and insertion points of each muscle or muscle subdivision, thus helping the student remember where they are located and, in most cases, how they function. After reviewing numerous articles and current textbooks, I have pretty much stuck with terms still current according to the TERMINOLOGIA ANATOMICA (Whitmore, 1998) with the exception of adopting the term "pubovisceral," as explained below.

There are three primary muscles that are part of the levator ani complex. From the most central muscles outward, these are:

•The most medial of the levator ani muscles is the **puboviisceral** (classically called the **pubococcygeus**). It is clearest to think of the term "puboviisceral" as referring collectively to several groups of muscles fibers that attach or insert into various soft tissues in the midline and onto the coccyx posteriorly. These four components are as follows:

-**Puboanalis muscle**: This, the primary U-shaped part, originates at the pubic bone and sends a cuff-shaped extension of fibers downward that blends with others in the anorectal wall to form the longitudinal anal muscle. It is from this U-shaped part that the other fibers extend.

-**Puboperinealis muscle**: A narrow, U-shaped layer of fibers, this part originates at the pubic bone and loops through the perineal body.

-**Pubovaginalis region**: The part of the puboanalis that reaches from the pubic bone to the yoni canal at the level of the midurethra. At that level, the **vaginolevator attachments** fibers form a bridge between the medial puboanalis wall and the anterolateral yoni wall on either side.

-**Pubococcygeal fibers:** The most lateral fibers, these are the ones for which the puboviisceral complex was originally named because they reach from the pubic bone along the upper, outer edge of the U-shaped puboanalis muscle and extend a tail beyond the posterior midline of the U that attaches to the coccyx.

•Next is the **puborectalis muscle**, a rounded, strap-shaped muscle that runs along the lower edge of the puboanalis muscle, like a very thick piece of cording on fabric. It has fibers that originate near the lower border of the pubic bone and wrap behind the rectum, forming a continuous sling. There is some debate as to whether this important muscle is truly a component of the levator ani complex. DeLancey considers it so (Kearney et al., 2004), and Garavoglia and colleagues (1993) did embryologic tissue studies that confirmed it. For these reasons, I discuss it as a part of the levator ani complex.

•The broadest muscle in the levator ani complex is the **iliococcygeus**. This is a paired muscle with fibers that originate at the tendinous arch of the levator ani on either side. In the midline, these fibers decussate into the anococcygeal ligament and attach to the coccyx. This paired, convexly cupped muscle fills in the space between the upper edge of the U-shaped part of the pubovisceral muscle complex and the sidewalls of the pelvis.

- Some sources also include the two **coccygeus (ischiococcygeus) muscles** as a fourth member of the levator ani complex. These paired muscles originate on either side at the posterior surface of the ischial spines, fan out and insert into the lower sacrum and coccyx, where they close the most posterior part of the pelvic cavity.

Some authors (Baggish & Karrem, 1999) have pointed to various additional connections between levator ani components and other structures, connections that other authors did not find (DeLancey, 2002a; Yucel & Baskin, 2004). Since reviewing every hypothetical connection would further complicate an already confusing topic, I will stick to the designations outlined above as the most "official" understanding as of this printing. You should be aware that other attachments (for example, attachments at other points where the puboanalis muscle meets the yoni wall and at the level of the proximal urethra) may also be mentioned in the literature and may, indeed, be eventually accepted.

Levator ani muscle fibers: In early life, slow-twitch striated muscle fibers predominate in the levator ani complex, providing tonic support for the pelvic organs. A smaller number of type II (fast-twitch) muscle fibers allow a quick response to increases in intra-abdominal pressure (Lukban & Whitmore, 2002). In women with normal pelvic floor function, the slow-twitch fibers are larger than the fast-twitch fibers, a finding that may be hormonally mediated and have functional implications (Beersiek et al., 1979). As humans age, smooth muscle fibers start to replace striated fibers.

Most of the muscles of the levator ani complex are digastric, allowing each muscle half to contract simultaneously and to function as a single sheet of muscle. For this arrangement to work properly, each muscle half must be intact and functioning. If one half is scarred, torn, partially separated from its normal attachment along the pelvic wall, or paralyzed due to levator ani nerve damage, the undamaged half of the muscle will tend to pull the anococcygeal ligament toward the intact side, straining the adventitial tissues that attach the organs to the pelvic walls on the damaged side. This type of nerve injury appears to result only from childbirth (van Houten, 2006).

Pubovisceral/pubococcygeus muscle: The traditional term for the central muscle fibers in the levator ani complex is "pubococcygeus" because most of its fibers originate at the pubic bone and a few reach back to attach to the coccyx, the only other bony attachment. But to label all these fibers the "pubococcygeus" obscures the complexity of this fiber group and implies that its primary function is to move the coccyx, when its primary functional parts attach to the anal canal, the perineal body and the walls of the yoni. Therefore, Kearney and colleagues (2004) favored adopting Lawson's (1974) term "pubovisceral muscle" as this makes clear that the muscle's primary functional attachments are to pelvic organs. Here, I will follow this recommendation.

This complex is often simply referred to as the "pubovisceral muscle" when collectively referring to its various groups of fibers and their function in organ support. Keep in mind, however, that, although the term "pubovisceral muscle" is used more and more in the current urogynecological literature, it has not yet been formally adopted as an anatomical term and its various parts are still collectively referred to as the "pubococcygeal muscle" in many sources.

We will start with an overview of the general shape of the primary component of this complex: the large U-shaped portion that is made up mostly of the puboanalis muscle. Dickinson (1889) and Curtis and colleagues (1939) were the only authors I could find that quoted specific measurements from adult dissections (remember that the relaxed muscle is probably larger than its toned, living counterpart). Other excellent and detailed descriptions derived from infant specimens were given by Lawson (1974), who found infant muscle fibers to be more distinct than those of adults.

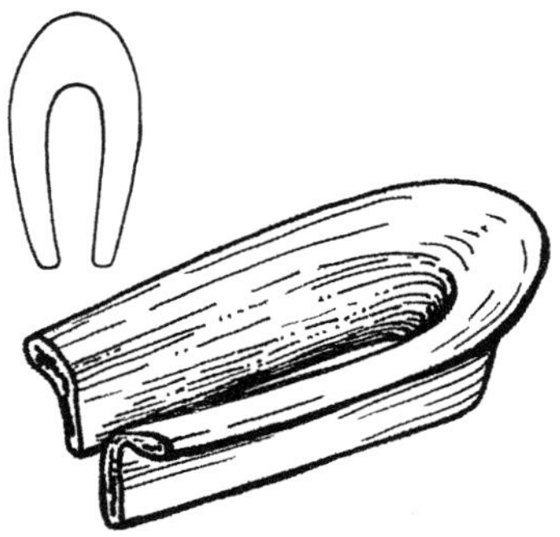

Antero-oblique view of the U-shaped part of the puboanalis muscle (extended "cuff" of puboanalis fibers not shown)

In cadavers, each side of the medial U-shaped part ranges from 3 to 4.5 cm wide along its anterior border. The most medial edge of each half originates about 3.5 cm below the upper border of the pubic bone and 1.25 cm lateral to the symphysis pubis (meaning Dickinson [1889] found a 2.5 cm midline gap between the medial tips of each side). From here the lines of origin follow a convexly curved, cranially directed path along the pubic bone. At its posterolateral end, the origin of the puboanalis muscle overlaps, or is overlapped by, the part of the tendinous arch of the levator ani that lies anterior to the obturator canal (Lawson, 1974).

On standing, the puboanalis muscle is oriented nearly horizontally. It consists of a variably tall U-shaped strap (with the tips of the U toward the pubic bone) that has convexly curved upper borders that flare to either side. The posterolateral walls of the strap wrap around the sides and back of the rectal canal. In the posterior midline, these fibers are covered by an extension of the pelvic adventitiae, forming a longitudinal ridge as they decussate with fibers of their opposite half, as observed on MRI scans. Some fibers blend into the anal wall. MRIs also indicate that the right half of the puboanalis layer is often thinner than the left (why this is so is not known). The mean thickness of the right side is 4.9 mm (± 2.3 mm) and of the left side is 6.5 mm (± 2.04) (Singh et al., 2002).

The true pubococcygeus portion of this complex consists of the uppermost lateral fibers of the puboanalis part that extend from the pubic bone, pass along its upper edges and conjoin in the posterior midline where they form an uplifted tail that reaches to the coccyx (these fibers are explained in more detail on page 89).

This U-shaped part keeps the urogenital hiatus narrow and tight, compressing the anterior yoni and urethra against the pubic bone. Active contraction draws the organs to which each part is attached upward and forward. Now we will discuss the various subdivisions of the pubovisceral complex in more detail.

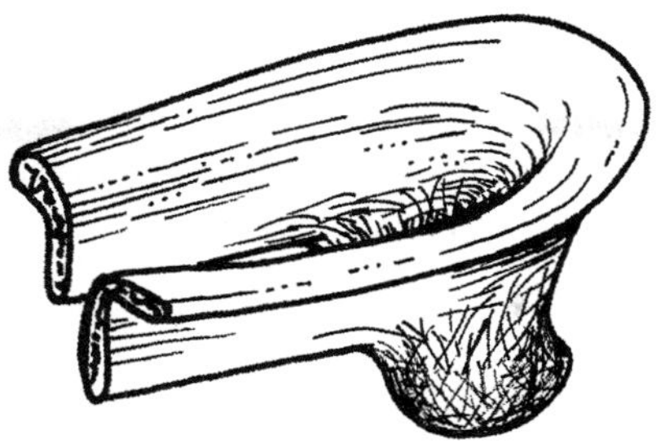

Pubeanalis muscle with cuff

Puboanalis muscle: Lawson's study (1974) offers by far the most detailed description of this part. He found that fibers of this part pass continuously from their curved line of origin to either side of the symphysis to the anal canal, which is why the entire medial U-shaped part is here referred to as the puboanalis. As the more inferior (lower) fibers reach the anorectal canal they encircle it and extend downward, forming a cuff around the anal canal below the level of the rectal hiatus (where the rectum passes through the U shape). In some sources, the U-shaped part may be called the "pubovisceral" or "pubococcygeus muscle" and this cuff may be the only part referred to as the "puboanalis muscle" (Lawson, 1974; Wendell-Smith & Wilson, 1991).

As this cuff of fibers encircles the rectal canal, the fibers split (and look much like the split ends of a hair) as they merge with the rectal wall. The topmost fibers reach up to fuse with the rectal fascia while the lower fibers pass downward through the intersphincteric groove (between the internal and external anal sphincters), reaching all the way to the anal skin. These downwardly directed fibers blend with others that form the longitudinal anal muscle coat of the anal canal. By virtue of these attachments, the anorectal canal is connected to the pubic arch (Lawson, 1974; Garavoglia et al., 1993).

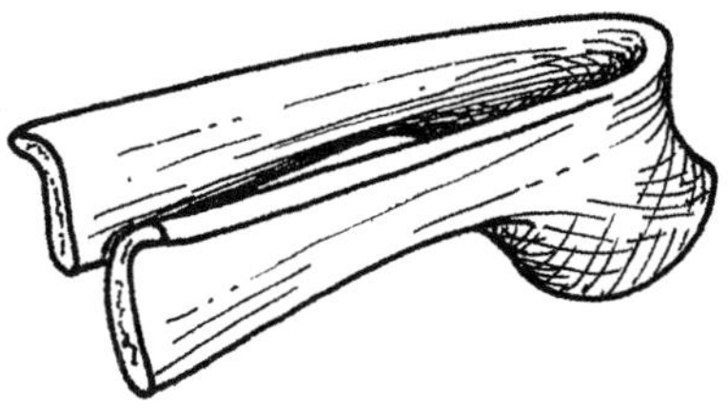

Puboanalis muscle with a narrow posterior region

The size, location and curvature of the line of origin of the puboanalis varies widely among individuals. In MRI studies, Tunn and colleagues (2003) could see no pubic insertion in 10% of the normal nulliparous women they studied. In these women, the puboanalis attachments were seen to originate only from the tendinous arch of the levator ani. Limitations of MRI notwithstanding (they could have missed a narrow attachment), these same women also had larger urogenital hiatus measurements.

Lawson's report (1974), based on infant specimens, illustrates the origin of this muscle as more lateral in relation to the pubic bone than is illustrated here; resembling a horizontal parenthesis mark with the convex side up. The fibers sweep straight back to the anal canal, and the posterior portion of the puboanalis is shown to be almost flush with the puborectalis, with the medial edge of the iliococcygeus reaching to the rectoanal junction, where it meets the puboanalis and the upper edge of the puborectalis muscle. My illustrations follow those from other MRI sources (especially Barber, 2005) that show the line of origin to be more vertical and the posterolateral edges of the puboanalis extending a variable distance up along the sides and back of the rectum before meeting the iliococcygeus (Curtis and colleagues quoted a posterior border height of 1.5 cm). Naturally, the accuracy of any of these drawings is limited because they show dissected tissue, which is flaccid. Unfortunately, most sources did not include a description of the dimensions of this part and those that did were often incomplete and failed to mention normal variations. Just be aware that the line of origin and height of the strap can vary widely among individuals.

During defecation, the puboanalis contracts, widening and shortening the anal canal, making way for the fecal bolus. At the same time, the puboanalis fibers that reach down to the anal skin help to stabilize the anal canal during fecal descent, preventing prolapse of the anal wall (Shafik, 1975a).

Pubovaginalis (PEW-bow-VAJ-ih-NALISS) region (DeLancey, 1986), (fibers of Luschka [Luschka, 1864]; pubovaginalis muscle [Macchi et al, 2008]): The portion of the puboanalis muscle that spans the space between the pubic bone and the vaginolevator attachments is often referred to as the "pubovaginalis muscle" (DeLancey, 2002a). Others use this term to refer to the vaginolevator attachments themselves (Macchi et al., 2008).

Seeking to better understand how the puboanalis muscle and the yoni wall are connected, DeLancey and Starr (1990) identified a 0.5 cm thick × 1 cm long attachment that spans the space between the puboanalis and the yoni wall either side. They called these the "vaginolevator attachments."

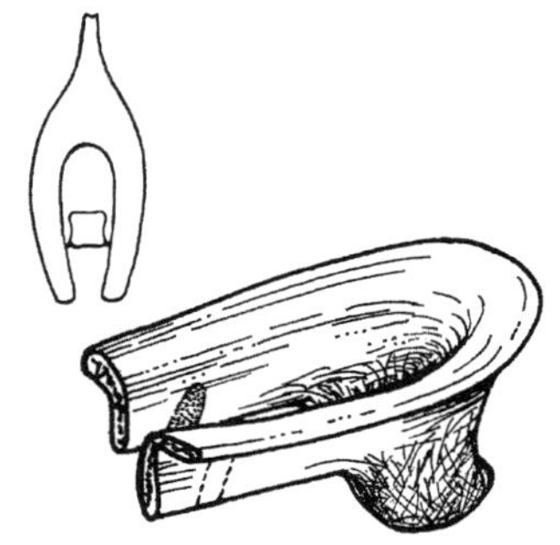

Location of vaginolevator attachments (shaded and dashed lined areas)

Each attachment begins where the urethra exits the bladder and forms a steep postero-oblique angle as it extends for about 1 cm along the medial side of the puboanalis muscle and the upper, outer yoni wall at the level of the anterior sulci on either side. The distal end stops at the lower border of the puboanalis muscle, just before reaching the deep fibers of the perineal membrane complex. These dense muscular attachments lie just beneath the tendinous arch of the pelvic fasciae and parallel the deepest and most mobile region of the urethra (roughly paralleling the 20 to 60% segment of its length), which is covered by the striated urethral sphincter muscle. Clinically, the distal end of each vaginolevator attachment lies just deep to the hymenal ring at the level of the paraurethral sulci, which are visible as dimples on either side of the urethral carina in the upper "corners" of the yoni when looking into the introitus with a posteriorly weighted speculum in place. (In a more recent study of the same anatomy, Macchi and colleagues (2008) found two fan-shaped attachments linking the medial puboanalis muscle and distal and midthird of the lateral yoni wall and the lateral thirds of the posterior yoni wall.)

The vaginolevator attachments consist of yoni wall fibers, including smooth muscle, collagen, and elastin, as well as fibers from the surrounding adventitiae, that reach out and attach directly to the puboanalis muscle, rather than puboanalis fibers that insert into the yoni wall, which would create a true pubovaginalis muscle. The yoni wall fibers involved have a higher concentration of elastin than do the surrounding tissues and interdigitate as they enter the puboanalis muscle. Some fibers pass through the muscle and insert into the inner surface of the obturator internus fasciae on either side in the area of the anterior recess of the ischiorectal fossa (DeLancey & Starr, 1990).

Even though no puboanalis fibers are directly attached to the female urethra, that the urethral canal is embedded in the ceiling of the yoni allows the vaginolevator attachments, along with other tissues classified as urethral supports, to form a hammock for the urethra. This hammock arrangement helps control the position of the upper urethra and supports it when the pelvic floor is at rest. During urination, the pelvic floor and urethral supports relax, allowing the urethra to descend, straightening the urethrovesical angle. This angle is immediately restored once the pelvic floor returns to its normal resting tone (DeLancey & Starr, 1990). The vaginolevator attachments also compress the yoni and anorectal canals from either side, anchoring the pelvic organs within the urogenital hiatus and maintaining the angles between those parts of the canals above and below the hiatus. The merging of striated and smooth muscle fibers in the vaginolevator attachments allows for shortening and widening of the canals during expulsive efforts and at the same time resists extrusion of the canals and pelvic organs when abdominal pressure is increased.

Puboperinealis muscle: The puboperinealis fibers form the most distal extension of the pubovisceral complex. They consist of a narrow, U-shaped strap that originates at the pubic bone below the inferior margin of the puboanalis part, passes just posterior to the hymenal ring and wraps around the lateral and posterior walls of the yoni. In the midline, the fibers pass through the anterior region of the perineal body (Lawson, 1974), where they contribute to those making up the central point of the perineum.

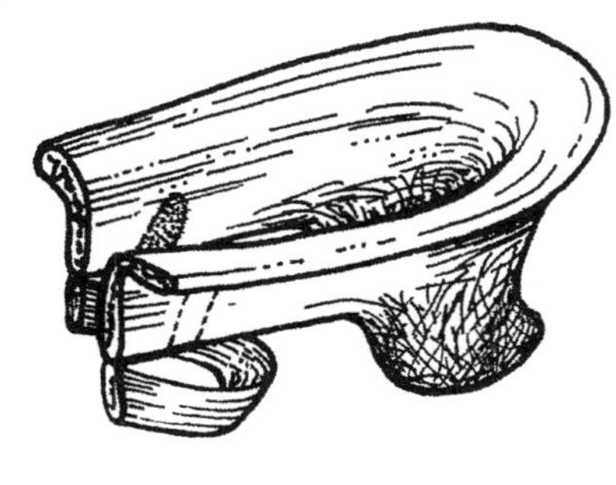

Puboperinealis muscle

Garavoglia and colleagues (1993) found it difficult to see these sparse fibers in the perineal body during dissections, particularly in females, and most sources do not mention this subdivision at all.

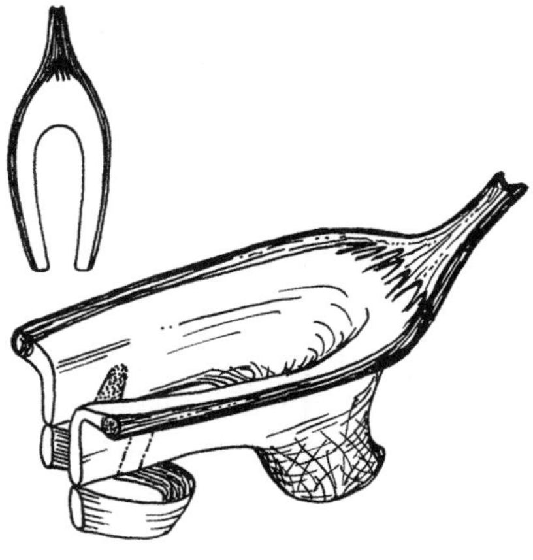

Pubococcygeus fibers with tendinous plate of the pubococcygeus muscle (overview and antero-oblique view)

The tonic activity of these fibers pulls the perineal body toward the pubis. Not surprisingly, Lien and associates (2004) found that, relative to the rest of the levator ani muscles, these midline fibers undergo the greatest degree of stretch during birth. Because these fibers lie just beneath the yoni wall, they may be involved in birth-related tears.

Pubococcygeus fibers (PEW-bow-COCK-sij-ee-us): Along the upper, outermost edges of the of the puboanalis part, run narrow bands of fibers that flow from the most lateral attachments at the pubic bone, around and behind the rectum on either side (Curtis et al., 1939; DeLancey, 2003b). A few of these fibers continue posteriorly to form a tail (up to 2 cm-wide) that, in 60% of women, passes over (is superior to) the iliococcygeal raphe. These posterior fibers become tendinous as they insert on the pelvic surface of the last two segments of the coccyx, where they blend with fibers from above, contributed by the presacral fascia. This tail is classically referred to as the **tendinous plate of the pubococcygeus muscle**. These lateral and posterior puboanalis fibers, along with the iliococcygeus and coccygeus muscles, make up the pelvic diaphragm proper (Wendell-Smith & Wilson, 1991).

Puborectalis (PEW-bow-WRECK-tahl-iss): The strap-like puborectalis muscle is about 1.5 cm wide in cadavers, but is tighter and more bundled in life. Each end originates from the lowest part of the medial (inner) surface to either side of the symphysis pubis and the adjacent pubic bone, immediately overlying the origins of the puboperinealis muscle (as illustrated in Lien et al., 2004). The antero-inferior surface of the puborectalis muscle is also attached to the cranial side of the perineal membrane complex.

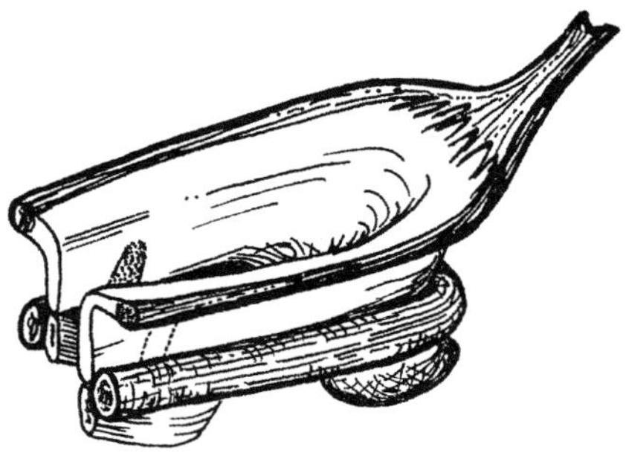

Puborectalis muscle

The medial surfaces of the puborectalis pass by the yoni, and the lateral walls of the yoni are attached to it (DeLancey, 2002b). The puborectalis then continues posteriorly, forming a rounded, U-shaped cord that runs along the bottom edge of the puboanalis muscle, where the superior fibers of the puborectalis muscle merge with the inferior fibers of the U-shaped part of the puboanalis muscle (DeLancey, 2002b; Shafik, 1975a). It then wraps behind the rectal canal just above the level of the anorectal junction (Shafik, 1975a).

This muscular sling is thicker and more condensed than the rest of the muscles in the levator ani complex, appearing as a rounded, rope-shape on MRI scans. Shafik (1975a) found a continuous muscle band, with no fibrous raphe in the posterior midline, although other sources do report a raphe in this area.

Many sources report that the puborectalis merges with the fibers of the external sphincter. Fucini and colleagues (1999), however, found that the inferior fibers of the puborectalis are fused to a layer of connective tissue that is sandwiched between it and the U-shaped part of the winged portion of the external sphincter (deep external sphincter).

Nonetheless, the most obvious division between the puborectalis and winged part of the external sphincter is provided by the anococcygeal ligament. In a study of female specimens, Fucini and associates (1999) found fibers from the sphincter attached to the anococcygeal ligament in the posterior midline, but none from the puborectalis muscle. This contradicts GRAY'S ANATOMY (Bannister, 1999), which states that the puborectalis does contribute fibers to the anococcygeal raphe. It is likely that whether this occurs varies among individuals, although the reference to such an attachment may well have been derived from studies done only on male specimens.

You may be wondering why this muscle, with its pubic attachment and visceral insertion, is not considered part of the pubovisceral muscle complex and, indeed, it is categorized as such in some sources. Some sources even refer to only a puborectalis muscle, combining it with the pubococcygeus (puboanalis part). However, it is formally considered as a separate structure so I am sticking with that designation.

When the pelvic floor muscles are well toned, the attachment of the puborectalis to the winged (deep) part of the external anal sphincter allows the two to work together to pull the rectal canal and the anococcygeal ligament toward the pubic bone, creating an anteriorly oriented midline bend at the anorectal junction averaging nearly 90° (ranging between 60 and 105°) called the **anorectal angle** (Aronson et al., 1990). (MRI studies suggest that the puborectalis does not actually contact the anorectal junction in living subjects [Guo & Li, 2007].)

The anorectal angle makes a major contribution to anorectal continence by helping to prevent rectal contents from constantly entering the anal canal. This angle becomes less extreme as the puborectalis relaxes during defecation.

The puborectalis muscle and the internal anal sphincter are in a state of constant tone when at rest, and both can be contracted voluntarily, working together to delay bowel evacuation. The function of the puborectalis in rectal continence is still being studied. It obviously plays an important role, because women can remain continent of solid stool even though their anterior anal sphincters are torn and left unrepaired. It is also known that atrophy of the puborectalis may be associated with fecal incontinence (Schorge et al., 2008).

The lowermost puborectalis muscle fibers extend down along the anal canal to join and mingle with others that contribute to the longitudinal anal muscle. These conjoined fibers end just above the superficial external anal sphincter, where they become fibrous before penetrating the subcutaneous external anal sphincter. When the puborectalis is properly contracted, it helps to close the anourogenital hiatus, compressing the anterior and posterior walls of the yoni together, keeping them closed when at rest (DeLancey, 1999).

Urogenital hiatus: The **urogenital** or **genital hiatus** is the U-shaped space created by the medial surfaces of the puboanalis and puborectalis muscles. Through this space the urethral, yoni and anorectal canals pass. The exact definition of the hiatus varies, depending upon which of these canals are included. The hiatus is generally said to encompass the urethral and yoni canals as they pass to the surface of the body. Oelrich (1983), on the contrary, defined the female hiatus as being smaller than in males and transmitting only the urethra and its muscles because of the attachment of the puboanalis muscle to the sidewalls of the yoni (the vaginolevator attachments); thus, in his view, the ceiling of the yoni comprises the inferior border of a **urethral hiatus**.

DeLancey and Hurd (1998) defined the external boundaries of the hiatus as the pubic bones anteriorly, the medial margins of the puboanalis part laterally, and the anterior border of the perineal body below (they do not include the rectal canal). This is a handy definition because it can be clinically assessed during a digital yoni exam. They found the mean size of this space to be 5.4 cm^2 in women who had no evidence of organ prolapse and a size of 8.4 cm^2 or smaller to be within a normal range.

Many authors, however, include the urethra, yoni walls, *and* the entire anorectal canal when they use the term "urogenital hiatus," defining it as the space encompassed by the lateral and posterior borders of either the puboanalis or the puborectalis muscle. Technically this would be the **anourogenital hiatus**.

The literature does not always make clear to which hiatus it refers, and the use and definition of these terms overlap. However, regardless of what landmarks are used to define the hiatus, it is generally agreed that toned levator ani muscles keep the space narrow and tight.

When the pelvic contents are under increased tension, the attachment of the puboanalis muscle to the perineal membrane complex helps redirect abdominal pressure and disperse gravity, responses that also prevent undue expansion of the urogenital hiatus. In nulliparous women, the anterior opening in the urogenital hiatus widens 4 to 14 mm at the level of the yoni during bearing down. This change is either less dramatic or absent in women who have recently given birth. Researchers suspect that the widening of the hiatus requires intact nerves and that childbearing may result in some temporary nerve impairment, since many women do recover most or all of their function as time passes after they give birth (Hjartardóttir et al., 1997).

If the hiatus becomes lax or damaged, some of the weight of the yoni and cervix will be transferred from the levator ani complex to the endopelvic adventitiae. A constant downward pull on these connective tissues over time causes the organs to drop down to fill the space and eventually a cystocele, a rectocele or both may develop. A weak pelvic floor may also result in uterine prolapse. Ultimately, the perineal body is the only part guarding against organ prolapse in such cases.

Iliococcygeus (ILL-e-oh-COCK-sij-ee-us): The two halves of the iliococcygeus muscle form the lateroposterior parts of the levator ani muscle complex. The iliococcygeus forms a broad-sided, U-shaped muscle. Each half consists of a wide, thin sheet of gently convexly cupped muscle that is about 5 cm wide at its line of origin, which runs from the medial surface of the ischial spine and across the pelvic sidewalls along the tendinous arch of the levator ani. Fibrous tissues are interspersed among the muscle bundles along this line of origin (Singh et al., 2002). In the posterior midline, fibers from the two halves converge and decussate as they form the iliococcygeus raphe (explained in more detail next). Their line of decussation forms a small midline ridge on the inferior surface of the muscle when at rest. The medial edges of the iliococcygeus muscles usually underlie (are inferior to) the lateral edges of the pubococcygeal fibers of the puboanalis muscle. The posterior fibers of the iliococcygeus muscles insert into the last two segments of the pelvic aspect of the coccyx on either side.

The iliococcygeus is the most purely diaphragmatic portion of the levator ani complex, providing upward lift when at rest and during active contraction. When the properly toned muscle is at rest, the two unattached posterior edges are convex. The muscle's halves then slope forward and downward as they approach the midline. Each muscle half is about 2.8 mm thick at each ischial spine (± 0.80 mm). During straining, each half thickens to around 3.9 mm (± 0.89). Straining produces no uniform pattern of change, with elevation of the muscle occurring in some women (who may have high-tone pelvic floor dysfunction) and descent in others. This muscle, being more posterior than the pubovisceral parts of the levator ani complex, is more prone to damage during the first phase of labor or from any condition, such as obesity or constipation, that produces persistently increased intra-abdominal pressure (Singh et al., 2002).

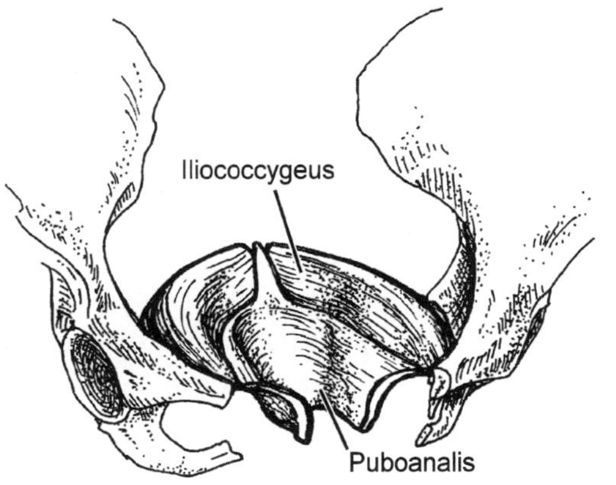

Antero-oblique view of iliococcygeus and puboanalis muscles. The puboanalis cuff and puboperinealis have been left out to better depict the U shape of the puboanalis muscle. Puborectalis not shown

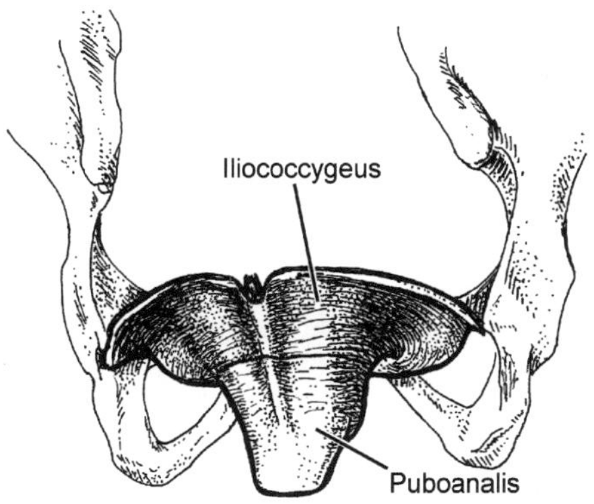

Postero-oblique view shows Iliococcygeus and puboanalis muscles with the puboanalis cuff extension

(Both views show pubic bone and sacrum removed.)

When the sides and posterior border of the puboanalis muscle are short, the medial edges of the iliococcygeus reach further down to meet the lateral borders of the puboanalis.

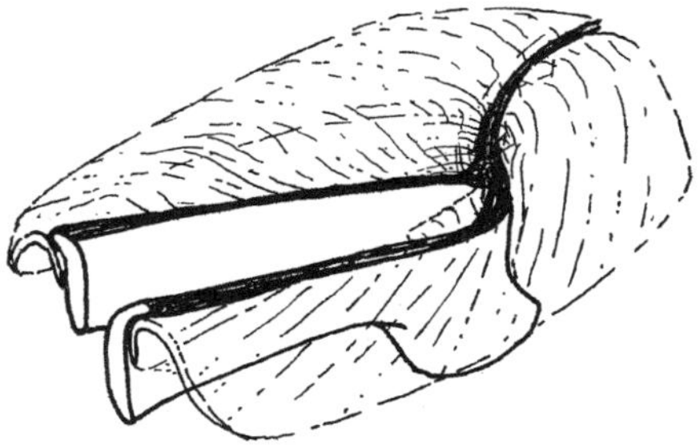

Short posterior edge of puboanalis with extended medial edge of the iliococcygeus muscle: oblique view

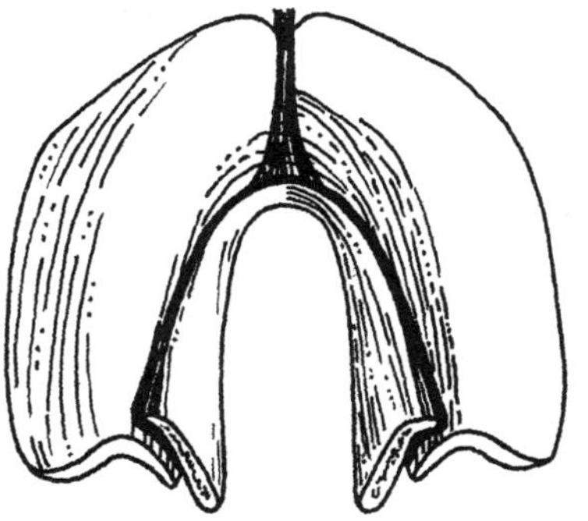

Anterosuperior view (cuff not shown)

Anococcygeal ligament or raphe (iliococcygeal raphe/levator plate/postanal plate): The anococcygeal ligament consists of a band of tissues that stretches between the posterior anorectum and the coccyx. The terms used to describe this structure vary among sources and are rarely specifically defined. Apparently, the term "raphe" is often applied to the entire structure, perhaps to emphasize the digastric nature of the levator ani components. At times, the term "iliococcygeal raphe" seems to refer to the entire structure, rather than just one layer. Contemporary sources tend to use the term "anococcygeal ligament" when discussing the contribution of the external anal sphincters, although this term technically refers to all the layers. The imprecise use of these terms is confusing and implies that there are several separate structures.

To clarify exactly what we are talking about here, I referred to the TERMINOLOGIA ANATOMICA (Whitmore, 1998), which defines the anococcygeal ligament as a single structure composed of several layers. The 38th edition of GRAY'S ANATOMY (Salmons, 1999) describes a multilayered, musculotendinous band. From the deepest layer to the most superficial, it is formed by and named for fibers contributed by the posterior midline parts of the following structures: the presacral fascia; the tendinous plate of the pubococcygeus muscle, the iliococcygeal raphe, posterior fibers from the puborectalis muscle (only in men?), and the tail-like extensions from the main and subcutaneous parts of the external anal sphincter. Fibers from all these layers come together before they attach to the coccyx. Here is a list of these layers with the connective tissue "spaces" interspersed: the presacral fascia (described on page 119), the tendinous plate of the pubococcygeus muscle, the muscular raphe of the iliococcygeus, fibers from the puborectalis muscle, the deep postanal space (which is filled with fatty tissue), and the tail-like extensions from the main and subcutaneous parts of the external anal sphincter, below which lies the superficial postanal space, (a part of the perianal space), which is filled with fatty tissue; superficial to that lies the skin.

The posterior, medial muscle fibers of the tendinous plate of the pubococcygeal fibers, as well as the midline fibers of the iliococcygeus muscle, meet behind the anorectal canal. In 60% of women, the posterolateral edge of the pubococcygeal fibers is superior to the most anterior medial edge of the iliococcygeus muscle. The same layering is present in the fibers as they enter the levator plate (discussed below). In 37% of women, the posterolateral edge of the pubococcygeal fibers and the anterior medial edge of the iliococcygeal muscle lie edge to edge. In only 3% of women, are the edges of iliococcygeus superior to those of the pubococcygeal fibers (Wendell-Smith & Wilson, 1991).

The pubococcygeal and iliococcygeal muscle fibers decussate as each layer meets in the midline to form their contributions to the anococcygeal ligament. In most cases their fibers cross once (X), but they may cross up to three times (XXX) as they join the deep, fleshy bundles from the other side. This digastric arrangement of fibers allows for a wide range of changes in both the length and breadth of the raphe and allows both sides of the muscles to contract simultaneously as a single sheet. When the anococcygeal ligament is contracted, the fibers of the levator plate shorten and broaden, widening the sidewalls of the anourogenital hiatus laterally while reducing its anteroposterior diameter (Shafik, 1975a).

The levator plate: When discussing the way the anococcygeal ligament works to support the pelvic organs it is often referred to as the "levator plate," a term first introduced by Halban and Tandler in 1907. They wrote of the posterior segment where the levator ani muscles unite and intertwine as strengthening the pelvic diaphragm behind the rectum. This term has been adopted by some contemporary researchers when studying pelvic prolapse.

When the muscles are at rest, the levator plate, along with the medial portion of the U-shaped part of levator ani complex, is normally convexly arched. A well-toned levator plate underlies and supports the rectal wall and, above that, the upper third of the yoni wall and, above that, the bladder. The tone and angle of the levator plate contributes to the angle created by the puborectalis and pubovisceral muscles, causing the upper third of the yoni to incline toward S3 or S4.

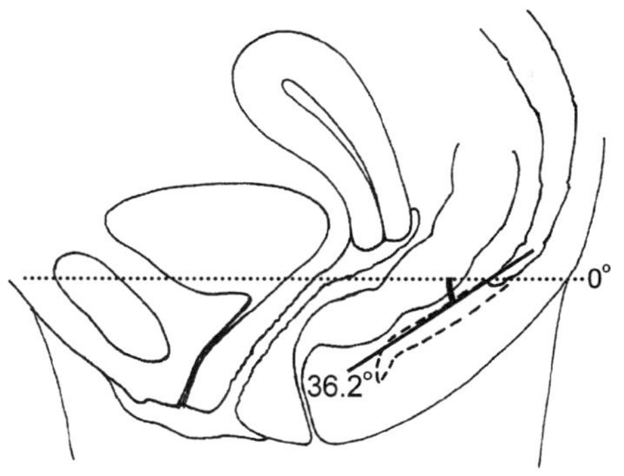

Measuring the levator plate angle

At rest, Hsu and colleagues (2006) found that the normally toned levator plate has a mean angle of 36.2° (ranging between 23.8 and 48.5°). This angle was obtained using a sagittal MRI scan of the pelvis and measuring from the point where the iliococcygeal raphe is attached to the coccyx relative to a horizontal (zero) line drawn from the tip of the coccyx, or a little higher, straight through the pubic bone. This angle becomes less acute during periods of increased abdominal pressure, when the mean angle widens to 44.3° (ranging between 29.1 and 59.5°). In women with some degree of pelvic prolapse, the levator plate is more vertically inclined when at rest (33.4 to 58.2°) and during straining (37.4 to 69.4°). (Previous studies described the normally toned levator plate as being nearly horizontal [Nichols et al., 1970].)

It is postulated that the levator plate functions like a flap valve (valve flap or clack valve, defined as a valve that opens and closes on one hinged side). In this case, the flap is the upper end of the yoni and the "hinge" is the gentle bend in the yoni tube. When abdominal pressure increases, as occurs during bearing down, the abdominal contents compress the upper third of the yoni against the levator plate. This action prevents undue stress on the adventitial support tissue, thus helping to prevent prolapse.

The normal baseline activity of the pubovisceral complex keeps the urogenital hiatus closed by compressing the yoni, urethra and rectum against the pubic bone and by lifting the organs upward (DeLancey, 2002a). When the levator plate is weakened, its angle is more vertical during rest and during straining, resulting in a longer hiatus length. During straining, the perineal body is also displaced further down than is normal in these women. Thus, the at-rest levator plate angle is probably a good indicator of levator ani damage. Any weakness in the levator plate that results in the straightening of the upper portion of the yoni will eventually lead to slippage of the yoni canal down over the anterior edge of the levator plate, resulting in prolapse of the yoni, the uterus or both.

As the levator plate is primarily made up of iliococcygeal muscle fibers, the iliococcygeal raphe plays a different role than the tendinous plate of the pubococcygeus muscle. Damage to the pubococcygeal component may result in widening the angle of the levator plate, but not to the same degree as when the iliococcygeal raphe is damaged, a problem that occurs in only 10% of those with levator ani damage. It is also possible for organ prolapse to result solely from abnormally weak connective tissues (because these tissues stabilize the organs), as might occur in women with connective tissue disease (Hsu et al., 2006).

Coccygeus/ischiococcygeus (IS-key-ho-COCK-sij-ee-us): The triangularly shaped coccygeus muscles are the most posterior component of the levator ani complex. They originate from the tip and posterior surface of the ischial spines laterally and insert along the lateral margins of the pelvic aspect of the coccyx and the fifth (lowermost) sacral segment posteriorly, filling in the rest of the posterior region of the levator ani diaphragm, where they provide a minimal amount of supplemental support. They are, however, relatively minor muscles in humans, forming a thin, nonfunctional covering over the strong sacrospinous ligaments, which are embedded within them. Because they overlie ligaments, they remain the same basic shape after death. There is disagreement as to whether these muscles are part of the levator ani complex. Those that believe them to be note that they complete the most posterior region of the pelvic diaphragm.

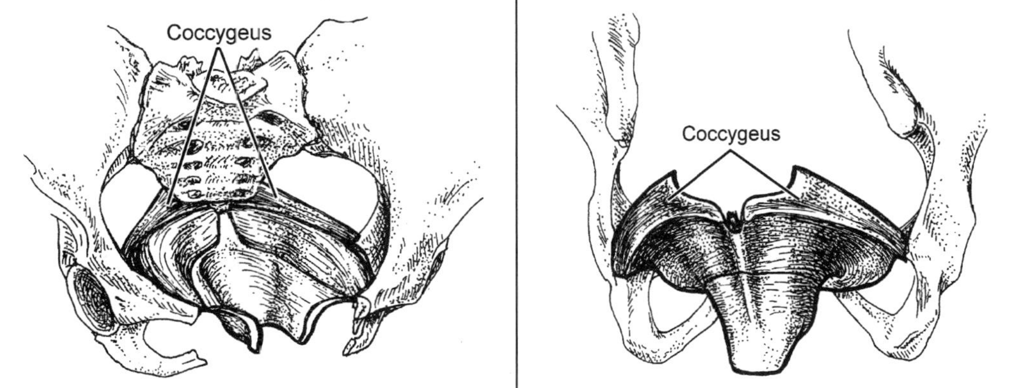

Coccygeus muscles filling in the levator ani complex with pubic bone removed (puboanalis extension, puboperinealis and puborectalis muscles not shown)	Postero-oblique view of coccygeus muscles in the pelvis with the sacrum removed

In the APPENDICES you will find instructions to make a model of the levator ani muscle complex. For those of you who are still having trouble visualizing the parts, this should help a lot.

Racial differences in the levator ani muscles

Compared to Caucasian American women, differences in pelvic type result in African American women having a 10.4% smaller posterior pelvic floor area and a 5.1% smaller total pelvic floor area (Baragi et al., 2002). Thus, African American women are less prone to developing pelvic floor prolapse problems than Caucasian women because the larger the pelvic floor, the more stress the tissues are subjected to when resisting downward pressure.

Ischiorectal/ischioanal fossa

The ischiorectal fossa, or "depression," lies below the skin to either side of the anal sphincters and canal. Its superficial boundary consists of the dorsal surface of the banded

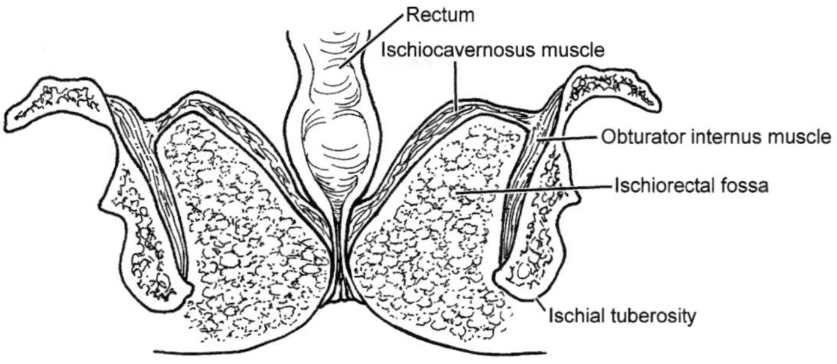

Ischiorectal fossa

part of the perineal membrane tissue complex. Its superior boundary is formed by the inferior fasciae of the levator ani muscles. The fasciae of the lower parts of the obturator internus muscles form its lateral boundaries.

The anal triangle contains the main part of the fossa that lies between the inferior side of the levator ani muscles and to either side of the external anal sphincters. The fossa's most posterior region extends above the gluteus maximus muscles of the buttocks. The pudendal neurovascular trunk passes through the ischiorectal fossa (DeLancey, 2003b).

The ischiorectal region is filled with mostly fatty tissue that provides cushioning for the organs, while still allowing them to expand and contract.

THE ANAL TRIANGLE AND RELATED STRUCTURES

This chapter covers the anal or posterior triangle, which primarily consists of the internal and external anal sphincters and other anal structures. Some sources also include the puborectalis muscle in this region (described on page 86).

The anal canal is the last part of the large intestines and forms the outlet for the gastrointestinal tract. It begins at the anorectal junction, where the rectal wall abruptly narrows as the rectal canal passes through the anogenital hiatus. The anal canal is highly expandable, conforming to the size and shape of the fecal mass. It normally varies between 2.5 to 4 cm in length and 1.2 to 3.5 cm in diameter during defecation. The lumen forms a slit when empty and at rest. Two sphincter muscles surround this canal. Together, these anal sphincters, the puborectalis muscle, the puboanalis fibers and possibly the levator plate all contribute to bowel continence. The tissues of the anal canal and its sphincters can be damaged during childbirth.

The anatomy of the anal sphincters has been the subject of much debate regarding subdivisions of the muscles and how they function, the degree to which they encircle the anal canal in females, the extent to which they contribute to rectal continence, and other morphologic and sexual differences. The variations between one study and another can leave one wondering how such vastly different findings could result from research done by experienced anatomists studying the very same structures. Once again, a large part of the problem stems from distortion of tissues in embalmed cadavers and the complex three-dimensional structures involved as well as significant sex-related differences. Because of this, and because, here too, there is little consensus regarding the basic configuration of this anatomy, particularly with regard to sexual differences, I will continue to describe the structures while pointing out differences of opinion as I go.

Fritsch and colleagues (2002) did extensive work to try to clear up some of the confusion using sagittal, coronal and axial dissections of cadavers, as well as MRI studies of living subjects. They found the sphincter complex to differ significantly from what is presented in anatomic texts: it consists of a thick internal sphincter, the longitudinal muscle layer, and the external sphincters. They also found the entire complex to be thicker in men than in women. These findings have been confirmed and refined by other researchers. The following description will proceed from deep to superficial structures, focusing on muscles and fasciae.

Internal anal sphincter

The muscular component of the rectal wall consists of two layers or coats: an inner layer of circular, smooth muscle fibers and a more superficial layer of longitudinal muscle fibers.

The lower end of the inner muscle layer becomes the internal anal sphincter. Beginning at the level of the anorectal junction, bundles of circular smooth muscle fibers thicken to a depth of 5 to 8 mm, forming a cuff around the upper three-quarters of the anal canal. Bollard and associates (2002) found the internal sphincter to be thicker in the anterior midline in women than in men and postulated that this may compensate for the narrower midline band of external sphincter in women (described on page 98). The overall height of the internal sphincter averages 32.9 mm and is always taller than the external anal sphincter by more than 10 mm, with an average difference of 17 mm in the anterior midline. The level of its lower boundary lies, on average, 3.7 mm above the external anal orifice (DeLancey et al., 1997).

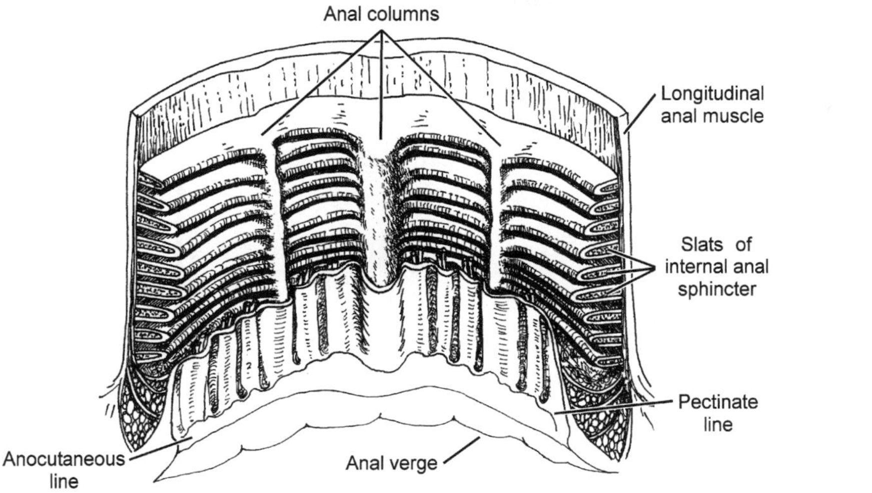

Dissected view of the Venetian blind–like slats that make up the internal sphincter, showing one large (center) and two smaller rectal columns between the sections

Uz and colleagues (2004) performed dissections of the internal anal sphincter and found no significant differences between the sexes as far as the detailed anatomy was concerned, although they only studied three female specimens. At the level of the anal canal, the circular smooth muscle bundles of the internal smooth muscle coat thicken to form stacks of flat, horizontally oriented, ring-shaped muscular slats averaging 6 mm in width that resemble the open slats of a Venetian blind. The widest slats are found near the center and the narrowest are located at the top and bottom of the muscular cuff. On average there are 20 to 30 of these rings.

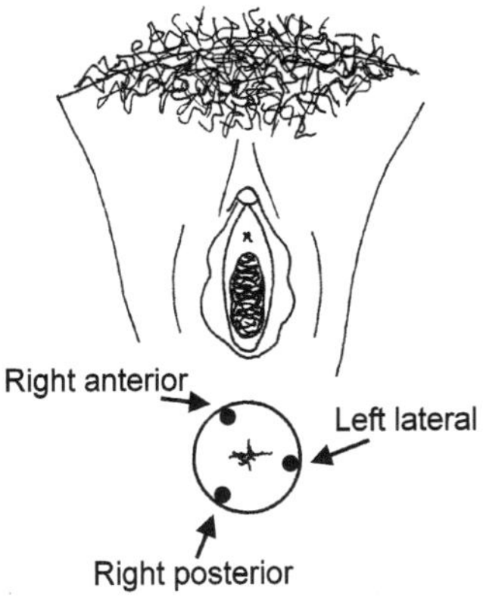

Locations of the three largest rectal columns

Around the circumference of the anal lumen, the rings are divided into three sections by three large, longitudinally oriented, fibromuscular columns that are located at equidistant points and that project into the lumen of the anal canal. (There are, altogether, approximately six to 10 anal columns in the mucosa around the lumen of the anal canal; these three are larger than the rest.) These three large columns overlie the vascular anal cushions and play an important role in anal continence. Each ring is entirely covered by its own fascia. The ends of each section of slats are attached by fascia to a column from either side. The rest of the fascial layer of each ring is attached to the submucosa of the anal canal, leaving the midportion of each section of slats freely mobile (again, similar to the way that slats of a Venetian blind are attached at either end but still movable). The slat-like sections of the internal sphincter may play a role in ensuring adequate venous flow in the anorectal region.

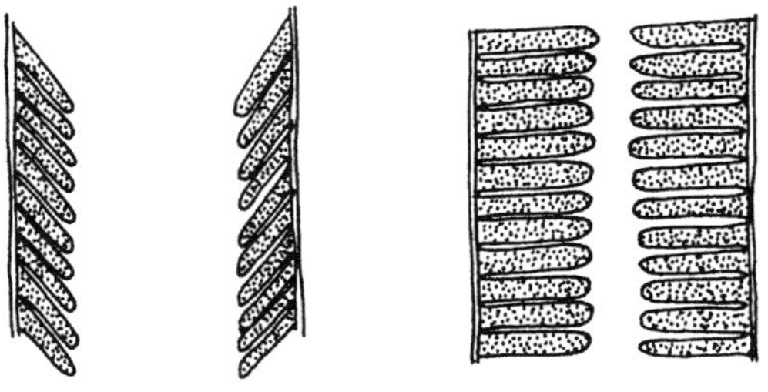

Longitudinal schematics of the slats in the down position (left) and in the horizontal at rest position (right)

The internal sphincter is innervated by autonomic fibers and provides 70 to 85% of the resting tone of the anal canal. During defecation, Uz and colleagues (2004) postulated that fibers of the longitudinal coat of the rectal canal pull the anal canal upward as the upper part of the canal relaxes, allowing feces to pass downward. Descent of the fecal bolus stimulates the smooth muscle fibers of the internal sphincter to relax. As the bolus presses against the slats, their edges are pushed downward (like closing a Venetian blind). Flattening the slats puts tension on the columns as well, flattening them against the sidewalls of the anal lumen. This widens the canal and allows stool to pass more easily.

Once the anal canal is empty, the internal anal sphincter resumes its normal resting tone, and the slats return to a horizontal position (like opening a Venetian blind), allowing the columns to reexpand toward the center of the anal lumen, which relieves pressure on the blood vessels underlying them. The expansion of the slats and columns into the lumen narrows the canal, aiding in continence. Damage to the slats, the columns, or their overlying mucosal folds may thus compromise the internal sphincter and affect the way it functions.

Longitudinal anal muscle (conjoined longitudinal muscle coat/rectococcygeus muscle/ retractor of the anus [of Treiz]/tensor fascia pelvis [of Kohlrausch]/ligamentum suspensorium [of Berau]/levator ani proprius [of Lesshaft]/everter ani muscle)

At the level of the anorectal junction, the external longitudinal muscle coat of the rectum becomes the longitudinal anal muscle, which consists of a cuff of muscle sandwiched between the internal and external anal sphincters, helping to bind together and support them. It has been called the "conjoined coat" because at the level of the anorectal junction it is augmented by muscle fibers contributed by adjacent muscles. This muscle has been sparsely studied and poorly understood for many years. In 2008, dissections of 8 male and 8 female specimens by Macchi and associates shed new light on this anatomy.

The outer fibers of the longitudinal anal muscle are primarily striated fibers from the puboanalis muscle and the innermost part of the puborectalis. The inner layer is composed of smaller numbers of smooth muscle fibers contributed by the longitudinal muscle of the rectal wall. No sex- or age-related differences were noted in the specimens studied.

The anterior portion of the longitudinal anal muscle extends along the anal canal, receiving fibers from the innermost part of the puborectalis muscle. It is composed predominantly of vertical muscle fibers. At its lower end, the anterior quadrant splits into seven to nine fibroelastic septa that pass through the external anal sphincter and attach to the deep dermis.

The posterior quadrant of the longitudinal anal muscle receives striated fibers from the innermost part of the puborectalis muscle and from the medial part of the puboanalis muscle. Fibrous septa course through the posterior quadrant to its distal end, some of which run toward the separation between the deep (likely the main part) and superficial (likely the subcutaneous part) parts of the external anal sphincter (terms for the parts of the external anal sphincter given later in this chapter are unique to the article quoted and it is not entirely clear how to correlate this new understanding of female sphincter anatomy with the work of Macchi et al., 2008). Other very thin septa pass through the internal anal sphincter to the submucosal tissue. The muscle fibers of the posterior quadrant follow a predominately oblique course. Along the sides the muscle fibers were more densely packed and follow a more oblique or transverse course (rather than being strictly longitudinal).

The anterior and posterior quadrants are significantly thinner than the sides, being found by Macchi's team to be only 1.36 mm (± 0.2) and 1.28 mm (± 0.27) thick, respectively, while the lateral quadrants of this muscle layer are thicker than its anterior or posterior quadrants, with a mean of 1.92 (± 0.24) mm on the right and 2.18 mm (± 0.46) on the left. The mean thickness of the longitudinal anal muscle coat was 2.09 mm (± 0.32) at its proximal end, 1.38 mm (± 0.38) at midlevel and 1.23 (± 0.05) mm at its distal end.

While studying living subjects using MRIs, Fritsch and colleagues (2002) found that the lowermost end of the external sphincter turns inward to wrap underneath the lower edge of the longitudinal muscle, and becomes continuous with the internal sphincter, thus enclosing the lower end of the longitudinal muscle layer. I could find nothing to corroborate this finding. They mentioned nothing about any fibers extending to the perianal skin (although this may not have been visible on MRI). They found the longitudinal coat to be rather thin in the anterior midline.

Due to its attachment to the puboanalis muscle, contraction of the longitudinal anal muscle shortens and widens the anal canal in an upward and lateral direction, everting the anal and perianal skin and opening the anal orifice. It may also help to angulate the cuff-shaped portion of the puboanalis downward, to create the anorectal angle (Petros, 2004). The conjoined longitudinal coat is believed to control eversion of the anal canal during defecation (Lunniss & Phillips, 1992).

Intersphincteric groove

This is the space between the internal and external sphincters, through which the longitudinal anal muscle passes as it descends to the perianal skin.

External anal sphincter

When exposed, the external sphincter is the most visually distinct muscle in a torn perineal body. For centuries there has been no consensus in the literature regarding whether or how to subdivide the different regions of the external sphincter, although it is generally agreed that it has different parts. Indeed reports of two, three and rarely four subdivisions have been published (Dalley, 1987). Many authors go with three layers (deep, superficial, and subcutaneous). Fritsch and colleagues (2002) proposed that the female external sphincter be divided into two layers: the deep or anorectal part and the superficial or subcutaneous part. As imaging technology continues to improve, structures are being noted in various anatomical studies that have not been observed in cadaveric specimens or earlier scans (Hsu et al., 2005). Hsu and associates (among them, DeLancey) did MRI studies on female subjects to better define the undistorted anatomy of the anal region. They came up with three subdivisions (which I will follow here) based on visible separation of the parts on MRI as well as differing origins and insertions of each component part. Please note that I could not find a similar description in any textbook, that this is not the final word on the subject, and that it pertains only to female anatomy.

Winged external sphincter (deep external sphincter): Hsu and associates (2005) refer to the deepest portion of the external sphincter as "winged." The muscle fibers in this part lie immediately below the puborectalis muscle. Like the puborectalis, this portion is U-shaped (rather than circular) in at least 75% of women, with fibers that parallel those of the puborectalis muscle in the back and alongside the rectal canal (Bollard et al., 2002; Fritsch et al., 2002; Oh & Kark, 1972). (Whether women in whom the U shape could not be identified have anatomically circumferential deep sphincters or whether the apparent absence of this feature is merely due to the limitations of MRI technology is not known.) The two flared ends (the wings) originate near each ischiopubic ramus and extend posteriorly on either side, passing around the sides of the anal canal and decussating in the posterior midline. In some women, a few anterolateral sphincter fibers merge with the superficial transverse perineal muscle. In most MRI images, there was a clear separation of the lateral sphincter fibers from the adjacent puborectalis fibers. Anterior wing anatomy after Netter.

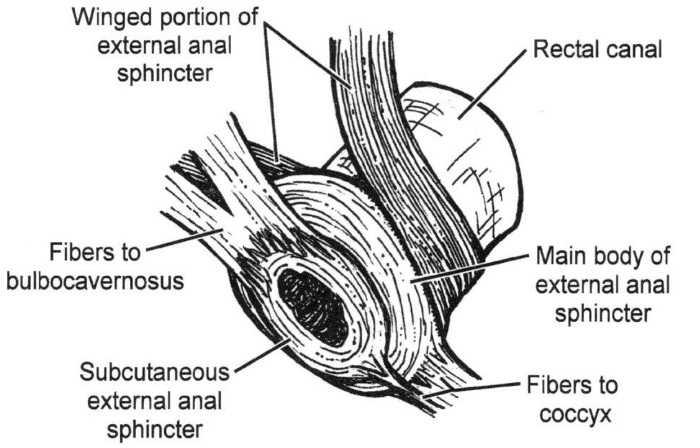

The external anal sphincters as described by Hsu et al. in 2005, with upward-reaching subcutaneous fibers that blend with those of the bulbocavernosus muscle (Shafik et al., 2007a). On MRI, there was no visible separation between main and winged parts.

The "gap" in the female external anal sphincter: Hsu and colleagues confirm the work of others regarding the presence of an anterior "gap" or narrowing in the deep external sphincter in women (no such gap exists in men). Here is a little history and more details on this finding.

In 1972, Oh and Kark were the first to identify what they described as an anterior gap in female cadaver specimens. They noted that the external sphincter was taller along the sides and posteriorly than in the anterior midline. Oh and Kark described fibers that approach the anterior midline, where they converge to form a single, shorter, muscle bundle. As external sphincter muscle fibers approach the midline from either side, they pass through the fibromuscular mass in the perineal body.

Bollard and colleagues (2002) confirmed an anterior gap below the level of the puborectalis muscle in 43 out of 57 (75%) nulliparous pregnant women under their care. In the same study, an additional 18 healthy volunteers (9 male, 9 female) were examined with an endoscopic probe. All nine males had a complete ring of external sphincter muscle throughout its length while all nine women had a natural anterior gap in the deep external anal sphincter inferior to the puborectalis muscle.

Natural gaps were characterized by uniform hypoechogenicity with smooth, regular edges. Gaps produced by previous trauma, in contrast, presented irregular edges and mixed echogenicity, which is often seen with scarred tissue. Trauma-related gaps were usually associated with defects in the internal anal sphincter as well.

The median transverse width of these natural anterior gaps was 2 cm. The longer the anal canal, the wider the gap tended to be. The longitudinal extent (up and down the sphincter) of the natural gaps varied between 0.75 to 1.5 cm. Gaps that were wider in their transverse dimension tended to also be taller in their longitudinal dimension (gaps that exceeded 90° transversely had a mean height of 1.33 cm; those that were smaller than 90° transversely had a mean height of 1.16 cm). The size of the anterior gap was associated with the degree of squeeze pressure that women can produce, with larger gaps, not surprisingly, being associated with weaker squeeze pressure.

The confirmation of natural gaps in the deep external sphincters of fully continent nulliparous women suggests that the apparent finding of widespread "occult" sphincter damage among parous women (Sentovich et al., 1997) needs to be reevaluated (Bollard et al., 2002).

The lack of anterior midline fibers helps the deep external sphincter withstand the pressures and stretching that accompany yoni distention during pushing that result in anal dilation. Since it seems the majority of women have a natural anterior gap, their deep external sphincter would not be damaged from a deep midline tear that extends past the perineal body. However, more lateral tears or cuts, if extensive enough, may damage the deep external sphincter or its wings as well as the puborectalis muscle (Fritsch et al., 2002).

The winged part of the external sphincter is primarily an involuntary muscle that works with the puborectalis to help achieve continence of feces and flatus by pulling the anal canal forward, which compresses it and helps maintain the anorectal angle. The puborectalis and winged external sphincter must relax in order for feces to be evacuated. The integration of smooth and striated fibers within the muscle enables the winged external sphincter to function even though these natural gaps exist (Fritsch et al., 2002).

Main external sphincter: Next, Hsu and associates (2005) identified a part they call the "main body of the external anal sphincter." It is composed of obliquely oriented fibers that fully encircle the anal canal. In the posterior midline, a tail of fibers passes straight back toward the coccyx, where they decussate as they blend into the anococcygeal ligament. The most posterior part of this tail consists of a tough, triangular extension that is attached to the underside of the last segment of the coccyx.

The concentricity of the main part suggests a constrictive function in closing the anal canal. Although there is no visible separation of the winged part from the main part on MRI scans, the differing directions of their fibers denote differing origins and insertions.

Subcutaneous external sphincter: Finally, Hsu and associates (2005) identified the subcutaneous external sphincter as the most shallow layer of the muscle, lying under a thin layer of skin, parallel with the surface of the perineal body. Thanks to the minimal tissue distortion produced on MRI studies, they could see that the main external sphincter forms a shorter outer cuff that surrounds the subcutaneous external sphincter, which forms an inner cuff. The subcutaneous cuff projects slightly beyond the lower border of the main cuff. These two parts are separated slightly by a space filled with loose connective tissue that they named the **external sphincter space**. The posterior midline fibers of the subcutaneous part pass backward, where they decussate as they enter the anococcygeal ligament.

The fibers of the subcutaneous part become increasingly fibroelastic as they approach its lower border. It is generally accepted that fibers from the conjoined longitudinal coat split this muscle into 9 to 12 little teardrop-shaped sections (similar in appearance to the pith that separates the smallest segments within an orange wedge) that radiate out and then attach to the dermis of the perianal skin, an arrangement that separates the subcutaneous part from the rest of the external sphincter (Lunniss & Phillips, 1992).

Shafik and colleagues (2007a) studied the relationship between the external anal sphincter and the bulbocavernosus muscle. They report that the more superficial "looped" fibers of the subcutaneous part of the sphincter pass uninterrupted, straight up though the perineal body. At the level of the fourchette, these fibers split into two groups that then proceed superolaterally. At the level of the clitoral bulbs, each group of sphincter fibers blends with those of the ipsilateral bulbocavernosus muscle as they continue upward toward the clitoral body. Simultaneous contraction of the external sphincter and the bulbocavernosus muscle may compress the clitoral bulbs, sending blood to the clitoral body; thus, the external sphincter appears to contribute to venous engorgement of the clitoral body and glans.

Although figure-eight interweaving of the fibers of the external anal sphincter and the bulbocavernosus muscle in the center of the perineal body is widely described and illustrated, dissections done by Shafik and associates (2007a) found external anal sphincter fibers decussating in the perineal body in only three female specimens out of 20. This means that a midline superficial tear will usually run parallel with the fibers as it divides them, increasing the likelihood of optimal healing. When interweaving was found, it consisted of only a few superficial fibers crisscrossing the perineal body; the right-sided fibers passed to the left and the left-sided fibers to the right. Interweaving may enhance the constrictive action of the external anal sphincter upon the clitoral bulbs.

Fritsch and colleagues (2002) proposed that the subcutaneous external sphincter regulates internal closure (controlled by mucous and submucous layers) as well as external closure of the anus to maintain bowel continence.

Fascial coverings of the external sphincter parts: Finding specific information about the fascia that overlies the sphincter muscles is difficult, but it appears to be typical parietal fascia that forms a tight membrane over each muscle part (Bannister, 1999). However, Oh and Kark (1972) described fibers that grossly encapsulate the "bundled" (main) part of the external sphincter that consist of a mixture of fibers from the conjoined longitudinal muscle and from the internal sphincter. The fascia surrounding the external sphincter is often referred to as the "capsule of the sphincter."

External anal sphincter function: The external anal sphincter consists of striated muscle fibers that are primarily innervated by somatic fibers from the inferior rectal fibers of the pudendal nerve. This multilayered muscle provides the anal canal's squeeze pressure, preventing the loss of bowel contents under pressure. Squeeze pressure occurs involuntarily or as a result of increased intra-abdominal pressure. The external sphincter may also contribute as much as 25% of the anal resting tone as it is in a constant state of contraction when at rest and must relax to allow the passage of stool (Schorge et al., 2008).

Multiparous external anal sphincters: In an effort to find out how the parts of the external sphincters are affected by previous childbirth, Frudinger and colleagues (1999) studied nulliparous and parous women. In parous women, the main and subcutaneous parts of the external sphincter tend to descend. The main portion becomes more horizontal and is partially overlapped by the flattened subcutaneous part. The problem with this and similar studies is that it employed an endoscope, which involves inserting a probe into the anal canal. The probe distorts the tissues and these findings may not reflect normal tissue relationships (Hsu et al., 2005).

Anococcygeal ligament of the anal sphincters

The posterior fibromuscular extensions from the main and subcutaneous parts of the external anal sphincters extend from the posterior sides of the sphincters and attach to the very tip of the coccyx. They contribute the two most superficial layers of the anococcygeal ligament. Contraction of the normally toned levator ani muscles draws the anococcygeal ligament upward; bearing down causes it to descend.

Deep postanal space (retrosphincteric space [of Courtney])

This is the space between the fibers contributed to the anococcygeal ligament from the levator plate or puborectalis muscle above and by the anal sphincters below. It is filled with fibrous, fatty tissue (Courtney, 1949). There is a similar anterior or preanal space in men, but such a space is uncommon in women (Garavoglia et al., 1993).

Structures and landmarks within the anal lumen and canal wall

The following brief descriptions of structures that form parts of the lining of the anal lumen are taken from contemporary anatomical descriptions. Although terminology does overlap somewhat, the description of these structures is fairly consistent from source to source. From my research they appear to be more or less accurate (but, as we have seen, future research may reveal very different findings). These structures are listed from deep to superficial and are illustrated in a full-page drawing at the end of the chapter.

Anorectal line: The anorectal line runs along the tops of the anal columns, 4 to 5 cm above the anal orifice. It marks the transition zone between the rectal wall and the anal canal. This is also the location of the 90° bend in the anorectal canal that occurs at the level of the puborectalis muscle. The anorectal line marks the upper limit of the "surgical" anal canal (here "surgical" refers to the area that can be examined digitally and with sonography).

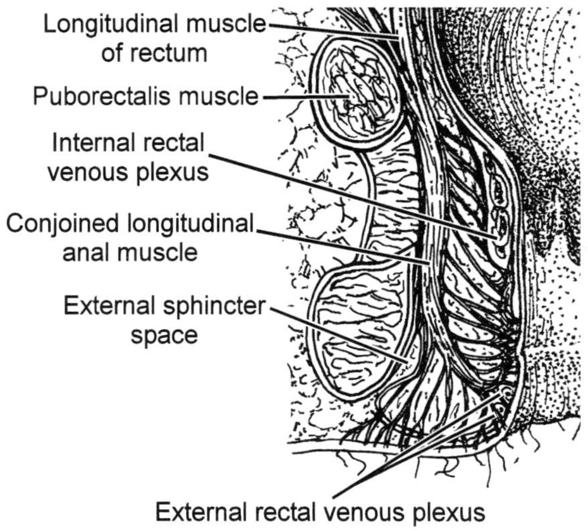

Dissected coronal section: detail of right side (see note on page 106)

Anal or rectal columns (columns of Morgagni): Below the level of the anorectal line, the diameter of the anorectal canal is sharply reduced. Narrowing of the passage creates six to 10 ridges that present as 1.5 to 2 cm tall vertical columns in the mucous membrane lining the upper half of the lumen of the anal canal. These columns change size; puffing up with blood when the anal canal is in a state of resting tone and flattening against the lumen as the canal fills with stool. Histologically, these columns consist of a somewhat denser muscularis mucosa, with a more elaborate lymphatic, vascular, and nerve supply than is found underlying the grooves that lie between them. Each column contains a terminal system of tiny vein radicles (roots) from the superior rectal artery and vein. This rich vascular supply renders the columns plum colored.

Three of these columns are larger than the others and are consistently located in the left-lateral, right-posterior and right-anterior regions of the canal lumen. These three columns are sometimes called the **anal cushions**.

Each anal cushion contains submucosal vascular plexuses formed by the anastomoses (connections) between the rectal veins within the anal columns. Similar vascular plexuses are located at two levels along the length of each of these three columns. The internal plexuses are located just above the **dentate line**, which is discussed below. **Internal hemorrhoids** are formed when these vascular cushions become enlarged. If quite enlarged, the distended internal plexus may prolapse outside the anal opening. The external vascular plexuses are located just inside the margin of the anal orifice. Distention of these plexuses results in **external hemorrhoids**, which may prolapse outside the anal orifice. A **mixed hemorrhoid** is present when there are enlarged vessels in both the internal and external plexuses (Fry & Kodner, 1985).

Anal sinuses (sinuses of Morgagni/sinus anales): The vertical depressions or grooves in the rectal wall that lie between the anal columns are sometimes called "sinuses." The anal crypts are located at the lower end of each of these grooves.

Anal valves (valvulae anales): The anal valves are crescent-shaped folds of mucous membrane that bridge the lower end of adjacent anal columns and form the free outer wall of the anal sinuses. Histologically, the valves have a thickened or cornified epidermis, which becomes continuous with the rectal columnar epithelium projected distally between the anal columns into the blind end of the sinuses. Tearing of these valves by hard stools leads to anal fissures, a painful injury that is difficult to heal.

Anal crypts or pockets (Morgagni crypts/saccules of Harner): Sometimes called "anal or rectal sinuses," the anal crypts are the tiny pockets formed by the folds of the anal valves. They vary in number, depth and shape. There are typically several larger crypts along the posterior wall of the anal lumen that may retain fecal matter and become infected. The closed lower ends of the crypts extend into the dentate line, and the superior ends open in the direction of the rectum (Gorsch, 1960).

Pectinate or dentate line (pectin): The scalloped pectinate line lies 2.5 to 3 cm above the anal verge. The **pectin** is a 1 to 1.5 cm **transition zone** where the simple columnar epithelium (the endoderm) of the rectal lumen gradually changes to the stratified epithelium of the anal canal (the ectoderm) that marks the anocutaneous junction, below which lies the anatomical anal canal. The pectinate line follows along the anal valves at the bases of the anal sinuses and overlies part of the rectal venous plexus, rendering it shiny and bluish. The region between the pectinate line and the anal verge is referred to as the **anoderm**. When the wall of the anorectal canal is severed, it is usually does not extend higher than the anoderm, although such a tear is commonly referred to as a simply a "rectal mucosa" tear.

The transition zone ends about 0.5 to 1 cm above the anal verge at the level of the **anocutaneous line** or **junction** (classically referred to as the "white line of Hilton"). In the living, this line is barely visible and appears bluish-pink. A digital exam finds an **intersphincteric groove** at this level, marking the lower border of the internal sphincter. Below the intersphincteric groove, the anal canal is lined with true skin that ranges in color from dull white to brown and contains sweat and sebaceous glands. These lines of demarcation vary greatly among individuals; they frequently overlap and are often poorly defined.

Anal glands: The terminology for and the descriptions of different types of glands in the human anal region have been a matter of much debate and considerable confusion in large part because there is a great deal of individual variation in number, form and size of these glands. Although vestigial in humans, these glands are clinically significant as pathologic sites.

Eglitis and Eglitis (1961) are among the few who have attempted to describe these glands in detail. They reported four different types of glands in the anal region

(1) Holocrine-secreting sebaceous glands (Holocrine glands release secretions consisting of disintegrated cells from the gland itself.)
(2) Eccrine-secreting merocrine sweat glands (Merocrine glands release an acellular secretory product. Eccrine refers to the flow of sweat from glands unconnected to hair follicles).
(3) Apocrine-secreting merocrine scent glands (Apocrine denotes that process of glandular secretion in which the apical portion of secretory cells is shed and

incorporated into the secretion.)

(4) Specialized eccrine sudoriferous (sweat) glands in the region of the anal columns; these are often referred to specifically as "anal glands."

Van der Putte (1994) described a fifth type, the mammary-like glands (see page 25) (Scurry & Melville, 2007; STEDMANS, 2007).

Sebaceous glands (No. 1 above) are found in the skin around the anal orifice and internally in the area below the dentate line. Three kinds of sebaceous glands have been found in the pectin: some with well-developed hairs, some with rudimentary hairs and some lacking hairs.

Common sweat glands (2) are found only in the skin around the anal orifice. Apocrine scent glands (3) are located all around the anus and in the region below the anocutaneous line inside the canal. These glands resemble those of the axillary region, but the ones below the anocutaneous line are modified: some are simple tubules whose secretory portions are not coiled, in others the secretory portions consist of ampulla-like sacs.

In the connective tissue zone between the sphincter ani muscles and the epithelial lining of the anal lumen are located what are commonly referred to as "anal glands" (4). These glands arise from the crypts of the rectal sinuses at the foot of the anal columns. Each consists of one to six spiral or straight tubules that may be branched and are lined with two or three layers of mucus secretory cells with ducts that open into the anal crypts. Some tubules branch up and down into the submucosa; others penetrate the internal sphincter muscle or even reach the ischiorectal fossa. These glands may be more numerous along the posterior lumen of the canal. The intramuscular portions of these glands appear to be eccrine types and are usually distended in pear-shaped sacs. According to Klosterhalfen and colleagues (1991), in fetuses, neonates and children, more than half of the anal sinuses are accompanied by intramuscular glands that penetrate the internal anal sphincter, whereas in adult specimens anal intramuscular glands are rare.

In contrast, Seow-Choen and Ho (1994) found that the median number of these secretory anal glands in adults to be 6 six (the range is 3 to 10). Eighty percent of the anal glands are submucosal, 8% extend to the circular internal sphincter, 8% reach to the longitudinal internal sphincter, 2% reach the intersphincteric space, and only 1% penetrate the external anal sphincter. Ampulla-like dilation of the anal glands occurs about two-thirds of the time, either at the submucosal level or the circular internal sphincter level. Lymphocytic infiltrations have been noted around the glands. Mucus-secreting cells are usually present, and many of these glands produce intraluminal secretions. One to two cell layers of smooth muscle fibers surround these types of anal glands (Seow-Choen & Ho, 1994). Occasionally these glands do not have an opening and a cyst may form. Infection of an anal gland may produce an abscess or a fistula (Bannister, 1999).

Anal verge: The anal verge is the skin immediately surrounding the anal opening where the moist, hairless, modified skin of the anal canal changes to the perianal skin that surrounds the anal orifice.

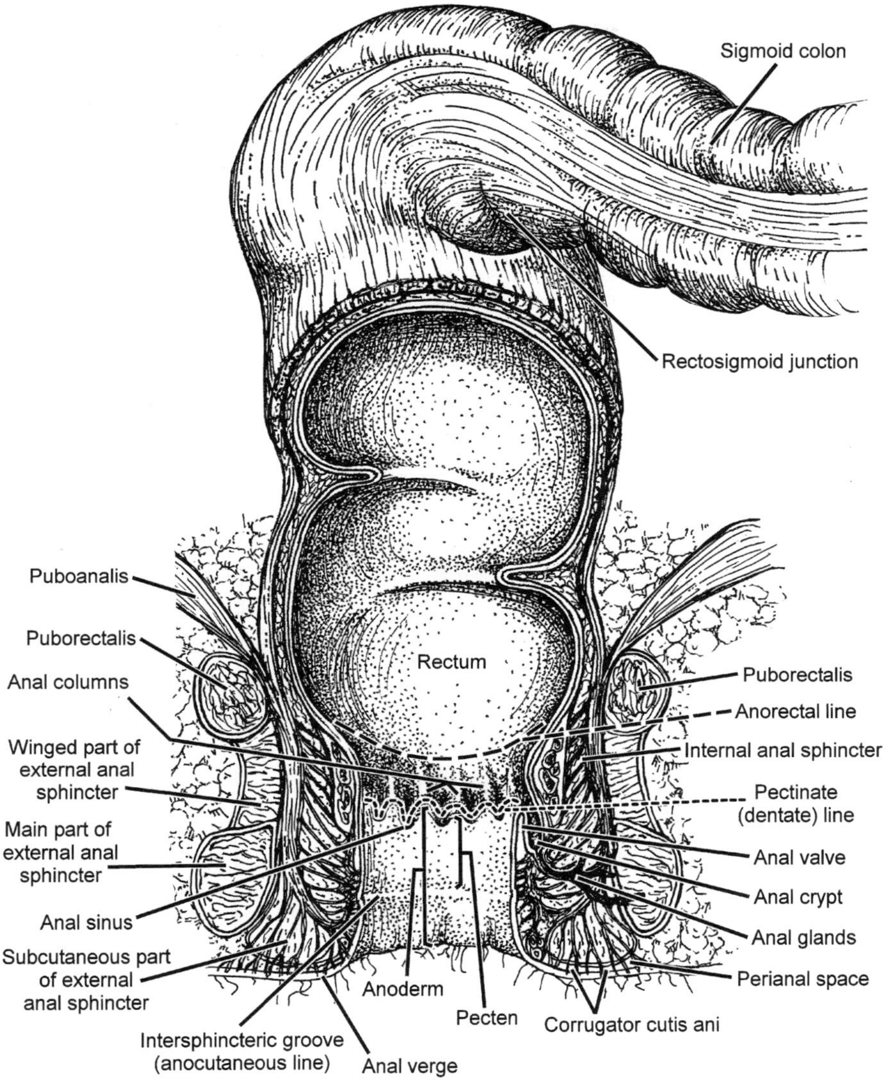

Detailed coronal section of the anorectal canal and sphincters from dissection
(see note on page 106)

Corrugator cutis ani: The corrugator cutis ani is the distinctive, purse-string puckering around the perimeter of the anal opening that extends into the upper part of the anal canal as the anal columns (Ellis & Dussek, 1999). The nature and even the existence of an underlying muscle to create this effect is a matter of much debate (Lunnis & Phillips, 1992). Depending upon the source, either elastic (Wilde, 1949) or smooth muscle (Goligher et al., 1955) fibers are said to radiate from the lowermost edge of the longitudinal anal muscle and pass through the subcutaneous sphincter to the perianal dermis. They then attach to the perianal dermis and radiate outward around the perimeter of the orifice. This arrangement of fibers is thought to produce the corrugated appearance. The puckering is believed to contribute to the watertight seal of the anal canal. Fowler (1957) found no such muscle fibers and ascribed the puckering to the combined effects of the levator ani and the subcutaneous part of the external sphincter on the skin around the anal orifice, although it is generally accepted that some sort of muscle fibers exist to create this effect.

Perianal or circumanal region: The perimeter adjacent to the external anal orifice.

Age-related changes in the anal muscles

As healthy women who are completely rectally continent age, the thickness of the longitudinal muscle decreases and the internal sphincter becomes hypertrophied to compensate. The thickness of the external sphincters, the puborectalis muscle and the levator ani muscles also decrease with age, but not significantly (Rociu et al., 2000).

Anorectal sensation and function

The function of the anorectum and the process of defecation and anal continence are not well understood. The rectum and anal canal are innervated by branches from the superior, middle and inferior rectal autonomic nerve plexuses, which contain both sympathetic and parasympathetic fibers, and by intrinsic nerves that are found in the rectoanal canal. The lower anal canal and the anal skin receive sensory input from the inferior rectal branch of the pudendal nerve. These receptors can detect rectal contents and distension.

The **rectoanal inhibitory reflex** produces transient relaxation of the internal anal sphincter and contraction of the external sphincter in response to rectal distension as stool first enters the rectum. This reflex, in turn, prompts the **sampling reflex**, whereby the internal anal sphincter relaxes, with or without distension, allowing some of the rectal contents to contact the anal wall so it can distinguish if the material is solid, liquid or gas. As this information is processed, the woman can decide when and where to evacuate her bowel. If rectal sensation is impaired, contents may pass into the anal canal and leak before the external sphincter can contract.

Normally, if evacuation is not convenient, **accommodation** occurs as the rectal wall expands to hold its contents. As rectal volume increases, an urge to defecate is perceived. If the puborectalis and external sphincter are voluntarily contracted to prevent defecation, the rectum continues to relax to hold the stool in a process known as **compliance**. Impairment of these processes interferes with the ability of the rectal wall to respond appropriately. This can lead to high rectal pressures that increase demand on the sphincters (Schorge et al., 2008).

Notes on the anorectal illustrations: The coronal sections included in this chapter that appear on pages 102 and 105 were originally based on a cadaver specimen of unspecified sex, but likely male. They show the anatomy of the anal canal adapted from Netter (2003). They are included to give you a specific idea regarding the more detailed internal and topical anatomy. The depiction of the structures of the bowel lumen are correct for both sexes. Unfortunately, no similar drawing is available that reflects the new understanding of the female external anal sphincter complex in living subjects as discussed in this chapter (you will recall that MRI studies are finding structures and relationships that are obliterated upon death). Given the lack of reference illustrations based on this new understanding, it was impossible to be sure how to alter these drawings, so the relationship between the main and superficial parts of the anal sphincter is our best guess based on available descriptions and images.

As these are coronal sections, they show the winged portion of the external sphincter on either side; the winged nature of this part is not obvious from a coronal section.

Primary Innervation of the Levator Ani Complex and the Perineal Muscles

The pudendal nerve has been widely regarded as contributing to the innervation of the levator ani muscles in women, and many texts still describe the innervation this way. At this point, it should come as no great shock that this has not been confirmed in careful dissections. That an accessory rectal branch of the pudendal nerve does supply the levator ani in men (Shafik & Doss, 1999) has clouded the understanding of the true female anatomy.

Levator Ani Nerve

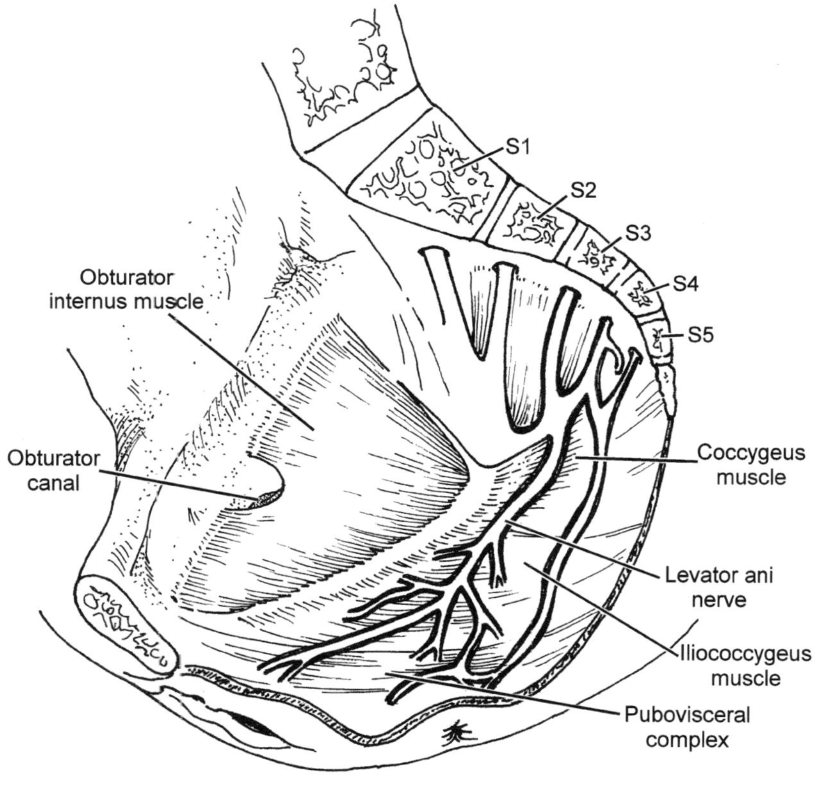

Course of the levator ani nerve (from dissection)

In women, the levator ani muscles appear to be innervated solely by the levator ani nerve (LAN), which originates variously from S3, S4 or S5 (sometimes from more than one foramen but never all three) and crosses the superior surface of the coccygeal muscle 1.2 to 4.2 cm medial to the ischial spine. The coccygeal muscle is innervated by small nerve branches, on the superior surface of the muscle, that originate from S3 and from either S4 or S5, or from both. The LAN then travels along the superior surface of the levator ani muscles before sending off one or more branches that penetrate the iliococcygeus muscle at a point halfway between the pubic bone and the ischial spine 2 to 3 cm below the tendinous arch of the levator ani. The nerve then continues to enter the puboanalis and the puborectalis muscles at a point halfway between the inferior pubis and the coccyx (Barber et al., 2002). In some specimens, a small independent branch from S4 or S5 innervates the midportion of the puborectalis muscle. In all, the levator ani nerve gives off 1 to 5 major branches. The nerve is sometimes firmly enmeshed in the levator ani fasciae and in other cases is only loosely applied to the fasciae and more firmly attached to the medial organs.

The levator ani nerve appears to be the primary nerve supplying this muscle group in females. The levator ani and pudendal nerves lie above and below the levator ani muscle respectively. They are both very near the ischial spine, at a distance of approximately 6 mm from each other. This means that anesthetic blockage of the pudendal nerve would likely also affect the activity of the levator ani nerve, which has helped foster the notion that both nerves supply these muscles in females (Wallner et al., 2006).

Pudendal Nerve

The pudendal nerve originated from a group of nerve roots that exit from S2, S3 and S4 (with S3 providing the largest of these). Looking into the pelvis from the front, it traveled over the anterior (ventral) surface of the piriformis muscle and behind (posterior to) the sacrospinous ligament (which is encased within the coccygeus muscle) just medial to the ischial spine. From here, it entered the gluteal region inferior to the piriformis muscle and just medial to the origin of the superior gemellus muscle. Along its course, the nerve divided into upper and lower trunks. The upper trunk passed just medial to the ischial spine, and the lower trunk crossed 1 to 2 cm medial to the ischial spine. Both trunks then divide further either just before or upon entering the pudendal (Alcock) canal (which is 2.8 to 3.6 cm in length), located in the fascia overlying the inner surface of the obturator internus muscle that lines the inner pelvis near the ischium. (The triangularly shaped piriformis muscle originates along the anterior margins of S1, S2, S3 and S4 and greater sciatic notch of the ilium on either side, passes through the gluteal region and inserts onto the upper border of the greater trochanter. The superior gemellus muscle originates at the ischial tuberosity and inserts on the greater trochanter. Both muscles help to rotate the thigh outward [STEDMANS, 2007].)

Although Barber and colleagues (2002) did not completely rule out the possibility that small branches from the pudendal nerve may exist that provide some minor innervation to the levator ani complex in women, in spite of diligent searching, they could find no such branches in their specimens, even though branches of the pudendal artery and vein were found to enter the levator ani muscles.

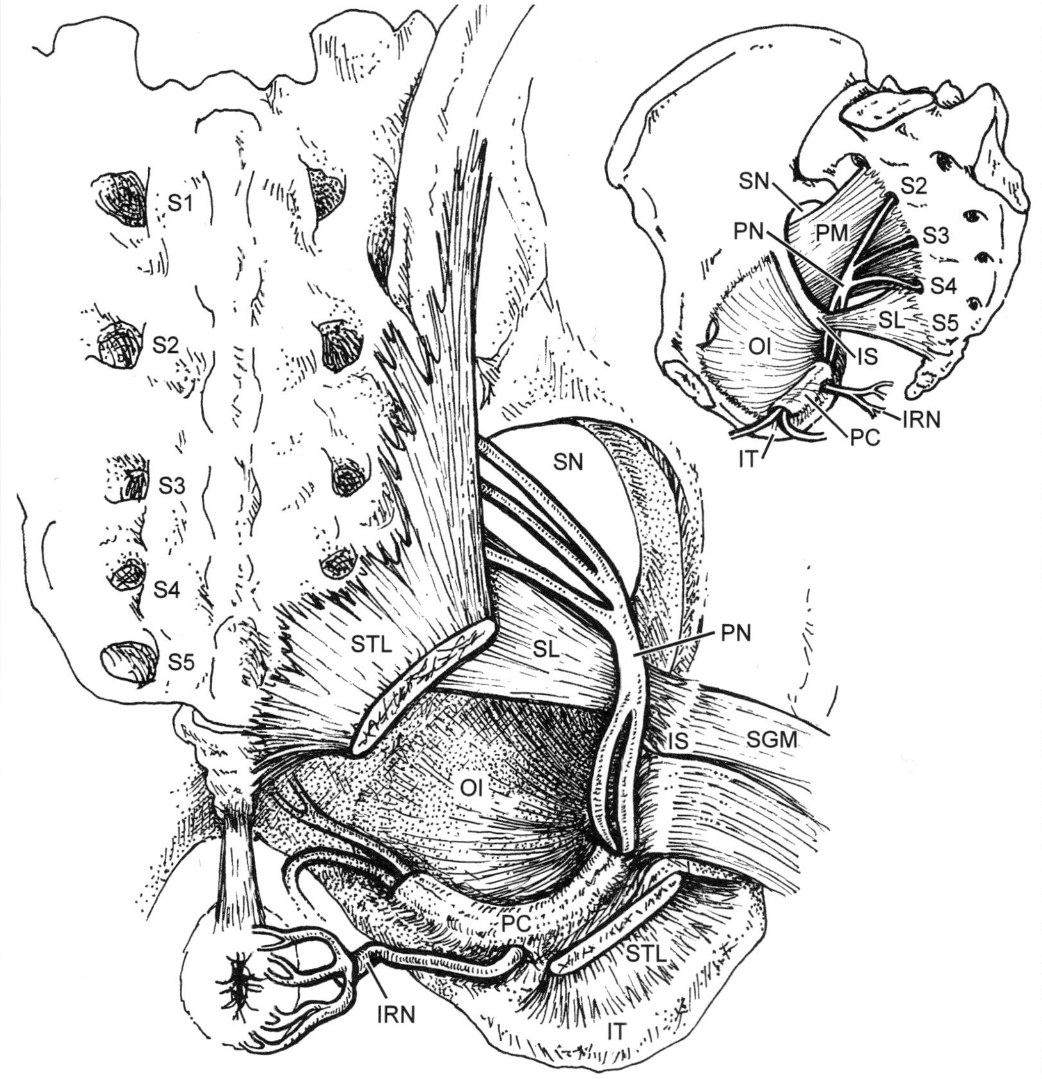

Course of the pudendal nerve on a woman's right side
(left: posterior view [piriformis muscle not shown]; upper right: anterolateral view)

Key: IRN=inferior rectal nerve; IS=ischial spine; IT=ischial tuberosity; OI=obturator internus muscle; PC=pudendal (Alcock) canal; PM=piriformis muscle; PN=pudendal nerve; S1 etc.=sacral foramina; SGM=superior gemellus muscle; SL=sacrospinous ligament (coccygeus muscle); SN=greater sciatic notch; STL=sacrotuberous ligament (cut)

Perineal innervation

Barber and associates (2002) found that, in most specimens (78%), within or just before entering the pudendal canal the upper and lower pudendal branches further divided into smaller ones. Within the canal, the lower pudendal trunk branched to form the inferior rectal nerve, which penetrated through the medial wall of the pudendal canal at its midpoint, then crossed the ischiorectal fossa in an inferomedial direction and divided into several small branches that supplied the external anal sphincter and perianal skin. Less often (22%), the inferior rectal nerve branched from the lower pudendal trunk and crossed the ischiorectal fossa, never entering the pudendal canal. In all dissections, the lower trunk of the pudendal nerve supplied at least one additional branch that exited the pudendal canal and passed forward to provide cutaneous innervation to the area lateral to that supplied by the inferior rectal nerve.

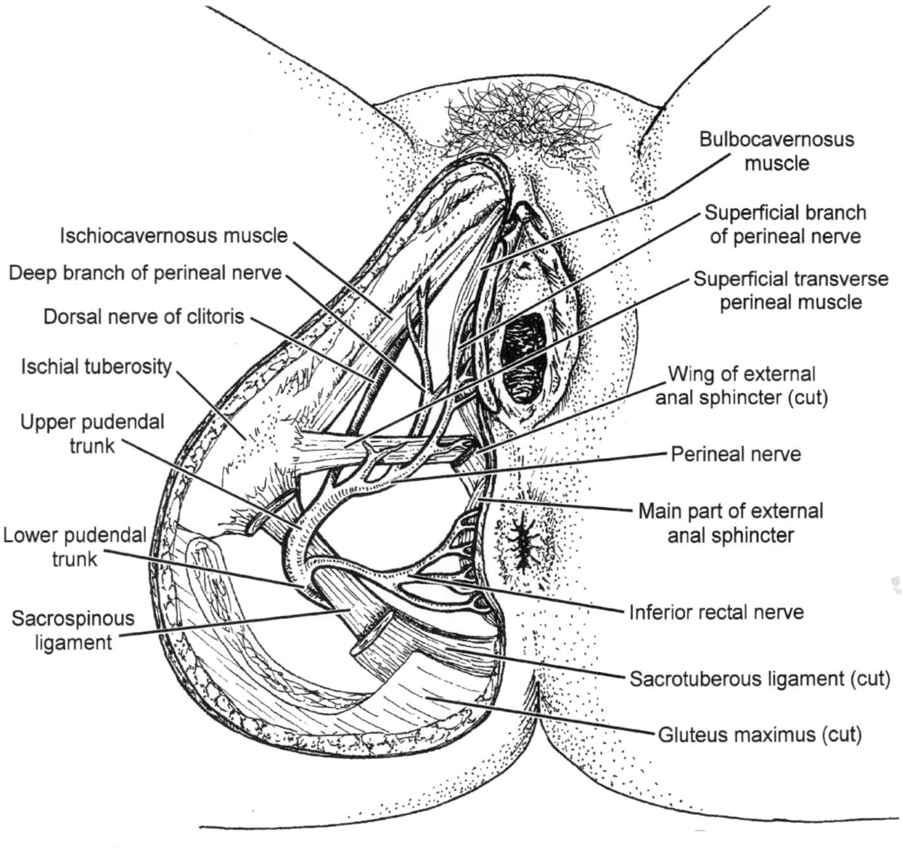

Perineal branches of the pudendal nerve (many other nerves are left out)

As it left the pudendal canal, the upper trunk extended a branch along the margin of the inferior pubic ramus. This branch became the dorsal nerve of the clitoris, which was the deepest of all the pudendal nerves branches, directly overlying the perineal membrane complex and beneath the perineal muscles. The remaining branch, the perineal nerve, arose from either the upper trunk (22%), the lower trunk (11%) or both (66%). After exiting the pudendal canal, it sent two or three major branches to supply the ischiocavernosus muscles, the bulbocavernosus muscles, the superficial transverse perineal muscles, the striated urethral sphincter and the labial skin. These nerves were more superficial than the dorsal nerve of the clitoris and, in most cases, ran along the superior surfaces of the perineal muscles they supply. The nerve to the striated urethral sphincter passed superomedially on the surface of the bulbocavernosus muscle and then penetrated deeply to supply the sides of the urethral sphincter.

Birth-related injuries

Damage to the pudendal or levator ani nerves from either injury sustained during chronic or acute stretching or as a result of neurologic disease can weaken the muscles that they supply, although such injury usually accompanies mechanical damage (O'Dell & Morse, 2008).

More about the Pelvic Connective Tissues

This chapter gives some more information on the pelvic connective tissues, but is, by no means, a complete description for several reasons. Due to difficulty in getting clear MRI scans and difficulty in reading them for the untrained eye, these tissues are, if anything, even harder to visualize in their live state than are the muscles. As with the levator ani muscles, definitions of structures and the terminology assigned to them vary among researchers, making the comparison of different articles extremely difficult. In all my research, I found no really excellent illustrations of this anatomy. Finally, midwives do not need the in-depth understanding of these tissues that urogynecological surgeons require.

Those midwives who are interested in more details on this anatomy should do a Medline search for the most current research and should refer to the articles listed in the bibliography of this part of the book, particularly Ercoli et al., 2005; Otcenasek et al., 2008; Pit et al., 2003 and Yabuki et al., 2005.

The role of the connective tissues in pelvic organ support

According to the research of Fritsch and colleagues (2004), Liu (2008) and others, many surgeons have attributed too much functional significance to the pelvic connective tissues. Although some of these tissues do attach to the levator ani complex and contraction of these muscles does affect these connections and thus the organs, these connective tissues are not formed in such a way that they can function as active supports; it is the pelvic floor muscles that provide virtually all the sustained support that the pelvic organs receive. DeLancey (1993) found that, when the levator ani muscles are normal and undamaged, they hold the pelvic floor closed, compressing the yoni and urethra against the pubic bone and supporting the organs in place, resulting in tension-free ligaments and connective tissues.

Debate continues over whether excessive stretching (attenuation) or actual breaks in the support system are what lead to pelvic organ support failure. For many decades, it has been thought that extremely stretched connective tissues alone could result in pelvic support failure. The contemporary concept held by many, however, is that the adventitiae stretch somewhat and finally break, and that the breaks are what result in clinically important defects (Rogers & Richardson, 2003).

DeLancey (1993) explained that the endopelvic adventitiae are not designed to provide support under tension. These relatively loose tissues are poorly suited to withstand the constant load from gravity and intra-abdominal pressure that is placed on the pelvic floor. Thus, the ligaments, fasciae and adventitiae that are attached to the uterus, the walls of the yoni, and the outside of the cervix stabilize, but are not normally called upon to completely suspend, these organs. These stabilizing tissues are relatively lax, like tethers attached to a boat that is docked. If the water level (the pelvic floor) drops, the tethers will be called upon to suspend the boat over the water by themselves, resulting in tension, stretching and eventual breakage. Depending upon the intrinsic strength of the woman's connective tissues, the organs will be held in place for a period of time but are likely to eventually descend as the connective tissues stretch and prolonged tension causes them to tear. Women with unusually weak connective tissue may experience organ prolapse even though the pelvic floor muscles are normal. In most cases, however, the strength and integrity of the muscles of the pelvic floor are of primary importance in maintaining the normal positioning of the pelvic organs.

Parietal fascia

As reviewed previously (page 37), sheets of well-defined parietal fascia enclose each muscle. The parietal fascia found in the pelvis is continuous with the fascial sheaths covering the transverse abdominal and iliopsoas muscles and blends with the periosteum covering of the bones. (The iliopsoas is a compound muscle consisting of the iliacus musculus and psoas major musculus that insert via a common tendon into the anterior surface of the lesser trochanter of the femur.) The presacral fascia overlying the sacrum also anchors structures of the pelvic floor and endopelvic adventitiae.

Specific regions of parietal fascia are named for the muscles they cover. As far as midwives are concerned, the most clinically important of these is the layer that clothes the levator ani muscles, which is attached to the pelvic brim. The superior fascia of the levator ani complex is continuous as it wraps around the free edges of the muscles to cover the underside, forming the bottom, or inferior, layer of the levator ani fascia (Moore & Dalley, 2006).

Tendinous arches of fascia

Connective tissues condense to form three sets of ridges or tendinous arches of fascia that are discussed later in this chapter. One of these is the line of origination for the levator ani muscles (see page 79). The other two sets are cord-like condensations of tissues that run along the upper and lower outer "corners" of the yoni that serve as attachment sites for the visceral adventitiae.

Endopelvic adventitia

The endopelvic adventitia mostly consists of loosely arranged **areolar tissue**, made up of fibroblast cells and an extracellular matrix composed of collagenous and elastic fibers, in which glycosaminoglycans and proteoglycans form a hydrated gel-like material. The predominant glycosaminoglycan is **hyaluronic acid (HA)**, a viscous polymer that organizes the structure of the connective tissue (Laurent & Fraser, 1992). This loose connective tissue is the most widely distributed in the body, serving as a packing material between other tissues and organs. In the pelvis it forms a continuous, three-dimensional web that fills the space between the pelvic organs, connecting them to the other pelvic fascia and to the peritoneum lining the abdominopelvic cavity. It serves as scaffolding between the organs and the pelvic walls, sacrum, and midline connective tissues of the pelvic outlet. The muscles of the pelvic floor and these connective tissue supports work together to facilitate the positioning, stability, expansion and movement of the pelvic organs. The uterus and the yoni are surrounded by membranous adventitial connective tissue only, without any other connective tissue coverings (Bergls & Rubin, 1953; Fritsch et al., 2004; Koster, 1933; Uhlenhuth & Nolley, 1957).

The remaining connective tissue that lies between the parietal and visceral membranous layers is also part of the endopelvic adventitia, although many authors label parts of it as parietal fascia. This extraperitoneal or subperitoneal endopelvic adventitia is continuous with the adjacent parietal and visceral connective tissues and contributes to the web of connective tissues that surround the pelvic organs. Much of it is soft and fat-filled, allowing for expansion of the bladder, yoni and rectum (Moore & Dalley, 2006).

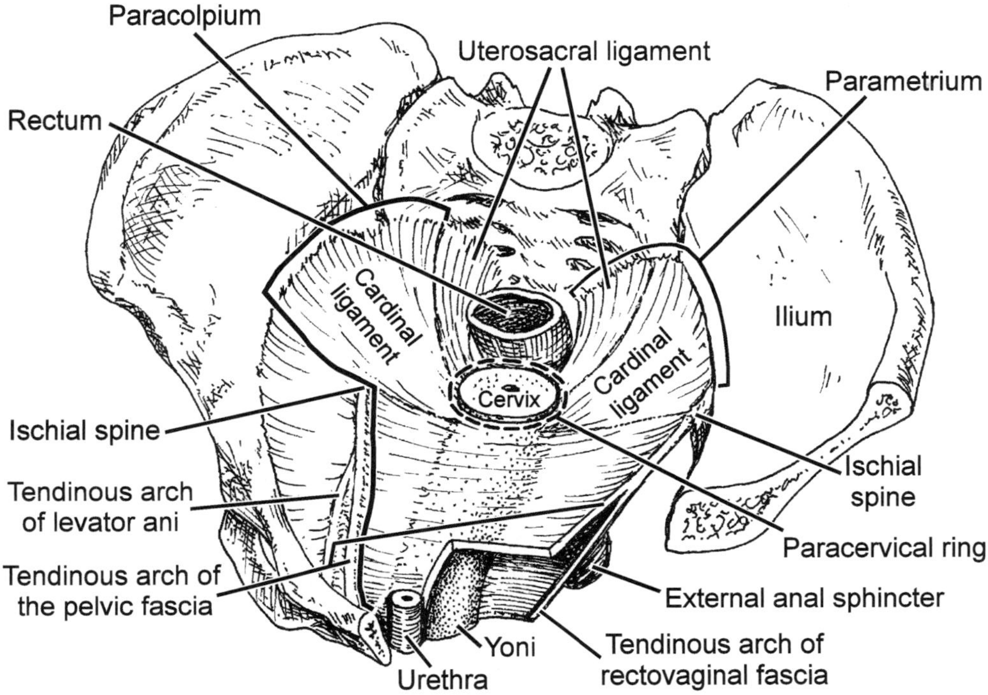

Simplified view of the connective tissues of the pelvic cavity in a cadaver (tissues are slack)

Within this matrix of tissue, the yoni, cervix and urethra are held in place by a variety of attachments. The endopelvic adventitia drapes over the uterus and yoni and attaches the cervix and yoni to the pelvic wall, forming a continuous, loosely woven, sheet-like mesentery extending from the uterine artery at its upper margin to the point where the yoni fuses with the puboanalis muscle below. All parts of this mesentery that attach to the uterus are called the **parametrium** and include both the cardinal and uterosacral ligaments (the dorsal [or posterior] parts of the parametrium are sometimes referred to as **rectal pillars**). The part of this mesentery that attaches to the yoni is called the **paracolpium (para-CAUL-pee-um)** and also includes the cardinal ligament. The endopelvic adventitia attaches to a variety of surrounding structures including the pubic bone, the perineal body and the ischial spines.

Levels of yoni support

DeLancey (2002b) defined three levels or regions of connective tissue support for the yoni and attached structures that have been widely adopted by urogynecologists.

Level I suspends the upper or proximal yoni. **Level II** attaches the upper "corner" of the midyoni walls to the arcus tendineus fasciae pelvis. **Level III** is a product of the fusion of the lower third of the yoni to adjacent structures. Defects at each of these levels result in various types of prolapses of attached structures. Depending upon the structure involved and the degree of defect, identifiable changes can be detected in either the proximal region of the yoni (in the vicinity of the fornices), at various levels along either the anterior or posterior yoni walls, or at a combination of sites if multiple or severe defects exist. Normal anatomy and the types of defects that can occur at each level are described in more detail below. How to examine for them is covered in the chapter entitled "Assessing Pelvic Organ Prolapse."

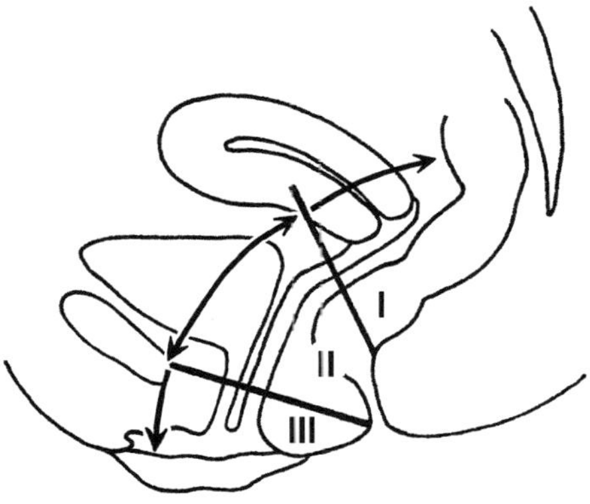

DeLancey's 3 levels of pelvic support

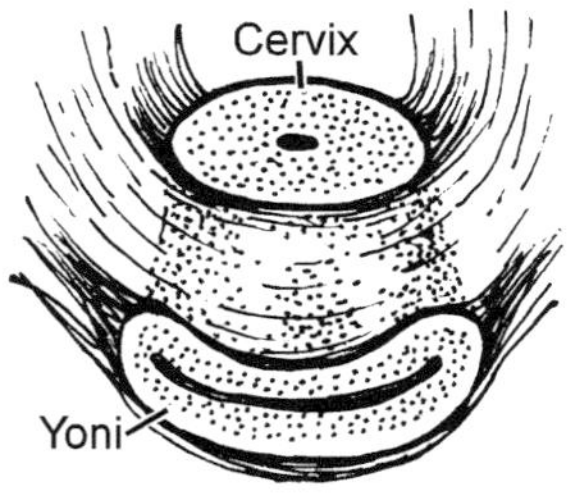

Shape of yoni canal at Level I

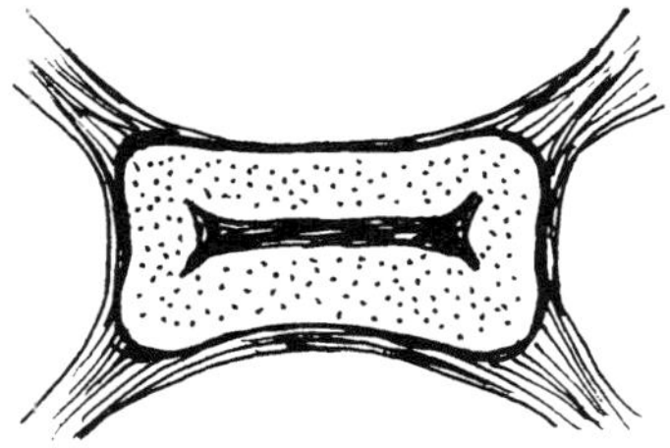

Shape of yoni canal at Level II

(The shape of the yoni at Level III is visible on examination of the introitus.)

Level I, the deepest layer, consists of the cardinal and uterosacral ligaments, which are two parts of the same connective tissue complex. The two ligaments coalesce into two long sheets of tissue that form the parametrium. The cardinal ligaments consist of a superior layer that forms a broad, webbed, fan-shaped sheath that attaches to the parietal fasciae of the obturator internus and piriformis muscles and then runs along the anterior border of the greater sciatic foramen to the ischial spines on either side. Layers of the cardinal ligaments envelope the internal iliac artery and vein. These layers fuse to form a vertically oriented sheath that follows the uterine artery and vein into the dense adventitia that encircles the cervix that is known to surgeons as the **paracervical** (or **pericervical**) **ring**. (The **paracervix** is the inferior portion of the parametrium, specifically the connective tissue extending on both sides of the cervix, sandwiched within layers of the broad ligament [Dox et al., 2000].) The attachment of the cardinal ligaments to the posterolateral cervix at the level of the internal os pulls on the tissues, forming the lateral yoni fornices.

In life when standing, the cardinal ligaments are vertically oriented. The widely held perception that they are transversely oriented is an artifact of the study of specimens prepared by injection embalming in the supine position and makes no sense from a mechanical point of view (DeLancey, 1996).

Posteriorly, the uterosacral ligaments consist of denser tissue located medial and inferior to the cardinal ligament sheath. The uterosacral ligaments thicken and narrow as they insert into the posterior and lateral aspects of the paracervical ring. The ligaments then pass to either side of and behind the rectum and attach to the presacral fascia overlying S2, S3 and S4. Together, these ligaments help to maintain the length and normal axis of the yoni canal and suspend the upper yoni over the levator plate so that the cervix is suspended in the hollow of the sacrum just above the level of the ischial spines. (Like the cardinal ligaments and for the same reasons, drawings frequently depict these ligaments as being horizontal [DeLancey, 1996].) Damage to these ligaments leads to descent of the yoni vault, which is frequently seen with enterocele (small bowel herniation into the yoni wall) as well as uterine prolapse.

At **level II**, the central layer, the sides of the midyoni and the rectum are suspended from the pelvic sidewalls by connective tissues that are continuous with the cardinal-uterosacral complex, where they meet at the ischial spine. This is the central portion of the paracolpium, which is called the **pubocervical (fasciae) adventitia** by surgeons. It arises from the superior fascia of the levator ani muscles and stretches across the pelvis in a postero-oblique direction, pulling upward in a parasagittal plane. It attaches along the sidewalls of the yoni, linking it to the pelvic walls via its attachment to the tendinous arch of the pelvic fasciae anteriorly and to the tendineus arch of the rectovaginalis posteriorly. It passively supports the bladder, the midyoni and the portion of the rectum that directly underlies the yoni. When the levator ani muscles contract, the pubocervical adventitia rises, providing evidence that they work together.

The pubocervical attachments prevent downward descent of the midyoni during periods of increased abdominal pressure. Detachment of the connective tissues from the tendinous arch of the pelvic fasciae leads to lateral or paravaginal prolapse of the anterior yoni wall. Damage to the anterior end of these tissues results in cystocele. Damage to the central part of the level II supports results in distention cystocele, while damage to the lateral attachments between the sidewalls of the yoni and the tendinous arch of the pelvic fasciae result in displacement cystocele. The rectovaginal space also falls within level II. The loose connective tissues that lie between the wall of the yoni and the wall of the rectum help prevent the rectum from bulging forward, blocking the formation of a rectocele.

Level III, the most shallow layer, includes the perineal body, the superficial and deep perineal muscles, and the connective tissues interwoven among them that are directly attached to adjacent structures without any intervening layer of paracolpium. Together, these tissues support the distal third of the yoni and urethra, as well as the introitus.

The lower 2 to 3 cm of the posterior yoni wall is attached to the perineal body, which itself is linked to the pubic rami. These connections hold the urethra, lower third of the yoni and the anal canal at steep angles when a woman is standing.

These links stabilize the perineal body and prevent the rectal wall from protruding into the lumen of the yoni. Damage to level III supports is associated with anterior and posterior yoni wall prolapse, a gaping introitus and perineal descent. Such damage can lead to urethrocele, hypermobility of the bladder neck, and urinary stress incontinence (Valaitis, 2000). Because the distal inferior surface of the pubovisceral muscle is directly connected to the superior surface of the perineal membrane complex, tearing of the banded part of the perineal membrane complex into two halves can cause the pubovisceral muscles to move apart, widening the urogenital hiatus and causing the introitus to gape (DeLancey, 1999).

Level II and III supports are continuous. Force applied to the anterior rectal wall at level II is resisted by the posterior yoni wall at level III and by its attachments to the pubovisceral muscle. Downward pressure applied to the perineal body from level II is resisted by both the inferior surface of the perineal membrane complex and the connection of the upper yoni wall to the level II attachments that help support the perineal body (DeLancey, 1999).

Tendinous arch of the pelvic fasciae

Sheets of pelvic fibroareolar connective tissue are intermingled with some smooth muscle fibers. They follow the main blood vessels from the pelvic sidewalls to the organs, comprising what amounts to a retroperitoneal mesentery. As these sheets approach the midline, they attach separately to the urinary, genital and lower intestinal tract, forming ligament-like bands that provide lateral attachments for the pelvic organs. On either side, these bands converge, forming two thick fibrous ropes of tissue that run across the superior fascia of the iliococcygeus muscle called the **tendinous arch of the pelvic fasciae** (Peters, 2000) (more rarely called the "arcus tendineus telae endopelvina" and classically referred to as the "fascial white line"). These bands run between the pubic bone and ischial spine on either side and lie in close proximity to the tendinous arch of the levator ani (a.k.a. "muscle white line"), where they function as a sort of suspension cable. The overall length of the tendinous arch of the pelvic fasciae averages 8.55 to 10 cm (Albright et al., 2005; Occeli et al., 2001). It can be subdivided as follows:

- The well-defined anterior end originates about 1 cm lateral and 1 cm above the midline of the inferior border of the pubic symphysis (DeLancey, 1994). From here, it passes in a posterior direction for about 3 cm. This part has adventitial attachments to the upper urethra and anterior yoni wall. As the arch proceeds posteriorly, it fuses with surrounding structures and widens to become a broad expanse of connective tissue where the endopelvic adventitiae are applied to the superior surface of the levator ani muscles.
- The midportion is about 3 cm long. The white line that is visible here is the margin of the endopelvic adventitiae, which continues medially as a broad sheet. The anterior part of this sheet attaches to the anterolateral yoni wall. Branches from the internal iliac artery run laterally through the central part of this section. The fascial attachments of the levator ani muscles and of the fibromuscular layer of the yoni are located at the posterior end of this section.
- The posterior segment of the tendinous arch is 2 to 2.5 cm long. As it proceeds posteriorly, the broad sheet once again becomes a well-defined ridge that merges with the tendinous arch of the levator ani before inserting into the ischial spine (DeLancey, 1994). Its attachment to the ischial spine anchors the adventitiae and all of their attachments (Albright et al., 2005).

The illustrations in this chapter show the tendinous arches (this one and the one described next) in dissected specimens. Trying to understand how these bands are arranged in life was impossible and could not be found illustrated well in any references as of this writing.

Tendinous arch of the rectovaginal fasciae

The rectovaginal adventitia extends laterally beyond the space between the anal and yoni canals as a very loose, web-like mesentery that also attaches to the pelvic sidewalls. These sidewall attachments consist of a fusion of this rectovaginal adventitia with the parietal fascia of the iliococcygeus muscle. These attachments follow a posteriorly oriented path that begins at the perineal body and is about 4.15 cm long. It does not form a thickened ridge-like the tendinous arch of the pelvic fasciae. Half-way between the symphysis and the ischial spine, it meets with the tendinous arch of the pelvic fasciae; this connection point forms an inverted Y that follows the yoni wall, with the open end of the Y toward the pubic bone. In relation to the pelvic sidewall, this meeting point is located where the muscles of the levator ani become wider than the yoni (Leffler et al., 2001). While Leffler's group stated that this connection is the only thing suspending the yoni from the pelvic sidewall in this area; others disagree and have emphasized that this tissue is too fragile to provide such support by itself (Kleeman et al., 2005).

Presacral fascia

The presacral fascia fills in the space between the sacrum and the rectum, forming the anterior boundary of the retrorectal space. It is the pelvic continuation of the visceral abdominal fascia, following the curve of the pelvic walls laterally and the sacrum dorsally, forming a hammock-like sheet that extends between the tendinous arches of the pelvic fascia on either side. Below, it extends to the anorectal junction, where it fuses with the sheath of the rectum; above it extends to the origin of the superior hypogastric plexus (Salmons, 1999).

The presacral fascia fuses ventrally with the parametrium and paracervix; laterally and dorsally with the uterosacral and rectovaginal ligaments and the rectal pillars; and caudally with the rectosacral fascia. The presacral fascia supports the rectum. It encloses the adnexal vessels, the ureters, the hypogastric and sacral splanchnic nerves, and the inferior hypogastric plexus and efferent branches. The perirectal fat that lies between the presacral fascia and the visceral peritoneum is referred to as the "mesorectum." Within the presacral fascia, one finds a thin, sagittally oriented connective mesentery enveloping the ureters that Ercoli and colleagues (2005) called the "mesoureter."

Notes on soft-tissue ligaments in the pelvic cavity

As summarized by Bastian and Lassau (1982), a variety of ligaments have been said to exist in the adult female pelvis. Fritsch and colleagues (2004) concluded that, other than the uterosacral and round ligaments, there are no other true uterine ligaments to be found in conventional anatomical specimens, in histological tissue sections or on MRI. The only tissues "fixing" the position of the uterus are the uterosacral ligaments running in a dorsocranial direction. They are connected to the fasciae covering the pelvic muscles at the same level as the sacrospinous ligaments and lift the entire uteroyoni complex upward. The remaining paracervical and paravaginal regions do contain adipose tissue, numerous blood vessels, nerves and connective tissue septa. Together, some of these structures converge to form cord-like bands that may be misinterpreted as true ligaments, especially in elderly females. While these bands are still referred to as "ligaments," they are not the same as those associated with cartilage or bones, which are typically what is meant when this term is used.

MORE ABOUT PELVIC SPACES

The pelvic spaces, or cleavage planes, are located between organs and other structures. Some of these are potential spaces that are normally filled or loosely covered with connective tissue that can be easily peeled apart, thus creating surgically developed "spaces." Others are regions created by a fold of tissue, such as the anterior and posterior cul-de-sacs. The rectovaginal space and, much less commonly, the rectouterine space, are the ones most likely to be encountered by midwives. The rectovaginal space is explained on page 48. The other pelvic spaces are described here because they are frequently not well described elsewhere and you may encounter mention of them as you study other sources; they are particularly relevant to an understanding of urogynecologic surgery. DeLancey (2003b) explained them as follows:

- **Vesicouterine pouch (anterior cul-de-sac):** The vesicouterine pouch is the region within the fold formed by the peritoneum where the anterior surface of the uterus overlies the posterolateral part of the bladder dome (when the uterus is anteverted or tipped forward); the deepest part of this fold lies a few centimeters above the yoni. The peritoneum is loosely applied over these surfaces, which allows the bladder to fill.
- **Rectouterine pouch (posterior cul-de-sac/pouch of Douglas):** This pouch is bordered by the yoni anteriorly, the rectosigmoid colon posteriorly and the uterosacral ligaments laterally. Its overlying peritoneum extends along the posterior yoni wall for about 4 cm to where the posterior fornix attaches to the cervix. The rectouterine pouch is the lowermost portion of the abdominal cavity and may contain loops of bowel. Very deep and serious tears can open into the lower end of this pouch, which may allow loops of small intestine to prolapse into the yoni vault.
- **Prevesical space (of Retzius):** This space is bounded anteriorly and laterally by the bones and muscles of the anterior pelvic wall. Above, it is bounded by the abdominal wall. The upper urethra and the bladder lie in the lower part of this space. The lower, lateral boundary is formed by the attachment of the bladder to the cervical ligament and by the attachment of the pubocervical adventitia to the tendinous arch of the pelvic fasciae. These lateral attachments separate this space from the vesicovaginal and vesicocervical spaces. Structures found within this space include many blood vessels and nerves: the dorsal clitoral vessels, the obturator nerve and vessels as they enter the obturator canal, and a dense plexus of vessels and nerves that lies at the border of the lower urinary tract.
- **Vesicovaginal and vesicocervical spaces:** The space between the lower urinary tract and the yoni and uterus can be divided into two regions. The lower part is the vesicovaginal space, which can be created when the upper and middle third of the posterior urethral wall is peeled from the surface of the anterior yoni wall, to which it is fused; it extends up under the peritoneum to the level of the vesicocervical peritoneal reflection or fold. The vesicocervical space begins at that point, extending laterally to the pelvic sidewalls, separating the vesical and genital sides of the cardinal ligaments.

•**Region of the sacrospinous ligament:** The region of the sacrospinous ligament has become an important area for surgeons addressing yoni support. The rectal pillars separate this region from the rectovaginal space. The sacral nerve plexus lies on the upper border of the sacrospinous ligament, wrapping to the side of the ligament as it traverses the greater sciatic foramen. The pudendal nerve splits off from the sacral plexus just before it enters this foramen. The pudendal nerve, along with its accompanying vessels, then passes alongside the sacrospinous ligament's connection to the ischial spine. The levator ani nerve lies nearby, on the inner surface of the midpart of the coccygeal muscle.

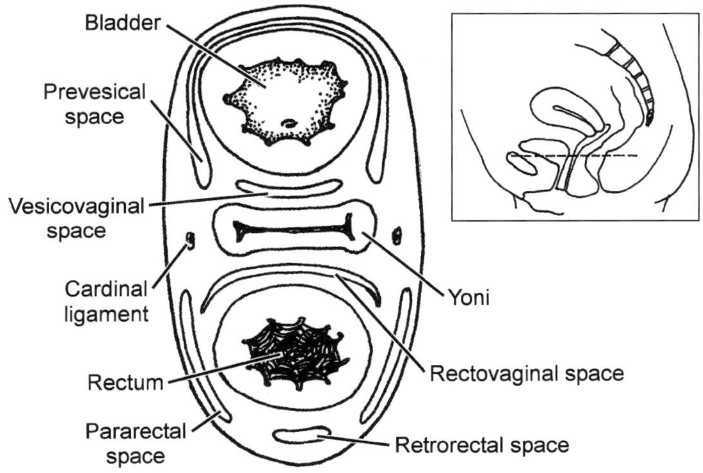

Transverse section showing some pelvic spaces

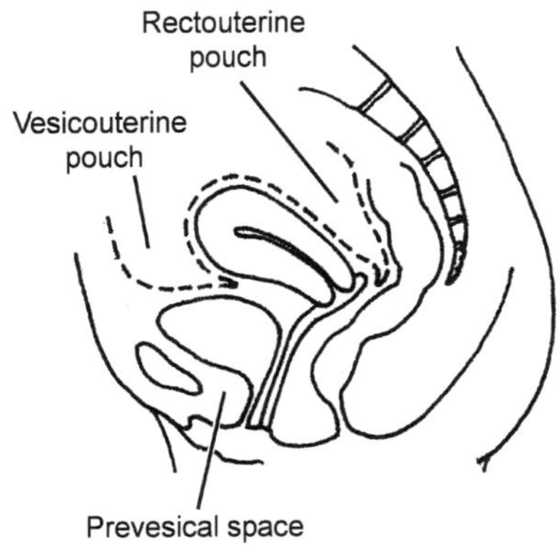

Peritoneal regions of the pelvis

Color-by-Number Illustrations of Pelvic Anatomy

Study the explanations, cross-sections, and full perineal views together. First, choose which color to assign to each number. Color the diagrams using colored pencils (pencils work best because they take a fine point and won't bleed through the paper). In the United States, Crayola™ makes nice sets of pencils that are not too expensive. When you decide on a color, fill in a patch beside the corresponding number on the list, so you don't use that color for two numbers. You may need to combine two colors to create enough of them to have a different color for each part, or you may decide to use the same color for two very dissimilar parts (to avoid confusion). Numbering is consistent in the drawings that follow, but the structures are listed in no particular order. Therefore, it will be easiest to first refer to the numbers from the drawings and then the list to find a structure. Not every structure is listed and not every listed part is illustrated in every drawing. Read about a structure and then go to each drawing and color it in, in order to learn its position from different perspectives. Doing the coloring will help you learn. It is a good idea to photocopy this list so you can refer to it as you draw without constantly turning back to these pages.

1. Clitoral body (1); crura (1a)
2. Clitoral glans
3. Clitoral bulbs
4. Urethra (4a); urethral orifice (4b)
5. Yoni canal
6. Clitoral root
7. Hymenal ring
8. Yoni fornices
9. Ischiocavernosus muscles
10. Superficial transverse perineal muscle
11. Perineal membrane connective tissue complex: banded parts (11a); 3-D part (11b)
12. Internal anal sphincter
13. Winged part of the external anal sphincter
14. Main part of the external anal sphincter
15. Longitudinal anal muscle
16. External sphincter space
17. Subcutaneous part of the external anal sphincter
18. Deep postanal space
19. Bulbocavernosus muscle
20. Puboanalis muscle component of pubovisceral complex
21. Pubococcygeus fibers of pubovisceral complex and tendinous plate of pubococcygeus
22. Puboperinealis muscle of pubovisceral complex
23. Vaginolevator attachments of pubovisceral complex
24. Fascia
25. Puborectalis muscle
26. Iliococcygeus muscle
27. Ureter

28. Vestibule of the vulva
29. Labia minora
30. Labia majora
31. Perineal body
32. Bladder
33. Uterus
34. Cervix
35. Ovary
36. Uterine or egg tube (Fallopian tube)
37. Baby's head crowning
38. Obturator internus muscle
39. Tendinous arch of the pelvic fascia
40. Anococcygeal ligament contribution from external anal sphincters
41. Bony structures of the pelvis (41); pubic bone (41a); pelvic brim (41b); ischiopubic rami (41c); sacrum (41d); ischial tuberosity (41e); coccyx (41f); ilium (41g). (Color coding does not apply to these alphabetical designations)
42. Rectal canal
43. Retrouterine pouch
44. Urethral sphincter
45. Compressor urethra
46. Urethrovaginal sphincter
47. Deep suspensory ligament of the clitoris
48. Pubourethral ligament
49. Urethral carina
50. Detrusor muscle of bladder
51. Cut edges of tissue (not always numbered)
52. Vestibular gland and duct
53. Anus
54. Gluteus maximus muscle
55. Sacrotuberous ligament
56. Round ligament
57. Suspensory ligament of the ovary
58. Ischiorectal fossa
59. Superficial perineal space
60. Perineal artery
61. Dorsal vein of the clitoris
62. Mons veneris
63. External coat of rectal canal
64. Ovarian ligament

Notes on these anatomical drawings: Some structures are left out to clarify the position of those being illustrated. This does not make them less important. The drawings in this part of the book have been adapted from illustrations based on dissected cadaver material. In some, an attempt has been made to show approximate tissue relationships in life, based on information derived from study as well as MRI images. For other drawings, we stuck strictly with what was true for cadavers, as noted. Keep in mind the differences in tissue relationships between a live woman and a cadaver as you go through this chapter.

I. This coronal (frontal) section is cut on a somewhat posterior angle. It shows the depth relationship of the more shallow pelvic structures. Note that the plane of this section is through the longitudinal center of the yoni, not through the central point of the perineum, and that the uterus is lifted up and out of the way. It was drawn from a cadaver specimen with levator ani muscle tone suggested.

II. This median sagittal section of the pelvic organs shows the muscles within the other soft tissue in a cadaver, with an attempt to demonstrate tone in the levator ani complex.

III. This parasagittal section focuses on the relationship between the muscles of the anterior and posterior compartments in a cadaver.

IV. Perineal view of the muscles of the pelvic floor in a cadaver. Tone is absent and thus pelvic floor components are flatter, broader and the entire pelvic floor is bowl-shaped.

V. Perineal view of the pelvic muscles at crowning, with an average amount of thinning. The mother is in a supine position. This view was chosen simply because reference images showing the muscles when the mother is pushing in other-than-supine positions could not be located.

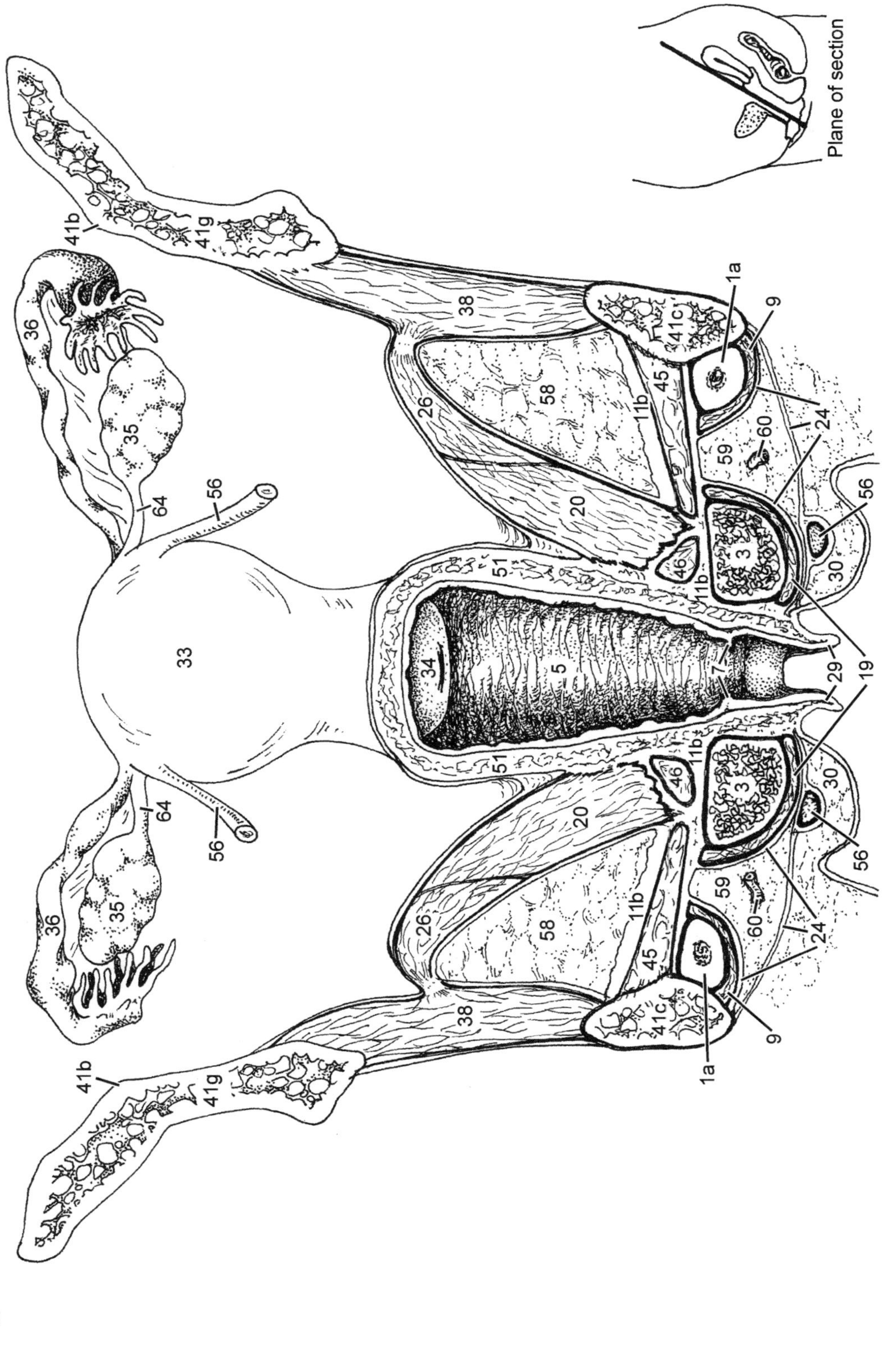

Plane of section
1a
3
5
7
9
11b
19
20
24
26
29
30
33
34
35
36
38
41b
41c
41g
45
46
51
56
58
59
60
64

I.

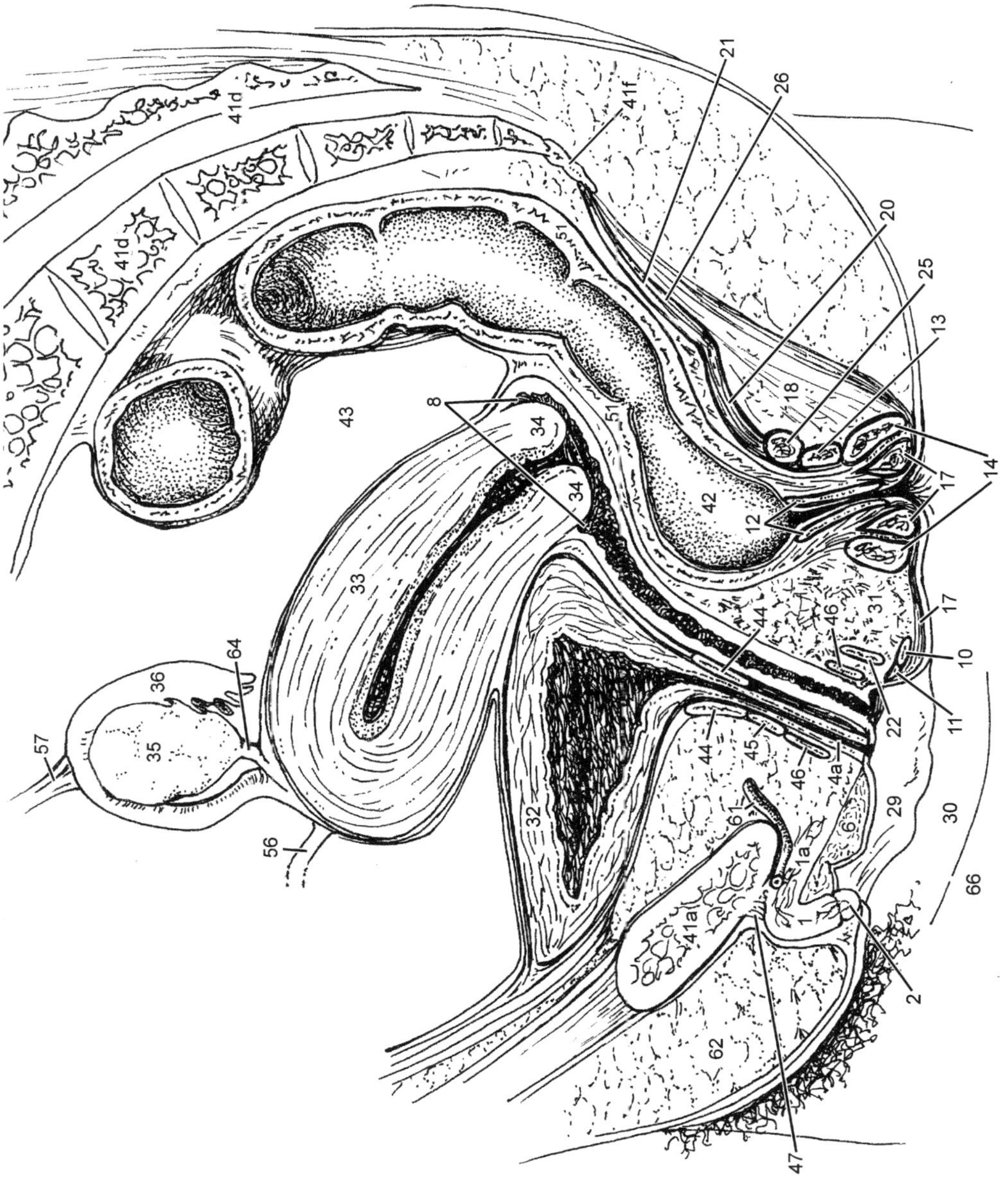

1
1a
2
4a
6
8
10
11
12
13
14
14
17
17
17
18
20
21
22
25
26
29
30
31
32
33
34
34
35
36
41a
41d
41d
41f
42
43
44
44
45
46
46
47
51
51
56
57
61
62
64
66

II.

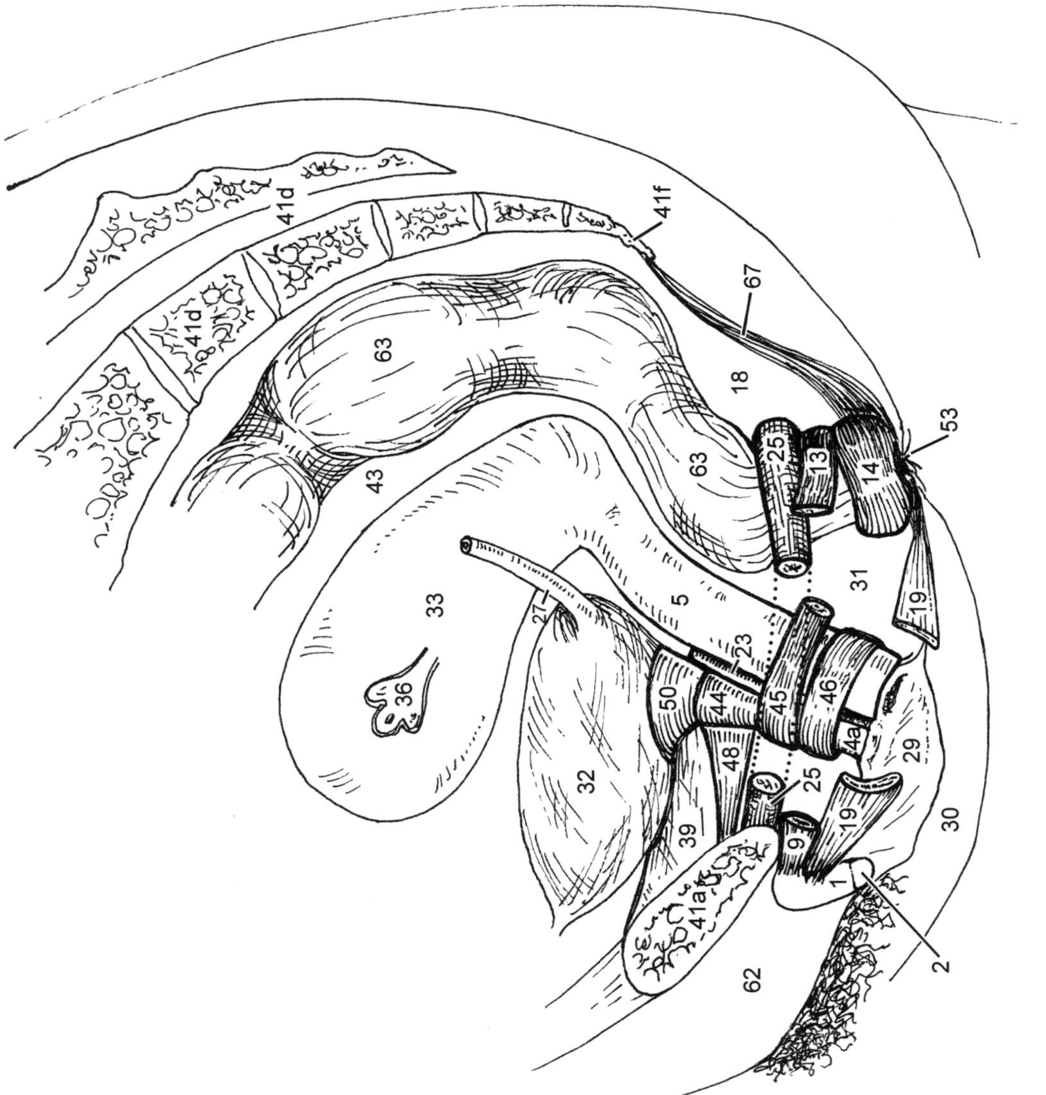
41d
41f
41d
67
63
18
53
43
25
13
14
63
31
33
27
5
19
23
36
50
44
45
46
4a
29
48
25
32
19
30
39
9
1
2
41a
62

III.

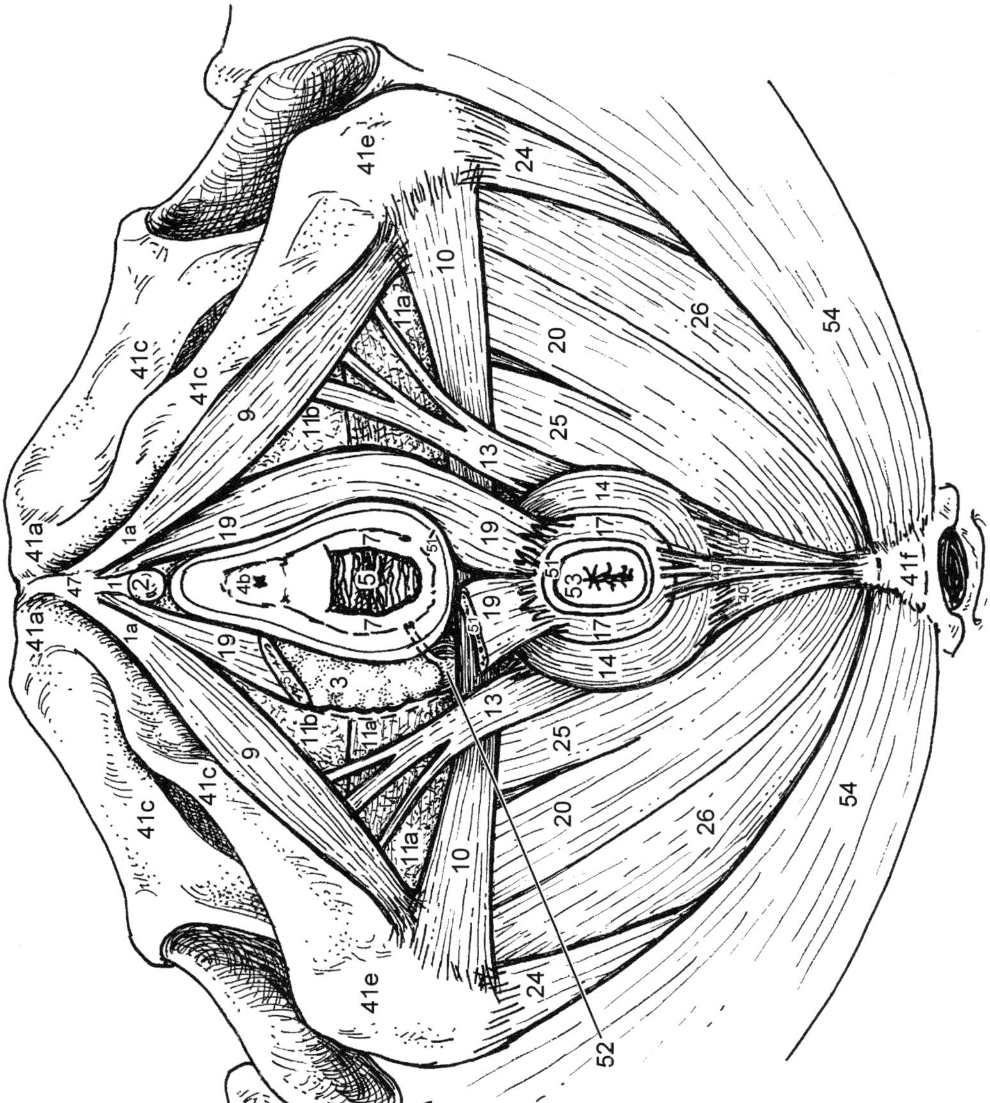
41e
24
10
11a
20
26
54
41c
9
11b
25
13
14
41a
1a
19
7
51
17
40
47
1
2
4b
5
53
41f
3
52

IV.

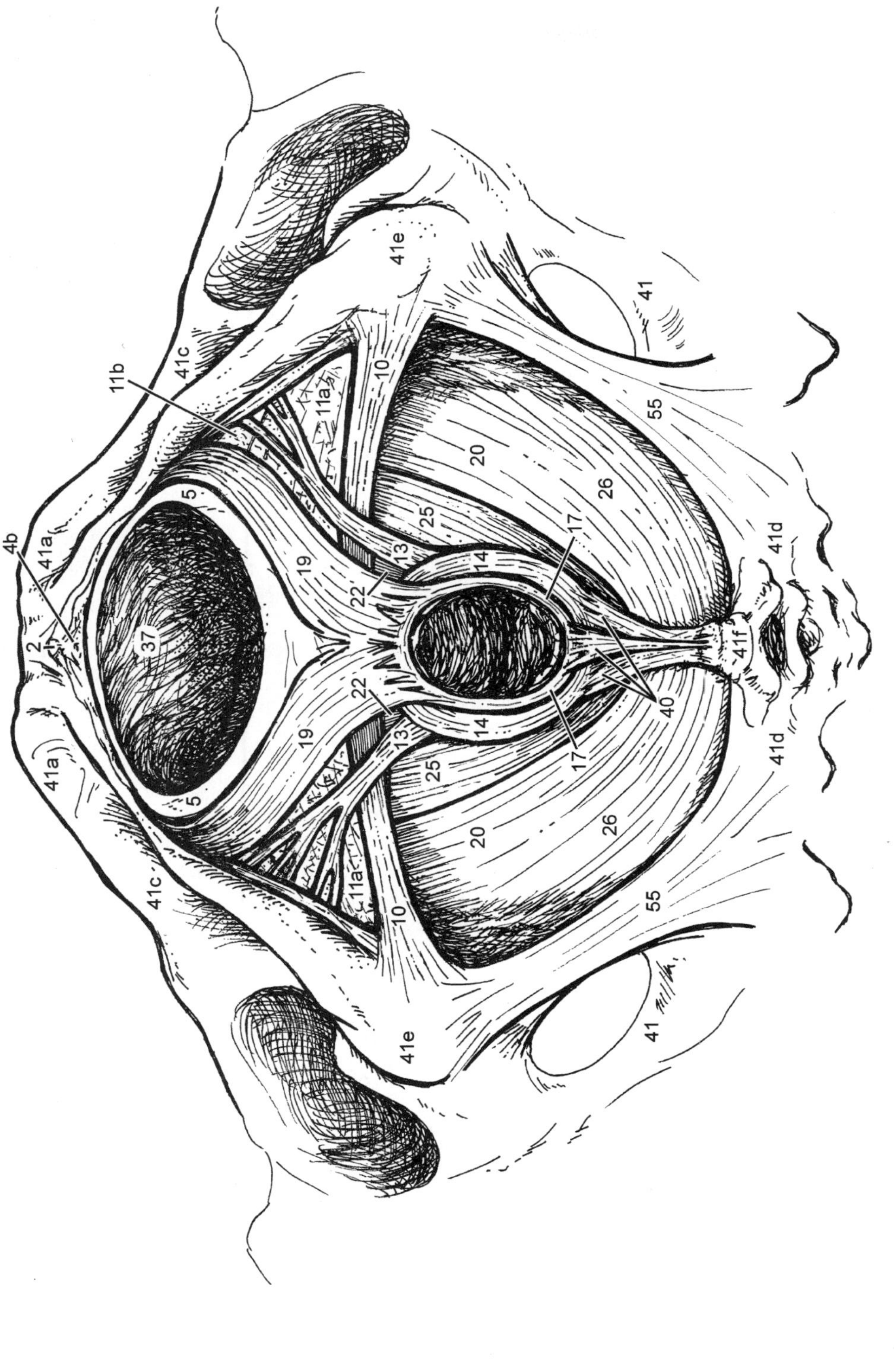
4b
41a
2
1
37
5
11b
41c
41e
10
11a
19
22
13
14
17
25
20
26
55
41
40
41d
41f

V.

REFERENCES AND FURTHER READING ON PERTINENT ANATOMY

REFERENCES USED IN MULTIPLE CHAPTERS

Baggish M, Karrem M. "A new perspective on the anatomic relationships of the perineum, vagina, urethra, and urethral vesical junction," J GYNECOL SURG, 15(3):119-125, 1999.

Bannister L. Chapter 12: "Alimentary system," in Williams P, et al., eds. GRAY'S ANATOMY: THE ANATOMICAL BASIS OF MEDICINE AND SURGERY, 38th ed. Churchill Livingstone, New York NY, 1999.

Barber M. "Contemporary views on female pelvic anatomy," CLEVE CLIN J MED, 72(Suppl. 4)S3-S11, Dec, 2005.

Basmajiam J. GRANT'S METHODS OF ANATOMY, 10th ed. Williams & Wilkins, Baltimore MD, 1980.

Benson R. HANDBOOK OF OBSTETRICS AND GYNECOLOGY, 5th ed. Lange Medical Pub., Los Altos CA, 1974.

Berglas B, Rubin I. "Histologic study of the pelvic connective tissue," SURG GYNECOL OBSTET, 97(3):277-289, Sep, 1953.

Bloom M, van Dongen L. CLINICAL GYNAECOLOGY–INTEGRATION OF STRUCTURE AND FUNCTION. JB Lippincott Co, Philadelphia PA, 1972.

Burkitt H, et al. WHEATER'S FUNCTIONAL HISTOLOGY: A TEXT AND COLOUR ATLAS, 3rd ed. Churchill Livingstone, Edinburgh, Scotland, 1993.

Clark-Collar T, CNM, PhD. Editing comments on anatomy material, Spring, 1990.

Clemente CD. ANATOMY: REGIONAL ATLAS OF THE HUMAN BODY, 3rd ed. Urban & Schwarzenberg, Baltimore MD, 1987.

Curtis A, et al. "The anatomy of the pelvic and urogenital diaphragms, in relation to urethrocele and cystocele," SURG GYNECOL OBSTET, 68(2):161-166, Feb 1, 1939.

DeLancey J. Chapter 1: "Anatomy of the female bladder and urethra," in Bent A, et al. OSTERGARD'S UROGYNECOLOGY AND PELVIC FLOOR DYSFUNCTION, 5th ed. Lippincott, Williams & Wilkins, Philadelphia PA, 2003a.

DeLancey J. Chapter 5: "Surgical anatomy of the female pelvis," in Rock J, Jones H, eds. TE LINDE'S OPERATIVE GYNECOLOGY, 9th ed. Lippincott, Williams & Wilkins, Philadelphia PA, 2003b.

DeLancey J. "Fascial and muscular abnormalities in women with urethral hypermobility and anterior vaginal wall prolapse," AM J OBSTET GYNECOL, 187(1):93-98, Jul, 2002a.

DeLancey J. Section 2A, chapter 2: "Anterior pelvic floor in the female," in Pemberton J, et al., eds. THE PELVIC FLOOR: ITS FUNCTION AND DISORDERS. WB Saunders, London UK, 2002b.

DeLancey J. "Structural anatomy of the posterior pelvic compartment as it relates to rectocele," AM J OBSTET GYNECOL, 180(4):815-823, Apr, 1999.

DeLancey J. "Standing anatomy of the pelvic floor," J PELV SURG, 2(5):260-263, Sep, 1996.

DeLancey J. "The anatomy of the pelvic floor," CUR OPIN OBSTET GYNECOL, 6(4):313-316, Aug, 1994.

DeLancey J. Chapter 1: "Anatomy of the urethral sphincters and supports," in Drife J, et al., eds. MICTURITION. Springer-Verlag, London UK, 1990.

DeLancey J. BASIC EXERCISES: SURGICAL TECHNIQUE. Davis-Geck, Wayne NJ, 1987.

DeLancey J. "Correlative study of paraurethral anatomy," OBSTET GYNECOL, 68(1):91-97, Jul, 1986.

DeLancey J, Hurd W. "Size of the urogenital hiatus in the levator ani muscles in normal women and women with pelvic organ prolapse," OBSTET GYNECOL, 91(3):364-368, Mar, 1998.

DeLancey J, Starr R. "Histology of the connection between the vagina and levator ani muscles," J REPRO MED, 35(8):765-771, Aug, 1990.

Dickinson R. ATLAS OF HUMAN SEX ANATOMY, 2nd ed. Williams & Wilkins Co., Baltimore MD, 1949.

Downer C, et al., eds. A NEW VIEW OF A WOMAN'S BODY: A FULLY ILLUSTRATED GUIDE BY THE FEDERATION OF FEMINIST WOMEN'S HEALTH CENTERS. Feminist Health Press, Los Angeles CA, 1991.

Drake R, et al., eds. Chapter 5: "Pelvis and perineum," in Drake, et al., eds. GRAY'S ANATOMY FOR STUDENTS. Elsevier, Philadelphia PA, 2005.

Drenth J. THE ORIGIN OF THE WORLD: SCIENCE AND FICTION OF THE VAGINA. Reaktion Books, London UK, 2005.

Ellis H, Dussek J, eds. Chapter 16: "Surface Anatomy," in Williams P, et al., eds. GRAY'S ANATOMY: THE ANATOMICAL BASIS OF MEDICINE AND SURGERY, 38th ed. Churchill Livingstone, New York NY, 1999.

Ercoli A, et al. “Terminologia Anatomica versus unofficial descriptions and nomenclature of the fasciae and ligaments of the female pelvis: a dissection-based comparative study,” AM J OBSTET GYNECOL, 193(4): 1565-1573, Oct, 2005.

Federation of Feminist Women’s Health Centers. A NEW VIEW OF A WOMAN’S BODY: A FULLY ILLUSTRATED GUIDE. Simon & Schuster, New York NY, 1981.

Fielding J, et al. “MR-based three-dimensional modeling of the normal pelvic floor in women: quantification of muscle mass,” AJR AM J ROENTGENOL, 174:657-660, Mar, 2000.

Fritsch H, et al. “Clinical anatomy of the pelvic floor,” ADV ANAT EMBRYOL CELL BIOL, 175:III-IX, 1-64, 2004.

Fucini C, et al. “Anatomic plane of separation between external anal sphincter and puborectalis muscle: clinical implications,” DIS COLON RECTUM, 42(3):374-378, Mar, 1999.

Garrey M. OBSTETRICS ILLUSTRATED. Churchill Livingstone, New York NY, 1980.

Garrey M, et. al. GYNECOLOGY ILLUSTRATED. Churchill Livingstone, New York NY, 1978.

Goldberg S. CLINICAL ANATOMY MADE RIDICULOUSLY SIMPLE. MedMaster, Miami FL, 1984.

Guo M, Li D. “Pelvic floor images: anatomy of the levator ani muscle,” DIS COLON RECTUM, 50(10):1647-1655, Oct, 2007.

Kapit W, Elson L. THE ANATOMY COLORING BOOK. Harper & Row, New York NY, 1977.

Kleeman SD, et al. “Rectoceles and the anatomy of the posterior vaginal wall: revisited,” AM J OBSTET GYNECOL, 193(6):2050-2055, Dec, 2005.

Kobelt, GL. “The female sex organs in humans and some mammals.” Translated from the German by Bernays H, in Lowry T, ed. THE CLASSIC CLITORIS: HISTORIC CONTRIBUTIONS TO SCIENTIFIC SEXUALITY. Nelson-Hall, Chicago IL [1844] 1978.

Krantz KE. “The gross and microscopic anatomy of the human vagina,” ANN NY ACAD SCI, 83(2):89-104, Nov 18, 1959.

Krantz KE. “Innervation of the human vulva and vagina. A microscopic study,” OBSTET GYNECOL, 12(4): 382-396, Oct, 1958.

Last RJ. ANATOMY, REGIONAL AND APPLIED, 7th ed. Churchill Livingston, New York NY, 1984.

Last RJ. ANATOMY, REGIONAL AND APPLIED. Little, Brown, Boston MA, 1954.

Lukban J, Whitmore K. “Pelvic floor muscle re-education treatment of the overactive bladder and painful bladder syndrome,” CLIN OBSTET GYNECOL, 45(1):273-285, Mar, 2002.

Luschka H. DIE ANATOMIE DES MENSCHLICHEN BECKENS. Leapp & Sibeck, Tübingen Germany, 1864.

Masters W, Johnson V. HUMAN SEXUAL RESPONSE. Little, Brown & Co., Boston MA, 1966.

Miller C. “Surgeons respond to pelvic reconstruction column,” OB/GYN NEWS, Mar 1, 2005, http://findarticles.com/p/articles/mi_m0CYD/is_5_40/ai_n13472461/print, accessed Jun 14, 2008.

Moore K, Dalley A. “Introduction to clinically oriented anatomy,” in their CLINICALLY ORIENTED ANATOMY, 5th ed. Lippincott, Williams & Wilkins, Philadelphia PA, 2006.

Mouchel T, Mouchel F. “Basic anatomic features in perineology,” PELVIPERINEOLOGY, 27(4):156-159, Dec, 2008.

Netter F. ATLAS OF HUMAN ANATOMY, 4th ed. Saunders Elsevier, Philadelphia PA, 2003.

Netter F. THE CIBA COLLECTION OF MEDICAL ILLUSTRATIONS: VOL 2, REPRODUCTIVE SYSTEM. CIBA Pub., Summit NJ, 1954.

Nichols DH, et al. “Significance of restoration of normal vaginal depth and axis,” OBSTET GYNECOL, 36(2): 251-256, Aug, 1970.

O’Connell H, Sanjeevan K. Chapter 4.1: “Anatomy of the female genitalia,” in Goldstein I, et al., eds. WOMEN’S SEXUAL FUNCTION AND DYSFUNCTION: STUDY, DIAGNOSIS AND TREATMENT. Taylor & Francis, New York NY, 2006.

O’Connell H, et al. “The clitoris: a unified structure. Histology of the clitoral glans, body, crura and bulbs,” URODINAMICA, 14:127-132, 2004.

O’Dell J, Morse A. “It’s not all about birth: biomechanics applied to pelvic organ prolapse prevention,” J MWH, 53(1):28-36, Jan-Feb, 2008.

Oelrich TM. “The striated urogenital sphincter muscle in the female,” ANAT REC, 205(2):223-232, Feb, 1983.

Otcenasek M, et al. “Endopelvic fascia in women: shape and relation to parietal pelvic structures,” OBSTET GYNECOL, 111(3):622-630, Mar, 2008.

Peters W. Chapter 2: "Anatomy of female pelvic support and continence," in Lentz G, ed. UROGYNECOLOGY. Oxford U Press, New York NY, 2000.

Rees MA, et al. "The suspensory ligament of the clitoris: connective tissue supports of the erectile tissues of the female urogenital region," CLIN ANAT, 13(6):397-403, 2000.

Rociu E, et al. "Normal anal sphincter anatomy and age- and sex-related variations at high-spatial- resolution endoanal MR imaging," RADIOLOGY, 217(2):395-401, Nov, 2000.

Salmons S. Chapter 7: "Muscle," in Williams P, et al., eds. GRAY'S ANATOMY: THE ANATOMICAL BASIS OF MEDICINE AND SURGERY, 38th ed. Churchill Livingstone, New York NY, 1999.

Schorge J, et al., eds. WILLIAM'S GYNECOLOGY. McGraw-Hill Medical, New York NY, 2008.

Scurry J, Melville R. Chapter 2: "Normal vulva and developmental anomalies," in Heller D, Wallach R, eds. VULVAR DISEASE: A CLINICOPATHOLOGICAL APPROACH. Informa, New York NY, 2007.

Sevely J. EVE'S SECRETS: A NEW THEORY OF FEMALE SEXUALITY. Random House, New York NY, 1987.

Shafik A. "A new concept of the anatomy of the anal sphincter mechanism and the physiology of defecation. II. Anatomy of the levator ani muscle with special reference to puborectalis," INVESTIGATIVE UROL, 13(3):175-182, Nov, 1975a.

Shafik A, et al. "A novel concept for the surgical anatomy of the perineal body," DIS COLON RECTUM, 50(12):2120-2125, Dec, 2007a.

Shafik A, et al. "Physioanatomical relationship of the external anal sphincter to the bulbocavernosus muscle in the female," INT UROGYNECOL J, 18(8):851-856, Aug, 2007b.

Shafik A, et al. "Surgical anatomy of the perineal muscles and their role in perineal disorders," ANAT SCI INTERNAT, 80(3):167-171, Sep, 2005.

Snell R. CLINICAL ANATOMY FOR MEDICAL STUDENTS, 3rd ed. Little, Brown & Co. Boston MA, 1986.

Sobotta, F. ATLAS OF HUMAN ANATOMY, VOL 2, 9th ed. Urban & Schwarzenberg, Baltimore MD, 1977.

Soga H, et al. "A histopographic study of the perineal body in elderly women: the surgical applicability of novel histological findings," INT UROGNECOL J PELVIC FLOOR DYSFUNCT, 18:1423-1430, Dec, 2007.

SOURCEBOOK OF MEDICAL ILLUSTRATIONS, Medical College of St. Bartholomew's Hospital, London UK, Parthenon, Park Ridge NJ, 1989.

STEDMAN'S ELECTRONIC MEDICAL DICTIONARY, Version 7.0. Lippincott, Williams & Wilkins, Baltimore MD, 2007.

Stilwell D. Chapter II: "Anatomy of the human clitoris," in Lowry T, et al. THE CLITORIS. Warren Green, Inc., St. Louis MO, 1976.

Sutton J. LET BIRTH BE BORN AGAIN: REDISCOVERING AND RECLAIMING OUR MIDWIFERY HERITAGE. Birth Concepts UK, Middlesex UK, 2001.

Uhlenhuth E, Nolley G. "Vaginal fascia, a myth?" OBSTET GYNECOL, 10(4):349-358, Oct, 1957.

van der Putte SC. "Mammary-like glands of the vulva and their disorders," INTER J GYNECOL PATH, 13(2): 150-160, 1994.

van Houten T. Chapter 4.4: "Anatomy of the pelvic floor and pelvic organ support system," in Goldstein I, et al., eds. WOMEN'S SEXUAL FUNCTION AND DYSFUNCTION: STUDY, DIAGNOSIS AND TREATMENT. Taylor & Francis, New York NY, 2006.

Weber A, Walters M. "Anterior vaginal prolapse: review of anatomy and techniques of surgical repair," OBSTET GYNECOL, 89(2):311-318, Feb, 1997.

Wendell-Smith C, Wilson P. Chapter 8: "The vulva, vagina and urethra and the musculature of the pelvic floor," in Philipp E, et al., eds. SCIENTIFIC FOUNDATIONS OF OBSTETRICS AND GYNAECOLOGY, 4th ed. Butterworth-Heinemann, Oxford UK, 1991.

Whitmore I, Chairman. TERMINOLOGIA ANATOMICA: INTERNATIONAL ANATOMICAL TERMINOLOGY. FCAT: Federative Committee on Anatomical Terminology, New York NY, 1998.

Woodburn R, Burkel W. ESSENTIALS OF HUMAN ANATOMY, 8th ed. Oxford U Press, New York NY, 1983.

Yucel S, Baskin L. "An anatomical description of the male and female urethral sphincter complex," J UROL, 171(5):1890-1897, May, 2004.

UNDERSTANDING FEMALE PELVIC ANATOMY: AN INTRODUCTION

Erickson J, Montana W. "New observations on the anatomical features of the female genitalia," J AM MED

Womens Assoc, 27(11):573, Nov, 1972.
Kolder V, MD. Editing comments, Aug, 1990.
Thompson P. "On the arrangement of the fasciæ of the pelvis and their relationship to the levator ani," J Anat Physiol, 35(N.S. Vol 15):127-150, Jan, 1901.

The External Genitalia

Apgar B, Cox T. "Differentiating normal and abnormal findings of the vulva," Am Fam Physician, 53(4):1171-1180, Mar, 1996.
Berg R, Davis C. Chapter 4: "Microbial ecology of the vulva," in Farage M, Miabach H, eds. The Vulva: Anatomy, Physiology and Pathology. Informa Healthcare USA, New York NY, 2006.
Bharucha A. "Pelvic floor: anatomy and function," Neurogastroenterol Motil, 18(7):507-519, Jul, 2006.
Carter R, ed. A Dictionary of Dermatologic Terms, 4th ed. Williams & Wilkins, Baltimore MD, 1992.
Cohen B, Taylor J. Chapter 6: "The skin in health and disease," Memmler's The Human Body in Health and Disease, 10th ed. Lippincott, Williams & Wilkins, Baltimore MD, 2005.
Deliveliotou A, Creatsas G. Chapter 1: "Anatomy of the vulva," in Farage M, Miabach H, eds. The Vulva: Anatomy, Physiology and Pathology. Informa Healthcare USA, New York NY, 2006.
Dennerstein G, et al. The Vulva and Vagina Manual. Gynederm Publishing Pty Ltd., Fitzroy Victoria Australia, 2005.
Dua A, et al. "Perineal length: relationship between the length of the perineum and ethnic origin," Study conducted at Queens Park Hospital, Sep 2005-Mar 2007, Blackburn, UK. www.icsoffice.org/ASPNET_Membership/Membership/Abstracts/Publish/46/000161.pdf, accessed Oct 21, 2008.
Elsner P. "What textile engineers should know about the human skin," Curr Probl Dermatol, 31:24-34, 2003.
Erickson J, Montana W. "New observations on the anatomical features of the female genitalia," J Am Med Womens Assoc, 27(11):573, Nov, 1972.
Farage M, Maibach H. Chapter 2: "Tissue structure and physiology of the vulva," in Farage M, Miabach H, eds. The Vulva: Anatomy, Physiology and Pathology. Informa Healthcare USA, New York NY, 2006.
Farage M, et al. Chapter 3: "Changes in the vulva and vagina throughout life," in Farage M, Miabach H, eds. The Vulva: Anatomy, Physiology and Pathology. Informa Healthcare USA, New York NY, 2006.
Faria DE, et al. "Perineal skin injury: extrinsic environmental risk factors," Ostomy Wound Manage, 42(7):28-30, 32-34, 36-37, Aug, 1996.
Fischer B, Margesson K. "Normal anatomy of the vulva," in Fisher B, Margesson L. Genital Skin Disorders: Diagnosis and Treatment. Mosby Pub., St. Louis MO, 1998.
Göttlicher S. "The labium tertium pudenid feminae: A prospective study of 1180 patients." (article in German), Zentralbl Gynacol, 116(7):419-421, 1994.
Gray M. "Preventing and managing perineal dermatitis: a shared goal for wound and continence care," J WOCN, 31(Suppl. 1):S2-S12, Jan-Feb, 2004.
Harper W, McNichol E. "A histological study of normal vulval skin from infancy to old age," Br J Dermatol, 96(3):249-253, Mar, 1977.
Hoyt R. Chaper 4.2: "Innervation of the vagina and vulva," in Goldstein I, et al., eds. Women's Sexual Function and Dysfunction: Study, Diagnosis and Treatment. Taylor & Francis, New York NY, 2006.
Humphrey P. Chapter 1: "Genital skin and urethral anatomy," in Brandes S, ed. Current Clinical Urology: Urethral Reconstructive Surgery. Humana Press, Totowa NJ, 2008.
Jones IS. "A histological assessment of normal vulval skin," Clin Exp Dermatol, 8(5):513-521, Sep, 1983.
Joseph J. A Textbook of Regional Anatomy. Macmillian Press, London UK, 1982.
Kalis V, et al. "The perineal body length and injury at delivery" (article in Czech), Ceska Gynekol, 70(5):355-361, Sep, 2005.
Nauth H. "Anatomy and physiology of the vulva," in Elsner P, Marius J, eds. Vulvovaginitis, Vol I. Marcel Dekker, New York NY, 1993.

O'Connell HE, DeLancey J. "Clitoral anatomy in nulliparous, healthy, premenopausal volunteers using unenhanced magnetic resonance imaging," J UROL, 173(6):2060-2063, Jun, 2005.

Rees MA, et al. "The suspensory ligament of the clitoris: connective tissue supports of the erectile tissues of the female urogenital region," CLIN ANAT, 13(6):397-403, 2000.

Ridley C. THE VULVA. WB Saunders Co, Ltd. London UK, 1975.

Sargeant P, et al. "Ultrastructural study of the epithelium of the normal human vulva," J SUBMICROSC CYTOL PATHOL, 28(2):161-170, 1996.

Skandalakis L, et al. Chapter 1: "Skin, scalp and nail" in their SURGICAL ANATOMY AND TECHNIQUE: A POCKET MANUAL, 3rd ed. Springer, New York NY, 2009.

Spence A. BASIC HUMAN ANATOMY, 3rd ed. Benjamin/Cummings Pub. Co., Redwood CA, 1990.

Tarcan T, et al. "Histomorphometric analysis of age-related structural changes in human clitoral cavernosal tissue," J UROL, 161(3):940-944, Mar, 1999.

Toesca A, et al. "Immunohistochemical study of the corpora cavernosa of the human clitoris," J ANAT, 188(Pt 3):513-520, Jun, 1996.

Trott A. WOUNDS AND LACERATIONS: EMERGENCY CARE AND CLOSURE, 3rd ed. Elsevier Mosby, Philadelphia PA, 2005.

van der Putte SC. "The development of the perineum in the human. A comprehensive histological study with a special reference to the role of the stromal components," ADV ANAT EMBRYOL CELL BIOL, 177:1-131, 2005.

Wilkinson E, Hardt N. Chapter 39: "Vulva," in Mills S, ed. HISTOLOGY FOR PATHOLOGISTS, 3rd ed. Lippincott, Williams & Wilkins, Philadelphia PA, 2007.

Wisegeek.com. "What is keratin?" www.wisegeek.com/what-is-keratin.htm, accessed Feb 15, 2008.

Woodman PJ, Graney DO. "Anatomy and physiology of the female perineal body with relevance to obstetrical injury and repair," CLIN ANAT, 15(5):321-334, Aug, 2002.

Yucel S, et al. "Neuroanatomy of the human female lower urogenital tract," J UROL, 172(1):191-195, Jul, 2004.

INTRODUCING THE PELVIC SUPPORT SYSTEM AND SOFT TISSUES

Bodyandfitness.com. "Sports nutrition: fast-twitch and slow-twitch muscle fibers," www.bodyandfitness.com/Information/Training/twitch.htm, accessed Jan 23, 2008.

Derry D. "Pelvic muscles and fasciæ," J ANAT PHYSIOL, 42(1st Pt):107-111, Oct, 1907.

Kurtz AB, et al. "Ultrasound evaluation of the posterior pelvic compartment," RADIOLOGY, 132(3):677-682, Sep, 1979.

Quinn E. "Fast and slow twitch muscle fibers," http://sportsmedicine.about.com/od/anatomyandphysiology/a/MuscleFiberType.htm, 2008, accessed Jan 23, 2008.

Wipff PJ, et al. "Myofibroblast contraction activates latent TGF-beta1 from the extracellular matrix," J CELL BIOLOGY, 179(6):1311-1323, Dec 17, 2007.

THE UROGENITAL TRIANGLE AND RELATED STRUCTURES

Baskin L, et al. "Anatomical studies of the human clitoris," J UROL 162(3, Pt 2):1015-1020, Sep, 1999.

Bazhenov DV, Blinova NV. "Morphological and functional characteristics of the urogenital diaphragm in women" (article in Russian), MORFOLOGIIA,122(4):64-67, 2002.

Betschart C, et al. "Histomorphological analysis of the urogenital diaphragm in elderly women: a cadaver study," INT UROGENECOL J PELVIC FLOOR DYSFUNCT, 19(11):1477-1481, Nov, 2008.

Brandon C, et al. "Anatomy of the perineal membrane as seen in magnetic resonance images of nulliparous women," AM J OBSTET GYNECOL, 200(5):583-588, May, 2009.

Chalker R. THE CLITORAL TRUTH: THE SECRET WORLD AT YOUR FINGERTIPS. Seven Stories Press, New York NY, 2000.

The-Clitoris.com. www.the-clitoris.com, accessed June 23, 2008.

DeLancey J. "Structural aspects of the extrinsic continence mechanism," OBSTET GYNECOL, 72(3, Pt 1): 296-301, Sep, 1988.

Danesino V, Martella E. Chapter V: "Modern conceptions of corpora cavernosa functions in the vagina and clitoris," in Lowry T, et al. THE CLITORIS. Warren Green, Inc., St. Louis MO, 1976.

Dorschner W, et al. "The dispute about the external sphincter and the urogenital triangle," J UROL, 162(6):1942-1945, Dec, 1999.

Funt M, et al. "Normal vaginal axis," SO MED J, 71(12):1534-1535, 1552, Dec, 1978.

Goff BH. "An histologic study of the perivaginal fascia in a nullipara," SURG GYNECOL OBSTET, 52:32-42, Jan, 1931.

Gräfenberg E. "The role of the urethra in female orgasm," INT J SEXOL, 3(3):145-148, Feb, 1950.

Helstrom K, Lundberg P. "Vibratory perception thresholds in the female genital region," ACTA NEUROL SCAND, 86(6):635-637, Dec, 1992.

Henle J. HANDBUCH DER SYSTEMATISCHEN ANATOMIE DES MENSCHEN, Bd II. Druck und Verlag von Fredrich Vieweg un Sohn, Braunaschweig Germany, 1873.

Hilliges M, et al. "Innervation of the human vaginal mucosa as revealed by PGP 9.5 immunohistochemistry," ACTA ANAT (BASEL), 153(2):119-126, 1995.

Hines T. "The G-spot: a modern gynecologic myth," AM J OBSTET GYNECOL, 185(2):359-362, Aug, 2001.

Hirst BC. A TEXTBOOK OF DISEASES OF WOMEN. WB Saunders & Co., Philadelphia PA, 1903.

Hudson CN, et al. "The anatomy of the perineal membrane: its relationship to injury in childbirth and episiotomy," AUST N Z J OBSTET GYNAECOL, 42(2):193-196, May, 2002. (Comment in AUST N Z J OBSTET GYNAECOL, 42(5):577-578, Nov, 2002.)

Huffman J. "The detailed anatomy of the paraurethral ducts in the adult human female," AM J OBSTET GYNECOL, 55(1):86-101, Jan, 1948.

Jannini E, et al. Chapter 4.3: "Histology and immunohistochemical studies of female genital tissue," in Goldstein I, et al., eds. WOMEN'S SEXUAL FUNCTION AND DYSFUNCTION: STUDY, DIAGNOSIS AND TREATMENT. Taylor & Francis, New York NY, 2006.

Jocelyn H, Setchell B. "Regnier de Graaf on the human reproductive organs: an annotated translation of TRACTATUS DE VIRORUM ORGANIS GENERATIONI INSERVIENTIBUS (1668) and DE MULLIRUM ORGANIS GENERATIONI INSERVIENTIBUS TRACTATUS NOVUS (1672)," J REPRODUCTION FERTIL (Suppl. 17), 1972.

Kato M, et al. "Female perineal membrane: a study using pelvic floor semiserial sections from elderly nulliparous and multiparous women," INT UROGYNECOL J PELVIC FLOOR DYSFUNCT, 19(12):1663-1670, Dec, 2008.

Kuhn R, Hollyhock V. "Observations on the anatomy of the rectovaginal pouch and septum," OBSTET GYENCOL, 59(4):445-447, Apr, 1982.

Lowry T, ed. THE CLASSIC CLITORIS: HISTORIC CONTRIBUTIONS TO SCIENTIFIC SEXUALITY. Nelson-Hall, Chicago IL, 1978.

Lowry T, et al. THE CLITORIS. Warren Green Inc., St. Louis MO, 1976.

Lukban J, Whitmore K. "Pelvic floor muscle re-education treatment of the overactive bladder and painful bladder syndrome," CLIN OBSTET GYNECOL, 45(1):273-285, Mar, 2002.

Milley PS, Nichols DH. "A correlative investigation of the human rectovaginal septum," ANAT REC, 163(3): 443-451, Mar, 1969.

Mirilas P, Skandalakis JE. "Urogenital diaphragm: an erroneous concept casting its shadow over the sphincter urethrae and deep perineal space," J AM COLL SURG,198(2):279-290, Feb, 2004. (Erratum in J AM COLL SURG,198[5]:858, May, 2004.)

Moore L, Clarke A. "Clitoral conventions and transgressions: graphic representations in anatomy texts," FEMINIST STUDIES, 21(2):255-302, Sum, 1995.

Narjani A (pseudonym of Marie Bonaparte), "Considérations sur les causes anatomiques de la frigidité chez la femme," (article in French) BRUXELLES-MÉDICAL, 42:768-778, 1924, cited in Drenth J. THE ORIGIN OF THE WORLD: SCIENCE AND FICTION OF THE VAGINA. Reaktion Books, London UK, 2005.

Nichols DH, Milley PS. "Surgical significance of the rectovaginal septum," AM J OBSTET GYNECOL, 108(2):215-220, Sep 15, 1970.

O'Connell H, DeLancey J. "Clitoral anatomy in nulliparous, healthy, premenopausal volunteers using unenhanced magnetic resonance imaging," J UROL, 173(6):2060-2063, Jun, 2005.

O'Connell H, et al. "The anatomy of the distal vagina: towards unity," J SEXUAL MED, 5(8):1883-1891, Aug, 2008.

O'Connell H, et al. "Anatomy of the clitoris," J UROL,174(4 Pt. 1):1189-95, Oct, 2005.

O'Connell H, et al. "Anatomical relationship between urethra and clitoris," J UROL, 159(6):1892-1897, Jun, 1998.

Perry J, Whipple B. "Pelvic muscle strength of female ejaculators: evidence in support of a new theory of orgasm," J SEX RES, 17:22-39, 1981.

Ricci J, et al. "The relationship of the vagina to adjacent organs in reconstructive surgery," AM J SURG, 74:387-410, Oct, 1947.

Richardson AC. "The rectovaginal septum revisited: its relationship to rectocele and its importance in rectocele repair," CLIN OBSTET GYNECOL, 36(4):976-983, Dec, 1993.

Riley A, Trimmer E. Chapter 15: "Physiology of human female sexual response," in Philipp E, et al., eds. SCIENTIFIC FOUNDATIONS OF OBSTETRICS AND GYNECOLOGY, 4th ed. Butterworth Heinemann, Oxford UK, 1991.

Schultz W, et al. "Magnetic resonance imaging of male and female genitals during coitus and female sexual arousal," BMJ, 319(7225):1596-1600, Dec 18-25, 1999.

Shafik A, et al. "Surgical anatomy of the perineal muscles and their role in perineal disorders," ANAT SCI INTERNAT, 80(3):167-171, Sep, 2005.

Shaktini N. ON MONIQUE WITTIG: THEORETICAL, POLITICAL AND LITERARY ESSAYS. U of Illinois Press, Chicago IL, 2005.

Siegal H. "Clinical significance of the rectovaginal septum," AM J PROCTOL, 15:386-395, Oct, 1964.

Skene A. "The anatomy and pathology of two important glands of the female urethra," AM J OBSTET DIS WOMEN CHILDREN, 13:265-270, 1880.

Stein T, DeLancey J. "Structure of the perineal membrane in females: gross and microscopic anatomy," OBSTET GYNECOL, 111(3):686-693, Mar, 2008.

Stepp K, Walters M. Chapter 2: "Anatomy of the lower urinary tract, rectum and pelvic floor," in Walters M, Karram M, eds. UROGYNECOLOGY AND RECONSTRUCTIVE PELVIC SURGERY, 3rd ed. Mosby Elsever, Philadelphia PA, 2007.

Suh DD, et al. "Magnetic resonance imaging anatomy of the female genitalia in premenopausal and postmenopausal women," J UROL, 170(1):138-144, Jul, 2003.

Tarcan T, et al. "Histomorphometric analysis of age-related structural changes in human clitoral cavernosal tissue," J UROL, 161(3):940-944, Mar, 1999.

Tepper SL, et al. "Homology between the female paraurethral (Skene's) glands and the prostate: immunohistochemical demonstration," ARCH PATHOL LAB MED, 108(5):423-425, May, 1984.

Thorek P. Chapter 36: "Female perineum," in ANATOMY IN SURGERY, 3rd ed. Springer-Verlag, New York NY, 1985.

Toesca A, et al. "Immunohistochemical study of the corpora cavernosa of the human clitoris," J ANAT, 188(Pt 3):513-520, Jun, 1996.

van Turnhout A, et al. "The female corpus spongiosum revisited," ACTA OBSTET GYNECOL SCAND, 74(10):767-771, Nov, 1995.

Verkauf B, et al. "Clitoral size in normal women," OBSTET GYNECOL, 80(1):41-44, Jul, 1992.

Wimpissinger F, et al. "The female prostate revisited: perineal ultrasound and biochemical studies of female ejaculate," J SEX MED, 4(5):1388-1393, Sep, 2007.

Woodman PJ, Graney DO. "Anatomy and physiology of the female perineal body with relevance to obstetrical injury and repair," CLIN ANAT, 15(5):321-334, Aug, 2002.

Yucel S, et al. "Neuroanatomy of the human female lower urogenital tract," J UROL 172(1):191-195, Jul, 2004.

Zaviacic M, Ablin F. "The female prostate and prostate-specific antigen. Immunohistochemical localization, implications for this prostate marker in women, and reasons for using the term 'prostate' in the human female," HISTOL HISTOPATHOL, 15(1):131-142, Jan, 2000.

Zaviacic M, et al. "The female prostate: history, functional morphology and sexology implications" (French with English translation), SEXOLOGIES, 11(41):38-49, 2002.

THE LEVATOR ANI MUSCLE COMPLEX AND RELATED STRUCTURES

Aronson MP, et al. "Anatomy of anal sphincters and related structures in continent women studied with magnetic resonance imaging," OBSTET GYNECOL, 76(5, Pt. 1):846-851, Nov, 1990.

Ashton-Miller J, DeLancey J. "Functional anatomy of the female pelvic floor," ANN NY ACAD SCI, 1101: 266-296, Apr, 2007.

Ayoub S. "The anterior fibres of the levator ani muscle in man," J ANAT, 128(3):571-580, 1979.

Azpiroz F, et al. "The puborectalis muscle," NEURO GASTROENTEROL MOTIL, 17(Suppl 1):68-72, Jun, 2005.

Baragi R, et al. "Differences in pelvic floor area between African American and European American women," AM J OBSTET GYNECOL, 187(1):111-115, Jul, 2002.

Beersiek F, et al. "Pathogenesis of anorectal incontinence: a histometric study of the anal sphincter musculature," J NEUROL SCI, 42(1):111-127, Jun, 1979.

Curtis A, et al. "The anatomy of the pelvic and urogenital diaphragms, in relation to urethrocele and cystocele," SURG GYNECOL OBSTET, 68(2):161-166, Feb 1, 1939.

D'Auglignac D, et al. "A shell finite element model of the pelvic floor muscles," COMPUTER METHODS IN BIOTECH BIOMED ENG, 8(5):339-347, Oct, 2005.

Dickinson R. "Studies of the levator ani muscle," AM J OBSTET DIS WOMEN CHILD, 22(9):897-917, Sep, 1889.

Garavoglia M, et al. "Arrangement of the anal striated musculature," DIS COLON RECTUM, 36(1):10-15, Jan, 1993.

Goh V, et al. "Dynamic MR imaging of the pelvic floor in asymptomatic subjects," AJR AM J ROENTGENOL, 174(3):661-666, Mar, 2000.

Goldberg R. Chapter 3: "Effects of pregnancy and childbirth on the pelvic floor," in Culligan P, Goldberg R, eds. UROGYNECOLOGY IN PRIMARY CARE. Springer-Verlag, London UK, 2007.

Halban J, Tandler J. ANATOMIE UND ATIOLOGIE DER GENITAL PROLAPSE BEIM WEIBE [ANATOMY AND ETIOLOGY OF GENITAL PROLAPSE IN WOMEN] (text in German). Willheln Braumüller, Vienna Austria, 1907.

Handa V, et al. "Architectural differences in the bony pelvis of women with and without pelvic floor disorders," OBSTET GYNECOL, 102(6):1283-1290, Dec, 2003.

Herschorn S. "Female pelvic floor anatomy: the pelvic floor, supporting structures, and pelvic organs," REV UROL, 6(Suppl 5):S2-S10, 2004.

Hjartardóttir S, et al. "The female pelvic floor: a dome–not a basin," ACTA OBSTET GYNECOL SCAND, 76(6):567-571, Jul, 1997.

Hulme J. BEYOND KEGELS: FABULOUS EXERCISES AND MORE, 2nd ed. Phoenix, Missoula MT, 2002.

Hsu Y, et al. "Levator plate angle in women with pelvic organ prolapse compared to women with normal support using dynamic MR imaging," AM J OBSTET GYNECOL, 194(5): 1427-1433, May, 2006.

Hoyte L. "MR-based 3-D female pelvic floor anatomy: the asymptomatic case, genuine stress incon-tinence, prolapse," slide presentation. www.spl.harvard.edu/archive/spl-pre2007/pages/ppl/lennox/tutorial/img0.html. Accessed Jun 7, 2009.

Hugosson C. "Morphology of the pelvic floor," LANCET, 337(8737):367, Feb 9, 1991.

Janda S, et al. "Measuring morphological parameters of the pelvic floor for finite element modelling purposes," J BIOMECH, 36(6):749-757, Jun, 2003.

Kearney R, et al. "Levator ani muscle anatomy evaluated by origin-insertion pairs," OBSTET GYNECOL, 104(1):168-173, Jul, 2004.

Lawson J. "Pelvic anatomy: 1. pelvic floor muscles," ANN ROYAL COL SURG ENG, 54:244-252, Jan-Jun, 1974.

Lien K-C, et al. "Levator ani muscle stretch induced by simulated vaginal birth," OBSTET GYNECOL, 103(1):31-40, Jan, 2004.

Macchi V, et al. "Histopographic study of the pubovaginalis muscle," PELVIPERINEOLOGY, 27(8): 7-9, Mar, 2008.

Margulies RU, et al. "Origin and insertion points involved in levator ani muscle defects," AM J OBSTET GYNECOL, 196(3):251.e1-5, Mar, 2007.

Margulies RU, et al. "Appearance of the levator ani muscle subdivisions in magnetic resonance images," OBSTET GYNECOL, 107(5):1064-1069, May, 2006.

Martins J, et al. "Finite element studies of the deformation of the pelvic floor," ANN NY ACAD SCI, 1101:316-334, Apr, 2007.

Noakes KF, et al. "Anatomically based computational models of the male and female pelvic floor and anal canal," CONF PROC IEEE ENG MED BIOL SOC,1:3815-3818, 2006.
Oh C, Kark AE. "Anatomy of the perineal body," DIS COLON RECTUM,16(6):444-454, Nov-Dec, 1973.
Parikh M, et al. "Three dimensional virtual reality model of the normal female pelvic floor," ANN BIOMED ENGIN, 32(2):292-296, Feb, 2004.
Piloni V, et al. "Dynamic imaging of the normal pelvic floor," INT J COLORECTAL DIS, 12(4):246-253, 1997.
Roberts W, et al. "The levator ani muscles and the nerve supply of its puborectalis component," CLIN ANAT, 1:267-283, 1988.
Singh K, et al. "Magnetic resonance imaging of normal levator ani anatomy and function," OBSTET GYNECOL, 99(3):433-438, Mar, 2002.
Smith W. "The levator ani muscles; its structure in man, and its comparative relationships," ANAT REC, 26(3):175-203, Oct, 1923.
Snooks S, Swash M. "The innervation of the muscles of continence," ANN ROYAL COL SURG ENG, 68(1):45-49, Jan, 1986.
Strohbehn K. "Normal pelvic floor anatomy," OBSTET GYNECOL CLIN NO AM, 25(4):683-705, Dec, 1998.
Strohbehn K, et al. "Magnetic resonance imaging of the levator ani with anatomic correlation," OBSTET GYNECOL, 87(2):277-285, Feb, 1996.
Tunn R, et al. "Anatomic variations in the levator ani muscle, endopelvic fascia, and urethra in nulliparas evaluated by magnetic resonance imaging," AM J OBSTET GYNECOL, 188(1):116-121, Jan, 2003.
Wall L. "The muscles of the pelvic floor," CLIN OBSTET GYNECOL, 36(4):910-925, Dec, 1993.
Wilson P. "Understanding the pelvic floor," SO AF MED J, 47(26):1150-1167, Jul 7, 1973.

THE ANAL TRIANGLE AND RELATED STRUCTURES

Andrews V, et al. "Occult anal sphincter injuries–myth or reality?" BR J OBSTET GYNAECOL, 113(2):195-200, Feb, 2006.
Bollard R, et al. "Normal female anal sphincter: difficulties in interpretation explained," DIS COLON RECTUM, 45(2):171-175, Feb, 2002.
Chaliha C. "Anal function: effect of pregnancy and delivery," AM J OBSTET GYNECOL, 185(2):427-432, Aug, 2001.
Cook T, Mortensen N. Chapter 5: "Colon, rectum, anus and anal sphincter and the pelvic floor," in Pemberton J, et al. eds. THE PELVIC FLOOR: ITS FUNCTION AND DISORDERS. WB Saunders, London UK, 2002.
Cornella J, et al. "Three-dimensional reconstruction of magnetic resonance images of the anal sphincter and correlation between sphincter volume and pressure," AM J OBSTET GYNECOL, 189(1):130-135, Jul, 2003.
Courtney H. "Anatomy of the pelvic diaphragm and anorectal musculature as related to sphincter preservation in anorectal surgery," 79(1):155-173, Jan, 1950.
Courtney H. "The posterior subsphincteric space, its relation to posterior horseshoe fistula," SURG, GYNECOL OBSTET, 89:222-226, Aug, 1949.
Dalley A. "The riddle of the sphincters: the morphophysiology of the anorectal mechanisms reviewed," AM SURG, 53(5):298-306, May, 1987. (Erratum in: AM SURG, 53(7):398, Jul, 1987.)
DeLancey J, et al. "Internal and external anal sphincter anatomy as it relates to midline obstetric lacerations," OBSTET GYNECOL, 90(6):924-927, Dec, 1997.
Eglitis J, Eglitis I. "The glands of the anal canal in man," OHIO J SCI, 61(2):65-69, Mar, 1961.
Fenner D, et al. "Anatomic and physiologic measurements of the internal and external anal sphincters in normal females," OBSTET GYNECOL, 91(3):369-374, Mar, 1998.
Fowler R. "Landmarks and legends of the anal canal," AUST NZ J SURG, 27(1):1-18, 1957.
Fritsch H, et al. "Anal sphincter complex: reinterpreted morphology and its clinical relevance," DIS COLON RECTUM, 45(2):188-194, Feb, 2002.
Frudinger A, et al. "Changes in anal anatomy following vaginal delivery revealed by anal endosonography," BR J OBSTET GYNECOL,106(3):233-237, Mar, 1999.
Fry R, Kodner I. "Anorectal Disorders," CIBA CLINICAL SYMPOSIA, 37(6):1-32, 1985.
Funt M, et al. "Normal vaginal axis," SO MED J, 71(12):1534-1535, 1552, Dec, 1978.
Garavoglia M, et al. "Arrangement of the anal striated musculature," DIS COLON RECTUM, 36(1):10-15, Jan,

1993.
Goligher J, et al. "The surgical anatomy of the anal canal," BR J SURG, 43(177):51-61, 1955.
Gorsch R. "The sigmoid, rectum and anal canal: relations, attachments and pelvic spaces," CLIN SYMP, 12:35-61, Mar-Apr, 1960.
Hsu Y, et al. "Magnetic resonance imaging and 3-dimensional analysis of external anal sphincter anatomy," OBSTET GYNECOL,106(6):1259-1265, Dec, 2005.
Hussain S, et al. "Endoanal MRI of the anal sphincter complex: correlation with cross-sectional anatomy and histology," J ANAT, 189(Pt. 3):677–682, Dec, 1996.
Klosterhalfen B, et al. "Anatomic nature and surgical significance of anal sinus and anal intramuscular glands," J DIS COLON RECTUM, 34(2):156-160, Feb, 1991.
Lee S-J, Meager A. Chapter 2: "Structure and function of the lower gastrointestinal tract," in Brubaker L, et al., eds. THE FEMALE PELVIS: DISORDER OF FUNCTION AND SUPPORT. FA Davis, Philadelphia PA, 1996.
Lunniss P, Phillips R. "Anatomy and function of the anal longitudinal muscle," BR J SURG, 79(9):882-884, Sep, 1992. (Comment in BR J SURG, 80[2]:262, Feb, 1993.)
Macchi V, et al. "Histo-topographic study of the longitudinal anal muscle," CLIN ANAT, 21(5):447-452, Jul, 2008.
Milligan E, Morgan C. "Surgical anatomy of the anal canal with special reference to anorectal fistulae," LANCET, 2:1150-1156, Nov 24, 1934; LANCET, 2:1213-1217, Dec 1, 1934.
Oh C, Kark AE. "Anatomy of the external anal sphincter," BR J SURG, 59(9):717-723, Sep, 1972.
Petros P. THE FEMALE PELVIC FLOOR. Springer, Heidelberg Germany, 2004.
Schäfer A, et al. "Anatomy of the anal sphincters: comparison of anal endosonography to magnetic resonance imaging," DIS COLON RECTUM, 37(8):777-781, Aug, 1994.
Sentovich S, et al. "Diagnosing anal sphincter injury with transanal ultrasound and manometry," DIS COLON RECTUM, 40(12):1430-1444, Dec, 1997.
Seow-Choen F, Ho J. "Histoanatomy of anal glands," J DIS COLON RECTUM, 37(12):1215-1218, Dec, 1994.
Shafik A. "A new concept of the anatomy of the anal sphincter mechanism and the physiology of defecation. VIII. Levator hiatus and tunnel: anatomy and function," DIS COLON RECTUM, 22(8):539-549, Nov-Dec, 1979.
Shafik A. "A new concept of the anatomy of the anal sphincter mechanism and the physiology of defecation. III. The longitudinal anal muscle: anatomy and role in anal sphincter mechanism," INVESTIGATIVE UROL, 13(4):271-277, Jan, 1976.
Shafik A. "A new concept of the anatomy of the anal sphincter mechanism and the physiology of defecation. The external anal sphincter: a triple-loop system," INVESTIGATIVE UROL, 12(5):412-419, Mar, 1975b.
Uz A, et al. "Internal anal sphincter: an anatomic study," CLIN ANAT, 17(1):17-20, Jan, 2004.
Wilde R. "The anal intermuscular septum," BR J SURG, 36(143):279-285, Jan, 1949.

PRIMARY INNERVATION OF THE LEVATOR ANI COMPLEX AND THE PERINEAL MUSCLES

Barber M, et al. "Innervation of the female levator ani muscles," AM J OBSTET GYNECOL, 187(1):64-71, Jul, 2002.
Guaderrama NM, et al. "Evidence for the innervation of pelvic floor muscles by the pudendal nerve," OBSTET GYNECOL. Oct 106(4):774-781, Oct, 2005.
Perchers U, et al. "Cross-sectional imaging anatomy of the anal sphincters," OBSTET GYNECOL, 90(5):839-844, Nov, 1997.
Shafik A, Doss S. "Surgical anatomy of the somatic terminal innervation to the anal and urethral sphincters: role in anal and urethral surgery," J UROL, 161(1):85-89, Jan, 1999. (Erratum in J UROL, 164[3, Pt. 1]:784, Sep, 2000).
Swash M. Chapter 2: "Innervation of the bladder, urethra and pelvic floor," in Drife J, et al., eds. MICTURITION. Springer-Verlag, London UK, 1990.
Wallner C, et al. "Innervation of the pelvic floor muscles: a reappraisal of the levator ani nerve," OBSTET GYNECOL, 108(3, Pt 1):529-534, Sep, 2006.

MORE ABOUT THE PELVIC CONNECTIVE TISSUES

Albright TS, et al. "Arcus tendineus fascia pelvis: a further understanding," AM J OBSTET GYNECOL, 193(3, Pt 1):677-781, Sep, 2005.

Bastian D, Lassau J. "The suspensory mechanism of the uterus: anatomical basis for the statics and dynamics of the normal uterus," SURG RADIOL ANAT, 4(2):147-160, Jun, 1982.

Berglas B, Rubin I. "Histologic study of the pelvic connective tissue," SURG GYNECOL OBSTET, 97(3):277-289, Sep, 1953.

Boreham M, et al. "Morphometric analysis of smooth muscle in the anterior vaginal wall of women with pelvic organ prolapse," AM J OBSTET GYNECOL, 187(1):56-63, Jul, 2002.

DeLancey J. "Anatomy and biomechanics of genital prolapse," CLIN OBSTET GYNECOL, 36(4):897-909, Dec, 1993.

Dox I, et al. MELLONI'S ILLUSTRATED DICTIONARY OF OBSTETRICS AND GYNECOLOGY. Parthenon Pub., New York NY, 2000.

Ghoniem G, Davila W, eds. PRACTICAL GUIDE TO FEMALE PELVIC MEDICINE. Taylor & Francis Group, London UK, 2006.

Koster H. "On the supports of the uterus," AM J OBSTET GYNECOL, 25:67-74, Jan, 1933.

Laurent T, Fraser J. "Hyaluronan," FASEB J, 6(7):2397-2404, Apr, 1992.

Leffler KS, et al. "Attachment of the rectovaginal septum to the pelvic sidewall," AM J OBSTET GYNECOL, 185(1):41-43, Jul, 2001.

Liu C. "Laparoscopic pelvic reconstructive surgery: part I," http://findarticles.com/p/articles /mi_m0CYD/is_19_39/ai_n6260211/print, OB/GYN NEWS, Oct 1, 2004. Accessed Jan 14, 2008.

Occelli B, et al. "Anatomic study of arcus tendineus fasciae pelvis," EUR J OBSTET GYNECOL, 97:213-219, 2002.

Olinger A. PhD. Discussion about path of pudendal nerve. Western States Chiropractic College, Portland, OR, Oct 12, 2009.

Pasley W. "Sacrospinous suspension: a local practitioner's guide," AM J OBSTET GYNECOL, 173(2):440-445, Aug, 1995.

Petros P. "Vault prolapse I: dynamic supports of the vagina," INT UROGYNECOL J, 12(5):292-295, 2001.

Pit M, et al. "Anatomy of the arcus tendineus fasciae pelvic in females," CLIN ANAT, 16(2):131-137, Mar, 2003.

Rogers R, Richardson C. Chapter 8: "Clinical evaluation of pelvic support defects with anatomic correlations," in Bent A, et al. OSTERGARD'S UROGYNECOLOGY AND PELVIC FLOOR DYSFUNCTION, 5th ed. Lippincott, Williams & Wilkins, Philadelphia PA, 2003.

Smith E. "Studies in the anatomy of the pelvis, with special reference to the fasiæ and visceral supports: Part 1," J ANAT PHYSIOL, 42:198-218, Jan, 1908.

Yabuki Y, et al. "Discrepancies between classic anatomy and modern gynecologic surgery on pelvic connective tissue structure: harmonization of those concepts by collaborative cadaver dissection," AM J OBSTET GYNECOL, 193(1): 7-15, Jul, 2005.

Valaitis S. Chapter 8: "Anterior compartment prolapse, urinary incontinence, and the effects of anterior colporrhaphy and paravaginal repair," in Lentz G, ed. UROGYNECOLOGY. Oxford U Press, New York NY, 2000.

MAINTAINING PERINEAL INTEGRITY DURING LABOR AND BIRTH

PREPARING THE PERINEAL TISSUES FOR BIRTH

Ethnicity and the Risk of Sustaining Tears at Birth

In a study of 17,216 women, Hopkins and colleagues (2005) found that ethnicity and racial background influence the risk of tearing. Caucasian women, who represented the largest group in this study, were considered the baseline population to which other groups were compared (other groups are listed in descending order of risk). In general, the greatest variation in risk existed for second-, third-, and fourth-degree perineal lacerations, with or without a clitorotomy. There was little difference in the risk of yoni floor laceration and the risk of cervical laceration was the same across all races and ethnicities studied.

Chinese, Filipino and other Asian women had a higher frequency of third- and fourth-degree tears. Chinese, Filipino, other Asian and Latina women showed a slightly higher than average rate of yoni laceration. Only Chinese and Filipino women were at a higher than average risk for all types of lacerations considered. Among the 8951 women who did not receive a clitorotomy, Chinese, Filipino, Japanese, other Asians and Latina women still had a greater frequency of second-, third- and fourth-degree lacerations. Potential reasons for these differences include maternal tissue strength and anatomy, variation in fetal weight, socioeconomic (i.e., nutritional) status, the type of care received at the time of birth and, perhaps most significantly, the position of the women as they pushed their babies out, a detail that was not mentioned in these studies.

Preventive Measures for the Prenatal Period

Good Nutrition

Good nutrition is your first line of defense against almost every complication, and tearing is no exception. This isn't to say that healthy, well-nourished women don't tear; they do. But strong, elastic tissue will usually tear less extensively and will always heal better than the tissue of a poorly nourished woman. During pregnancy, a high protein, whole-food, preferably organic diet with fresh fruits and vegetables and adequate salt, calories and fluids is ideal. When such high-quality food is not affordable, help women to make the best food choices possible. JuicePlus+ food concentrates can provide nutritional backup without the worry of imbalanced supplements or overdosing on any one nutrient. See my HOLISTIC MIDWIFERY: VOL. I: CARE DURING PREGNANCY for more information on nutrition.

Assessing and preparing the pelvic floor for birth

Pelvic floor health affects us for a lifetime. Like other muscle groups, the pelvic floor can be adversely affected when used improperly and weakened when proper exercise is neglected. The pelvic muscles are more vulnerable to damage during birth if they are not functioning normally.

Understanding normal and dysfunctional pelvic floor tone: Before advising a woman regarding pelvic floor preparation, it is important to assess her baseline tone. Pelvic floor tone is characterized as normal, high or low. While proper strengthening exercises are appropriate to help maintain normal tone and for women with low tone, those with high tone need to learn to relax their pelvic floor. Once normal function has been restored, they can learn to work with their muscles properly to avoid recreating the problem all over again.

Normal tone: A healthy pelvic floor has both tone and elasticity. Normal tone is demonstrated when women are completely continent of urine, feces and flatus. Urine flows easily without discomfort in a steady stream without pushing or straining until the bladder is empty. Urination takes place four to six times daily and not at all or only once at night. Each voiding produces at least 300 to 400 mL of urine, indicating that the bladder can easily retain this much urine without discomfort or leakage. Aging results in a slight reduction in bladder capacity, with older adults normally urinating up to eight times a day. Initially, the first urges to urinate signal that the bladder is stretching and may be felt even before the bladder is full. Normally, these initial sensations can be controlled, and a full bladder can be tolerated for a while before it must be emptied.

Healthy pelvic tone is also characterized by a pain-free pelvis with pelvic organs that are normally positioned and well supported. Women with healthy tone can identify when their muscles are tight and when they are relaxed and can contract and relax their pelvic muscles without recruiting adjacent muscles in their buttocks, abdomen or legs. Their pelvic muscles exhibit normal resting tone and contours on MRI studies.

At the time of birth, normal tone greatly increases the likelihood that a woman's perineum will stretch rather than tear and that it will return to an optimal postbirth condition. Properly toned muscles help prompt and maintain optimal positioning of the presenting part and anterior rotation of the occiput. When the toned pelvic floor is well applied to the presenting part, receptors in the yoni are stimulated, leading to a spontaneous urge to push.

Dysfunctional tone: Pelvic floor dysfunction describes any impairment of tone, contractile force or both within the muscles. The nuances of these conditions vary widely among individuals. Dysfunctional tone may be initially caused by some sort of abuse and may be induced or enhanced by regular jumping, running or fast walking, all of which increase downward pressure on the pelvic floor (Chaitow, 2006). Repeated episodes of intense pressure can either create or aggravate low-tone conditions or contribute to the development of high-tone dysfunction, depending upon the baseline condition of the tissues and how a woman uses her pelvic floor and adjacent muscles when responding to the stress.

While, as a general rule, exercise tends to strengthen muscles, it is equally important to know when and how to relax muscles or overly tense muscles may develop. Exercise enthusiasts understand the importance of stretching at the end of a session. Unfortunately, while tightening the pelvic floor is easy, relaxing it is far less so because the muscles normally retain tone when at rest. Stretching the pelvic floor directly during normal exercise is virtually impossible because it is contained within the bony ring of the pelvis. Leg, spinal and abdominal stretches indirectly act to stretch and relax the pelvic floor.

Urinary symptoms may be associated with either high- or low-tone pelvic floor dysfunction, even without prolapse, because the tone and contractility of the pelvic floor muscles influence lower urinary tract function and perceptions of bladder filling and storage.

One such symptom is **urinary incontinence**, defined as the involuntary loss of urine. There are several types. **Stress incontinence** occurs during exertion (such as coughing). **Urge incontinence** results in urinary leakage preceded by a strong, sudden urge (due to contraction of the bladder wall). Some women have **mixed incontinence** (both kinds). Another symptom, **urinary frequency**, occurs when the urge to urinate arises often and usually reflects a reduction in bladder capacity, a problem that can be induced by voiding too frequently, before the bladder is really full.

Low tone: Low pelvic floor tone, leading to conditions such as incontinence and organ prolapse, is the most recognized type of pelvic floor dysfunction. It is characterized by an impaired ability to isolate and contract the pelvic floor muscles in the presence of weak or atrophic musculature. Low-tone dysfunction is associated with habitual straining, trauma (especially that associated with childbirth), denervation, connective tissue laxity and aging. Overactive bladder symptoms such as urgency, frequency and stress incontinence are frequently seen as well. Fecal incontinence may also occur (Lukban & Whitmore, 2002).

Women with low tone may experience malposition of the fetal presenting part prior to or during labor but seldom have problems pushing their babies out, as the muscles are lax. They may, however, develop increasingly weak muscle tone with each pregnancy or as they age unless they are taught how to strengthen their pelvic floor and how to work with the muscles properly during normal daily activities.

High tone: High-tone pelvic floor dysfunction can be equally debilitating, although it has been discussed less frequently in the medical literature. High-tone dysfunction has been recognized for some time under a variety of names: coccygodynia (Thiele, 1937); tension myalgia of the pelvic floor; coccygeus-levator spasm syndrome; levator syndrome and levator spasm syndrome.

High-tone dysfunction is the product of hyperclonic or spastic pelvic floor musculature. It is most often found in young, very active, nulliparous women, many of whom engage in strenuous exercise such as running, aerobics, balance ball work, bicycling, gymnastics or dance, or practice Pilates, yoga or similar strengthening exercises with insufficient emphasis on relaxation and flexibility. Other factors include stress and the general body tension that accompanies it. Prolonged sitting with poor posture or sacroiliac dysfunction may also be contributory and can aggravate symptoms because these conditions distort the relationship of the pelvic bones, resulting in unequal tension on the pelvic muscles. The muscles that attach to the pelvis may be extremely shortened, especially the adductors (muscles of the groin and inner thigh), the hip flexors and the "core stabilizing" muscles of the abdomen. Indiscriminately recommending pelvic floor exercises to every woman will result in worsening the symptoms of women with high-tone dysfunction, with increased spasm and uncoordinated muscle contraction, neither of which will help during labor.

Associated signs and symptoms include urinary urgency or frequency (overactive bladder). Painful bladder syndrome (interstitial cystitis) may also occur, perhaps due to the guarding and tension that develops in the bladder wall. This can present with painful urination, voiding dysfunction, sexual dysfunction, or fecal retention. Other symptoms include stress incontinence; vulvar, rectal or pelvic pain; pain in the coccyx or lower sacrum;

pain with sexual or other forms of penetration (such as inserting a speculum); orgasmic dysfunction; low back pain; and a "heavy feeling in the pelvis" (Lukban & Whitmore, 2002). Hypertonus may be severe enough to cause urinary retention with enlargement of the bladder to the point that the yoni canal becomes obstructed, leading to pain upon yoni penetration or even blockage of the menstrual flow (Chaitow, 2006).

A high-toned, unyielding pelvic floor can hold the pelvic bones rigidly in place during labor and resist fetal descent or stretching, promoting asynclitism of the fetal head. It may impair or even prevent fetal descent, posing a real obstacle to normal birth. Forcing a baby through an unrelaxed pelvic floor also strains and can damage the pelvic connective tissues. Performing a clitorotomy to eliminate muscle resistance can work to get the baby out, but it leaves the woman with an incision through thick, undilated tissues.

***Mixed tone*:** Women can also have mixed-tone dysfunction, where only some muscles are either too tense, excessively relaxed or both. This can lead to unilateral findings of excessive tension, laxity or pain, a weak urine stream; urinary frequency, urgency or retention; constipation; or pain with yoni penetration or even from external sexual stimulation.

Assessing pelvic floor tone: Everyone can benefit from a screening evaluation of their pelvic floor tone, especially those experiencing urinary or fecal continence problems, since various types of dysfunction can lead to similar signs and symptoms.

To assess the tonicity of the pelvic floor, begin by taking a careful history. When women report problems that suggest pelvic floor dysfunction, other causes of pelvic or genital discomfort such as urinary tract or yoni infection, a low-fiber diet leading to constipation and other similar conditions need to be ruled out or resolved as appropriate.

If a muscle tone issue is suspected, next perform an internal digital exam to assess the pelvic floor muscles for tone, sensitivity to pressure, and voluntary contractile abilities. The following description combines assessments from several sources. It is important to assess both muscle contractility as well as impaired relaxation, indicated by tenderness, to determine the type of tone dysfunction that may be present. Be sure to evaluate both sides of the pelvic cavity. The parenthetical references are explained in the tables that are found on the following page (Lukban & Whitmore, 2002).

1. Begin by inserting one gloved finger into the yoni; apply light pressure against one inferolateral yoni wall and then the other to assess the general condition of the muscles.
2. Then insert two fingers and ask the woman to squeeze your fingers by contracting or lifting her pelvic floor. Observe her abdomen, buttocks and legs for activity in the abdominal, gluteal and adductor muscles to determine if and to what extent she recruits these muscle groups in this effort (Table 2-D). Ideally, she can contract her pelvic floor while leaving these other muscles groups relaxed (i.e., she can isolate and contract her pelvic floor). Assess the degree of squeeze pressure during a contraction (Table 1-A).
3. As she tightens, note the degree of displacement of your examining fingers (Table 1-C) and the length of time she can maintain voluntary pelvic floor contraction (Table 1-B), with at least 5 seconds as the goal.
4. While the pelvic floor muscles are contracted, assess the degree of tightening of the right and left sides separately on a scale of 0 to 4 (Table 2-D). An imbalance in tension from

side to side may indicate a mixed-tone problem if the woman also has signs and symptoms of dysfunction. Slight differences in the thickness of the muscles on either side is very common among women with normal function.

5. Tenderness (Table 2-E), a measure of hypertonicity (impaired relaxation), is assessed next. Ask the woman to completely relax her pelvic floor. As she does so, note if the muscles feel any different to your examining fingers. Once she reports full relaxation, apply pressure to first one and then the opposite inferolateral yoni wall with the pad of your fingers. If the muscles are normally toned or lacking in tone, direct finger-pressure into the relaxed muscle belly should not produce pain. However, if the woman's ability to relax is impaired, pressure will produce varying degrees of pain, which can be severe.
6. Assess the number of sequential, one-second contractions a woman can perform, with 10 being ideal. She should tighten completely and fully relax before tightening again.

The following tables consolidate the findings from these assessments. In each table, normal findings are shown in bold. Table 1 shows findings during voluntary muscle contraction. A value of 3 for each assessment is normal, unless the woman cannot relax her muscles. In Table 2-D, a contractility score of 3, 2, 1 or 0 indicates increasingly severe weakness. In Table 2-E, a tenderness score of 2, 3 or 4 indicates increasingly severe impairment of a woman's ability to relax her pelvic floor. These are all subjective assessments and no standards have been set to establish these diagnoses.

TABLE 1: PELVIC FLOOR MUSCLE CONTRACTION ASSESSMENT PARAMETERS

Score	1-A. Pressure	1-B. Duration	1-C. Displacement of finger
0	None	None	None
1	Weak: examiner feels pressure on sides of fingers, but not all around	< 1 second	Slight incline, base of fingers moves upward
2	Moderate: examiner feels pressure all around finger	1 to 3 seconds	Greater incline, fingers move up along their total length
3	**Strong: fingers come together or overlap**	**> 3 seconds**	**Fingers move up and are drawn in**

TABLE 2: PELVIC FLOOR MUSCLE ASSESSMENT PARAMETERS

Score	2-D. Contractility	2-E. Tenderness (hypertonus)
0	Unable to isolate muscles, or no perceived tightening	No sense of pressure and no pain with exam
1	Light contraction, unable to retain exam finger	**Comfortable pressure with exam**
2	Light contraction, unable to sustain tightening for 1 second	Uncomfortable pressure with exam that gets worse during tightening
3	Moderate contraction, sustained for 3 seconds	Moderate pain with exam that gets worse during tightening
4	**Strong contraction, sustained for 5 seconds or longer**	Severe pain with exam; attempts at tightening the pelvic floor produce pain

(Normal reference parameters are shown in bold.)

Typical findings: Here is what you are likely to find with different conditions.
Normal tone: Women with normal tone can isolate their pelvic floor muscles from other groups of muscles during contraction (although they cannot necessarily selectively contract specific muscles within the pelvic floor, which is generally a learned response). On palpation, their urogenital hiatus is tight, and their pelvic floor feels firm and resilient when at rest. Direct digital pressure is painless. They have normally placed pelvic organs and are free of pelvic symptoms.

Low tone: Women with low-tone pelvic floor dysfunction cannot isolate their pelvic floor muscles when they attempt to contract them, instead they also tighten adjacent muscles, such as those in the abdomen, buttocks and legs. Volitional levator ani contractions are weak and cannot be sustained for long. This is because the muscles are lax; they or their nerve supply may be damaged; rendering the muscles unable to contract normally. The pelvic muscles may feel thin and atrophied with a longer or wider urogenital hiatus and, in severe cases, a lax anal sphincter (Fletcher, 2005).

High tone: Those with high-tone dysfunction also exhibit poor pelvic floor muscle isolation as well as impaired contractility, tenderness or pain with pressure, spasticity and impaired relaxation on digital exam. Voluntary contractility is reduced as is the ability to sustain a contraction. This is so because the muscles are already so tense that they cannot be tensed any more (Chaitow, 2006). Attempts at contraction may actually cause these tense muscles to descend rather than rise up. High-tone pelvic floor muscles may feel thick, boggy or hypertrophied with taut bands in the belly of the muscle (Fletcher, 2005).

Other methods of evaluating pelvic floor tone require a variety of devices that midwives will not typically have access to. Women who require further assessment, for example those with complex or severe symptom pictures, can be referred to a urogynecologist, a physical therapist who works with the pelvic floor, or both, for more sophisticated evaluations.

Therapy for those with high-tone pelvic floor dysfunction

Once you have done a preliminary assessment and have determined that a woman may have high-tone dysfunction, she can start working to correct it right away. Advise women to read Tami Kent's book WILD FEMININE: FINDING POWER, SPIRIT AND JOY IN THE ROOT OF THE FEMALE BODY, which explores emotional and psychological issues associated with pelvic floor dysfunction. Refer her to a psychotherapist for any emotionally-related causes and to a physical therapist who specializes in pelvic floor disorders (and hopefully is aware of emotionally related causes). The physical therapist will evaluate her for pelvic misalignment, lumbar and hip range of motion and the strength and flexibility of the spinal and pelvic-stabilizing muscles, and will perform an internal evaluation of her pelvic floor.

Appropriate physical therapy should then be applied for whatever conditions are identified. Once normal skeletal relationships are restored, the internal exam is repeated. Sometimes this resolves high-tone dysfunction without further therapy.

Full recovery may require a commitment to becoming aware of the pelvic floor and breaking old habits of holding tension in the pelvis. For many women, high-tone dysfunction is a product of habitually holding tension in the pelvic floor that may be a physical expression of a psychologically defended state related to a history of traumatic toilet training, unhealthy habits such as prolonged postponing of urination or defecation, or related to abuse, either physical, sexual or emotional. These women may have both physical relearning and emotional healing to do before the problem is resolved.

Treatment options include a variety of approaches to balance pelvic floor tone. Overactive bladder can be addressed by dietary changes such as limiting bladder irritants including acidic foods and caffeine, timed voiding to achieve a predictable bladder volume and a regime to promote urge inhibition to extend voiding intervals and reduce episodes of incontinence. Other approaches include stabilization of the external pelvis; manual therapy such as massage or trigger point work; electrical stimulation with a yoni or rectal probe to desensitize nerves or to contract and relax pelvic floor muscles; biofeedback to help a woman learn to identify, relax and contract these muscles; and acupuncture as well as home exercise and therapy. A constitutional homeopathic remedy may help; if the woman is interested, she should see a skilled constitutional prescriber. The goal is to help the woman learn how to relax her muscles and not strain them (Lukban & Whitmore, 2002).

While ordinarily hands-on pelvic muscle preparation is postponed until the last six weeks of pregnancy, when high-tone dysfunction is the problem, massage, if appropriate, can begin at any time to restore normal function. Then, in the last trimester, perineal stretching can be done to prepare the tissues for further relaxation and expansion during fetal descent.

Thiele (1937) originated a massage technique that helps to deal with certain types of high-tone pelvic floor dysfunction. During an internal exam, the pelvic floor muscles are firmly stroked in a longitudinal direction from origin to insertion points while the woman relaxes into the pressure as much as possible. Ten to fifteen sweeps of maximally tolerated pressure are performed on each side.

Myofascial massage is also helpful. Steady pressure is applied to areas of tenderness for 10 to 15 seconds, working up to 60 to 90 seconds. Alternatively, a tender spot is found, massaged in a circular motion and then pressure is applied. The pressure helps release and thereby reduce or eliminate tension in the associated muscle, at least temporarily.

These areas of tenderness are referred to as **trigger points**. Trigger points are defined as taut bands either on the surface of or within the belly or the attachment of the muscle. Pressure on a trigger point usually elicits a twitch response that can felt by a sensitive therapist. When a trigger point is touched, the woman will often startle due to pain felt at the point or that is referred to a site remote from it, a frequent occurrence. Pain in the groin, rectum, labia, perineum and other adjacent parts may be referred from tense pelvic muscles. Active trigger points both refer pain and recreate it upon palpation. Latent trigger points may become sources of pain (i.e., become active), but usually the woman does not complain of ongoing pain from latent points (Wise, 2008).

At the end of each treatment session, time should be allotted for the woman to rest and relax before resuming her daily activities. Ongoing awareness and relaxation of the pelvic floor and quieting the nervous system are necessary to avoid undoing the work of the physical therapist. In severe cases muscle relaxants may be prescribed, but these should be avoided during pregnancy.

Recommended activities may include general relaxation techniques such as consciously relaxing her pelvic floor in a warm bath twice daily; stretching her leg and back muscles, which will help to stretch the pelvic floor to the extent possible; maintaining good posture; visualization of her pelvic floor and, eventually, pelvic floor exercises emphasizing control, proper muscle activity and use, and relaxation rather than just strengthening.

Thiele (1937) recommended massage treatments every day for 5 to 6 days and then every other day for 7 to 10 days initially, with follow-up treatments as needed. Lukban and Whitmore (2002) reported success using massage once or twice weekly for 6 to 8 weeks.

When massage or trigger point therapy is indicated, a woman's partner may be able to perform the massage for her at home after she has been properly evaluated and she and her partner have been shown what to do by the physical therapist. These women can also be taught abdominal breathing (see the entry entitled "Abdominal or 'happy baby' breathing" on page 151) as they work to restore normal pelvic floor tone.

Pelvic floor activities and exercises to create more awareness of proper muscle function for those with normal- or low-tone pelvic floor muscles

To begin with, it is important to grasp that the pelvic floor muscles do not work in isolation. Their activity must be coordinated with the muscles of the diaphragm and the deep abdomen.

Rhythmically tightening and consciously relaxing the low-tone or normal-tone pelvic floor helps maintain strong, resilient muscles with good genital sphincter control. When appropriate, teach women to work with their pelvic floor, beginning early in prenatal care. This, along with perineal stretching during the last six weeks of pregnancy, encourages elasticity. Learning how to properly care for the pelvic floor may take practice. It starts with tuning in to how these muscles are being used daily, understanding the baseline condition of the pelvic floor (normal, high, or low tone) and changes that may be needed in the daily relationship to the pelvic floor muscles. Learning proper use of the pelvic floor can retrain a woman with high-tone dysfunction so that she does not recreate the problem. For parous women whose pelvic floor has become lax, these recommendations can help restore normal function and guard against further weakening.

Anatomical review pertinent to learning proper pelvic floor activity: Pelvic floor therapists emphasize that the abdominal muscles and the diaphragm are all involved in pelvic floor function. The abdominal muscles consist of several broad pairs of muscular sheets arranged in more or less horizontal layers. There are three layers of flat muscle sheets that originate posterolaterally, pass anteriorly, stopping short of the midline on either side. Between the medial edges of these sheets are the longitudinally-oriented rectus abdominis muscles, which are encased in an **aponeurosis** (A-po-neurosis), which is a sheetlike fibrous membrane, resembling a flattened tendon, that functions as a type of fascia to bind muscles together or as a means of connecting two muscle parts. The parietal fascia of the three horizontal layers contribute to that which makes up the aponeurosis.

The deepest of the horizontal sheets is the **transverse layer**, which has fibers that are the most horizontally oriented. This layer originates along the thoracolumbar fascia of the spine, the iliac crest and the lateral third of the inguinal ligament on either side, wraps around the torso to the midline, where each half contributes to the aponeurosis from behind the rectus abdominis muscles. The middle layer is the **internal oblique**, which also originates from the fascia of the thoracolumbar spine, the anterior two-thirds of the iliac crest and the lateral half of the inguinal ligament. These muscles fibers pass to the midline (at a gently upwardly inclined angle above the level of the iliac crest), where their fascial coverings contribute to the aponeurosis. They support the lumbar spine and sacroiliac joints. The most superficial of these three layers are the **external obliques** that originate from the outer surfaces of the lower eight ribs and insert into the lateral edge of the iliac crest. They pass from these points at a declining angle as their fascia merges with the aponeurosis to either side of the midline.

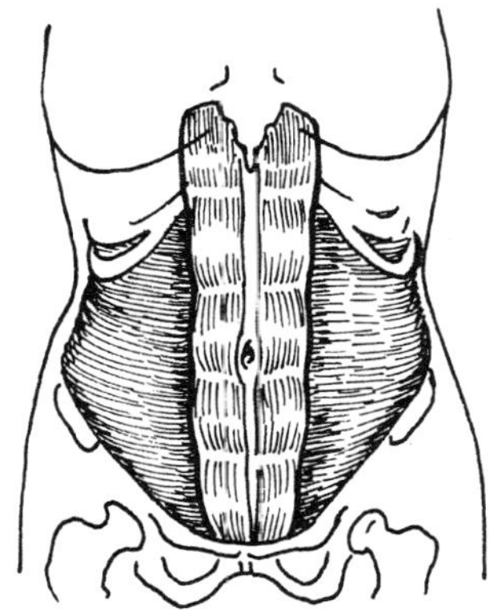

Transverse muscles with unsheathed rectus abdominus muscles in the midline

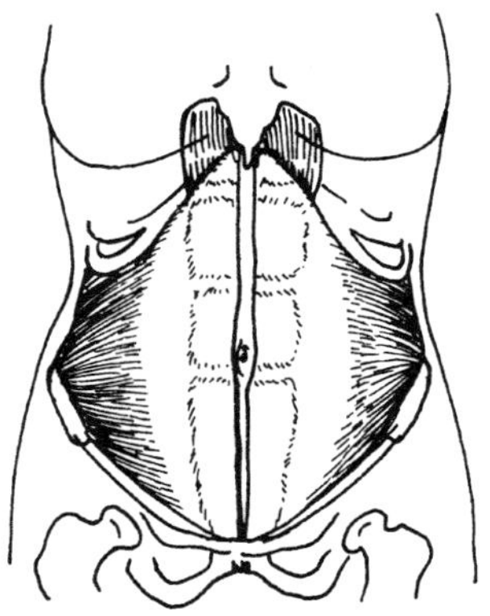

Internal oblique abdominal muscles with aponeurosis enclosing rectus abdominus muscles in the midline

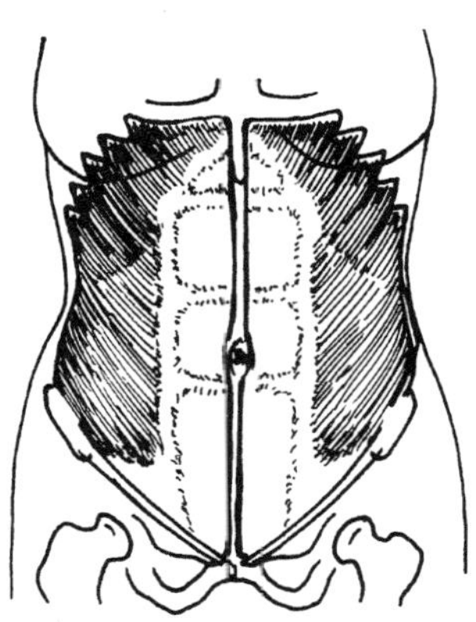

External oblique muscles

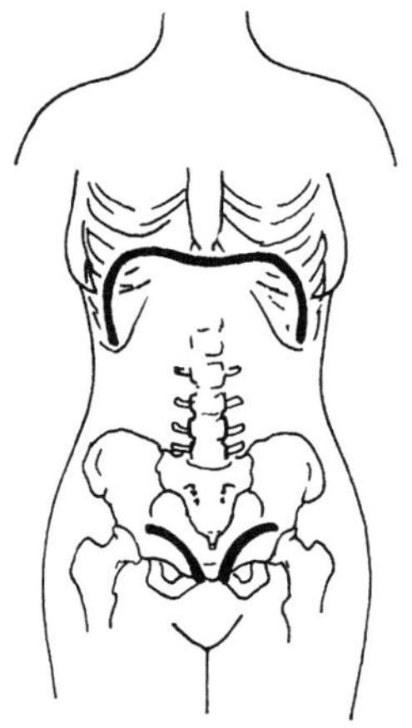

The two diaphragms

To either side of the midline, two vertical muscle bands are enclosed within the aponeurosis; these **rectus abdominis** muscles are the strongest of all the abdominal muscles. (The other pair is the small, sometimes absent, pyramidalis muscle, which is not important to this discussion.) The rectus abdominis muscles originate along the top of the pubic bone and insert into the costal cartilages of the 5th through the 7th ribs. The rectus abdominis muscles work to flex the spine forward and are often recruited to compensate for weakness in the others as well as in the pelvic floor.

The **thoracic diaphragm** is the dome-shaped sheet of musculomembranous tissue that underlies the lower ends of the lungs. It divides the abdominal and thoracic cavities and flexes up and down to move air in and out of the lungs. Humans cannot breathe without a functional diaphragm. The diaphragm is the upper-body compliment to the diaphragmatic activity of the pelvic floor, and these two diaphragms tend to move synchronously during respiration in women with normal pelvic floor tone.

Teaching pelvic floor awareness: Mary O'Dwyer, an Australian pelvic floor physio-therapist, offered some valuable exercises you can share with women to teach them how to tune into their pelvic floor (2008). Her book, MY PELVIC FLAW, (referring to the flaw of not understanding proper pelvic floor care) is available through her web site (www.mypelvicfloor.info) and is worth recommending to your clients. Women who have normal tone or minimal to moderate low-tone dysfunction can begin these exercises right away. Those with high-tone dysfunction should see a specialist and get treatment to restore normal tone before beginning these exercises. For your own reference, FITNESS FOR THE PELVIC FLOOR by Beate Carrière is an excellent addition to your library. The step-by-step explanation of what to teach your clients that follows relies primarily on O'Dwyer, Carrière, my own experience and a few other sources.

For some women, the following exercises are challenging. With practice, the exercises will teach women to breathe more physiologically as well as work with their pelvic floor to avoid or correct prolapse and continence issues and to restore function in those who have low tone.

Anatomy review: Begin by using a model of the pelvic bones to show a woman where her ischial tuberosities, pubic bone and coccyx are located. Describe the linked tissues that reach from the pubic bone to the coccyx, forming a bridge of support. Use illustrations to explain the relevant abdominal muscles and the pelvic and thoracic diaphragms.

Correct sitting posture: Have the woman sit upright in a straight-backed, flat-seated chair, with her weight centered on her tuberosities, not her sacrum. Good sitting posture helps activate the transverse and internal oblique abdominal muscles, which helps to activate the pelvic floor. Slumping forward shifts weight to the sacrum and also recruits the rectus abdominis muscles, which tend to compress the abdominal contents, transferring pressure to the pelvic floor. This results in perineal bulging in women, which is most pronounced in women with low-tone dysfunction.

Abdominal or "happy baby" breathing: This is the way a relaxed baby breathes, which most adults have forgotten how to do (Hendricks & Hendricks, 1991). Ask the woman to lie on the floor with her knees bent and her back pressed flat against the floor. Ask her to spread her hands over her lower abdomen, with her thumbs level with her navel and to breathe slowly and gently. As she inhales, she fills her abdomen with air so that her belly expands under her hands. At the same time, her spine should arch gently upward and her lowermost ribs and abdomen expand to either side and forward, while her shoulders and the rest of her rib cage remain relaxed. Upon exhalation, the abdomen flattens gently and the spine relaxes as her thoracic diaphragm moves up, compressing the lungs to expel the air. Have her breathe like this for a minute or two.

Now direct her attention to her pelvic floor, reminding her that these muscles form her pelvic diaphragm. As she breathes, the pelvic floor should move synchronously with her thoracic diaphragm, gently relaxing with inhalations, as both diaphragms move down, and gently rising with exhalations, as both diaphragms move upward. If she has trouble feeling movement in her pelvic floor while lying supine, have her lie on her side. Women who cannot feel any pelvic muscle movement in either position may be simply unfamiliar with tuning in to their pelvic floor or they may have pelvic floor dysfunction (those with low tone may not sense receding and those with high tone may not sense expansion).

Identifying the pelvic floor muscles: Once a woman has learned abdominal breathing, teach her how to contract her pelvic floor. She can start by going to urinate and contracting her muscles to stop the flow of urine to help her identify the muscles.

After she uses the toilet, have her lie on her back with her knees up. O'Dwyer suggests directing the woman to focus on her urethral meatus, using her finger to identify it if necessary. Guide her finger to her symphysis pubis, down the midline, over and below her clitoral glans to her urethral meatus. Then assist her to find the tip of her coccyx with her other hand.

When she has clearly identified these landmarks, O'Dwyer suggests that she place one hand just above her pubic bone, with her little finger touching the pubic symphysis. Ask her to rest the other hand in the center of her abdomen at the level of her navel.

Have her relax the muscles of her legs, abdomen and anal sphincter. Since the anal sphincter is the pelvic muscle most people can readily identify, if she focuses on exercising the muscles around the urethra and yoni while releasing her anal sphincter, she is more likely to learn to differentiate them.

Now ask her to exhale as she slowly and gently tenses her pelvic floor (doing so gently helps avoid recruiting her rectus abdominis muscles) and to visualize using her pelvic floor muscles to bring her pubic bone in contact with the tip of her coccyx. You can also ask her to place her finger lightly over her urethra and have her pull away from it using the surrounding muscles. When done correctly, she will feel tension in her pelvic floor and in her lower abdomen under her pubic hand. O'Dwyer points out that the lower abdominal tension is subtle, as it is taking place in the internal oblique and transverse abdominal layers that underlie the external oblique and rectus abdominis muscles. The abdominal muscles under her other hand should remain relaxed. Trying too hard tends to recruit muscles in the buttocks, legs and waist and will interfere with identifying the more subtle action of the deeper abdominal muscles.

When a woman is in the habit of tensing her rectus abdominis muscles when she is contracting her pelvic floor, or if her other abdominal muscles or her pelvic floor muscles are weak, she may have to practice awhile before she masters these exercises. When a woman is in the habit of using her rectus abdominis muscles inappropriately, she also contracts these muscles during lifting and coughing, resulting in downward pressure on the pelvic floor.

If she has not been able to identify her transverse abdominal muscles during this exercise and her stage of pregnancy will allow it, she can try lying face down on a padded surface or bed to perform this exercise with her hands under her lower abdomen. The tension in the deep abdominal muscles is often more noticeable in this position.

Once she has a working idea of all the preceding steps, send her home to practice what she has learned so far about breathing and identifying tension in her lower deep abdominal muscles and in her pelvic floor.

Holding tension and relaxing exercises (Kegels): Once a woman has identified her pelvic floor muscles, she can continue to breathe gently while holding tension in her pelvic floor for 5 to 10 seconds, fully relaxing (without bearing down) for 5 to 10 seconds and then repeating this four times. (Noble [1995] recommends holding a contraction for no longer than five seconds at one time, while O'Dwyer recommends 10 seconds.) She can repeat this series three or four times daily for three weeks either in a side-lying position or a supine, knees-up, feet-flat on the floor position. Once she can confidently identify the proper muscles and their appropriate actions, she can move to practicing while sitting and then standing. Since standing puts more pressure on the pelvic floor, many women with low tone find these exercises to be most challenging to do while standing.

Elevator exercises: Once women have mastered the basic tension–relaxation exercise, they can move on to more elaborate elevator exercises. The pelvic floor muscles can be tightened progressively, layer by layer, in an attempt to exercise each one as individually as possible, and then released slowly, one by one, to full relaxation. Since the muscles are all connected, complete isolation of individual muscles is impossible. However, the muscles will be better toned with elevator exercises than if simply tightened and relaxed. Elevator exercises should take place in cycles of 15 for each session (Noble, 1995).

Pushing out: The woman should also note how her perineum feels when she is at rest, and should practice gently exaggerating the relaxation into a bulge (pushing out); this is essentially the action needed for effective pushing. Unless she has high-tone dysfunction, she should only do this enough to become aware of what the muscles feel like while doing this. This instruction is difficult for many women to grasp. Have the woman imagine ejecting a tampon from her yoni, using only her muscles to assist her.

Devices to help retrain the perineal muscles: A variety of tools are available to help women retrain their pelvic floor muscles. These devices can be used by the woman at home to help her identify her muscles and receive feedback regarding whether she is doing her exercises correctly.

Several brands of weighted cones (Step Free, Lady Care, Aquaflex) are available. These generally consist of cone-shaped forms with graduated weights. Each cone has a string that can be used to remove it. Starting with the largest, lightest one first, the cone is inserted with the tip pointing out. While it is in place, the woman exercises her pelvic floor in an attempt to prevent the cone from falling out. Smaller cones with heavier weights are used as her pelvic floor tone improves. This is an excellent remedy for stress incontinence and can help any woman become more aware of and strengthen her pelvic floor. These cones are available in the US from Medgo (www.medollc.com/zen/vaginal-weights, 888-918-9489).

The Pelvic Muscle Educator is a device designed on the same principle as the cotton swab test for urinary muscle tone (discussed on page 191). It consists of a contoured form attached to a long handle. The form is designed to follow the movements of the pelvic floor. It is inserted into the yoni, and the woman then exercises her pelvic floor. If she is exercising her muscles correctly, the handle should move away from her body (down). Such a tool can be helpful to women who are having trouble identifying which muscles to contract. It also gives the midwife a hands-off indication regarding whether the woman is contracting her muscles correctly. It is available from Medgo as well.

The EPI-NO Birth trainer can also be used to help strengthen the pelvic floor. It is discussed on page 158. Other inflatable devices that are inserted into the yoni to provide pressure and feedback on correct performance are also available. Many of these products can be found at the same Medgo website.

The Kegelmaster is a resistance exercise device with adjustable resistance settings that is inserted into the yoni. The woman uses her pelvic muscles to squeeze the device closed. This can be a very effective tool, particularly if a woman is having trouble identifying which muscles to exercise (available from www.kegeltoner.com).

Healthy pelvic floor habits

While teaching women these pelvic floor and abdominal muscle awareness exercises, you can share with them these healthy pelvic floor habits as well (O'Dwyer, 2008).

1. Review her history regarding bowel habits; her intake of fruits and vegetables, fiber and water; and her exercise level to ensure that obvious reasons for irregularity and constipation are addressed. She should try to have uninterrupted time to have a bowel movement so that she does not feel rushed.
2. Show her how to simulate a squatting position for bowel movements, if she uses a Western toilet. Have her sit in a straight-backed chair. Place a foot stool under her feet and have her straighten her lower back and lift her sternum. O'Dwyer points out that raising the knees helps open the anus and rectum. Have her spread her knees widely apart and lean forward from her hips, keeping her back straight; stools should pass easily in this position (curling the spine and pushing with the abdominal muscles tends to close the anal sphincter). Have her practice deep abdominal breathing as she totally relaxes her belly outward. Next, she should focus her attention on the muscles of the pelvic floor and anal sphincter and how they respond in this position.

   She should avoid sustained straining at any time, as this will only stress the pelvic floor and tends to work against, rather than with, the muscles. If she feels she needs to work with her body to facilitate a bowel movement, advise her to use a series of several short pushes from her abdomen while relaxing her pelvic floor; then rest, then several more short pushes. She can keep this up until her bowels take over. Show her your felt model of the pelvic floor so she can see how substantial the puborectalis muscle is and that this muscle must be relaxed, along with the anal sphincters, in order to allow feces to pass. Short pushes work with the fast-twitch muscle fibers of the pelvic floor most efficiently and allow the tissues to gradually dilate, lessening discomfort and minimizing tissue trauma. They also help to stimulate the rhythmic contraction of the colon walls. Her sphincter and pelvic floor muscles will tend to return to their normal resting state of tone between pushes, so she must carefully work with them to keep them relaxed and open between pushes. Tuning into all these nuances of pelvic floor activity during bowel movements will serve her well when she is ready to give birth.

After a bowel movement O'Dwyer recommends tightening the anal sphincter, slowly bring the tension up through the rectum and holding for 10 seconds and then consciously relaxing to restore the normal, baseline tone of the pelvic floor.

A woman can tune into the sensation of involuntary bearing down by becoming aware of the peristaltic action of her colon during bowel movements. Ask her to notice that her bowels are pushing and that she can choose to bear down with them or not. The uterine sensations associated with pushing, are similar to this but much more intense and the outward force is centered in the birth passage, not in the anal canal. She can also practice consciously tuning into what her pelvic floor is doing as stool is passed and how she can work with the muscles to relax them to let it out.

3. When the pelvic floor is not being actively stressed, it should be relaxed, remembering that the relaxed pelvic floor retains tone and the organs are fully supported in women whose tone is normal.
4. During activities that increase intra-abdominal pressure, such as lifting, sneezing, pushing, and coughing, the transverse and internal oblique abdominal muscles and the pelvic floor should be gently contracted upward all together to support the pelvic organs and the spine. Very often, women (and men) use only their rectus abdominis muscles during lifting, which pushes the abdominal contents down against the pelvic floor, straining both sets of muscles.

   Proper lifting involves squatting with the knees apart, with the object to be lifted between the legs. Grasp the object and rise from the knees, using the strength in the quadriceps muscles (the ones overlying the anterior thighs). As a woman lifts, she should use all her abdominal muscles, exhale and contract her pelvic floor to protect herself from prolapse. If she cannot tense her pelvic floor properly while lifting an object, she should not lift it. Once her pelvic floor is no longer under stress, she should consciously relax it to restore normal resting tone.
5. Urge her to participate in regular strengthening exercises, remembering to place equal emphasis on flexibility and stretching after sessions and to cultivate an awareness of pelvic floor status. Swimming, biking, Pilates and balancing activities using a large blow-up exercise ball are good options. If a woman's pelvic floor is currently weak, she should avoid any exercise that causes her abdomen to bulge forward or that pushes her pelvic floor down, such as sit-ups or leg-lifts. These types of exercises are only appropriate for those who can maintain tension in their pelvic floor while doing them. If she leaks urine during impact exercise, such as running, have her discontinue it until her pelvic floor has normalized and she has mastered the ability to tense her pelvic floor during exercise and to relax it afterward. This may take five to six months. After that

point, if she still leaks, she needs to find another regular exercise program. If she does not leak, she needs to keep up her pelvic floor exercises followed by relaxation to maintain this level of continence.

6. Emphasize the need to maintain a normal body weight. No woman should be instructed to actively lose weight during pregnancy, however, as this is dangerous. Visceral fat (the fat around internal organs) puts pressure on her pelvic floor, and continence improves when overweight women lose as little as 5% of their excess body weight. This is something she can focus on after pregnancy, although making better food choices may result in a spontaneous loss of weight during pregnancy. Should this occur, it is not harmful as long as her nutritional needs are adequately met and the baby is growing normally.
7. Daily pelvic floor exercises should always be followed by conscious relaxation.
8. Advise her to discontinue heavy exercise during her menses. Hormonal shifts create heaviness in the pelvis, and any pelvic floor weakness may be exaggerated.
8. Help her develop good urination habits. First, learn to control urgency. Urgency is a sudden, compelling need to urinate. It occurs when the bladder starts to contract. Urgency is fostered when people empty their bladder more often than is really necessary. When drinking proper amounts of water (four to eight 8 oz glasses daily), she should urinate at least every four hours and no more often than every two. Emptying the bladder too often, before it is really full, reduces its capacity and creates a frequency problem. Women with normal bladder muscles will still be comfortable initially, even when the bladder is full.

   During urination, relax the urethra and let the urine flow without force. This lets the bladder walls contract to push the urine out. Forcing urination by using the abdominal muscles can lead to lazy bladder walls and puts undue pressure on the pelvic floor. While voiding, she should be able to count at a moderate pace to at least 20. If she can't, she has gone to the bathroom too soon.

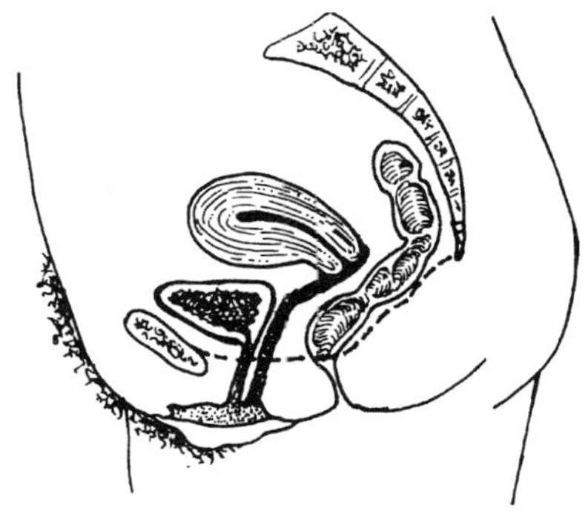

A well-supported pelvic floor

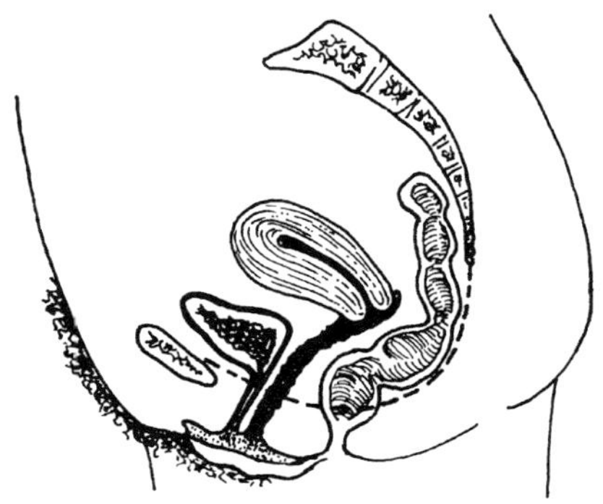

Compromised pelvic floor tone

Pelvic floor exercises should not be done during urination except on rare occasions as a test of muscle strength by stopping the flow of urine once or twice. Regular pelvic floor exercise during urination can confuse the contractility of the bladder muscle, which can encourage urgency or even urinary tract infections. A confused bladder muscle may eventually become overactive. Over activity occurs when the bladder wall contracts spastically, resulting in sustained pressure and urgency. If urgency is already a problem, have her reduce or eliminate her intake of caffeine (coffee, sodas, chocolate and tea) as well as citrus foods, all of which irritate the urinary tract. Alcohol should also be avoided. It is a diuretic that increases urine production and decreases bladder control.

10. Walk on a regular basis, not just around the house, but as an exercise. Traditional Mexican midwives swear by walking as one of the best preventative measures to ensure a strong, elastic, tear-resistant perineum as well as to restore these attributes after a tear (Rosenberg, 2005).

Perineal stretching: In my experience, apart from good nutrition, general fitness, pelvic floor awareness and good toning habits, the biggest factor in preventing tears has been a daily, five-minute session of perineal stretching, starting six weeks before the due date. Stretching is appropriate for women with normal or high pelvic floor tone and for those who have nasty perineal scarring from a previous birth. It is intended to encourage elasticity and to help the mother learn to relax and integrate the sensations of stretching and burning that occur as the head distends the perineum. Pelvic floor exercises should continue through the last six weeks as well, so that resilient elasticity (not laxness) is encouraged.

Note that I am recommending stretching, *not* perineal massage. It is often recommended that the introitus be massaged back and forth in a semicircular motion, which, in my experience, produces more irritation than elasticity. The technique I have found successful involves helping women prepare their tissues while learning to deal with the sensations of fetal descent and emergence.

Regardless of what kind of perineal preparation you recommend (stretching or massage), it should not be started too early in pregnancy. The hormones will not have sufficiently softened the tissue, and stretching too soon is more traumatic than helpful. Thirty-four weeks is a good time to begin with daily sessions, each lasting no less than five minutes and no longer than fifteen. You may find it best to explain the stretching technique during the prenatal visit before stretching should begin so that it is fresh in the woman's mind. Giving her a handout is also very helpful. Show the woman's partner, if any, what needs to be done as well, unless the mother does not want the partner involved for any reason.

The partner should use either a water-based product (such as K-Y, Astrolube or Replens) or a pure vegetable oil for lubrication. Lansinoh cream, a pharmaceutical-grade hypoallergenic lanolin, is highly viscous and could also be used. If the woman has a tendency to develop yeast infections, water-based lubricant is probably best. Petroleum-based products (mineral oil or petroleum jelly) should not be used; they clog pores and leach vitamins from the tissue.

A hot bath before each session will help soften and relax the tissues. The woman should then lie comfortably on her back with her knees up and spread and her feet flat on the bed. Have her partner place lubricated fingers or thumbs in both sides of the introitus to the depth of the solid band of tissue (the pubovisceral muscle) at about the level of the hymenal ring. The woman should then tighten her muscles around her partner's fingers to ensure that the proper muscular landmark has been identified.

Now have the stretcher direct bilateral pressure down and outward toward each ischial tuberosity or "sit bone" (toward 4 and 8 o'clock) while the mother breathes deeply into her abdomen, consciously exaggerates the relaxation of her pelvic muscles and visualizes the tissues as being very elastic (stretching as much as possible and returning to their unstretched condition completely once the tension is released). When she begins to feel stretching or burning discomfort, or when her partner detects an area of resistance, the partner should hold the stretch for thirty seconds to a minute while the woman breathes into the tension to consciously relax the area. Then have the partner slowly apply more pressure, cycling between stretching, breathing, and pressure gradually to allow the woman to become accustomed to the changes. The stretch can then be held longer and more steadily. The stretcher can cross the forearms at the wrists to minimize shoulder discomfort when doing the stretching using both hands (Loprenzi-Kassel, 1995).

As practice continues and the tissues become more elastic, more fingers can be used and the stretch increased until the partner can insert an entire fist inside the band of muscles. This promotes familiarity with the sensations of crowning and really helps women get used to the burning they will experience during birth.

The woman can also stretch her perineum herself. While lying down with her knees up, she can reach around under her thighs on either side and stretch down and out toward her tuberosities with her index fingers. Many women find that hot baths are the perfect place to practice.

Occasionally a woman who has herpes will notice that yoni stretching causes flare-ups. Likewise, the presence of genital warts, if extreme, around the introitus. Should either of these conditions be an issue, postpone stretching and use supportive therapies to heal the lesions. (See my text UNDERSTANDING DIAGNOSTIC TESTS IN THE CHILDBEARING YEAR for a discussion of herpes and genital warts in pregnancy.)

Women who have previously had clitorotomies or epidural anesthesia should be warned that they will feel considerably more stretching and burning when no clitorotomy is performed. Unprepared women may be alarmed by these sensations during pushing, insisting that something is wrong. Explain the benefits of an intact birth and what to expect. Prenatal stretching will be immensely helpful in preparing them for these intense sensations.

Some women have previous scars that are thick or painful. They can massage a mixture of vitamin E and evening primrose oil from opened capsules directly into the scar tissue to make it more flexible. Oil from capsules is the most potent because it has been protected from exposure to air and light, both of which cause oxidation and breakdown of the oils.

All women (especially first-time and YBAC mothers) should visualize the head descending and stretching the yoni when they do their exercises. They need to maintain a strong image of birth (always including good tissue elasticity; a normal, healthy, pink and breathing baby; timely placental delivery; the uterus clamping down and the baby nursing after birth). Birth is a normal process, and they can do it!

After each stretching session, the woman should perform several rounds of pelvic floor tension–relaxation exercises to promote healthy tone.

EPI-NO perineal trainer: The EPI·NO Birth Trainer is a specialized balloon that consists of two ball-shaped ends connected by a fat middle, a hand pump to inflate the balloon and a pressure gauge.

It can be used in a variety of ways to train the perineal muscles. Before birth, if a woman can afford to buy one, it can be used in place of manual perineal stretching to gradually familiarize her with the sensation of birth. Because the balloon size is adjustable, smooth and round and because it enlarges uniformly, it provides a perfect tool to learn the sensations of birth by mimicking the baby's head. It has been found to be a very effective way to reduce perineal damage at birth (Ruckhäberle et al., 2010).

It is recommended to begin using the EPI·NO three weeks prior to the due date. Daily 20 minute exercise sessions should be performed, during which the perineal tissue is stretched by the balloon to promote elasticity.

To use the device the woman first makes herself comfortable. Lying down is probably the best way to begin, but as practice continues, it might be helpful to trying stretching in different positions. To insert the balloon, tighten the pressure release valve and inflate the balloon just enough to make it firm but still small enough to be introduced into the yoni without difficulty. If the balloon is too big, drain off some of the air by opening the release valve. Alternatively, completely deflate the balloon and fold it into 3 sections (right side in, then left side in) to make insertion easier; if necessary, the balloon can be moistened with a little water-soluble lubricant. Insert the balloon two-thirds of the way into the yoni. The balloon is stabilized by its contoured waist in this position in the introitus (if it starts to be expelled, a rolled towel can be placed between the legs to apply counter pressure, which should keep the balloon it in place during inflation). The balloon is then gently inflated with the hand pump to stretch the muscles, following the same suggestions for relaxation that were given for manual stretching. The device should be inflated a little more at each practice session. The pressure can be reduced at any time by opening the pressure release valve on the hand pump. Over time, the woman gets used to the pressure and stretching, just as with manual stretching.

Providing prostaglandin precursors and ensuring normal uterine activity

Evening primrose, borage seed and black currant oils are all high in linoleic acid, a prostaglandin precursor that is lacking in refined vegetable oils. Prostaglandins are hormones that, among other things, help prepare the soft tissues for birth. Supplemental capsules can be recommended to help enhance tissue elasticity. (Evening primrose oil is the type that has been used the longest in the midwifery community; black currant and borage oil capsules are less expensive alternatives.) Supplementation is especially useful for encouraging a soft and pliable cervix in first-time mothers.

Nulliparas may take one 500 mg capsule daily from 36 weeks until birth. Multiparas who have had long labors, extensive perineal scars or any cervical scars may also benefit from taking one 500 mg capsule daily for the last six weeks (otherwise multiparas do not usually need any help because their cervix has opened previously). Very thick scarring warrants 2 or 3 capsules daily. Anyone with a family history of cervical tears, those who have taken birth control pills or other hormone-based forms of contraception, and those who have had anovulatory cycles can take it as well.

Evening primrose, borage and black currant oils are contraindicated for those with a loose (incompetent) cervix, in those whose cervix is otherwise abnormal and in those with a history of premature birth unrelated to poor nutrition.

Be sure clients are not functioning on the "if a little is good, more is better" theory. One woman I worked with took evening primrose oil throughout her pregnancy without my knowledge and wound up with a very easy birth but one of the worst tears I'd ever seen.

Yoni infections and genital warts

Severe yoni infections leave the tissue irritated, making tearing more likely. Watch for and treat them prenatally, well before term whenever possible. Use prescription drugs, if necessary.

Certain strains of human papilloma virus can cause genital warts. A thick outbreak of warts in and around the introitus greatly increases the risk of tearing. It will leave the tissue unable to stretch. It usually shreds instead and may bleed profusely. Repair is a nightmare. If homeopathic remedies do not clear the warts, laser or cryo (freezing) surgery are the least noxious allopathic choices for wart removal during pregnancy. This should be done in plenty of time for the tissues to heal before labor begins (Frye, 2007).

Varicose veins

Varicose veins are enlarged blood vessels that have weakened valves. The valves normally assist in directing blood flow. Weakened valves lead to pooling of blood and subsequent enlargement of the vessels. These distended vessels can be painful. Blood pooling increases the risk of clot formation, especially after birth. Expansion of the blood volume in combination with indiscriminate hormonal relaxation of muscles during pregnancy accentuates the tendency for the blood to pool, where it may form clots. Varicosities may be located in the legs, vulva or yoni. When located in the anus, they are called "hemorrhoids." Due to the pressure of the pregnancy, women may have vulval or yoni varicosities that only become apparent then. (See HOLISTIC MIDWIFERY, VOL. I for details regarding care and treatment during pregnancy.)

If varicosities are not given proper support, venous distention can become aggravated during pregnancy and the likelihood of clot formation with accompanying pain and inflammation increases. Blood pooling can also eventually lead to infection. Stasis and infection may produce heat in the vessels. There is a risk of a clot becoming dislodged and entering the brain, heart, or lungs, any of which can be fatal. (To minimize this risk, warm or swollen vessels should never be massaged.)

Trauma to vulval, yoni, and rectal varicosities may occur during birth. Be sure to check for them prenatally. Sewing around them is tricky and, if one ruptures or is punctured during repair, a hematoma will be the likely result.

Pelvic herniations and uterine prolapse

Either a hernia or a uterine or cervical prolapse may cause uncomfortable dragging sensations in the back and pelvis during pregnancy. Assuming a knee–chest position several times daily during the first six months of pregnancy will encourage normal positioning of a prolapsed cervix or uterus as it enlarges. Pelvic floor exercises as described previously will help with all herniation problems and should begin prior to conception or as early in pregnancy as possible. (See the chapter entitled "Assessing Pelvic Organ Prolapse" for more details.)

Psychological factors

Helping women deal with their natural fears of an unknown process while fostering a close relationship and maintaining a sense of humor can be big assets throughout pregnancy and birth and can help prevent tearing as well. A solid, trusting relationship can help a woman listen to you when sensations are overwhelming her during crowning (Gaskin, 1992).

PROTECTING THE PERINEUM DURING LABOR AND BIRTH

The pelvic tissues during late labor and pushing

As midwives, we need to understand what happens to the pelvic tissues during fetal descent and where damage is likely to occur. This will help guide us to the best, least traumatic ways to support birthing women. In order to understand this chapter first study the part entitled "Pertinent Anatomy." The following explanation of how the process of birth affects the pelvic floor is based on DeLancey (2002) unless otherwise noted.

The baby's presenting part must dilate the cervix and then dilate and pass through the other complex layers of tissue in the pelvis. The presenting part is usually the head, which averages about 10 cm in diameter but can be considerably larger. The diameter of the baby's lower torso in a term frank breech presentation is actually a bit larger still, but is more compressible. The enormous stretching the pelvic tissues must undergo to accommodate the fetal parts is made possible by hormonal shifts that occur in late pregnancy that remodel the collagen in the tissues of the pelvic floor and cervix, causing them to become increasingly softened as term approaches so that they will yield to the pressure from uterine contractions by stretching rather than tearing.

Just prior to labor and until the baby starts to descend though the pelvis, the levator ani muscle complex maintains its normal at-rest shape. In a standing woman, the base of the bladder and the urethrovesical junction are normally located in the anterior pelvis, level with a line drawn between the lower border of the symphysis and the tip of the sacrum. Their position does not change significantly during thinning of the lower uterine segment or during active cervical dilation. In most women, the cervix is positioned at the level of the ischial spines at the onset of labor and remains at that level until birth.

Once the cervix is fully dilated, or nearly so, the resting phase of labor begins. During this time, the uterus continues to contract, taking up any slack in the fundus that is created as the baby's presenting part slips down past the cervix. Once the slack is taken up, the uterus begins involuntary bearing-down activity. Sometimes this happens quickly, so that the uterus moves right into bearing down, but it can take minutes to hours for some women to move through this phase. Added to the uterine forces are the mother's voluntary bearing-down efforts.

Upon complete dilation, the presenting part comes into direct contact with the yoni walls, opening them circumferentially. The pressure generated between the fetal presenting part and the yoni wall during pushing averages 100 mmHg and may reach as high as 230 mmHg (Goldberg, 2007). As the presenting part starts to descend through the pelvis, the bladder base moves upward in front of the presenting part, aligns with the urethra, and both continue to move up toward the upper border of the symphysis. In most women, neither the bladder neck nor the urethra become significantly elongated in this process. However, the degree of elongation that occurs varies widely among individual women. In those with a small pelvis who experience an arrest of fetal descent, the bladder can be pushed up as high as the upper level of the symphysis and the urethra may be elongated as well. It is not known at what point elongation of this kind results in injury.

As the baby moves down, the presenting part presses against the levator ani muscles, which descend into a bowl shape and begin to stretch. As the presenting part distends the perineal body, the elastic limit of the parietal fasciae covering the top and bottom of the levator ani muscles and the elastic limits of the connective tissues of the perineal membrane, are reached. Further descent depends on stretching these tissues even more, resulting in circumferential elongation of the connective tissues and muscles to a diameter averaging 10 cm, which equals a circumference of about 31 cm. The pubic attachments of the pubo-visceral muscle and the attachment of the perineal membrane to the perineal body limits downward descent of the perineal body. Thus, as the baby's body passes through the introitus, a great deal of stress is placed on the perineal membrane and on its midline connection to the perineal body. How much stress depends upon the degree to which the tissues resist stretching and thus the amount of force required to dilate them.

At any time during active descent, tissues may give way at their weakest point and tear. Whether a woman tears is influenced by her constitutional tissue integrity, nutrition and a host of other factors, but it is also very much influenced by the mother's position during pushing. Positions that accentuate the curve of the birth canal or (in most cases) that don't maximize the effects of gravity require excessive stretching and thinning of the perineal body, straining the tissues and encouraging tearing. Maternal positions that straighten the birth canal by rotating the sacrum up and out of the way and that work with gravity reduce the amount of perineal thinning that occurs, even in women who have a long perineal body. An upright, kneeling position with the woman leaning forward slightly with her pelvis tipped forward both straightens the birth canal and minimizes stress on the pelvic tissues (Sutton, 2001). Positions that minimize stress like this are even more critical for a woman whose perineal body is short, as she is at higher risk for tears that involve the anal sphincter.

Occult soft-tissue injuries: While obvious tearing of the skin and underlying tissues of the perineal body is the most recognized type of soft-tissue injury that results from childbirth, other types of damage can also occur. These invisible injuries are much more difficult to study. There is debate among researchers as to when and how various kinds of childbirth-related soft tissue damage occur and what their long-term impact may be on a woman's urinary and fecal continence and on her risk for pelvic organ prolapse.

The cervix starts out closed and dilates to 10 cm, a more than10-fold increase in size, and returns, more or less, to its nonpregnant size and shape by six weeks postpartum. The cardinal and uterosacral ligaments attach the cervix to the posterosuperior and lateral pelvic walls. As the cervix opens, its edges move ever closer to the pelvic walls, narrowing the distance between the cervix and these attachment points, which relieves strain on the ligaments. These ligaments could be stressed, however, if the partially dilated cervix is dragged down to the introitus or if fundal pressure is applied prior to complete dilation or after the birth to deliver the placenta or help expel clots from the uterus.

In contrast to the cervix, the upper end of the yoni starts with a diameter of about 5 cm prior to labor and must expand only another 5 cm or so to accommodate the baby, just a two-fold increase. Therefore, it is reasonable to expect that the birth process will not permanently stretch or damage the yoni canal.

Furthermore, there is little evidence to suggest that any pelvic floor damage occurs before the presenting part is actually pressed against it. The levator ani muscles do not receive direct pressure from the head until it reaches +1 station. From this point until the baby is out, the baby's body is in firm contact with the pelvic tissues. The presenting part pushes down on the muscles and all the surrounding, attached structures as the urogenital hiatus is dilated.

Dilation and thinning of the muscles also stretches the attached nerves, specifically the levator ani and the pudendal nerves. The pudendal nerves are attached to the ischial spines and then enter the pudendal (Alcock) canal on either side. Their location makes them vulnerable to traction injury, which can occur anywhere along the nerve's path from its origin at the sacral nerve roots at S2, S3 and S4 to the terminal branches that supply the external anal sphincter. Stretching and compression of the pudendal nerve seems to be most extreme as the baby passes between the ischial spines (Goldberg, 2007).

Once the presenting part enters the pelvis, especially when it is the hard fetal head, the resulting pressure that it applies against the pelvic sidewalls as descent proceeds could cause compression injury to the levator ani nerve or to the pudendal nerve. Generalized atrophy may result from levator ani nerve injury due to excessive stretching and can lead to diminished muscle function or alter the resting tone of the levator plate. Pudendal nerve injury may lead to failure of the pubovisceral muscle to reflexively contract and may increase sphincter pressure during a cough or sneeze; the perineal body may also be adversely affected (Aston-Miller & DeLancey, 2007; Goldberg, 2007). Such pressure can also result in a particular kind of compression nerve injury known as "maternal obstetrical paralysis." This type of injury is rare, however, and is usually associated with prolonged, arrested labor.

Excessive stretching of striated muscles is a well-known cause of injury. The best predictors are the magnitude of stretch, called **strain**, and the combined effects of **stress** (force on the muscle surface) and strain, called **work**. These two types of stretch are essentially equivalent in their predictive value (Brooks et al., 1995; O'Dell & Morse, 2008). Research consistently shows that pelvic floor strength decreases after yoni birth, and histologic studies find that a higher parity of yoni births is associated with the replacement of a significant amount of muscle tissue with fibrosis (Nygaard & Gregory, 2007). For more details, see the entry entitled "Biomechanical principles of tissue damage" later in this chapter.

Trauma to the levator ani muscles may include detachment of individual muscles from their points of origin along the tendinous arch of the levator ani. Damage tends to occur near the origin of the pubovisceral muscles at the pubic bone (Aston-Miller & DeLancey, 2007). DeLancey (1994) noted that the attachment of the tendinous arch of the pelvic fasciae to the ischial spine is torn in 96% of all parous women, but he did not tell us whether the women he studied received epidurals or other drugs that unduly relaxed the tissues, nor did he say anything regarding the position the women assumed or other details concerning the pushing phase of their labors.

If the urogenital hiatus is unusually narrow or if it strongly resists fetal descent, more force will be necessary to dilate the opening. The additional stretching against such resistance may also result in nerve injury. Instrumental delivery, using either forceps or vacuum extraction; the use of epidural anesthesia, which unduly relaxes the tissues while often prolonging the pushing phase of labor; or both can also result in nerve damage as well as anal sphincter injury. Successive births may result in cumulative injury, with altered continence presenting years later. Nevertheless, whether nerve disruption or compression is the cause of such problems is just theoretical, and it is not known for certain exactly how pudendal nerve dysfunction occurs.

Injury to the perineal body, whether due to an incision or a spontaneous laceration, may result in a loss of yoni or rectal muscle tone. Damage to the nerves that supply the anal sphincters may also occur, which explains why normal function is not always restored even when the anal sphincter is adequately repaired. The risk of anal incontinence is increased with prolonged labor, forceps use and clitorotomy (Goldberg, 2007).

Biomechanical principles of tissue damage

Biomechanics is the application of mechanical principles to living organisms. An understanding of biomechanics helps explain normal function and how tissues can be injured. The concepts of stress and strain are used to study tissue elasticity related to pressure and movement. "Stress" is a measure of pressure or force applied to the tissue surface. "Strain" is a change in the length of the tissue in any direction when force is applied, including shortening and twisting. Other factors include the direction of strain as the tissue is compressed, stretched or twisted; the timing of the stress or strain (abrupt versus slow stretching or repetitive pressure); and the duration and intensity of the stress. The biological condition of the tissues (variations in fluid content or permeability or both) cause some tissues, such as collagen, to have a steady response to deformity, while others develop "creep," or increasing deformity, even when stress is consistent. The temperature of the tissue may also be a factor because it influences the fluid content of the tissue. Extreme stress or strain can overwhelm tissue elasticity, resulting in tearing or rendering it unable to recover its original shape, resulting in permanent deformity (O'Dell & Morse, 2008).

Identified factors that increase the risk of tearing

Based purely on hospital data, it is estimated that over 85% of women will sustain some type of perineal trauma during a normal birth and that 60 to 70% of these women will require stitches (Head of Midwifery, 2009). Although any tearing at all is less than optimal, the literature has focused on studying tears and perineal incisions that involve anal structures. Thus, the incidence of more superficial tears (first and second degree) is harder to quantify, in large part because all types of providers often deem any damage that does not require repair as no damage at all; this imprecise method of record-keeping hides the true incidence of more superficial damage.

In contrast, third- and fourth-degree tearing has been studied extensively. The overall risk of such a tear in a normal (yoni) birth is only 1%. Certain associated factors that increase the risk have been identified in several retrospective studies of hospital births (Nygaard & Gregory, 2007; Power et al., 2006; RCOG, 2007). The following findings list these factors. The parenthetical comment shows how much over the background risk of 1% (1 in every 100 women) the risk is increased in each case. These risks are generally ranked from least to most risky.

- Baby's birth weight over 8 lb 8 oz (4 kg) (up to 2%) (odds ratio of 1.5 to 2.5)
- Persistent occipitoposterior position (2 to 3%) (odds ratio of 1.2 to 1.8)
- Induction of labor with pharmaceuticals (up to 2%)
- Epidural analgesia (1.5 to 3%)
- Previous anal sphincter tear (4%)

- •Midline clitorotomy (3 to 5%) (odds ratio of 4.9 to 16.5)
- •Nulliparity (3 to 4%) (odds ratio of 2.5 to 4.0)
- •Pushing for longer than 1 hour (up to 4%)
- •Shoulder dystocia (up to 4%)
- •Instrumental delivery: overall risk (3%) (operative delivery odds ratio of 2.5 to 3.5)
  - -Forceps–assisted delivery (3% to 7%)
  - -Vacuum–assisted delivery (3%)
  - -Forceps compared to vacuum extraction (2.88%)
  - -Forceps with midline clitorotomy (25-fold increase [Power et al., 2006])
- •Short perineal body (odds ratio of 8 [Power et al., 2006])
- •Mediolateral clitorotomy (1.4 to as high as 9%)

(An odds ratio is a way to compare whether the probability of a certain event is the same for two groups. An odds ratio of 1 implies that the event is equally likely in both groups. An odds ratio greater than one implies that the event is more likely in the first [intervened with] group. An odds ratio less than one implies that the event is less likely in the first group. Odds ratios are frequently used in medical statistics. Those given above are from Nygaard & Gregory, 2007, unless otherwise noted.)

Severe perineal tears that involve the one or both anal sphincters, the rectal mucosa, or all three occur in 0.6% to as many as 9% of births, even when a mediolateral clitorotomy has been performed. This high rate is likely to be related to mediolateral incisions that are made at an angle that does not avoid the sphincters. There is a 50% relative reduction in the risk of creating third-degree damage for every 6° away from the perineal midline that a mediolateral incision was made (more about the importance of the angle of the incision can be found in the chapter entitled "Clitorotomy ['Episiotomy'].")

Protecting the perineal tissues at the time of birth

Hands-off: In most cases, the best thing we can do is nothing but watch and wait for nature to take its course. When women are left as undisturbed as possible, their hormonal milieu is such that they are optimally prepared, both physically and psychologically, for the baby to descend with a minimum of tissue trauma. Allowing the mother to give birth in the position of her choice while you stand back and keep your hands off is absolutely the best thing you can do to facilitate an optimal birthing experience on all levels for both mother and baby. Waterbirth is one of the best ways to promote routine hands off birth and to support the mothers in using their own hands to provide support when it is needed.

Especially in cases where the mother has done some prenatal perineal preparation, a hands-off approach is unlikely to result in much of a tear, if any. However, although prenatal perineal preparation is the ideal, not every mother will have done it. In addition, some mothers will not allow themselves to go into an optimally internalized state during labor due to previous emotional or physical traumas that they bring to their birth experience.

Hands-on: Historically and today, many midwives have had a very hands-on approach to perineal protection at the time of birth. This focus has been fostered by midwifery practices that have taken pride in a very low tear rate and, in some cases, because they were also either unwilling or forbidden by law to suture. To avoid transports for stitches, midwives have been highly interventive and inventive in coming up with techniques that they swear prevent tearing at birth. While such techniques, in the proper hands, can help prevent tears, it is good practice to wean yourself away from hands-on techniques at the time of birth in particular because any such intervention tends to mess with the energy. We must remember that anything we do, regardless of how well intentioned or how seemingly necessary, constitutes an intervention. On the other hand, you are holding yourself out as an expert in normal birth and you should know what might help if a woman needs your hands-on assistance, so, while I am advocating a routine hands-off approach, I do recognize that hands-on assistance is called for in certain situations.

Talk to ten different midwives and you'll probably come away with ten different opinions about what hands-on techniques work to prevent tears. It is very individual. Keep in mind that attending births requires a flowing relationship between the mother, the baby, and the midwife as well as the Energy of Birth itself. Each birth is unique, and often midwives report a sense of being led to the proper approach at a given birth. We must always transcend techniques per se to tune into the needs of each individual woman and baby. Remember, what works in just one situation is valid for that circumstance, even if others said it would never work or if it never works again.

I shall offer some suggestions from my research as well as my experience. I do not find that all of these recommendations work for me, and neither will you. I am including a wide variety of suggestions because it is important to be aware of as many options as possible, particularly in difficult situations. Keep in mind that if a physical problem is dealt with via interventions while the underlying psychological issue goes unacknowledged, you may trade one problem for another further along in the birthing process. For more details about how to support a woman throughout labor and pushing, see my text HOLISTIC MIDWIFERY, VOL. II. There you will find chapters entitled: "The Resting Phase of Labor," "Active Pushing," "Maternal Positions during Pushing and at the Time of Birth" and "Assisting the Birth of a Vertex Baby." All of these chapters contain valuable information regarding normal labor and pushing. To make space for other information in this text, that information has not been repeated here.

What midwives think vs. what the research shows: Midwives have lots of ideas about how to reduce perineal trauma at the time of birth. Research, however, has not revealed clear advantages of any particular approach. Albers and colleagues (2005) studied the use of warm compresses, perineal massage during pushing and a hands-off approach until crowning and found no significant difference in the rate of tearing (defined as no tissue separation at any site). No damage occurred in 23% of these women. With a more lenient definition of trauma (none, minor or unsutured), 73% would were tear-free, with 40% of these women being primiparas, which is a pretty good percentage. The study identified two risk factors for trauma that will be no particular news to experienced midwives: first-time mothers and birthweight over 8 lb 13 oz (4000 g). Two factors that tended to reduce the incidence of trauma were sitting upright and birth of the head between contractions. Although mention is made of the women assuming different positions during pushing, "sitting upright" is not further defined.

Albers and colleagues looked again at birth related trauma in 2007. In this study they concluded that certain measures tend to reduce the risk of tissue injury and offered these key concepts for clinical practice:

- Teach perineal massage with lubricant to first-time mothers during the last 6 weeks of pregnancy.
- Avoid Valsalva pushing at the time of birth unless there is a clear reason to use it
- If an epidural is used, wait 1 to 2 hours after complete cervical dilation before commencing active pushing. This has been called "laboring down" because the uterus is being allowed to bring the baby down as much as possible before pushing begins.
- Encourage upright or lateral positions for pushing, help the woman identify and assume a position that she finds most comfortable.
- Use hands-on perineal support techniques only when clearly indicated, which includes the need to make her more comfortable or for distraction.
- Avoid clitorotomy unless a clear indication exists (such as severe fetal distress).
- Control the birth of the baby's head by using gentle hands-on techniques as the head emerges and by assisting the birth of the head to come out slowly, between contractions (in my experience, this often results in sticky shoulders if the mother is encouraged to actively push the head out between contractions; if the head slips out as the contraction finishes, that is not such a problem).

What happens to the perineal tissues during pushing and fetal descent: Unlike the cervix, which usually dilates over many hours, the perineal tissues are multilayered and must thin and open in a relatively short period of time. If you do an internal exam as the baby is descending, you can feel the pubovisceral and puborectalis muscles along either side and the tissues of the anterior compartment being thinned and dilated. Once the pubovaginalis and puboperinealis parts of the pubovisceral muscle are embracing the fetal head, the baby is well beneath the pubic bone and preparing to rock out from under it. At this point you can see the labia minora and the pads of fat beneath the labia majora being pressed forward. The anal sphincter will also thin out and become elongated in an anteroposterior direction, exposing a small portion of the anterior wall of the anal canal. As this process continues, the perineal body thins as the muscles are stretched around the presenting part (or pushed forward if the mother is supine). This continues until crowning, when the perineum suddenly retracts around and behind the presenting part as it emerges.

Most studies focus on women giving birth in a recumbent or semi-sitting position. When a woman pushes in either position, the dependent weight of the fetal presenting part pushes the soft tissues forward and the introital opening is stretched farther from the pelvic girdle. The baby must now pass across the soft tissues (rather than down and through them toward the opening). This causes gravity to pull the weight of the baby down against the increasingly thinned perineal and periurethral tissues, which then continue to stretch while bearing an increasingly large weight load at the same time. Even in a semi-sitting position, the mother is still pushing against gravity because the perineum stands between the earth and the force of pushing; leaving the perineum to redirect the force toward the introitus rather than the ground. The mother must also push the baby across the resistant perineum toward the introital opening without benefit of a mobile sacrum. Fixation of the sacrum helps direct the head around and forward toward the introitus as the mother pushes against gravity to move the baby down. This disproportionate downward distribution of increasing weight as the baby's body fills the perineum, along with the unequal forces involved in stretching under such conditions, maximally stresses the tissues. It's no wonder that tears frequently occur and that clitorotomies so often extend.

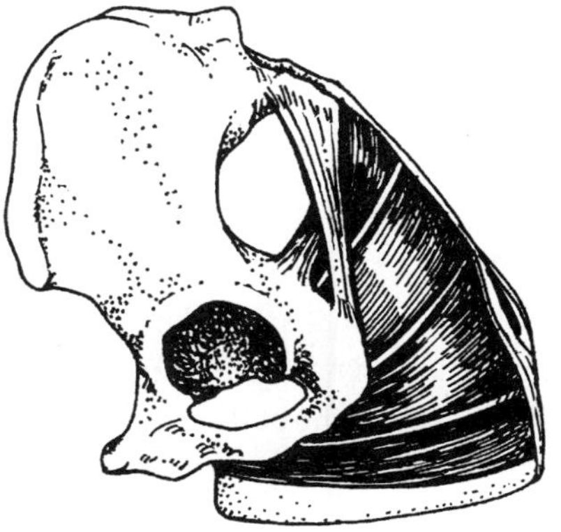

Stretching in an average length perineum (Woman is kneeling, brim tipped forward.)

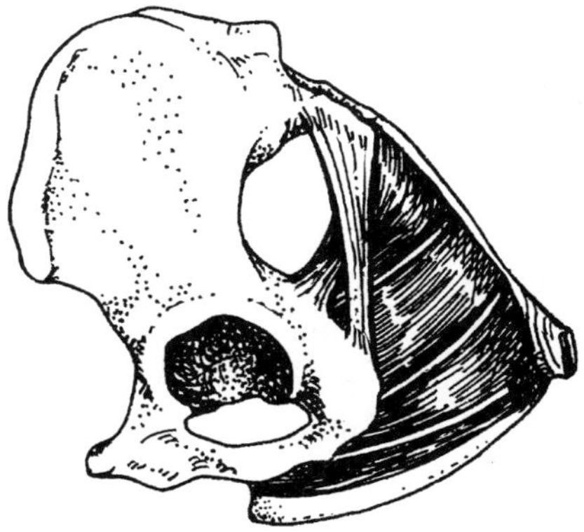

Stretching in a short perineum: note that the anus tends to jut outward.

The upright kneeling position with the pelvic brim tipped forward is ideal for pushing because it moves the sacrum up and out of the way, maximally straightening the birth canal and thus reducing the stretch that the tissues of the pelvic floor and perineum must undergo before the baby emerges. It also works optimally with gravity, lessening the amount of stress the tissues are subjected to before the baby comes out (Sutton, 2001). In this position, the perineum will not elongate as much as it might when the mother is lying supine with her knees up because the presenting part is centered over the introital opening and the pressure is distributed circumferentially around the pelvic and vulval tissues. The perineum is not subjected to the dependent weight of the fetal body and thus can stretch around the fetal presenting part and can retract behind it much more easily. The sacrum can move and rotate up and out of the way, maximally straightening the birth canal. These things help minimize trauma. While women who give birth upright do tear at times, the tears they sustain are likely to be less severe.

The short perineal body during fetal descent and pushing: It is generally accepted, and it has been my observation as well, that women with a short perineum are at increased risk for tearing into the anal sphincter, although very little formal research has been done to investigate this. Deering and colleagues (2004), after controlling for both clitorotomy and instrumental delivery, found that women with a perineal body length of 2.5 cm or less have a significantly higher chance of sustaining a third- or fourth-degree tear (40% versus 5.6%). Rizk and Thomas (2000) studied 221 primigravid women carrying a single baby to term. In their study, the mean perineal length was 4.6 cm (ranging between 3.7 to 5.5 cm) and the mean anal position index was 0.49 (ranging between 0.37 to 0.61). The anal position index is calculated by dividing the distance between the fourchette and the center of the anal opening by the distance between the fourchette and the tip of the coccyx. A short anal position index indicates anterior displacement of the anus. There were higher rates of clitorotomy, perineal tears and instrumental delivery among women whose perineal body lengths were less than 4 cm and whose anal position index was below 0.42.

In contrast, another study involving 318 women concluded that a short perineum (≤3 cm) may actually be associated with a lower risk of tearing, but there were very few women who got to prove it, as this study involved a clitorotomy rate of 75% (Kalis et al., 2005). The problem with these and most other hospital-based studies is that the women are subjected to so many interventions on top of the question that the researchers are trying to answer that the results are not really applicable to what can be achieved by low-intervention midwives practicing at home or in a birth center.

When the perineum is short, the perineal body is small as well. A small perineal body has less tissue to stretch and thin around the baby's head as it crowns. This leaves the perineal muscles and anal sphincter to take the brunt of the stretching without the additional cushion provided by a longer perineal body to help distribute the pressure. Anterior displacement of the anus only increases the risk that it will tear.

With a short perineum, you will see the sphincter jut forward more during crowning, although when women give birth in an upright position, perineal stretching does not occur to the extent that it can when birth occurs in the supine position. Neither the small perineal body nor the sphincter tolerate the pressure very well, especially if the woman is on her back and the perineum is forced to bear all the weight of the baby. Women with short perineal bodies benefit greatly from prenatal perineal stretching. They should be allowed to assume whatever position they find most comfortable during pushing, with an upright forward-leaning position being ideal for them as well.

I do not recommend a clitorotomy for these women. To do one almost assures anal sphincter damage unless you do a mediolateral cut, which involves more nerve, muscle, and blood vessel damage even if it doesn't extend (see the chapter entitled "Clitorotomy ['Episiotomy']").

If the perineal muscles are highly toned, they may give the impression that there isn't much to the perineal body because it is more concave than is typical due to the strength of the muscles. Only as the introitus begins to stretch during pushing will you see if the anus juts forward because the perineal body is lacking.

Things the midwife can do to help protect the perineum

Tell the mother what to expect in advance: Gloria Lamay (2005) emphasizes the importance of explaining to a woman what she can expect as the baby emerges: the increasingly intense intrayoni pressure, the sensation at crowning of splitting open, followed by a pins-and-needles feeling that quickly builds to a sensation of a "ring of fire" around the introitus; once the head is born, there is a great sense of relief and a brief rest period as the next contraction builds that will rotate and birth the shoulders and body with little additional effort. Explain the need for the mother to be intensely focused at this time and that you will be doing all you can, as the midwife, to quiet the environment so that she can remain centered. Advise her that her own hands are often the best ones to be touching her baby and perineum at this time and that you encourage her to do so (some women who have birthed in the hospital may have been forcibly prevented from touching in this manner at a previous birth, so it is always a good idea to tell women that this is okay). Once the baby is out, the last tasks include getting the placenta out, which feels more like a large, soft tampon coming out (than a baby), after which the uterus clamps down.

Positions for birth: As already reviewed, the amount of stretching the perineum must undergo is greatly influenced by the mother's position as the presenting part crowns. An ideal position allows maximal sacral mobility with the least amount of tension on the perineum, while encouraging strong, effective contractions. One option is to have the mother, regardless of whether she is upright, semi-sitting or on her hands and knees, position her legs so that her knees and feet are about 14 to 16 inches (33.6 to 40.6 cm) apart. This minimizes external stretching of the perineum and affords more give for the baby's head (Formato, 1985). When women assume an upright, kneeling position, they often naturally spread their knees in this way. If you are concerned about tearing, watch the perineum during pushing, using a mirror if necessary. If it seems unduly strained, consider having the mother change position.

If you feel that fetal descent needs to slow down or that downward pressure is not desirable (as in women with vulval varicosities or hemorrhoids), side-lying is a much better choice than either a supine or a seated position. Side-lying allows full sacral mobility, which greatly relieves perineal stress, and although the perineum must still stretch sideways quite a bit, the thighs and the way the pelvis is shaped help to support the tissues better than when the mother is upright with counterpressure on her sacrum.

Massage vs. perineal support: I have worked with many women who hate internal yoni massage during birth, although I know midwives who do quite a bit of it. Yoni massage often produces edema and makes the tissue more friable.

Instead, I have either left the perineum entirely alone or, if the mother is having a hard time, I have used hot herbal compresses, which seem to counterbalance the sensation of burning that occurs as the tissues stretch. The compresses are kept warm in a crock pot placed nearby. (Herbal bath solution or fresh ginger or comfrey leaf or root infusion can be used, although plain water or saline solution [¼ tsp salt to one cup water] is acceptable.) Once the head starts to crown, gently apply compresses to the entire periurethral and perineal area. Place the cloth in one hand and cup your hand over the vulva very lightly. You can also apply oil or a water-based lubricant to help the tissue stretch, but I do not thin the perineum manually, since that may irritate and traumatize tissues.

If you do decide to provide hands-on perineal support, take care not to apply pressure in such a way that you cause the head to deflex. It is best to hold the compress very lightly against the perineum so that it is touching the mother but you are not applying any pressure.

If the face is presenting, the baby must usually be chin-up to birth. Remove any hot compresses once the face is visible, and apply finger-pressure to the forehead to maximize extension until the chin is out. If the baby is presenting chin posterior, and progress is continuing, a face presentation can spin around even after the face has reached the perineum to bring the chin anterior. Some women's pelvises are even large enough to permit a posterior face presentation to emerge, but this is rare.

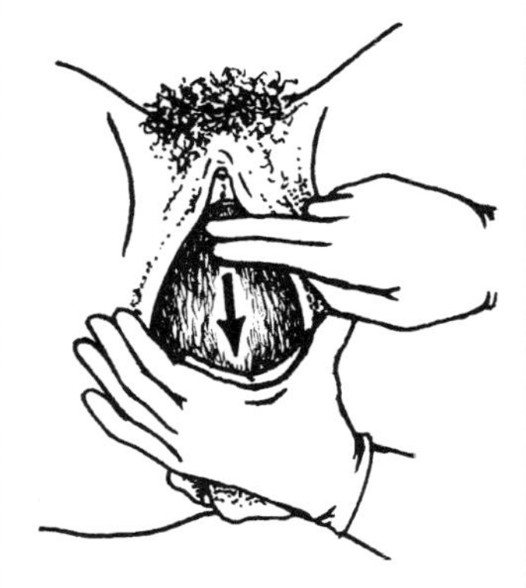

Flexing the head (occiput anterior presentation, woman semi-sitting)

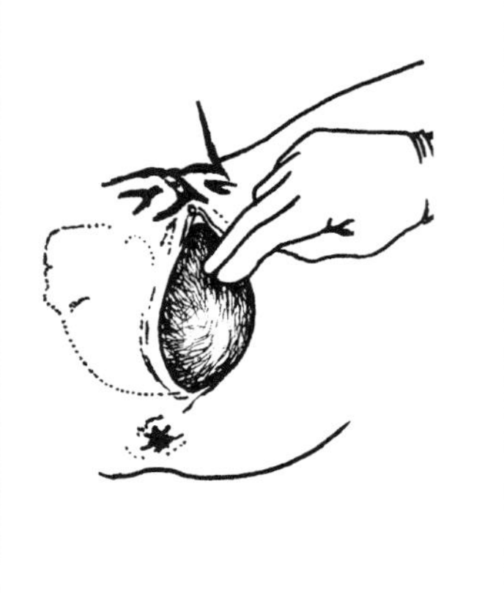

Sagittal view of flexing the occiput anterior head

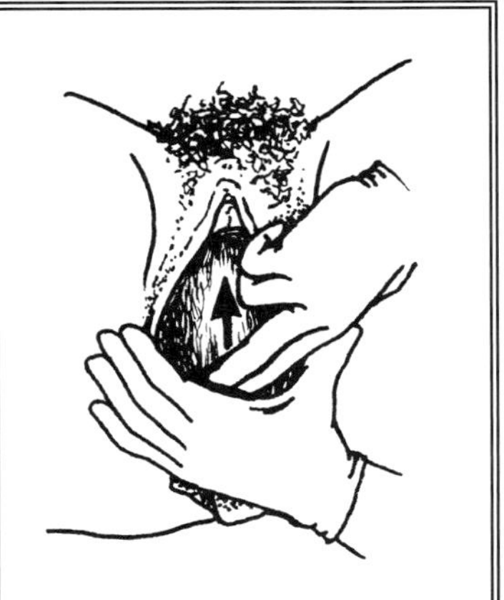

Flexing the head (occiput posterior presentation)

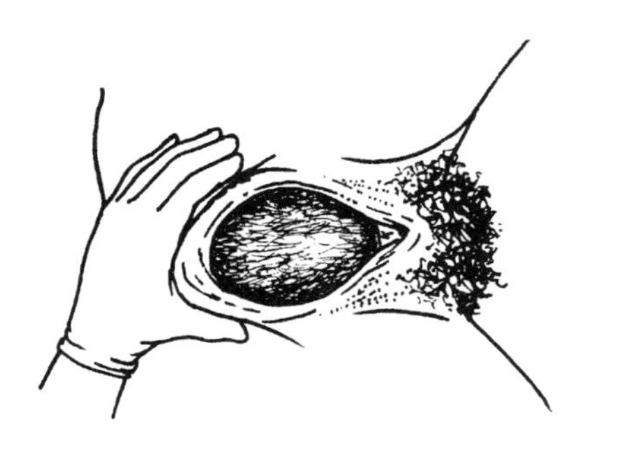

Creating perineal slack (woman side-lying, legs spread)

When women are birthing in a position that allows it, some midwives have found it helpful to "pinch" the perineal tissue to either side of the head to create slack around the opening of the yoni (Tritten, 1987). This may help to prevent perineal tears but be careful not to create extensive periurethral damage by transferring all the stress to the upper tissues in the process.

Relaxation throughout labor and pushing is another important component of a tear-free birth. If the woman is having difficulty, one way to help her relax is to use humor. Deep belly laughs can relax the mouth and yoni muscles. Remind her not to grimace or clench her jaw in resistance to the pressure as the baby comes down. Between pushes, try to help her relax as much as possible (Gaskin, 1992). Pillows, people supporting her legs if she is recumbent, and positioning can help accomplish this.

If pushing is resulting in a tightly stretched, taut and shiny perineum, have the mother refrain from pushing for several contractions. This can assist in reestablishing a more physiologic pattern and help ease the head out slowly. When offering verbal encouragement, emphasize a loose mouth and opening up the tissues rather than pushing through them (Kitzinger, 1990). Reminding her to visualize the tissues as very elastic can also help, especially if she has been using that image prenatally.

If a woman has painful hemorrhoids, she may involuntarily hold back and resist pushing because she fears increasing the pain. This tenses the perineum and makes tearing more likely. Applying counterpressure to the anus with a hot or cold compress (e.g., a gauze-covered ice cube) can help relieve the pain enough to get her past this resistance. Be especially careful not to contaminate the perineal compress solution or the yoni area with compresses used for this purpose.

The passage of stool during pushing is a good sign of progress. However, wiping it away can cause the woman to involuntarily tense her anal sphincter, which will also cause her to tense her genital sphincters. If she is upright, be sure a disposable pad or a piece of clean newspaper is beneath her bottom. Let any stool fall to the floor and remove the soiled pad. If you do need to wipe her bottom, be sure to warn her first ("I'm going to clean you up a little bit"), and then wipe very gently, directing your wiping efforts away from the yoni opening. Use toilet paper or facial tissue rather than gauze, since they are less abrasive. Applying a little oil to the paper before you wipe will ease discomfort. However, the best thing to use is unscented baby wipes, as they are made for this purpose and work very well. They can be warmed by removing them from their box, placing them in a zipper lock plastic bag and wrapping them in an electric heating pad.

If the head is not completely born by the end of the contraction, do not encourage the mother to birth the head with a few small pushes between contractions. This seems to increase the likelihood of sticky shoulders, because the next contraction has not been allowed to rotate them correctly. It is better for the crowning head to stretch the perineum between contractions and then allow the uterus to complete the birth of the head with the next contraction.

Another technique midwives find helpful is to ease the baby out. Ask the mother to blow lightly or pant or to use short pushes broken up by breathing. During controlled pushing, as the presenting part reaches a full crown, the precision and timing of pushes and breathing must be more carefully tuned. The more upright the mother is, the sooner you will need to have her slow her pushing down to avoid too rapid a birth. Watch the tissue and talk to the mother. If she reports burning, have her blow and then push again, bringing the baby out in little nudges. If the mother shouts or cries out, remind her that low, moaning sounds bring the energy down and will help her to relax as much as possible (Gaskin, 1992).

Pushing is an all-consuming task for most women. Some, however, can direct their attention to their vulva and will use their own hands to guide the head and massage their own tissue. Encouraging a woman to do this can help her center herself if she is overwhelmed with the sensations of birth.

Often after the head is born over an intact perineum, the shoulders, small and irregularly shaped as they are, cause a tear as they are born. Continue perineal support as the shoulders birth, but not so firmly that you inhibit rotation.

If shoulder rotation seems delayed, check for a very tight cord or a hand near the face or an impacted shoulder inhibiting birth. A little elbow can cause a very big tear. If you can manage it, guide the baby out so the arm is kept as close to the baby's body as possible. Bringing the hand and arm out as the shoulders begin to birth frequently jabs the elbow right down into the perineum, creating a deep pocket tear. This maneuver can cause the shoulders to malrotate as well.

Protecting the periurethral area: If you are providing hands-on support, take care not to focus so much attention on the perineum that your overzealous efforts push the head upward, causing major labial or periclitoral damage while the perineum remains intact.

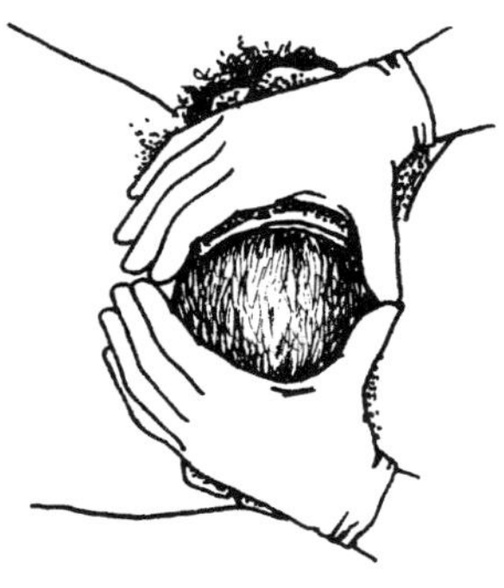

Supporting the upper tissues (woman semi-sitting)

If there is a low or very steeply angled pubic arch, the head will be pressed further down into the perineal body. This, in combination with a strong, resistant perineum, is a set-up for labial tears. Again, positions that allow maximal sacral mobility are an important factor in reducing the chances of tearing. If the head is large, if a cystocele or rectocele exists, or if the vulva is swollen or varicosed, check carefully after the birth to make sure that the periurethral area is intact. A side-lying position with the knees together and deeply flexed (like a side-lying squat) can help minimize periurethral damage, but should not be assumed until the head is nearly crowning because this position pinches off the brim. Side-lying like this helps the mother control her pushing urges and still relieves weight on the perineal tissues to an extent, while leaving the sacrum free to move. For all these reasons, it was a position frequently used by old time doctors and is the least stressful of any horizontal position. If necessary, the upper leg can be lifted slightly as the head emerges. Try to ease the shoulders out one at a time (Feral, 1988).

Birth with a birthing stool or support: Generally speaking, gravity works most effectively with the mother upright during pushing, and many midwives carry birthing stools for this reason. Nevertheless, most birthing stools and chairs have the unfortunate feature of putting pressure on the sacrum, so that (in my view) any benefit gained by being upright is lost by the inability of the sacrum to rotate backward as the head descends.

The deBy birth support is an exception. The deBy is constructed of two U-shaped pieces of pipe with three upright open-frame supports. It weighs about 14 pounds, and it is made entirely of plumbing pipe, giving it a narrow seat which, when padded, simulates a wide toilet seat that can suspend the entire pelvic girdle over an open space.

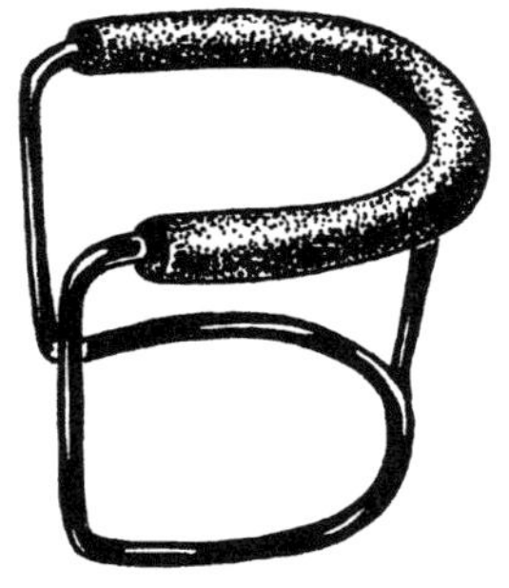

deBy birth support

The mother may lean forward or back to push and can lean back between contractions into someone's arms. Efficient contractions and spontaneous rotation from the posterior position during labor are but two of many reported benefits. This support affords continued pressure on the perineum between contractions, which facilitates stretching. Gravity helps the baby move under the pubic bone toward crowning and is especially helpful with first babies.

If support of the perineum seems necessary with a woman in the suspended upright position afforded by the deBy, apply a warm, wet, wrung-out washcloth or piece of old diaper to the entire vulval area. Use one hand to hold it over the tissue but apply no pressure.

Have the mother slow her pushing efforts when you can see about a third of the top of the head (i.e., sooner than usual). This signals that the biparietal diameter is beneath the pubic bone (or almost so). Have the mother blow through pushing to allow the uterus to complete the birth while you allow the head to emerge into the washcloth. Do not apply localized pressure to any part of the perineum, as this may produce irregular tension on the tissue and encourage tearing. Be ready to support the baby around the neck and shoulders and expect the body to deliver in short order (deBy product information, 2009).

Learning to support mothers to give birth without tearing while adapting to a more hands-off approach takes some adjustment. Midwives experienced with this stool report a significant reduction in perineal tears and a somewhat more frequent occurrence of minor labial tearing (which may be due to the pressure on the upper tissue from the mother leaning forward on the stool).

Hyaluronidase injections: (Before studying this section, read about hyaluronic acid on page 114). Hyaluronidase (HAase) is an enzymatic complex found in the skin, eyes, liver, kidneys, uterus, testicles, sperm, blood and other human organs and tissues. It has the ability to depolymerize and hydrolyze hyaluronic acid, which reduces the acid's viscosity and increases the permeability of cellular membranes and blood vessels. HAase has been studied extensively and used for years in a variety of medical applications either as an injection or a topical cream, usually to enhance the absorption of injected drugs.

Injectable HAase is synthesized from bovine testicles and sold as a water-soluble powder. Intracervical injections have been used to soften the cervix. Because the perineal body is also rich in hyaluronic acid, HAase has also been used to soften the connective tissues of the skin and subcutaneous muscles, rendering them less susceptible to mechanical stress during birth; this was a fairly common practice during the 1950s and 1960s to reduce the incidence of clitorotomy. The injection is given at some point during the pushing phase of labor (about 15 to 30 minutes prior to the birth of the presenting part), with a return to normal tissue consistency by the time the woman is discharged from the hospital. Several older studies point to the effectiveness of HAase when used like this, while others found no significant effect.

A more recent randomized, unblinded trial involving 139 primparous women by Scarabotto and Rieso (2008) also found a reduction in tearing among mothers who received perineal injections of HAase. Hyalozima (Apsen Farmacêutica SA, São Paulo, Brazil) in a dose of 20,000 turbidity-reducing units was reconstituted with sterile water and then administered immediately using a 5 cc syringe fitted with a 26 gauge, half-inch needle. At the time of pushing, the woman was asked to assume a dorsal position and her perineum was cleansed with a neutral liquid soap. HAase was then injected in a fan pattern, with 1 cc given in the perineal midline and 2 cc given on each side, to the left and right of the midline. Following injection the perineum was not massaged or otherwise manipulated and the woman was asked to give birth in the left lateral position. Hand maneuvers were used to guide the birth of the head and provide support to the maternal tissues. The average time till birth was 12.6 minutes, with a range of 4 to 35 minutes.

This procedure resulted in a statistically significant reduction in the rate of perineal trauma as well as the severity of any damage. No second-degree tears occurred in the treated group and third- or fourth-degree tears were not noted in either group. Most of the tears that occurred in the treated group were sustained in the periurethral area, suggesting a protective effect of HAase on local tissues. When those with intact perineums were removed from the analysis, however, the differences in trauma rate were no longer significant. While these results suggest that the use of HAase is associated with a reduction in the frequency and severity of perineal lacerations, especially when the perineum is not cut, the number of subjects in this study were not sufficient to establish whether treatment is benign, ineffective or helpful. No complications related to HAase injection were noted in this study. Additional studies are needed to look at the use of HAase in multiparas and in cream form as an alternative to injections.

All the studies to date have been done on women who were either lying laterally or supine during pushing. That HAase may reduce tearing when women give birth in these positions is good, but it is a better to get women off their backs during pushing. Given its history of benefit in other therapeutic applications, the (somewhat mixed) results of studies to prevent perineal tears, the expense and the highly interventive nature of the procedure it is certainly nothing to consider using routinely. However, it may be a reasonable option to discuss with women who have tough scar tissue from previous genital-altering surgery or some other factor that places them at very high risk for a very bad tear.

Preventing trauma to vulval varicosities: Minimize stress on vulval varicosities during birth by suggesting that the mother give birth in a side-lying position. If the varicosities are only on one side, a lateral position with the mother lying so that the most prominent veins are uppermost can work well. Most women with varicose veins are also multiparas; their babies will usually come out without intense pushing, which is an advantage. As the head begins to crown, apply compresses around the opening of the yoni, being sure to provide evenly distributed counter-pressure support over the varicosed vessels. Have the woman blow or breathe but not add to her uterus's pushing efforts, letting the uterus birth the baby's head and shoulders. After the birth, withdraw your hands and leave the mother as undisturbed as possible to allow her uninterrupted time immediately after the birth. During your postpartum stay, be alert to the possibility of a developing hematoma from deeper tissue damage.

If support hose have been helpful during pregnancy to cope with varicosed veins in the legs, they can be worn during labor and continued throughout the first six weeks postpartum until the veins reduce to their prepregnant size.

Protecting other soft tissues during labor: Certain preexisting medical conditions, such as cervical infection or cancer, may encourage tearing during labor. Cervical damage more commonly occurs when there is edema, an anterior lip, or scars from previous tearing or surgery (i.e., cerclage, surgical abortion, biopsies, cryosurgery, etc.) or when the birth is accomplished with instruments (forceps or vacuum extraction). Very rarely, previous cervical damage leaves such severe scarring that normal dilation is impossible. Please refer to the chapter entitled "Cervical and Other Soft Tissue Problems during Labor," in HOLISTIC MIDWIFERY, VOL. II, for a complete discussion of these problems and how to deal with them.

Avoiding bladder damage: Although it is widely believed that a full bladder can inhibit descent as well as uterine activity, this usually does not occur (Read et.al., 1980). The bladder may rarely present a problem if it is extremely distended and the baby not yet engaged. Even without obstructing descent, though, a full bladder can be painful during pushing. As the baby descends, the bladder can be damaged from pressure or by a small fold of tissue being caught between a low head and the pubic bone. Either can cause a vesicovaginal (VES-eh-koe-VAJ-eh-nahl) fistula (hole between the bladder and the yoni), even if other upper yoni wall damage does not occur. Damage is more likely if forceful, sustained pushing takes place before the head reaches the pelvic floor. Fortunately, the actual incidence of bladder damage from labor trauma is extremely rare.

A full bladder presents as a fluctuant mass above the pubic bone. There may be a slight dip just above the fundus of the bladder, which falls between the pubic bone and the navel, giving the abdominal contour the look of a posterior presentation.

To minimize the need for catheterization, be sure the bladder is emptied every hour or two throughout labor. Have the mother attempt to urinate, either on the toilet or lying in a hot bath. Sometimes a horizontal position helps reduce pressure on the urethra. Putting a few drops of spirits of peppermint in the toilet may stimulate urination, but not if the presenting part is low and obstructing the flow. Do not but spirits of peppermint directly on the vulva and not in bath water; it is the fumes that help relax the urethra.

If the mother cannot void and the bladder is obviously full, catheterization before the baby gets any lower is the best solution. With the mother lying flat, push the fetal head up slightly before you insert the catheter. If the head is too far down to allow this, place your fingers on either side of the urethra, between the fetal head and the pubic bone, as you insert the catheter. Otherwise, follow the basic instructions for catheterization as given in the chapter entitled "Repairing the Anterior Yoni Wall."

Pelvic prolapses and the progress of labor: Large prolapses into the yoni (cystoceles, rectoceles, etc.) may become trapped in front of the presenting part. If a woman already has an obvious prolapse of this type, be sure to check it periodically during labor. If it becomes trapped, replace it by pushing it above the presenting part. This allows the head to descend unimpeded, as well as avoiding further damage to the wall of the yoni.

When a tear seems likely: The appearance of a white line down the perineum frequently precedes a tear as the tissue becomes more strained. This line will usually appear along the line of a previous scar, if one exists. Assuming that the baby is fine, the first thing to do is to help the mother to stop actively pushing by having her take deep breaths. (If the baby is in distress, get him out as soon as possible.) Wait until the next contraction (or even for several contractions) to resume active pushing. This allows the perineum to adjust to the pressure and to stretch rather than tear. In the meantime, apply hot compresses and plenty of oil to assist this process. Changing maternal position may also help. If the perineum starts to tear, use the same tactics as well as supporting beneath the laceration to try to prevent more damage. Slow, gentle birth of the head and shoulders can minimize further trauma.

The same suggestions apply if periurethral or labial damage seems likely. These tears are often heralded by bright red bleeding that, at first, may appear to come from behind the baby, but is really from the labial area. A slight trickle of blood may also appear as the hymen is torn during the birth of a first baby. Bright red bleeding may also herald a tear beginning high up in the yoni. When this last occurs, the resulting tears are usually extensive. Bleeding, especially if darker in color, could also signal premature placental separation, so monitor the fetal heart carefully to ascertain if this is a factor.

When there is a crisis (such as shoulder dystocia), protecting the perineum must be set aside for the more urgent need to get the baby out without delay.

Unhealthy tissue

Unhealthy tissue is, of course, attached to an unhealthy woman. A lifetime of poor nutrition and inadequate health care can leave a woman with very fragile tissue at the time of birth. Such tissue is often the consistency of wet newsprint or rotten meat and may tear extensively, despite an easy birth. The tissue cannot withstand much stress either from birth or from your perineal inspection. Stitches pull through the tissue, resulting in a more difficult repair; healing may also be impaired.

Prenatal dietary improvement, food concentrates such as JuicePlus+ or, if the woman cannot afford JuicePlus+, vitamin supplements (C with bioflavinoids, E, and zinc), and postpartum herbal therapy using herbal poultices and sitz baths may help as well as drinking comfrey infusion. Nevertheless, don't expect miracles in nine months after a lifetime of deficiencies.

References and Further Reading on Maintaining Perineal Integrity during Birth

References Used in Multiple Chapters

Deering SH, et al. "Perineal body length and lacerations at delivery," J Reprod Med, 49(4):306-10, Apr, 2004.

Gaskin IM. "Ask the midwife," Birth Gazette, 8(2):38, Spr, 1992.

Shipman M, et al. "Antenatal perineal massage and subsequent perineal outcomes: a randomized controlled trial," Br J Obstet Gynaecol, 104(7):787-791, Jul, 1997.

Sutton J. Let Birth Be Born Again: Rediscovering and Reclaiming Our Midwifery Heritage. Birth Concepts UK, Middlesex UK, 2001.

Preparing the Perineal Tissues for Birth

Avery M, Burket B. "Effect of perineal massage on the incidence of episiotomy and perineal laceration in a nurse-midwifery practice," J Nurse-Midwifery, 31(3):128-134, May-Jun, 1986.

Buchanan A. "The abdomen," in his Buchanan's Manual of Anatomy, 7th ed. Jones FW, et al., eds. Baillière, Tindall & Cox, London UK, 1946.

Bruce E. Getting Through Childbirth in One Piece! How to Prevent Episiotomies and Tearing. Writers Club Press, Lincoln NE, 2001.

Carrière B. Fitness for the Pelvic Floor. Thieme, New York NY, 2002.

Chaitow L. "The pelvic floor paradox," Massage Today, 6(12): Dec, 2006. www.massagetoday.com/mpacms/mt/article.php?id=13515, accessed May 15, 2008.

Davidson K, et al. "Prenatal perineal massage: preventing lacerations during delivery," J Obstet Gynecol Neonatal Nurs, 29(5):474-479, Sep-Oct, 2000.

Fletcher E. "Differential diagnosis of high-tone and low-tone pelvic floor muscle dysfunction," J Wound Ostomy Continence Nurs, 32(Suppl 3):S10-S11, May-Jun, 2005.

Frye A. Understanding Diagnostic Tests in the Childbearing Year: A Holistic Approach, 7th ed. Labrys Press, Portland OR, 2007.

Gallagher PG. "Varicose veins of the vulva," Br J Sex Med, 13:12-14, Jan, 1986.

Hendricks G, Hendricks K. Radiance! Breathwork, Movement and Body-Centered Psychotherapy. Wingbow Press, Berkeley CA, 1991.

Hopkins L, et al. "Racial/ethnic differences in perineal, vaginal and cervical lacerations," Am J Obstet Gynecol, 193(2):455-459, Aug, 2005.

Hulme J. Beyond Kegels: Fabulous Exercises and More, 2nd ed. Phoenix, Missoula MT, 2002.

Interstitial Cystitis Association. "IC and pelvic floor dysfunction," www.ichelp.org/Default.aspx?tabid=229, accessed May 15, 2008.

Kent T. Wild Feminine: Finding Power, Spirit and Joy in the Root of the Female Body. Tami Kent MSPT LLC Publisher, Portland OR, 2008.

Knutson M. "Differential diagnosis of pelvic floor dysfunction and vulvar pain," Medscape Today, www.medscape.com/viewarticle/465853, 2004, accessed May 15, 2008.

Loprenzi-Kassel KB. Conversation regarding perineal stretching, 1995.

Lukban J, Whitmore K. "Pelvic floor muscle re-education treatment of the overactive bladder and painful bladder syndrome," Clin Obstet Gynecol, 45(1):273-285, Mar, 2002.

Miller J-J, Sand P. Chapter 6: "Kegel exercises, dietary and behavioral modifications: simple strategies for getting started," in Culligan P, Goldberg R, eds. Urogynecology in Primary Care. Springer-Verlag, London UK, 2007.

Noble E. Essential Exercises for the Childbearing Year : A Guide to Health and Comfort before and after Your Baby is Born, 4th ed. New Life Images, Harwich MA, 1995.

O'Dwyer M. My Pelvic Flaw: Preventing Pelvic Floor Problems Throughout Life. Redsok Pub., Buderim QLD, Australia, 2008.

Owen J, Hauth J. "Episiotomy infection and dehiscence." in Gilstrap L, Faro S., eds. Infections in Pregnancy, Alan R. Liss, New York NY, 1990.

Rosenberg J. "What if? Tearing, stitching and pelvic floor healing," in Midwifery Today Holistic Clinical Series, TEAR PREVENTION AND TREATMENT HANDBOOK. Midwifery Today, Inc., Eugene OR, 2005.

Ruckhäberle W, et al. "Prospective randomized multicentre trial with the birth trainer EPI-NO for the prevention of perineal trauma," MIDRS, 20(1):59-64, Mar, 2010.

Sand P, et al. "Pelvic floor electrical stimulation in the treatment of genuine stress incontinence: a multicenter, placebo-controlled trial," AM J OBSTET GYNECOL, 173(1):72-79, Jul, 1995.

Theofrastous J. "The clinical evaluation of pelvic floor dysfunction," OBSTET GYNECOL CLIN N AM, 25(4): 783-782, Dec, 1998.

Thiele G. "Coccygodynia and pain in the superior gluteal region and down the back of the thigh," JAMA, 109: 1271-1274, 1937.

Vodušek D. "Anatomy and neurocontrol of the pelvic floor," DIGESTION, 69(2):87-92, 2004.

Warnock J. CORRECT ASSESSMENT OF PELVIC FLOOR TONE: A NECESSARY COMPONENT OF INDIVIDUALIZED CARE (unpublished paper), Birthingway College of Midwifery, Winter, 2008.

Wise D. "Explaining the details of physical therapy used in Stanford protocol," www.pelvicpainhelp.com/physical_therapy.php, accessed May 15, 2008.

PROTECTING THE PERINEUM DURING LABOR AND BIRTH

Albers L, et al. "Midwifery care measures in the second stage of labor and reduction of genital tract trauma at birth: a randomized trial," JMWH, 50(5):365-372, Sep-Oct, 2005.

Ashton-Miller J, DeLancey J. "Functional anatomy of the female pelvic floor," ANN NY ACAD SCI, 1101: 266-296, Apr, 2007.

Brooks S, et al. "Injury to muscle fibers after single stretches of passive and maximally stimulated muscles in mice," J PHYSIOL (London), 488(Pt 2):459-469, Oct 15, 1995.

Childbirth Graphics. Slides: "The effect of giving birth on the muscles of the pelvic floor and episiotomy anatomy." Childbirth Graphics, Rochester NY, 1987.

Cohain J. Letters to the Editor: "Use of hyaluronidase to prevent perineal trauma during spontaneous delivery: a pilot study," JMWH, 54(1):92, Jan-Feb, 2009.

Davidson K, et al. "Prenatal perineal massage: preventing lacerations during delivery," J OBSTET GYNECOL NEONATAL NURS, 29(5):474-479, Sep-Oct, 2000.

deBy product information. www.birthchair.net, accessed Jan 13, 2009.

DeLancey J. Section 2A, chapter 2: "Anterior pelvic floor in the female," in Pemberton J, et al., eds. THE PELVIC FLOOR: ITS FUNCTION AND DISORDERS. WB Saunders, London UK, 2002.

DeLancey J. "The anatomy of the pelvic floor," CUR OPIN OBSTET GYNECOL, 6(4):313-316, Aug, 1994.

Dietz HP, Lanzarone V. "Levator trauma after vaginal delivery," OBSTET GYNECOL, 106(4):707-712, Oct, 2005.

Feral C. "Protecting the upper tissues," MIDWIFERY TODAY, 1(5):22-23, Win, 1988.

Formato LS. "Routine episiotomy: is it always necessary?" J NURSE-MIDWIFERY, 30(3): 144-148, May-Jun, 1985.

Fynes M, et al. Chapter 4: "Childbirth and pelvic floor injury," in Pemberton J, et al., eds. THE PELVIC FLOOR: ITS FUNCTION AND DISORDERS. WB Saunders, London UK, 2002.

Goldberg R. Chapter 3: "Effects of pregnancy and childbirth on the pelvic floor," in Culligan P, Goldberg R, eds. UROGYNECOLOGY IN PRIMARY CARE. Springer-Verlag, London UK, 2007.

Hastings-Tolsma M, et al. "Getting through birth in one piece: protecting the perineum," MCN AM J MATERN CHILD NURS, 32(3):158-164, May-Jun, 2007.

Head of Midwifery, Powy's Local Health Board, (PLHB) Mat 0013: "Policy for care of the perineum during and after birth–Powys Midwife Led Care," Approved: Clinical Governance and Risk Management Committee, Aug, 2006, www.wales.nhs.uk/sites3/docopen. cfm?orgid=501&id=62528, accessed Mar 26, 2009.

Hyde S. "Powerful pushing: new method promises safer, more efficient delivery," http://includes.iparenting.com/layout/article_print.php?aid=2143&type=1, accessed Nov 9, 2007.

Kalis V, et al. "The perineal body length and injury at delivery" (article in Czech), CESKA GYNEKOL, 70(5):355-361, Sep, 2005.

Kearney R, et al. "Obstetric factors associated with levator ani muscle injury after vaginal birth," OBSTET

GYNECOL, 107(1):144-149, Jan, 2006.
Kitzinger S. "Episiotomy," MOTHERING, (55):62-65, Apr-May-Jun, 1990.
Lamay G. "Midwife's guide to an intact perineum," in Midwifery Today Holistic Clinical Series, TEAR PREVENTION AND TREATMENT HANDBOOK. Midwifery Today, Inc., Eugene OR, 2005.
Lien K-C, et al. "Levator ani muscle stretch induced by simulated vaginal birth," OBSTET GYNECOL, 103(1):31-40, Jan, 2004.
Nygaard I, Gregory T. Chapter 13: "Obstetrics and pelvic floor disorders," in Walters M, Karram M, eds. UROGYNECOLOGY AND RECONSTRUCTIVE PELVIC SURGERY, 3rd ed. Mosby, St Louis MO, 2007.
O'Dell KK, Morse AN. "It's not all about birth: biomechanics applied to pelvic organ prolapse prevention," JMWH, 53(1):28-36, Jan-Feb, 2008.
Power D, et al. "Obstetric anal sphincter injury: how to avoid, how to repair: A literature review," J FAM PRAC, 55(3):193-200, Mar, 2006.
Rauli A. "The use of birth stools during second stage labour and the risk of perineal trauma," Centre for Clinical Effectiveness, Evidence Centre Evidence Report Series 2001: intervention, Jun, 2001. www.mihsr.monash.org/cce/res/pdf/c/655.pdf, accessed Aug 31, 2007.
Read J, et. al. "Urinary bladder distention: effect on labor and uterine activity," OB GYN, 56(5):565-570, Nov, 1980.
Rizk D, Thomas L. "Relationship between the length of the perineum and position of the anus and vaginal delivery in primigravidae," INT UROGYNECOL J PELVIC FLOOR DYSFUNCT, 11(2):79-83, 2000.
Rogers R, et al. "Obstetric anal sphincter lacerations: an evidence-based approach, Part 1: anatomy and risk factors," FEMALE PATIENT, 27(4):21-24, Apr, 2002.
Royal College of Obstetricians and Gynecologists (RCOG), "The management of third- and fourth-degree perineal tears," Green-tip Guideline no. 29, Mar, 2007.
Scarabotto L, Riesco M. "Use of hyaluronidase to prevent perineal trauma during spontaneous delivery: a pilot study," J MIDWIFERY WOMEN'S HEALTH, 53(4):353-361, Jul-Aug, 2008.
Shafik A, et al. "A novel concept for the surgical anatomy of the perineal body," DIS COLON RECTUM, 50(12):2120-2125, Dec, 2007a.
Shafik A, et al. "Physioanatomical relationship of the external anal sphincter to the bulbocavernosus muscle in the female," INT UROGYNECOL J, 18(8):851-856, Aug, 2007b.
Shafik A, et al. "Surgical anatomy of the perineal muscles and their role in perineal disorders," ANAT SCI INTERNAT, 80(3):167-171, Sep, 2005.
Sultan AH, et al. "Pudendal nerve damage during labour: prospective study before and after childbirth," BR J OBSTET GYNAECOL, 101(1):22-28, Jan, 1994.
Tritten J. "Preventing Tears," MIDWIFERY TODAY, 1(2):16, 44, Spr, 1987.

NOTES:

ASSESSMENT OF THE PELVIC TISSUES

Note: Study the part entitled "Pertinent Anatomy" and the chapter entitled "Preparing the Perineal Tissues for Birth" before studying this part.

LEARNING TO RECOGNIZE NORMAL PELVIC ANATOMY

Knowing what normal tissues look and feel like will help you to know when there is cause for concern, particularly when findings are subtle. Enlist the help of sister students to learn the range of normal and its many variations by performing thorough exams on each other. Discuss the specifics of the exam before you begin and talk her through what you are doing as you perform the exam, just as you would a woman in your care. Be sure to ask her permission before proceeding with the exam and to reconfirm permission at each point during the exam, especially before performing a rectal exam. You can try to perform a self exam with a mirror, and this can be informative, but you will find out more if you examine other women. You will need a cotton swab, gloves and water-based lubricant.

Neurologic function

- To elicit the bulbocavernosus reflex, stroke a cotton swab along one labia majora. This should trigger bilateral contraction of the bulbocavernosus muscle and the anal sphincter. (The sphincter response may not be obvious; ask the woman if she can feel her sphincter responding to this stimulation.)
- Use the same swab to stroke the skin beside the anus to elicit the anocutaneous or "anal wink" reflex. This should cause the anus to contract, suggesting neurologic integrity in this area. (See page 191 for more details on these two reflexes.)

Identifying pelvic soft structures and musculature

- Use the pad of your finger to gently palpate the symphysis, starting over the mons and moving down till you find the clitoral body. This will give you an idea of how much the clitoral structures project beyond the bones.
- Place two fingers inside the introitus with the finger pads facing either 3 or 9 o'clock. Use your thumb to gently palpate the tissue underlying the area lateral to the yoni wall. Notice the spongy feel? This is the clitoral bulb encased within the bulbocavernosus muscle. Remember that the bulbs originate posteroinferiorly to the clitoral body and fill the space laterally between the body and the crus on either side. They are consistently located in relation to the rest of the clitoral complex and the urethra, not to the vestibule. Have the woman tighten her introitus, and note the contraction of the bulbocavernosus muscle to either side as she does so.
- Ask the woman to constrict her yoni opening and note how that feels against your fingers. Ask her to relax. Now press down into the yoni floor and note the slight movement in the clitoral–urethral area as you press; this movement occurs because you are pulling on the bulbocavernosus muscle.
- Use the fingers inside the yoni to palpate the much firmer muscle inside the introitus on either side. This is the pubovaginalis portion of the pubovisceral complex.
- Note the location of the hymenal ring or tags and the location of the muscles in relationship to it. In particular, note the appearance of the hymen in the posterior midline (landmarks will vary somewhat from woman to woman).
- Note that, behind the hymenal ring and rising to either side of the middle third of the

yoni is another portion of the pubovisceral muscle. When tone is good, this part hugs the urogenital hiatus, creating an obliquely oriented opening approximately 2 to 3 finger-breadths deep (4 to 6 cm). The muscles should offer strong resistance even when relaxed, keeping the hiatus narrow and snug.

•Ask the woman to constrict her muscles. In nulliparous women, the levator muscles usually retract firmly, elevating them to form flat, lateral ledges on either side, over which one can easily hook a finger. Parous women often have less distinct ledges that lie further apart with sloping sidewalls (Baden & Walker, 1992). When the muscle is at rest, weakness is also indicated by the need to press more deeply into the lateral yoni wall before you run into the pubovisceral muscle. The borders of the urogenital hiatus will be less distinct. A lax inferior muscle boundary may cause the introitus to gape.

•Have the woman contract her pelvic floor muscles again. Place the tip of your dominant index finger about 4.5 cm inside, against the posterolateral yoni wall at 3 or 9 o'clock. Locate the puborectalis muscle and follow it up to its attachment behind the pubic bone; it should be firm. Now, locate the more shallow tissues just in front of the puborectalis muscle and try to insert your fingertip into the angle they form. Lack of muscular tension or an inability to locate this angle suggests muscular damage or weakness.

•Palpate the inferolateral skin surface to either side of the introitus and see if you can identify the superficial transverse perineal muscle. If you can, follow each muscle half to the midline where it meets the central perineal body. Note the length of the perineum from the yoni introitus to the anal opening.

•The muscle you feel surrounding the anal opening and behind the lower center of the perineal skin surface is the anal sphincter, not the bulbocavernosus. If the perineum is short, you will also feel the sphincter immediately beneath the floor of the yoni. (This is because a short perineum leaves very little perineal body.) In a short perineum, note how little of the perineal body there is to allow the muscles to thin during birth.

•Place your thumb in the center of the perineum and the index and ring finger of the same hand about 5 cm inside the yoni at the 6 o'clock point. Now pull down and forward with your yoni fingers while pressing into the perineum just above the anus with your thumb. Your yoni fingers will run into the perineal body. This will give you a good idea of how much perineal body exists between the surface of the yoni floor and the top surface of the anal sphincter and of where the posterior tip of the perineal body is located. Press into the perineum with your thumb and have the woman contract her muscles to further evaluate the tone of her perineal body. (Whitley, 1985)

Connective tissue supports

Next, evaluate the condition of the pelvic adventitiae. Only by examining normal, young, nulliparous women can you get a sense of the normal parameters of these tissues. You will need gloves, a speculum, lubricant, a ring forceps and a bright, glare-free light.

Examine each region of the yoni visually and by palpation, focusing this time on the thickness, tension and strength of the tissues and underlying adventitiae. Include the yoni walls, fornices, cervix, ureterovesical junction, urethra, levator hiatus, perineum and the anorectal canal. Women with normal anatomy have normally positioned organs, clearly demarcated sulci, no bulges and no other evidence of prolapse.

Yoni fornices and ectocervix: Insert a bivalve speculum, such as a Graves or a Pederson, into the yoni. This should require opening the introitus somewhat to insert the blades. Look at the cervix, which is normally located at the same level as and slightly anterior to the intraspinous diameter. When gentle traction is applied with a ring forceps, normal bilateral ligamentous attachments to the cardinal and uterosacral ligaments via the pericervical ring allow the cervix only limited lateral movement as well as limited downward mobility in the upper third of the yoni. Pulling down on the cervix tenses these attachments, which can then be felt to the side of and behind the ectocervix if you examine the area with your other hand (these attachments are easier to feel during a rectal exam).

The attachments of the cardinal ligaments cause the lateral fornices to be concave (from the examiner's point of view) when at rest. Ask the woman to bear down. You should see and feel limited downward movement of the cervix; there should be little movement in the lateral fornices and only slight movement in the anterior fornix. The posterior fornix is bounded by the uterosacral ligaments inserting into the posterolateral aspects of the paracervical ring. It may normally move a bit more than the others during bearing down.

Yoni walls: The anterior yoni wall is composed of a thick epithelium with a relatively thick fibromuscular coat. Pronounced transverse rugae are present when the underlying adventitiae is intact, thick and healthy. Normally, the posterior yoni wall is also well rugated but the underlying connective tissue is a bit thinner and more mobile than that of the anterior wall. The absence of rugae or rugae that display a geographic rather than transverse pattern both indicate underlying problems of connective tissue support Baden & Walker, 1992).

Detach the posterior blade of a Graves or Pederson speculum. Gently insert it into the center of the yoni lumen and then use it to slightly depress the posterior yoni wall (avoid downward traction, which can distort the tissues). Observe the grooves of the anterolateral yoni sulci running from about the level of the hymenal ring back toward the ischial spines. These grooves are formed by the attachment of the external yoni wall to adventitia that is itself attached to the tendinous arch of the pelvic fasciae. Ask the woman to bear down and study the movement of these sulci while she is straining. The walls of the yoni should remain in place and not collapse to the midline.

Ask her to relax. Palpate and visualize the entire length of the anterior yoni wall in the midline and over to each side, beginning at the cervical end and carefully moving along the wall until you are two-thirds of the way toward the introitus: this is the level of the urethrovesical junction. When this region is palpated or subjected to gentle traction with a ring forceps, there should be very limited lateral movement of the urethra in this area. Normally, if you insert your finger alongside the urethra and try to poke your fingertip up to the top of the interior pubic rami you are prevented from doing so by the firm connective tissue attachments to the tendinous arch of the pelvic fasciae on either side.

Starting at the ischial spines on one side, gently palpate along the lateral yoni wall toward the pubic arch. You should feel the tendinous arch of the pelvic fasciae as a taut band. In the midthird of the yoni wall, you should be able to feel (or in some women see) a fork in this underlying ropelike structure, separating the anterolateral sulci that proceed to the pubic arch on either side, which are formed by the attachment to the tendinous arch of the pelvic fasciae, from the posterolateral sulci that pass toward the perineal body that are formed by the less distinct attachment between the rectovaginal adventitiae and the parietal fasciae of the levator ani muscles (tendinous arch of the rectovaginal fasciae).

Urogenital hiatus: While the woman is relaxed, place two fingers in the introitus to the depth of the distal third of the yoni to appreciate the size, length, breadth and tone of her urogenital hiatus. Ask the woman to contract her hiatus, and note the difference in tone.

Perineum: When at rest, the normal perineum appears slightly concave because all the internal attachments that run through it are well toned.

Rectovaginal examination: Be sure to get permission from your student-partner before proceeding with a rectal exam.

Inspection of the surface anatomy: Look over the perianal area for lumps, ulcers, hemorrhoids, or any other abnormal features. Palpate for lumps or tenderness. Adult perianal skin is more pigmented and somewhat coarser than the surrounding skin. Use two fingers to gently part the anal orifice and search for lesions within the folds of the corrugator cutis ani.

Positioning for a rectal exam: The anus and rectum can be examined with the woman is one of several positions. Left-side-lying with the hips and knees flexed is one option; allowing adequate visualization of the perianal and sacrococcygeal areas. The lithotomy position, however, is probably best when you are performing a rectal exam to gain information about the uterus or cervix because it allows you to reach higher into the rectum and to perform a bimanual exam more easily when you are also searching for a pelvic or rectal mass.

Examine the anus and rectum: Double-glove one hand. Lubricate that index finger and ask the woman to relax her sphincters. If she has trouble with that instruction, ask her to cough into her pelvic floor. Inspect the anus during straining to see if any surface anatomy changes; it may cause prolapses to become evident or hemorrhoids to pooch out. Place the pad of your finger over the anal orifice and apply light pressure. Ask her to relax or bear down gently until the sphincters relax, admitting the curve of your fingerpad. Incline your finger toward her umbilicus as you fully insert it. If the sphincter tightens, pause and reassure the woman. If the exam is painful, withdraw your finger.

Note the tone of the sphincters; normally they close snugly with uniform pressure around your finger. Insert a finger in the yoni and perform a bimanual exam of the sphincters while the woman is relaxed and when she is contracting them.

Palpate the walls of the anal canal, which should feel incredibly soft and smooth. Check for any hardness (induration), irregularities or nodules. Advance your finger into the rectum as far as possible. Rotate your hand as you palpate as much of the rectal wall as you can reach in each quadrant.

If you feel something unusual, ask the woman to bear down again, which often brings the upper wall within easier reach. The cervix can be felt through the anterior rectal wall, so sometimes a retroverted uterus is palpable above that level (Bates, 1991). Palpate the rectovaginal wall and, above that, the rectovaginal pouch (posterior cul-de-sac).

When examining the posterior midline, advance your fingers into the larger rectal ampulla. Flex your finger, which should now rest on the levator plate. The coccyx and the lower part of the sacrum can also be felt. To either side lie the ischial tuberosities and spines and the ischiorectal fossa.

Perineal body: A bimanual rectovaginal examination will allow you to get a feel for the perineal body at rest. It should feel thick and broad between the anus and the introitus. Ask the woman to bear down and note the downward movement of the perineal body. The downward displacement of the perineal body should be no more than 1 cm.

Advance your rectal finger through the anal canal as you palpate the anterior rectal wall to feel how the pyramid-shaped perineal body tapers to a point at the level of the lower third and midthird of the yoni, beyond which the yoni and rectal walls are in much closer contact.

Anorectal canal: Palpate the walls of the rectal canal, which feel incredibly soft and mushy. These walls are adjacent to the rectovaginal wall anteriorly, the levator plate posteriorly and the downward extensions of the uterosacral ligaments on either side. Ask the woman to contract her pelvic floor. During this maneuver, it should be easy to feel her levator plate through her posterior rectal wall as a nearly vertical wall of tissue (vertical because she is supine). Then palpate the walls of the rectal canal to detect the puborectalis muscle embracing it on three sides (Rogers & Richardson, 2003). Check with the muscles at rest, during bearing down and during a strong pelvic floor contraction. Gently palpate about 1 cm inside for the intersphincteric groove.

Assessing pelvic floor tone

Study the chapter entitled "Preparing the Perineal Tissues for Birth." Using the description that begins on page 145 as a guide, practice assessing pelvic floor tone.

Checking Prenatally for Previous Damage

The initial pelvic exam is the ideal time to check the perineal region for evidence of damage or prolapse. Question the woman regarding any previous tears, clitorotomies or injuries from other sources and subsequent scarring. (Remember, she thinks of it as an episiotomy, so be sure she understands that clitoral structures are severed, which is not generally known.) Ask about the course of prior healing; inquire about pain, infection or any other long-term problems. If you suspect that difficulties with healing were caused by a suture reaction, or if she knows for sure that she had a reaction, make a note to use one of the several absorbable synthetic sutures if she requires a repair. (Also ask about other allergies, especially to iodine and local anesthetic.)

Note the location and shape of the hymen. In first-time mothers it will usually appear as a ring of tissue 0.5 to 2 cm inside the opening of the yoni. In multiparas it usually appears as ruffled tags of tissue on either side. The hymen is an important landmark when examining the yoni after birth and when approximating tissue.

Note any abnormal yoni discharge and the presence of venereal warts, so that treatment can begin without delay. Yoni discharge that smells of urine or feces indicates the likelihood of a fistula (for more details see the chapters that follow as well as the one entitled "Checking Tears and Repairs in the Weeks Postpartum").

Check previously repaired areas inside and out for scar tissue, sinus tracts or inclusion cysts that may be lurking beneath the path of the scar. Scar tissue may feel slightly lumpy inside the yoni and will often appear as a white line down the perineum, although such a line may not always be visible until the perineum is stretched at the time of birth. A cyst feels like a small, round, firm, fluctuant mass that may enlarge, or appear for the first time, with the hormonal stimulation of pregnancy. (For more details, see the chapter entitled "Inclusion Cysts.") Other lesions may be found as well and should be examined by your backup practitioner.

Access the length of the perineum by noting the distance between the introitus and the anterior margin of the anus. Does the puckering around the anal opening look uniform all around? Does the skin above the anal opening look normal? If the puckering is irregular or absent, or if the anterior anal opening consists of a small bridge of skin, prior anal sphincter damage is likely. These findings warrant a digital exam to determine the extent of the damage (for details, see page 480). Note the conformation of the woman's musculature, and any evidence of pelvic soft-tissue prolapse, and perform a more thorough exam whenever indicated. Look for varicosities or anything else out of the ordinary. Refer to the diagrams and explanations in the part entitled "Pertinent Anatomy" and to the chapter entitled "Learning to Recognize Normal Pelvic Anatomy" for instructions regarding the assessment of muscles and connective tissues.

The principle pelvic complaints include urinary or anal incontinence and pelvic prolapse. Any of these conditions can be related to pelvic floor weakness or damage. Identifying and classifying these conditions are discussed in the chapters that follow.

FUNCTIONAL DISORDERS OF THE URINARY TRACT

Urinary Incontinence

Causes and prevalence

Studies of urinary incontinence indicate a prevalence of 25 to 55% across all age groups. Presentation increases dramatically after age 50, irrespective of childbearing history. Contributing factors include obesity, an abdominal mass, menopause, childbirth, smoking, chronic lung disease and hysterectomy. The most common causes of urinary incontinence among women of childbearing age include high-tone or low-tone pelvic floor dysfunction and obesity. Pelvic floor dysfunction is discussed beginning on page 145. Normal innervation is also essential to normal continence and urinary incontinence can be the first symptom of a neurologic disorder such as multiple sclerosis (10% at onset), cerebral vascular accidents or Parkinson disease.

Voiding diary

If you have taken a history and examined a woman and if pelvic floor tone dysfunction does not seem to be the culprit, ask her to keep a voiding diary for at least three days. She should record her oral intake of fluids, amount of urine voided at each visit to the toilet, episodes of leakage and what precipitated it (if she can tell); she should also record when she sleeps and wakes.

Defining urinary symptoms

Frequency: In the absence of increased fluid intake, voiding more than eight times daily outside of pregnancy constitutes a frequency problem and may reflect urge incontinence, urinary tract infection, interstitial cystitis, calculi, urethral pathology such as a diverticulum, or even systemic fluid disorders such as congestive heart failure (especially nocturia).

Stress incontinence: This occurs when a physiological stress that puts pressure on the bladder causes a small amount of urine to leak out. Such stresses include coughing, sneezing, laughing, running or jogging.

Urge incontinence: This occurs when there is a strong need to urinate that cannot be controlled before voiding is appropriate. The usual cause is a sudden contraction of bladder, which is known as an "overactive bladder."

Volume of loss: If a woman is losing a large amount of urine with each incontinent episode, spontaneous detrusor muscle contraction may be the cause, although this typically causes the loss of smaller volumes of urine. Affected women can usually stop the flow by tightening their pelvic floor.

Dribbling after urination is most often associated with a urethral diverticulum; this condition may be mistaken for incontinence.

Urinary retention: Retention occurs when a woman is not fully emptying her bladder with each void; stress incontinence or urgency frequently follow.

Blood in the urine: Hematuria it is most commonly associated with urinary tract infection and more rarely malignancy. During pregnancy, it may reflect placenta percreta.

Physical examination

Examine the vulval area looking for evidence of atrophy (shriveling of tissue, asymmetric tone) and suburethral bulging, which may indicate a diverticulum.

Neurologic assessment: External urethral sphincter activity requires intact innervation at S2 and S3. The presence of both of the reflexes described here suggests that these sacral nerve pathways are normal; however, false negatives can occur.

The **bulbocavernosus reflex** is elicited to assess the integrity of the clitoral branch of the pudendal nerve, which constitutes the afferent limb of this reflex (receives signals to the nerve); and the inferior hemorrhoidal branch of the pudendal nerve, which forms the efferent limb (sends signals from the nerve). Both nerve branches are integrated at S2 and S3. To trigger the reflex, gently stroke down one labia majora with a cotton swab, or tap or stroke to the side of the clitoral body. Normally, one of these stimuli will cause these muscles, which underlie both labia minora, to contract equally. Absence of this reflex may indicate central or peripheral neurologic deficits.

Next, check for the **anocutaneous reflex** or "anal wink," indicated by a circumferential anal sphincter contraction. Elicit this response by using the swab to brush over the perianal skin to the side of the anal orifice.

Cotton swab test: When the urethra is poorly supported, it may become hypermobile when abdominal pressure increases. The woman lies supine with her legs spread, knees up, feet supported. The test is performed by applying 1% lidocaine jelly to the soft tip and shaft of a cotton swab and inserting it into the urethra up to the level of the urethrovesical junction (about 3 cm). Use a cotton swab with a paper or plastic shaft to avoid getting splinters in the urethra. Use a protractor or a goniometer to measure the angle of the swab handle at rest and then ask the woman to hold her breath and bear down while you measure the angle again. Normally, the handle of the swab moves within a range of 20 to 25°, demonstrating normal changes in the urethrovesical junction. A range of movement greater than 30° above the horizontal indicates hypermobility. This test can be uncomfortable and may introduce pathogens into the urethra. Explain the test fully to the woman before proceeding. If a woman is planning to see a urogynecologist, she can wait to have the doctor decide if this test is warranted.

Bimanual examination: An internal exam may find a mass or uterine enlargement due to fibroids that may prompt incontinence from increased external pressure that is transferred to the bladder. Palpate the urethra all along the anterior yoni wall, checking for bulges that may be from diverticula or prolapse of the wall. If the woman has reported constipation, palpate the posterior yoni wall for hard, impacted stool as this too can cause bladder urgency.

Urinalysis and culture: Perform a urinalysis to rule out infection and treat if appropriate.

If these simple screening evaluations are unrevealing, the woman can be referred to a urogynecologist for further testing using more sophisticated methods.

Treatment

Nonsurgical management depends on the specific diagnosis. Stress incontinence may respond to one or more of these therapies: dietary changes, pelvic floor therapy or strengthening, biofeedback or scheduled voiding. Any of these therapies could be used during pregnancy. Outside of pregnancy, electrical stimulation of the pelvic floor may also be helpful. In addition, weight loss may have a profoundly positive impact on simple incontinence, but should not be attempted during pregnancy.

The following nonsurgical therapies are more invasive and therefore probably not very good options during pregnancy. They include certain drugs (available for either stress or urge incontinence and often not very effective), pessaries (to provide support, when appropriate), a silicone urethral insert that acts as a plug, and periurethral bulking agents to puff up the urethral mucosa.

For those who do not respond to such interventions, surgery can be performed in certain cases. A specialist should be consulted.

Genitourinary Fistula

Although urinary fistulas can cause symptoms that mimic either urinary or anal incontinence they are unrelated to either. A **genitourinary fistula** is an abnormal communicating tract (usually due to a healed hole) between the urinary system and the genital tract. The communication may involve either the bladder, a ureter, the urethra or the uterus, and the uterus, cervix or yoni. A **rectovaginal fistula** occurs when there is a communicating channel between the rectal or the anal canal and the yoni. It is covered in the chapter entitled "Anorectal Disorders and Incontinence."

Although, among Western women, the incidence of genitourinary fistula is higher than for rectovaginal fistula, they are both relatively uncommon and the exact incidence of either is unknown. They both occur much more frequently in women in developing countries who have little or no access to appropriate medical care should their labor become obstructed.

Medical history

Your initial history should include screening questions to determine if a woman may have a fistula. Be alert for associated risk factors.

Risk factors: Obstetric trauma due to prolonged or obstructed labor is the most common cause among women of childbearing age and is the cause in 90% of affected women in developing countries. Associated factors include pregnancy at an early age and surgical alteration of the genitals (female genital mutilation) performed by untrained practitioners. Obstructed labor or malpresentation of the presenting fetal part can lead to pressure or ischemic necrosis of the anterior yoni wall or bladder that can result in vesicovaginal fistula.

Damage associated with the use of instruments, malnutrition and limited health care options are contributing factors in many cases.

In developed countries, iatrogenic injury sustained during surgery is the primary cause of 90% of the genitourinary fistulas that occur, with hysterectomy being the most common such surgery and with surgical birth playing a significant role as well. The typical timing of symptom onset after hysterectomy is 1 to 3 weeks. A variety of other things can lead to the development of a genitourinary fistula including injury inflicted during pelvic surgery, radiation therapy, malignancy and trauma from a foreign body. Rare causes include congenital defects, infection, inflammatory bowel disease and autoimmune disease. Conditions associated with impaired healing such as diabetes, smoking, peripheral vascular disease and chronic steroid use may also be related. Some fistulas remain unnoticed for years before symptoms appear.

Signs and symptoms: Women who enter pregnancy with an existing genitourinary fistula may complain of constant leakage of urine from her yoni. The amount of urine leaked varies with the size and location of the fistula. Intermittent leakage may be mistaken for urinary stress incontinence. Less specific symptoms include fever, pain, ileus (intestinal obstruction) and bladder irritability. Any woman who has had pelvic surgery, a history of a difficult birth or extensive tearing, or who complains of passive leakage should be examined for fistula.

Classification systems

Many systems have been used to classify the characteristics of a genitourinary fistula, but none have been standardized. Vesicovaginal fistulas can be classified by their size and location along the yoni wall. **High vaginal** fistulas are at the proximal end; **midvaginal** fistulas are in the center and **low vaginal** or distal fistulas are nearer the introitus. In obstetrics, high-risk vesicovaginal fistulas are classified by size (diameter larger than 4 or 5 cm); urethral, ureter or rectal involvement; proximity to the cervix with an inability to see the upper edge; and rehealing of the fistula tract after a failed repair (Elkins & Thompson, 1999).

The table that follows shows how fistulas are named and presents a classification system based purely on location.

Genitourinary Fistula Terminology Based on Site of Communication			
Genital Tract Involvement	Urinary Tract Involvement		
	Ureter	Bladder	Urethra
Yoni (Vagina)	Ureterovaginal	Vesicovaginal	Urethrovaginal
	Vesicoureterovaginal		—
Cervix	Ureterocervical	Vesicocervical	Urethrocervical
Uterus	Ureterouterine	Vesicouterine	Not reported

Goh and colleagues (2004) introduced a comprehensive classification system that categorizes genitourinary fistulas into four main types, depending upon the distance between the distal margin of the fistula and the external urethral meatus. These types are further subdivided by size, the extent of any associated scarring, whether the yoni's length is reduced due to scarring or fistula involvement, and other special considerations.

CLASSIFICATION OF GENITOURINARY FISTULA	
PRIMARY TYPE	DISTANCE BETWEEN DISTAL EDGE OF FISTULA AND EXTERNAL URETHRAL MEATUS
Type 1	> 3.5 cm
Type 2	2.5 to 3.5 cm
Type 3	1.5 to 2.5 cm
Type 4	< 1.5 cm
DIAMETER	SIZE OF FISTULA OPENING AT ITS' WIDEST DIAMETER
(a)	< 1.5 cm
(b)	1.5 to 3 cm
(c)	> 3 cm
OTHER FACTORS	DEGREE OF FIBROSIS/YONI LENGTH AND SPECIAL CONSIDERATIONS
i.	Little or no fibrosis around fistula or yoni or yoni length > 6 cm with normal capacity
ii.	Moderate to severe fibrosis around the fistula, the yoni or both; or reduced yoni length, capacity or both
iii.	Special situations such as postradiation, ureteric involvement, circumferential fistula or previous repair.

Physical examination

Most urinary fistulas can be detected during a careful visual inspection of the yoni wall. Use of a clear plastic speculum and good light will help. One bill of a speculum may be used to depress the anterior or posterior yoni wall to aid visualization of the opposite wall of the yoni or a Guardian retractor may be inserted. To view the upper wall, it may also be helpful to use an exam table and have the woman lie on her side with her body rotated forward and her upper leg supported by an assistant. Small fistulas are often hard to see, and may present an opening that looks like a depression or pit-like defect.

If you cannot find a fistula but symptoms are highly suspicious, have the woman take a large dose of Vitamin C before her next appointment and drink enough water to partially fill her bladder. This will result in bright yellow urine that may be easier to spot leaking. If you still cannot rule out fistula during a visual inspection, a urogynecologist can instill dye into the bladder via a catheter to increase the chance that leakage will be seen.

If only a small amount of fluid is leaking, you can have the yoni fluid checked for creatinine to see if it is urine or not. Although urinary levels of creatinine vary (the mean level is 113.5 mg/dL), a value exceeding 17 mg/dL in a sample of yoni fluid is considered positive for urine (Barr et al., 2005).

Another way to confirm either the presence of or location of a leak is to pack three pieces of gauze into the yoni in high, middle and low positions. A large tampon can also be used if it fills the canal sufficiently. Dye is then introduced into the bladder and the woman is asked to resume normal activities, such as walking, for 15 to 30 minutes. Then the tampon or gauze is removed piece by piece to determine if and where any leakage has occurred. If the distal gauze or tampon is stained, it is important to make sure it is from a fistula and not due to stress incontinence.

A urogynecologist can perform a few other tests to confirm location if these have failed and to check for ureteral involvement.

Treatment

Some small genitourinary fistulas will heal spontaneously. In the meantime, herbal compresses in the yoni won't hurt and may help the area heal together. Homeopathic remedies may also be of use in these cases. A 6-month period of observation prior to treatment is recommended. Expectant management should include the placement of an indwelling urinary catheter, to allow the hole to rest and heal. If the fistula looks like a fresh wound or is small (2 to 3 mm in diameter), try this first, especially in resource-poor countries where further medical evaluation is hard to come by. The time is takes to heal varies widely and may range from 2 to 8 weeks or sometimes longer.

Generally, however, large fistulas do not respond well to this, although in one study fistulas as large as 2 cm in diameter healed in 50 to 60% of women who had an indwelling catheter placed (Waaldijk, 1989). If it has not closed by 4 weeks, it is unlikely to do so.

Other conservative approaches may be offered by a urogynecologist. In some cases, surgery may be warranted and can be performed when the fistula is identified. If severe infection or inflammation is present, surgery will be postponed until the inflammation has cleared up. Surgical repair of obstetric fistulas is usually successful, with an 81% rate of correction on the first attempt and 65% on the second (Elkins, 1994; Hilton & Ward, 1998).

Urinary Diverticula

A urethral diverticulum (pl. diverticula) is a cystic enlargement of a female prostate (paraurethral) gland. Diverticula develop along the anterior yoni wall and open into the urethral lumen, with a reported incidence of 1 to 5% among the general female population. Among women who experience lower urinary tract symptoms, the incidence rises to 40%. Diverticula are most common in women aged 30 and into their sixties.

Urinary diverticula are often asymptomatic and may be first noted during a routine pelvic exam as an outpouching along the yoni wall. Although urinary diverticula may be congenital, most are acquired secondary to infection or birth trauma. Birth trauma may be associated with young age, prolonged labor, or injury during instrument use. Stones may develop in larger diverticula due to stagnation of urine with crystal precipitation. Rarely, diverticula become cancerous, usually among women in their 60s or older.

Classification

Accurate determination of the number, location and type of defects is critical, because surgery that fails to address all the diverticula may leave a woman symptomatic. Large lesions may require more complex surgical procedures. Due to the branching nature of the female prostate glands, diverticula may be singular or branched and may be simple, saddle shaped or encircle the urethra. Finally the location of the opening into the urethral lumen must be accurately identified.

A woman's urinary continence status and urethral hypermobility, if present, are also documented as many women with diverticula also have stress incontinence and each of these problems may require different surgical solutions.

Leach and colleagues (1993) came up with a comprehensive classification system (L/N/S/C3) that encompasses all these characteristics.

L (Location): the site of the diverticulum (i.e., distal, mid, or proximal urethra), with or without extension beneath the bladder neck

N (Number): how many diverticula are present.

S (Size): measured in centimeters (cm).

C3 (Configuration, Communication, and Continence Configuration)

C1 (Configuration): whether the diverticulum is single, multiloculated, or saddle shaped

C2 (Communication): the site of any communicating channel with the urethral lumen, i.e., distal, mid- or proximal urethra (differs from L in that L merely locates the bulge along the urethral canal).

C3 (Continence) continence status of the woman.

This format provides the surgeon a systematic means of approaching a urethral diverticulum and thus may minimize postoperative complications and allow accurate comparison of surgical results. For example, the practitioner might note: "distal, no extension into neck/two/1 & 2 cm/multi-loculated, no communication, no stress incontinence."

Signs and symptoms

Symptomatic women may report a variety of symptoms, usually related to the size, location and extension of the diverticula. Classic signs include postvoiding dribbling and a discharge of fluid from the urethra when the diverticulum is compressed. But a woman may present with nonspecific symptoms such as pain due to occlusion of the diverticular neck with dilation of the pouch or dyspareunia when the diverticulum is inflamed or infected. Diverse other symptoms are more common, including urinary incontinence (35 to 60%) due to interference of the diverticula with the urethral sphincter complex or with support at the urethrovesical junction. During urination, urine may enter the sac and spill out later. Urinary retention may also develop if the sac is large; in these cases cancer of the diverticulum or urethra should be ruled out. Infection is a common complication of diverticula. Diverticula may mimic Gartner duct cyst, yoni inclusion cyst, ectopic ureterocele or endometrioma.

A large diverticulum may be mistaken for early-stage pelvic organ prolapse, especially among women reporting yoni fullness, a bulge or pressure. The mass may mimic a cystocele or even a rectocele. In most cases, however, careful palpation of the yoni wall will distinguish prolapse from a discrete yoni wall cyst or diverticulum because the wall will feel normal except in the area where the sac emerges from the wall.

Physical exam

The most common physical finding (found in 50 to 90% of symptomatic women) is an obvious mass protruding from the anterior yoni wall that underlies the urethra. Compressing the mass may produce a purulent urethral discharge. Once one diverticulum is identified, the entire length of the urethra should be carefully inspected to see if there is more than one.

Additional sophisticated testing can be performed by a urogynecologist.

Treatment

Women with few to no symptoms require no treatment. They should be made aware of their diverticulum so they can be alert for changes that may indicate a problem. Surgical treatment carries the risks of urethrovaginal fistula and urethral sphincter damage and is reserved for women with persistent, debilitating symptoms.

ASSESSING PELVIC ORGAN PROLAPSE

Women who report sensations "as if their insides are falling out" may have a degree of organ prolapse, which involves the downward displacement of one or more of the pelvic organs from their normal positions that results in displacement of the yoni wall, usually presenting as a protrusion or bulge. The most common pelvic support defects involve uterine prolapse, yoni vault prolapse, enterocele, low and high cystocele, low and high rectocele, urethrocele (including urethral hypermobility), a gaping introitus and perineal descent (a discussion of these diagnoses begins on page 208). Prolapse may occur due to damage to the muscles, the support tissues or their innervations. Pelvic organ prolapse affects millions of women worldwide and is the third most common reason for women to seek a hysterectomy. Overall, 11% of US women seek some sort of corrective surgery for prolapse conditions.

Risk factors

Factors that affect the support of pelvic organs include genetics, nutrition and hormonal changes. Mechanical stresses include childbirth and high-impact exercise. The most common environmental stress is cigarette smoking, which is antiestrogenic and affects connective tissue integrity. Advancing age or connective tissue disease may be associated factors. Racial or ethnic differences in bony pelvic structure may play a role, with black and Asian women at lowest risk and Latina women at highest risk. Conditions associated with increased abdominal pressure such as obesity, chronic constipation, chronic coughing and repetitive heavy lifting can also play a role.

How damage occurs

When the urethra, bladder and rectum are normally supported, they do not descend below the level of the levator plate, even during maximal straining. Yoni wall prolapse may occur when the pelvic floor muscles or adjacent connective tissues are weakened or damaged. Once such damage occurs, ligaments and fasciae that normally stabilize the reproductive organs and yoni are called upon to provide support and suspension as well. While they can do so for a time, eventually they give way, allowing pelvic structures to drop from their normal position, resulting in prolapse. Such damage most often occurs as a result of childbirth.

While it is commonly believed that overdistention of the yoni by the fetus causes adjacent ligaments to become stretched and injured, this is probably not the case during most natural births. As DeLancey explains (1993), before labor begins, the diameter of the yoni is about 4 to 5 cm and the cervix is closed. During labor, both must open to about 10 cm to allow for birth. Cervical dilation requires far more stretching than does dilation of the yoni because of the initially smaller size of the cervical os. After birth the cervix closes sufficiently so that considerable effort is required to redilate it should a procedure such as curettage become necessary. Since the yoni undergoes less distention, it is unreasonable to conclude that stretching of adjacent endopelvic adventitiae would be any greater than the stretching that occurs in the cervix. Furthermore, tension on the cardinal ligaments is actually relieved as the cervix dilates, bringing their points of attachment between the pelvic walls and lateral cervical surfaces closer together as the cervix approaches complete dilation. Since, in the typical circumstance, the cervix doesn't descend markedly within the pelvis as labor progresses, it seems unlikely that the cardinal and uterosacral ligaments are stretched unduly by the normal process of birth.

The exception to this is when forceful, sustained pushing commences prior to complete dilation or when a cervical lip is stretched down to the introitus. Although physicians sometimes use ring forceps to pull the cervix down to the introitus to examine it after birth, this does not by itself seem to result in permanent prolapse. (While this often produces temporary prolapse, the cervix has usually returned to its normal position 6 months to 1 year later and additional traction does not result in abnormal descent.) The dramatic cervical descent that is often noted immediately after birth may be more due to hormonal softening of the tissue rather than actual damage.

While I don't mean to suggest that damage to the connective tissues is inconsequential, it is important to remember that it is the pelvic floor, not the surrounding ligaments and stabilizing adventitiae, that is primarily responsible for maintaining the pelvic organs in their proper positions. This underscores the importance of pelvic floor exercises, which can greatly reduce the chances of these types of damage.

Weaknesses in the pelvic floor are categorized by location. In the upper third to half of the yoni, weakness is caused by increased intra-abdominal pressure, resulting in weakening of the support provided by the cardinal and uterosacral ligaments. The resulting slack in these stabilizing ligaments results in prolapse of the upper yoni that may or may not involve the uterus. The ligaments become elongated and stretched, permitting the cervix and the apex of the yoni to slide down over the edge of the levator plate. Such descent may be accompanied by an enterocele and is frequently associated with some degree of cystocele. However, loss of upper support alone usually does not produce a rectocele by itself. Herniations of the middle and lower yoni vault are usually a direct result of weakness in the pelvic floor and can lead to cystocele, rectocele or both (Wexner & Bartolo, 1995).

Signs and symptoms

Signs and symptoms vary widely and do not correlate well with the degree or progression of prolapse conditions. Many affected women, even some with pronounced prolapses, have no bothersome symptoms. Women may report seeing a mass protruding from their introitus, or report symptoms such as a sensation of pelvic pressure, of a bulge, of a mass in the yoni, of "sitting on a weight," or of something falling out and rubbing against their clothes. These symptoms tend to worsen as prolapse becomes more extreme.

Symptoms of urinary incontinence, frequency or retention; recurrent urinary tract infections; and voiding dysfunction may also accompany prolapse. While these types of problems may be caused by or made worse by prolapse, they are not necessarily cured when the prolapse is corrected. Correction may even make urinary symptoms worse, especially irritative bladder symptoms (frequency, urgency and urge incontinence). For these reasons, urodynamic testing by a urogynecologist is recommended.

When the posterior yoni wall is weakened, constipation is a frequent complaint. The woman may have to apply pressure to her posterior yoni wall during a bowel movement to prevent the fecal mass from becoming trapped in the pocket formed by the prolapsed wall. Surgery often does not fix this problem either.

Women may also report sexual dysfunction of various kinds. If due to an obstructing bulge, nonsurgical forms of therapy may be the best treatment option because surgical procedures, especially those involving posterior repair, also alter the anatomy and frequently lead to postoperative pain during sexual penetration.

Pelvic and back pain are also often reported, but there is little evidence that these symptoms are a direct result of prolapse.

Some of these symptoms cannot predictably be improved, regardless of the interventions chosen to correct a prolapse.

Terminology

Classical references to conditions of prolapse have used a specific vocabulary. The terms "cystocele" (bladder), "cystourethrocele" (bladder and urethra), "uterine prolapse" (descent of the cervix and uterus down through the yoni canal), "rectocele" (rectum) and "enterocele" (small bowel) have been used to describe the visual impression of protruding tissues, with these assignments based purely on the location of the bulge. However, the use of these diagnostic terms to describe the mere appearance of a bulge in the yoni wall implies that one knows with certainty the cause of the bulge. This can be very misleading because it focuses on what is presumed to be prolapsed, rather than what can actually be confirmed by the examiner. Such uses of terminology lead to assumptions that may require revision when other factors are discovered to be contributing to the prolapse, as can occur during surgery.

For these reasons, it is more clinically useful initially to describe the prolapse in terms of what one can actually report from an external examination: "anterior yoni wall prolapse," "prolapse of the uppermost (apical or superior) yoni wall," "cervical prolapse," "posterior yoni wall prolapse," "perineal prolapse" or "rectal prolapse." These descriptors explain what part of the wall is prolapsed without assuming what is behind the protruding area.

Pelvic examination to detect support defects

To detect defects in the pelvic floor, you must first be completely familiar with the characteristics of healthy tissues in young, nonpregnant, asymptomatic, nulliparous women. To perform an exam, you will need good light and preferably an exam table or a bed for the woman to lie on with her bottom near the edge with chairs placed to either side for her feet. You will need either a Sims retractor or a Graves or Pederson speculum. In addition, a gentle instrument to grasp the cervix may be required, such as a ring forceps or an Allis clamp.

During the exam, the appearance and movement of the various areas of the anatomy should be observed with the woman relaxed and again while she performs a Valsalva maneuver (holding her breath while bearing down forcefully). You will also be palpating for the feel of the tissues, including qualities such as thickness, tension and the strength of the underlying adventitiae (baseline findings are reviewed in the chapter entitled "Learning to Recognize Normal Pelvic Anatomy." Women whose anatomy is normal have uniform rugae on all their yoni walls, no bulges and no other signs of prolapse. While this exam is easiest to perform with the woman recumbent, you may be able to appreciate changes more readily if she is upright. Prolapse symptoms generally do not occur when a woman is lying down, but only when gravity is engaged during sitting or standing.

Pelvic organ prolapse quantification (POP-Q): In 1996, the International Continence Society introduced a system to standardize communication about pelvic organ prolapse, the pelvic organ prolapse quantification or POP-Q (Bump, 1996). It consists of a series of site-specific measurements of a woman's pelvic organ support system. The point system will be explained first and then the exam procedure will be described.

Prolapse in each region is measured in relation to a fixed anatomical landmark that can be consistently identified: for most POP-Q measurements, this landmark is the posterior midline of the hymenal ring (this point may simply be referred to as the hymen in the text that follows). Six points are designated with reference to the hymen. Each point is assigned a two-letter code. The first letter is capitalized and designates a point or region within the yoni. As the first letters advance from A to D, the points are increasingly deep within the yoni. The second letter is lowercased and is used only with points A and B to indicate whether the point is located on the anterior (a) or posterior (p) yoni wall. There are two locations on the anterior yoni wall (points Aa and Ba), two in the superior yoni (points C and D) and two on the posterior yoni wall (points Ap and Bp).

Anatomic Landmarks Used in Assessing the POP-Q

Anterior wall Aa	Anterior wall Ba	Cervix or cuff C
Genital hiatus gh	Perineal body pb	Total vaginal length tvl
Posterior wall Ap	Posterior wall Bp	Posterior fornix D

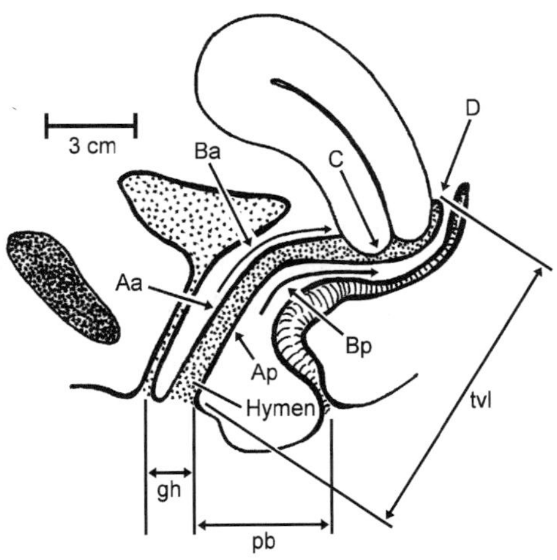

The yoni is first observed when the woman is at rest. To elicit full protrusion of any prolapsed tissues, the woman is then asked to engage in a maximum Valsalva effort as each point is measured. The anatomic position of each point is measured in centimeters using the plane of the hymen as the zero (0) point. Locations above the hymen are designated by a negative number and points below the hymen are designated by a positive number.

Anterior yoni wall points: A large diverticulum may be mistaken for early-stage pelvic organ prolapse, especially among women reporting yoni fullness, bulging or pressure. The mass may look like a cystocele or even a rectocele, but careful palpation will distinguish prolapse from a discrete yoni wall cyst or diverticulum in most cases because the wall will feel normal except in the area where the cyst or diverticulum protrudes. Diverticula are discussed on page 195.

***Point Aa*:** This point lies in the midline anterior yoni wall 3 cm above the external urethral meatus, the location of the posterior urethrovesical angle or crease. In relation to the hymen, this point's position may range from –3 (normal) to +3 (maximum prolapse of point Aa).

***Point Ba*:** This measurement evaluates the region that reaches from the anterior fornix (or yoni cuff if the woman has had a hysterectomy) to point Aa. The "point" is actually the distance between the deepest part of the anterior yoni fornix (or yoni cuff) to point Aa. It is normally –3 cm (that is, 3 cm above point Aa). It is a negative value because it is normally above the hymen. In a woman with total, post-hysterectomy eversion of the yoni, point Ba would be a positive figure equal to the level of descent of the cuff below the hymen in cm.

Superior (apical) yoni wall points: Two superior points, C and D, are located in the upper yoni vault and represent the deepest positioning of a normally supported lower reproductive tract. Descent of points C or D or both are related to uterine prolapse, which is characterized by descent of the uterus into the yoni canal with the cervix leading the way.

***Point C*:** Point C is the distance from the lowermost edge of the anterior exocervix (or the leading edge of the yoni cuff in women who have undergone hysterectomy) to the hymen.

***Point D*:** Point D is measured from the deepest point of the posterior fornix (which is where the uterosacral ligament attaches to the proximal posterior cervix) to the level of the hymen. It is omitted in women whose cervix has been removed. This assessment prevents confusing a prolapse due to failure of the uterosacral–cardinal ligament support with an apparent prolapse that is really the result of cervical elongation.

***Total vaginal length (TVL)*:** The TVL is the greatest depth of the yoni in centimeters when points C or D are normally located. If C or D or both are already prolapsed, use your fingers to support the tissues in a normal position while you measure the TVL. Manual support prevents including an abnormally elongated area of the yoni wall in the TVL measurement.

Posterior yoni wall points:
***Point Ap*:** Ap is located in the midline of the posterior yoni wall 3 cm above (proximal to) the hymen. The location of this point ranges from –3 cm in women with normal support to +3 in those with maximum prolapse of point Ap.

***Point Bp*:** Point Bp refers to the region of the posterior yoni wall from the posterior yoni fornix (or yoni cuff) to point Ap. This value is –3 cm in women with normal support.

***Genital hiatus (gh)*:** Measure the genital hiatus from the middle of the external urethral meatus to the posterior midline of the hymenal ring.

***Perineal body (pb)*:** The perineal body is measured from the level of the posterior margin of the genital hiatus (the posterior midline of the hymenal ring) to the center of the anus.

Recording your findings: As you assess each point, your findings can be organized on a three-by-three grid as shown on page 201. Write the value for each point in the appropriate box. Once all the point values are recorded, you can quantify your findings using a five-stage ordinal system as described below. Stages are assigned according to the most severe region of prolapse.

PELVIC ORGAN PROLAPSE QUANTIFICATION (POP-Q) STAGING SYSTEM	
STAGE	CHARACTERISTICS OF PROLAPSE
0	No prolapse. Points Aa, Ap, Ba and Bp are all at – 3 cm and either point C or D is between – TVL cm and – (TVL – 2 cm) (quantitation value for points C or D is ≤ – [TVL – 2] cm)
I	Slight prolapse. The most distal portion of the prolapse is > 1 cm above the hymen (its quantitation value is < – 1 cm).
II	The most distal part of the prolapse is ≤ 1 cm above or below the hymen. (i.e., quantitation value is ≥ – 1 cm but ≤ +1 cm).
III	The most distal part of the prolapse is > 1 cm below the hymen but protrudes no further than 2 cm less than the TVL in cm (i.e., quantitation value is > +1 cm but < + [TVL – 2] cm).
IV	Complete eversion of the total length of the lower genital tract. The distal portion of the prolapse protrudes to at least (TVL – 2) cm (its quantitation value is ≥ + [TVL – 2] cm). In most cases, the lowermost edge of the prolapse will be the cervix (or yoni cuff scar).

Examining for pelvic organ prolapse

Visible bulges along the yoni wall and the associated presence or absence of normal rugae in that area offer important indications that underlying breaks in the adventitiae or levator ani muscle weakness may have occurred. Breaks in the adventitiae typically occur at peripheral attachments sites and are less common at central locations.

Woman's description of prolapse: Before you begin to examine a woman who reports a problem, ask her to describe the extent of the prolapse and when is it most extreme (time of day, activities leading to most extreme presentation, etc.). Prolapse often becomes worse as the day progresses, especially when women are on their feet or when they engage in certain physical activities.

Neurological assessment: Ask the woman to assume a lithotomy position. Begin your physical exam by performing the neurological tests described on page 191.

Evaluate the anatomy: Next, evaluate the undisturbed anatomy when the woman is at rest. Look for evidence of bulges as well as irregular, indistinct or absent rugae in the yoni walls. Then ask her to perform a Valsalva maneuver. If she cannot do this, ask her to cough. While she does either of these, look for evidence of prolapse. This assessment helps determine if there is a visible prolapse. If so, does the protrusion descend past the hymen? What part of the anatomy is presenting (anterior, posterior, transverse or superior)? (You may not be able to tell just from looking.) Does the genital hiatus widen with increased abdominal pressure (noted by seeing the introitus gape)? Ask the woman to evaluate whether bearing down has elicited the maximal prolapse. If not, she should be reexamined in a standing position at rest and while performing a Valsalva maneuver. Symptoms are usually worse when a woman sits or stands, not when she lies down.

Site–specific defects: DeLancey has given the opinion that, in most cases, muscle weakness eventually results in connective tissue failure, as explained on page 113. Nichols and Randall (1989) proposed the term "distention cystocele/rectocele" for situations which the yoni wall gives way but the connective tissues are still attached, indicated by the presence of rugated walls. Anterior or posterior wall defects caused by a loss of connective tissue attachments between the lateral yoni wall and the pelvic sidewall are termed "displacement (paravaginal) cystocele/rectocele"; in these cases the yoni wall is smooth.

Performing a POP-Q assessment: To assess the POP-Q, a measuring device marked in 1 cm increments that is suitable for insertion into the yoni will be required. A closed ring forceps with 1 cm marks scratched into the surface on one side of the shaft can be used. You could also mark the shaft of a long-handled cotton swab with a permanent, fine-point marker or insert the cotton end of a couple of swabs into the open end of a Peri-Rule to use as a ruler (by inserting the swab padded-tip first, the Peri-Rule is less likely to slip off the swab during measurements). Assess each area while the woman is breathing normally with her pelvic area at rest. Then ask her to perform a Valsalva maneuver as you take each measurement.

Begin by identifying the hymenal ring or tags in the posterior midline; this is the stationary landmark you will use to take measurements. Then, measure the total length of the yoni by inserting your measuring device to the depth of the internal apex of the posterior fornix. Taking care not to stretch the canal, measure to the level of the hymenal ring. Then, measure the genital hiatus by placing the tip of the "ruler" in the middle of the urethral meatus and measuring to the hymenal ring. Finally, measure the length of the perineal body by placing the end of the measuring device at the level of the posterior hymen and measuring to the center of the anal opening.

Now, insert a bivalve speculum (such as a Graves) to displace the anterior and posterior yoni walls so you can measure points C and D. Slowly withdraw the speculum and assess whether and to what extent the yoni vault (apex) descends as you do so.

A split speculum is then created by disconnecting the blades of a Graves speculum and using only the lower blade. Insert it along the posterior yoni wall and displace it downward slightly to better visualize the anterior wall so you can measure points Aa and Ba. Sagging lateral sulci with rugae still intact suggest a loss of lateral support. A median bulge with absent rugae is called a "midline" or "central defect." Loss of support due to a detachment of the anterior yoni wall's superior (apical) segment from the anterior yoni apex downward is termed a "transverse defect." These defects are further assessed by using your fingers to support the anterosuperior tissues into a normal position and looking to see if the prolapse descends during a Valsalva maneuver.

To examine the posterior yoni wall the blade of the speculum is then removed, inverted and replaced so that it supports the anterior yoni wall so you can measure points Ap and Bp. If the posterior yoni wall bulges, attempt to determine if a rectocele or enterocele is present.

An enterocele is suggested if small bowel peristalsis is observed through the thinned yoni wall. As a general rule, bulges at the top of the posterior yoni wall are due to enteroceles, while bulges in the distal posterior yoni wall are more likely to be due to rectoceles.

Here are four examples of what you might find during such an exam. These diagrams show the uterus and cervix to your right, the central thin oval represents the hymen and the slanted shaded oval represents the pubic bone. Notes on each example follow.

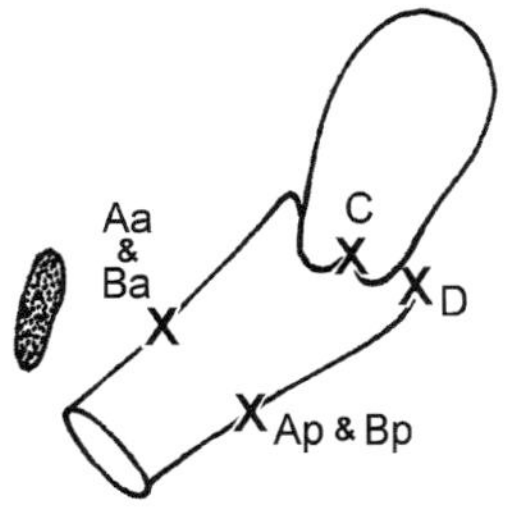

–3 Aa	–3 Ba	–8 C
2 gh	3 bp	10 tvl
–3 Ap	–3 Bp	–10 D

1. Normal support

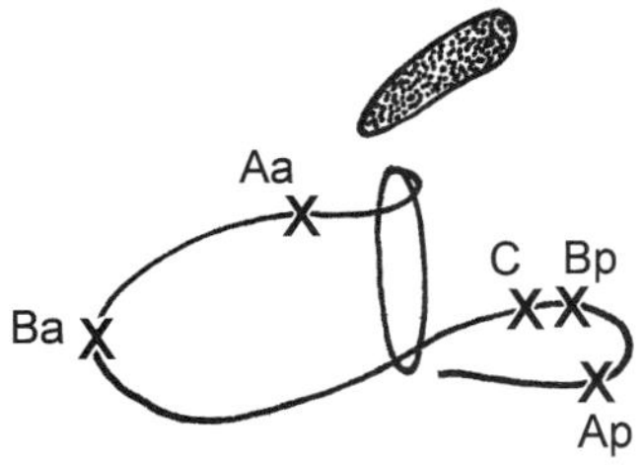

+3 Aa	+6 Ba	–2 C
4.5 gh	1.5 bp	6 tvl
–3 Ap	–2 Bp	— D

2. Predominant anterior support defect

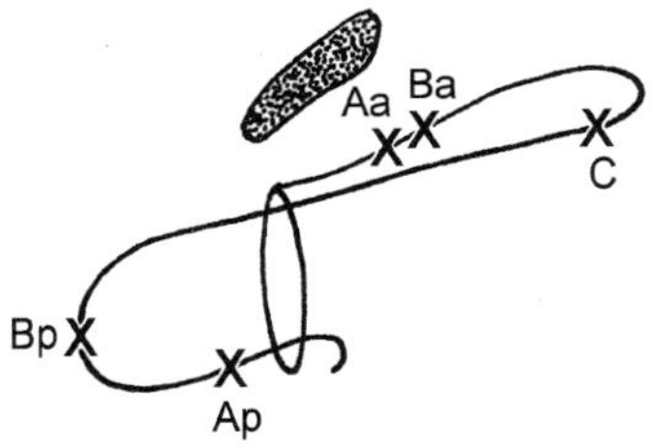

–3 Aa	–3 Ba	–6 C
4.5 gh	1 bp	8 tvl
+2 Ap	+5 Bp	— D

3. Predominant posterior support defect

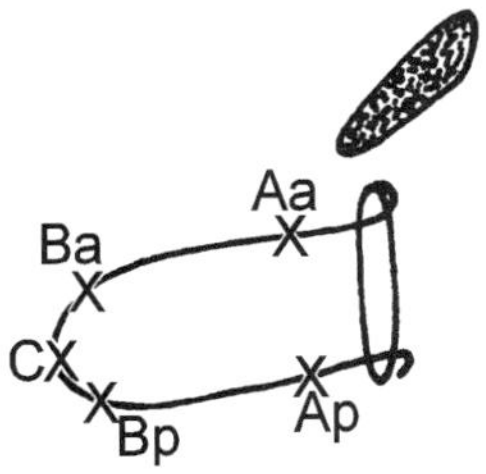

+3 Aa	+8 Ba	+8 C
4.5 gh	1.5 bp	10 tvl
+3 Ap	+8 Bp	— D

4. Complete eversion of the yoni

1. Points Aa, Ba, Ap and Bp are all –3 because the anterior and posterior yoni wall is normally supported. The lowest point of the cervix is 8 cm above the hymen (–8) and the posterior fornix is 2 cm above this (–10). Yoni length is 10 cm and the genital hiatus and perineal body measure 2 and 3 cm respectively.
2. In this post hysterectomy example, the leading point of this prolapse is the upper yoni wall,

point Ba (+6). There is significant elongation of the bulging anterior wall. Point Aa is maximally distal (+3) and the yoni cuff scar is 2 cm above the hymen (point C). The scar has descended 4 cm; it would be at –6 if it were perfectly supported. Here tvl is not the maximum depth of the yoni with an elongated anterior yoni wall maximally reduced, but rather the depth of the yoni at the cuff with point C maximally reduced. This example shows a stage III prolapse of point Ba.

3. Here we have another post hysterectomy example where the leading point of prolapse is the upper posterior yoni wall, point Bp (+5). Point Ap is 2 cm distal to the hymen (+2) and the yoni cuff scar is 6 cm above the hymen (–6). The cuff has undergone only 2 cm of descent because it would be at –8 tvl if it were perfectly supported. This represents a stage IIII Bp prolapse.
4. The most distal point of the anterior yoni wall (point Ba), cervix (C) and most distal point of the posterior wall (point Bp) are all at the same position (+10) and point Aa and Ap are maximally distal (both at +3). Because the tvl equals maximal protrusion, this is a stage IV yoni prolapse.

Standing exam: If the woman is symptomatic and nothing definitive is discovered during a supine exam, you may need to perform a repeat exam while the woman is standing to allow gravity to assist you in identifying a prolapse. This can be especially helpful when confirming an enterocele (prolapse of small bowel). Have the woman stand with one foot elevated on a small stool or step. Insert your well-lubricated index finger gently into her rectum and your thumb against her posterior yoni wall. Use both fingers to reach up toward the posterior fornix and feel for thinness, weakness or herniated intestines. An enterocele is confirmed if you can feel a loop of small intestines between your fingers.

Baden-Walker Halfway System

The Baden-Walker Halfway System (1992) for the evaluation of pelvic organ prolapse is a widely used alternative to the POP-Q. It is not as elaborate or as specific as the POP-Q but is adequate for clinical use if all three areas of the yoni wall are evaluated.

It consists of a descriptive grading system to classify the position of the superior (apical), anterior and posterior yoni walls using a number from 0 to 4 at each of six sites along the yoni canal (see diagram on the following page). There are two sites on each of the anterior, superior, and posterior walls of the yoni. The table on the next page lists each anatomical site with symptoms that the woman may report.

Each site is assessed by inserting two fingers, pads down, as far as possible into the yoni, and gently depresses the posterior yoni wall to obtain a good view. To elicit full protrusion of any prolapsed tissues, the woman is asked to engage in a maximum Valsalva effort as each point is measured. As the woman strains firmly, spread the fingers and slowly withdraw them as you observe what falls out and how far. For all the yoni sites, the hymen is used as a fixed point from which to measure. If the grade of an area is in doubt, assign the higher grade. If you are still unsure, examine her when she is standing (Baden & Walker, 1992).

PRIMARY AND SECONDARY SENSATIONS OR SYMPTOMS AT EACH SITE IN THE BADEN-WALKER HALFWAY SYSTEM		
ANATOMIC SITE	**PRIMARY SYMPTOMS**	**SECONDARY SYMPTOMS**
1. Urethra	Urinary incontinence	Falling out
2. Bladder	Voiding difficulties	Falling out
3. Uterus	Falling out	Heaviness, dragging or pulling sensation, etc.
4. Posterior cul-de-sac	Pelvic pressure (on standing)	Falling out
5. Rectum	True bowel pocket	Falling out
6. Perineum	Anal incontinence (gas/feces)	Too loose

BADEN-WALKER HALFWAY SYSTEM FOR EVALUATING PELVIC PROLAPSE		
GRADE	**FINDINGS FOR DIFFERENT SITES**	
	Urethral, bladder (vesical), uterine, cul-de-sac, rectal	**Perineal (lacerations)**
0	Normally positioned	None
1	Descent of site halfway to hymen	Halfway to anal sphincter
2	Descent of site to the level of the hymen	To anal sphincter
3	Descent of site halfway past the hymen	Involves anal sphincter
4	Maximum possible descent	Through rectal mucosa

Any persistent evidence of prior perineal damage is graded using the same system that is used to evaluate tears (further discussed on page 484). The woman is asked to contract her pelvic floor to evaluate whether and to what extent her muscles and connective tissues can compensate for any degree of prolapse that may be present when the tissues are at rest. Also record the site of the most severe prolapse, the location of any scars, palpable plications (folds in the walls) and the type of effort required to demonstrate maximum prolapse (this might be standing, holding the breath and pushing [Valsalva maneuver], etc.). The strength of pelvic floor contraction may also be evaluated with 0 being none and 3 being normal; 4 is high toned.

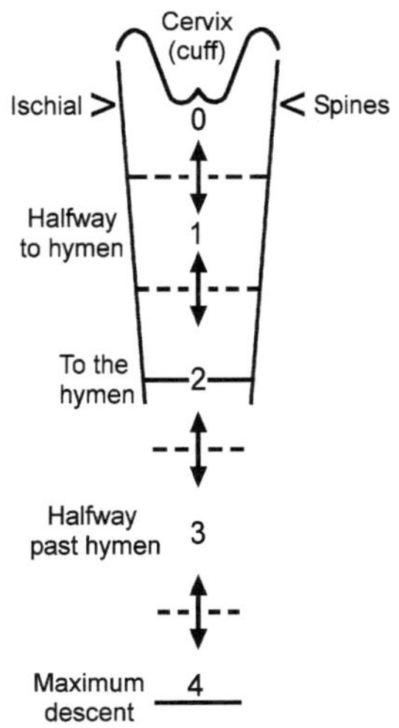

Baden-Walker grading system

Results are recorded by assigning values to each location in the three areas of the yoni, like so: the urethra and bladder on the superior wall/the uterus and cul-de-sac on the anterior wall/the rectum and the perineum on the posterior wall, according to the 0 to 4 grading system described in the above table. An example of this type of report is 12/44/32 (the numbers follow the same order as the table of symptoms, above, with 1 being the value assigned for the urethral wall, 2 the value assigned to the bladder/4 the value assigned to the location of the uterus, etc.). This example records a dominant complete prolapse in the upper third of the yoni, likely to be associated with an enterocele, significant cystocele and rectocele, plus perineal descent to the level of the anal sphincter. In this example, 2/4 levator strength is present (meaning that the woman scored 2 out of a possible 4 points). Although this system records many details in a very small space, it does not include the location of specific connective tissue defects (Zimmerman, 2003).

Referral and follow-up

Pelvic floor tone dysfunction can be evaluated and treated with biofeedback, physical therapy or, when indicated, pelvic floor strengthening exercises, or all three. However, significant degrees of actual prolapse should be further evaluated by a urogynecologist. Once a more definitive evaluation has been done, you can continue to follow the woman, help her learn pelvic floor strengthening exercises and explore other options for treatment.

Any of these defects should be repaired if they are severe enough to cause bothersome symptoms. In many cases, repair is postponed until childbearing is completed because surgical reconstruction may not tolerate a yoni birth without breaking down.

Diagnoses Related to Pelvic Prolapse

The POP-Q and the Baden-Walker Halfway System are both screening tests to narrow down the area of weakness in the pelvic cavity. Further investigations can diagnose the following problems.

Cystocele (vesicocele) and urethrocele

Cystoceles (SIS-toe-seals) are herniations of the bladder wall, usually into the yoni wall and sometimes through the introitus. A cystocele presents as a soft, elastic bulge that causes the urethra to appear more prominent. Small cystoceles are commonly seen in parous women, and some physicians consider them normal in that population. Symptoms include a bearing-down sensation and discomfort when sitting or walking. Large, exposed cystoceles may become irritated or ulcerated and may bleed. Descent of the anterior bladder below the vesical neck may result in incomplete emptying of the bladder as well.

Urethroceles (you-REE-throw-seals) are prolapses of the urethral wall and appear as smaller bulges at the vulvar end of the yoni ceiling. Even when severe, they usually do not protrude beyond the introitus and typically appear as spherical bulges that fill the opening of the yoni. By themselves, such weaknesses do not cause problems. A diverticulum can mimic a urethrocele and vis versa, and should be ruled out.

Problems do arise, however, when a urethral prolapse occurs at the urethrovesical junction. These prolapses are usually accompanied by a degree of cystocele. Such damage destroys the posterior urethrovesical angle (damage to the anterior angle does not cause problems). Urinary incontinence is the most common complicating factor. The mildest form is stress incontinence, which occurs when tiny amounts of urine are expressed during sneezing, coughing or laughing when the bladder is full or during exercise that exerts downward pressure, such as running. Symptoms, enlargement of the hernia or repeated urinary tract infections call for treatment.

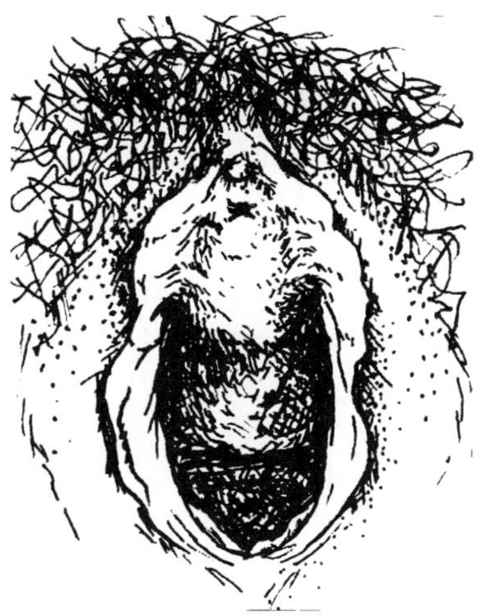

Urethrocele

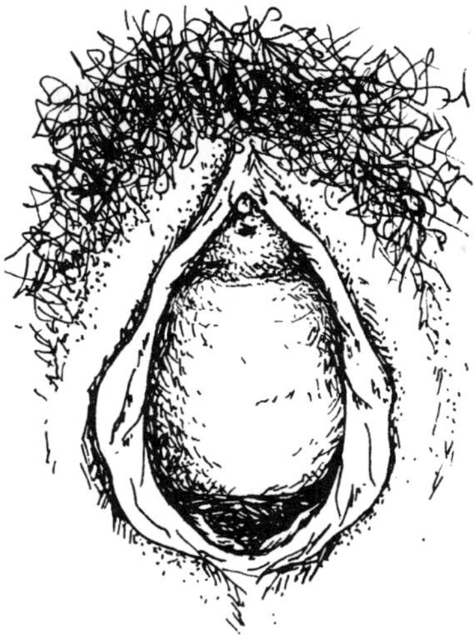

Central cystocele

Rectocele and enterocele

A **rectocele (WRECK-toe-seal)** is a prolapse or herniation of the rectum that protrudes into the yoni floor. A low rectocele appears as a bulge in the yoni floor right behind the perineum and is frequently the result of birth-related damage. This weakness occurs because of disruption of the perineal body and lower yoni. The yoni and rectal walls are still adherent. A rectocele is often associated with a cystocele, but not necessarily with uterine prolapse. If severe, it may impede the normal passage of stool, requiring the woman to support the bulging tissue when moving her bowels. Constipation is often associated with a low rectocele.

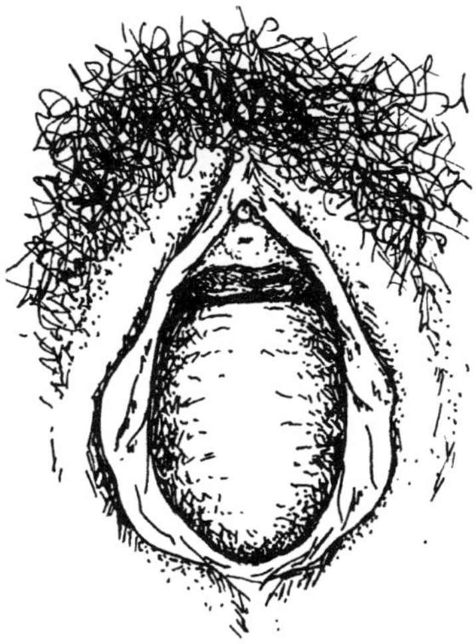

Rectocele

A midyoni rectocele is also frequently a result of childbirth. It forms due to pathologic overstretching or tearing of the adventitia that lies between the rectum and the yoni, resulting in detachment of the two walls. Associated symptoms include a sense of pressure or "bearing down," of incomplete rectal emptying and of discomfort after a bowel movement.

The high or upper yoni rectocele is associated with overstretching and often coexists in combination with a midyoni rectocele and uterine prolapse. Normally the uppermost portion of the wall of the rectoyoni space is attached to the lowermost wall of the rectouterine pouch. By itself, the high rectocele is not associated with rectal pressure or discomfort. Because of its proximity and thinning, a high rectocele often coexists with an enterocele.

An **enterocele (EN-ter-oh-seal)** is a prolapse of the rectouterine pouch (posterior cul-de-sac) that comes down between the rectum and yoni, thus separating them (Sorger, 1991). It is often mistaken for a high rectocele. It may contain loops of small bowel. It presents as a bulge behind the cervix, a fingerlike projection in the upper yoni that may expand and contract with breathing. Rectoceles and enteroceles often occur together. If enteroceles are not repaired they tend to enlarge.

To further investigate unusual findings that are outside the scope of this discussion and for details regarding other procedures included in a complete internal exam, refer to HOLISTIC MIDWIFERY, VOL. I.

Prolapses and pregnancy or birth

Mild to moderate degrees of pelvic organ prolapse may cause dragging pains in the lower back and abdomen during pregnancy and may make walking uncomfortable. Pelvic floor exercises may be done daily throughout pregnancy, but because the muscles are relaxed by pregnancy hormones, no dramatic improvement should be expected.

Large defects in the yoni wall may lodge themselves in front of the presenting part and impede the progress of labor. If this occurs, the defect should be carefully and gently replaced above the presenting part. Recheck as the baby moves down to be sure the prolapse does not recur.

Uterine and cervical prolapse that occurs during pregnancy or birth: After birth, the cervix and uterus may be found low relative to their normal position in the yoni. In many women, this is a temporary occurrence, with the organs returning to their normal positions within 6 months to a year after birth. (Descent of the uterus or cervix is not to be confused with uterine inversion, a serious complication that involves the uterus turning inside out after birth.)

Pushing with the head still high and no spontaneous urge (especially without progress) or vigorous fundal pressure to assist in placental delivery may weaken the uterosacral and cardinal ligaments and lead to at least a temporary degree of uterine prolapse. Perform an internal exam and note the position of the cervix in the yoni. True uterine prolapse may pull the bladder wall down with it, causing an accompanying cystocele. A rectocele is sometimes involved as well. Ultimately, surgery is the urogynecologist's answer to these problems.

Conception is rare when the uterus is totally prolapsed, and when it does occur, progress to term is unlikely. However, partial degrees of uterine prolapse are frequently associated with pregnancy. Early on, this may cause the cervix to protrude from the yoni opening. As pregnancy advances the situation may actually improve because uterine enlargement often draws the prolapsed portion of the lower uterine segment and cervix back into the yoni.

Incarceration (entrapment of an extremely retroflexed uterus in the abdominal cavity) may occur as the prolapsed uterus enlarges, which can lead to miscarriage. If the pregnancy continues, however, progress to term can be expected (Hellman & Pritchard, 1971). Assuming a knee–chest position for 20 minutes several times daily during the first 6 months of pregnancy will help to prevent incarceration. If the uterus has not become incarcerated, birth usually proceeds without problems. Be mindful that weak ligaments and muscles make a woman more likely to sustain additional damage during birth and that a prolapsed uterus may invert (turn inside out) more easily, especially during placental delivery.

What Women Can Do for Prolapse Conditions after Birth

The most important thing a woman can do is pelvic floor strengthening exercises (see the chapter entitled "Preparing the Perineal Tissues for Birth"). Some of these should be done in a knee–chest or headstand position to assist in returning the organs to their proper location. Minimizing constipation is also helpful.

Some women have good results using a pessary (a device inserted into the yoni to provide artificial support). Pessaries can be fitted by a midwife trained to fit them but are usually obtained through a urogynecologist. Their use is associated with infections, pain (if wrongly sized), abrasions, erosions, ulcers or granulation tissue; often these problems are heralded by bleeding. If there are no such problems, however, and the woman is comfortable removing, washing and replacing the pessary, it can be worn long-term. There are a variety of sizes and styles. Pessaries are sometimes recommended while a woman is awaiting surgical reconstruction but one can used during pregnancy as well, as long as there are no adverse side-effects.

A variety of devices have been developed to assist in strengthening the pelvic floor muscles such as weighted yoni cones (also discussed on page 153) that help teach and monitor the progress of pelvic floor exercises and a small vibrator, which helps strengthen the levator ani muscle. Inserting a diaphragm or a tampon during exercise may help a woman focus on which muscles she is using, although the use of any such devices, including biofeedback machines, should be delayed until six weeks after birth.

Herbal baths of uva ursi leaf, and taking certain homeopathic remedies may help strengthen the area. Consult a naturopath well versed in gynecological care for other suggestions. (Bent & Saint, 2003; Garrey, 1978; Kolder, 1990; McCool & Durain, 2004; Netter, 1954, 2003; Rogers & Richardson, 2003; Schorge et al., 2008; Snell, 1986; Whitley, 1985)

ANORECTAL DISORDERS AND INCONTINENCE

Incontinence

Anal incontinence is the involuntary loss of flatus (gas), stool (liquid or solid) that causes social or hygienic problems. Anal incontinence is common in both sexes and affects all age groups with an incidence ranging between 2 and 24% if flatal incontinence is included and 0.4 to 18% if it is not. **Fecal incontinence** is the loss of liquid or solid stool only. **Fecal urgency** is the inability to defer defecation for more than 5 minutes. **Anal mucoid seepage** is yet another designation, referring to leakage due to colonic disease or dietary sensitivities but with functional anal sphincters and intact cognition.

Risk factors

Fecal continence depends on an intact anal sphincter complex as well as normal stool delivery and consistency, intact sensation and motor innervation and a functioning puborectalis muscle (Rogers et al., 2002). Damage to this complex of tissues occurs most frequently during childbirth and can occur in three ways: by direct injury such as tearing; by neurologic injury to the pudendal nerve either from mechanical damage during an instrumental delivery or persistent nerve compression from the fetal head; by traction neuropathy, which may occur with a large baby or prolonged pushing in successive pregnancies or by prolonged stretching of the nerve due to persistently lax pelvic floor tone. Injured nerves often become demyelinated but usually recover over time. This type of nerve damage usually accompanies mechanical injury; isolated neurologic injury is believed to be rare (Power et al., 2006).

Consequently, among women of childbearing age, the most commonly associated risk of either fecal or flatal incontinence is increasing parity, especially among those who sustain either mechanical or neurological anal sphincter damage. Rates of childbirth-related sphincter injury in the US range from 6 to 18% (Fenner et al., 2003). Borello-France and associates (2006) compared women who had no such injury with those who sustained sphincter injury at birth. Those with injuries had twice the risk of fecal incontinence both 6 weeks and 6 months later. Nevertheless, in another study looking at 151 women who had various types of childbearing experiences 30 years prior, those that had a history of sphincter damage were more likely to have flatal incontinence, but were at no increased risk for fecal incontinence compared with women who had a history of isolated clitorotomy or surgical delivery (Nygaard et al., 1997). Thus other factors related to pregnancy and aging probably contribute to ongoing problems regardless of injuries sustained at the time of birth.

Other risk factors include obesity, advancing age, diabetes, chronic hypertension, chronic obstructive pulmonary disease, stroke, Scleroderma, a history of pelvic radiation therapy and certain drugs. Urinary incontinence or prolapse of pelvic organs may be associated factors. Gastrointestinal disorders may be contributory and can include chronic constipation with straining (because it can lead to neurologic or muscular damage), diarrhea, fecal urgency, food intolerance, irritable bowel syndrome, fistula or anal surgery. Neurologic conditions such as spinal cord injury or surgery, Parkinson disease, multiple sclerosis, myopathies, cognitive dysfunction or psychosis may also be related factors.

History

Always ask about anal continence, as most women are reluctant to volunteer that they have problems in this area. If the woman reports a problem, find out the duration, frequency, stool consistency, when it occurs (in social situations? during sex? at other times?), timing of episodes, use of sanitary protection and the social impact of the condition. A detailed record of these factors will not only help determine the severity of the problem but will assist with monitoring whether therapy is helping.

Urge-related incontinence must be distinguished from accidents that happen without her awareness, as these problems may have different causes. Urgency without incontinence may reflect an impairment of rectal compliance rather than anything wrong with the sphincter muscles themselves. The scale below can be used to help quantify the type of problems the woman is explaining.

FECAL CONTINENCE SCORING SCALE
SYMPTOMS 1. Passage of any flatus when socially undesirable 2. Incontinence of liquid stool 3. Need to wear a pad due to anal leakage 4. Incontinence of solid stool 5. Fecal urgency (inability to delay defecation for more than 5 minutes)
ASSIGN A SCORE TO EACH SYMPTOM AS LISTED ABOVE 0=Never 1=Rarely (less than once monthly) 2=Sometimes (once weekly to once monthly) 3=Usually (once daily to once weekly) 4=Always (more than once daily)
Obtain a total by scoring for each of the symptoms above and add them up. A score of 0 indicates complete continence and a score of 20 complete incontinence. A score of 6 is the cut-off for further evaluation (Mahony et al., 2004).

Physical exam

(It may also be helpful to review the suggestions about positioning the woman for a vesicovaginal fistula exam on page 194 before reading further.) Have the woman assume a lithotomy position. Carefully inspect the perineum and anus for soiling, scars, the length of the perineal body, hemorrhoids, warts, rectal prolapse or other anatomic abnormalities. Look for the **Dovetail sign**, the term employed for the characteristic appearance of the disrupted puckering of the corrugator cutis ani, usually present along the anterior anal verge. Disruption of the puckering may indicate an underlying torn sphincter or even a fistula (illustrated on page 480).

The **anocutaneous (anal wink) reflex** is elicited next. Stroke to the side of the anal orifice with the tip of a cotton swab. This should prompt an involuntary contraction of the external sphincter. A positive test provides a gross indication that the pudendal nerve is intact.

Next, with the woman's understanding and permission, perform a gentle digital rectal exam to assess the resting tone of the internal anal sphincter, to obtain a specimen of rectal contents so you can perform a test for gross or occult blood (if she has reported bleeding or has not had such a test in the past year) and to check for a fistula, masses or fecal impaction. A finding of rectal blood with no obvious source may indicate a source of bleeding higher in the gastrointestinal tract. This is only a screening test, however, and a definitive answer as to the source will require a referral for further testing. The entry entitled "Physical exam" under rectovaginal fistulas later in this chapter for more details about how to examine a woman when a fistula is suspected.

Enema: A simple test to evaluate the status of anal competence is a tap water enema. This can be performed by filling an ear syringe with tepid tap water and injecting it into her rectum (direct the tip of the syringe toward her navel). Since liquid stool is much more difficult to control than is solid stool, anyone who can successfully retain liquid in their rectum for several minutes is not likely to have significant fecal incontinence; other reasons for her symptoms should be investigated.

Other diagnostic methods: There are many diagnostic tests that can be performed. If more sophisticated testing seems warranted, refer women to a urogynecologist or a proctology specialist in women's health.

Treatment

Conservative treatments include high-fiber supplements, which can make the stool firmer and thus easier to control, and drugs that slow fecal transit time, which allows more time for water to be absorbed in the bowel and thus also helps to firm up the stool. Biofeedback and pelvic floor therapy may help many of these women restore normal awareness and function. For those with severe or unresponsive dysfunction, daily timed use of tap water enemas or a suppository can be incorporated into a schedule for planned bowel evacuation.

There are also a wide range of surgical approaches to the problem of anal incontinence. None are ideal, however, and surgery is reserved for only the most extreme structural abnormalities with severe symptoms that fail to respond to conservative treatment. You will need to refer women who want to be evaluated for surgery to a specialist.

Functional Anorectal Disorders

There are currently three recognized types of functional anorectal disorders. The first is **functional fecal incontinence**, defined as the recurrent, uncontrollable passage of fecal material that persists for more than three months in a person with abnormal functioning of anatomically normal defecatory muscles. Fecal retention or diarrhea is common in these individuals. Causes range from disorders of intestinal motility, poor rectal compliance, impaired sensation and low-tone pelvic floor dysfunction. There is often a psychological component. Treatment includes medical management using drugs or biofeedback therapy.

The second is **functional anorectal pain**, which is subdivided into two categories according to the duration of pain and the presence of tenderness in the puborectalis muscle on palpation. **Levator ani syndrome** or **levator ani spasm** is a type of high-tone pelvic floor dysfunction that presents with episodic sensations of pressure or aching in the upper rectum, lasting at least 20 minutes and persisting for more than 3 months. On exam, the puborectalis muscle is tender.

The second type is **proctalgia fugax**, defined as a spasm of the anal muscle of unknown cause. It presents with episodes of sudden severe pain in the anus or lower rectum lasting anywhere from a few seconds to a few minutes. Pain may be significant, but these episodes rarely occur more often than 5 times a year. The puborectalis muscle is not tender on palpation. The best thing to do for this condition is to reassure the woman that it is benign and to recommend that she pursue therapy with a Chinese doctor or a homeopath.

The third is **functional defecation disorders**, a category which includes **dyssynergic defecation**, also variously referred to as pelvic floor dyssynergia, anismus, outlet obstruction constipation or spastic pelvic floor syndrome. Another type of high-tone pelvic floor dysfunction, dyssynergic defecation is characterized by failure to relax the puborectalis muscle and external anal sphincter during attempts to defecate. As many as 25 to 50% of those who report chronic constipation have this problem. Symptoms include chronic straining and impaired or incomplete evacuation of the anal canal. Other causes of constipation should be excluded and the diagnosis confirmed by testing that can be done by a specialist. Treatment includes biofeedback sessions to retrain these women to relax their pelvic floor during bowel movements. Awareness exercises, a review of pelvic floor anatomy and instruction in positioning on the toilet for a bowel movement (see page 154) may be helpful as well.

Rectovaginal Fistulas

Rectovaginal fistulas may be either congenital or acquired epithelial-lined, tube-like passageways between the yoni and the rectum. The cause of the fistula is felt to be the most significant predictor of a successful treatment outcome as it takes into account the overall health of the woman's tissues.

Most rectovaginal fistulas occur as a result of traumatic, birth-related events. These fistulas are most commonly found in the distal third of the yoni, just above the hymenal ring. Defects can range from 1 mm to several centimeters in diameter, and most of them pass through to the rectum at or above the dentate line. The higher up the fistula is located, the harder it can be to identify it on visual inspection. An endoscopic study may be required. **Anovaginal** fistulas are similar defects that open below the pectinate line.

Classification

Fistulas are classified according to their location, size and etiology, a system that aids in selecting the appropriate treatment and in predicting the outcome of surgical repair. Various classification schemes have been proposed. No standardized system has yet been accepted that allows comparison of surgical results or that helps define the incidence of these fistulas. One system classifies fistulas as either "simple" or "complex." Fistulas that result from prolonged labor or that fail to heal after repair should probably always be classified as complex, regardless of their size or location.

CLASSIFICATION OF RECTOVAGINAL FISTULA		
CHARACTERISTICS	**SIMPLE**	**COMPLEX**
Location	Low to mid yoni wall	Upper third of yoni
Size	≤2.5 cm	>2.5 cm
Associated factors	Trauma or infection	Inflammatory bowel disease; irradiation; cancer; prolonged obstructed labor; failed prior repair

(Rothenberger & Goldberg, 1983)

Anatomic schemes have also been suggested that classify fistulas according to their location along the yoni wall: high third (where the yoni is covered only by peritoneum), middle third (where only a thin septum separates the yoni and rectum) or distal third (where the perineal body separates the yoni and rectum). High fistulas are located close to the cervix (or yoni cuff in women who have had a hysterectomy) and may open into the sigmoid colon.

History

Women with a rectovaginal fistula usually report that flatus or stool leaks from the yoni. They may have recurrent bladder or yoni infections, rectal or yoni bleeding, and pain. Birth-related fistulas are usually associated with a history of third- or fourth-degree laceration that was either unrecognized or that was repaired and then dehisced. These women commonly present with large defects of the anterior portion of the external sphincter accompanied by gross fecal incontinence. A woman whose fistula is the result of infection or inflammation may report diarrhea, abdominal cramping and fevers.

Physical examination

Most obstetric fistulas are located along a scar in the yoni wall or perineum following clitorotomy or a tear and can be often be seen during inspection of the perineum and distal portion of the posterior yoni wall, although identification can be difficult if the fistula is small. The most common fistula location on the rectal side is at the pectinate line or at the upper edge of the external anal sphincter. Dimpling or retraction of the epithelium is often present, indicating the opening of the fistula.

Bimanual exam of the rectum and yoni allows for palpation to assess the thickness of the perineal body and rectovaginal wall and may allow palpation and visualization of the fistula as well. Gentle probing with a cotton swab or tissue forceps can help locate the opening, but do not insert such a large object down into the tract (a small lacrimal probe can be used, if you have one). With a finger inserted into the rectum, the probe can be passed through the fistula to the rectal side. This exam is usually not painful unless the tract is infected.

If the fistula has not been located with these steps, methylene blue dyed lubricant can be placed in the rectum and the rectovaginal septum massaged with your rectal finger. This will push some of the blue dye through the tract to the yoni opening of the fistula, if one exists. If that doesn't work or there is no stained lubricant handy, some fistulas not otherwise apparent can be identified by using a needleless syringe to fill the yoni with water and noting air bubbles over the fistula's opening into the yoni wall.

If none of this is helpful, methylene blue stained fluid can be introduced into the rectum with a Foley catheter with a 30 cc balloon. The balloon is inflated to obstruct the anal canal and the yoni wall is then examined with a speculum or retractor to see if and where blue fluid is leaking. Or, insert a tampon in the yoni, wait 20 minutes and check the tampon. The leakage of blue dye onto the tampon confirms a fistula and the level of staining denotes the approximate location of the fistula along the posterior yoni wall. If no dye appears on the tampon, a rectovaginal fistula is unlikely; however, a fistula communicating between the yoni and a superior portion of bowel is still possible if there is fecal contamination in the yoni.

Diagnostic tests

Further evaluation can be obtained through a specialist. Unless there is a clear history that accounts for the presence of the fistula, a biopsy should be obtained from the fistula's tract to rule out malignancy or inflammation. A proctoscopy or colonoscopy should be performed if inflammatory bowel disease, cancer or infection cannot be excluded.

Treatment

Small fistulas that result from birth trauma are treated conservatively, as many will eventually heal on their own. Larger fistulas more often require surgical closure. A specialist should be consulted.

One approach to surgery involves cauterization of the sinus tract from the rectal side; a 1 cm flap of anal mucosa is then created by dissecting the tissue, and this flap is sutured over the rectal end of the opening (Orrom & Buls, 1992; Owen & Hauth, 1990).

Anal Fistulas

Fecal soiling and drainage after childbirth usually due to a rectovaginal fistula. However, fistulas that pass through or terminate in the anal sphincter muscle complex may also occur. With an anal fistula, the tract typically never epithelizes but remains at the granular stage of healing. Once feces or bacteria enter the tract, due to infection or trauma, an inflammatory process begins that may eventually erupt through the skin via one of several pathways. The simplest type results in direct division of tissue from the intersphincteric plane to the perianal skin. The most difficult fistulae to identify and treat are those that extend upward into the supralevator space before exiting. After clitorotomy, particularly one associated with a third- or fourth-degree extension, these planes might be disrupted, and the course of the fistula may not be easy to predict (Howard, et al., 1999).

Classification

The classification system devised by Parks and associates (1976) is widely accepted. It is based on the relationship of the fistulous tract to the external anal sphincter. He defined four main types, with many variations. In this system, the external sphincter muscle is designated as the "keystone," to which the prefixes "inter-," "trans-," etc. refer.

1. **Intersphincteric fistulas** are the most common type (45%). They occur when the tract of the fistula begins in the anal wall and traverses only the intersphincteric

space (the space between the internal and external sphincters where the longitudinal anal muscle is found) before turning down toward the skin.

2. **Trans-sphincteric fistulas** (30%) occur when the tract begins in the anal wall, passes through the intersphincteric space and the external sphincter complex at varying levels into the ischiorectal fossa before turning down toward the skin.
3. **Suprasphincteric fistulas** (20%) exist when the tract begins in the anal wall, passes through the internal sphincter, arches over the puborectalis, then down through the levator plate to the ischiorectal fossa and finally to the skin.
4. **Extrasphincteric fistulas**, the least common type (5%), occurs when the tract passes from the skin, through the ischiorectal fat and levator ani muscles and into the rectum. It is outside the external anal sphincter complex completely.

There are numerous variations on these types and many anal fistulas do not open onto the perianal skin or the anal canal but extend from abscesses within the perianal tissues. These lesions may remain completely internal. For more details, see Parks et al., 1976.

Risk factors

Risk factors for the development of obstetric-related fistula-in-ano are not well defined. They might be the same as those for rectovaginal fistulas, because these conditions are quite similar. Risk factors include fourth-degree lacerations, wound infection or dehiscence. Avoiding such complications might prevent the development of an anal fistula.

Physical exam

Women with an anal fistula usually present with pain and inflammatory drainage, in contrast to the relatively painless drainage of watery stool in those with rectovaginal fistulas. When the fistula opens on the perineum, the mouth will consist of beefy red granular tissue from which drains a purulent exudate. When the fistula does not open onto the perineum diagnosis will not be so straightforward. A hard, tender swelling in the region of the anal canal raises the suspicion that an abscess is present. Although you may suspect the presence of an anal fistula after a pelvic exam, it is often necessary to perform another exam under anesthesia to confirm the condition and plan treatment (Howard, et al., 1999).

Treatment

Anal fistulas, unlike rectovaginal fistulas, are not be treated by excision and primary repair. Because anal fistulas contain chronically infected tissue, they are best treated by incision and drainage. Fistulotomy and curettage should be done, ensuring that the entire tract is carefully traced and opened from internal to external sites. With the application of frequent moist dressings to the wound, healing occurs after several weeks by secondary intention. Unlike rectovaginal fistulas, which typically develop in the posterior midline of the yoni wall, anal fistula tracts can be complex and circuitous.

The long term outcome of anal fistulae is unknown. Potential sequelae include fecal incontinence if the sphincter is damaged either during fistulotomy or birth, dyspareunia, if significant perineal scarring results, continued drainage, if the fistulotomy is not successful, or other associated problems not identified at the time of surgery (Howard, et al., 1999).

References and Further Reading on Assessment of the Pelvic Tissues

References Used for Multiple Chapters

Borello-France D, et al. "Fecal and urinary incontinence in primiparous women," Obstet Gynecol, 108(4):863-872, Oct, 2006.

McCool W, Durain D. Chapter 14: "Common diagnoses in women's gynecological health," in Varney H, et al. Varney's Midwifery, 4th ed. Jones & Bartlett, Sudbury MA, 2004.

O'Dell J, Morse A. "It's not all about birth: biomechanics applied to pelvic organ prolapse prevention," J MWH, 53(1):28-36, Jan-Feb, 2008.

Rogers R, Richardson C. Chapter 8: "Clinical evaluation of pelvic support defects with anatomic correlations," in Bent A, et al. Ostergard's Urogynecology and Pelvic Floor Dysfunction, 5th ed. Lippincott, Williams & Wilkins, Philadelphia PA, 2003.

Rosenblatt P, Elkardy E. Chapter 5: "Diagnosing incontinence and pelvic floor problems: an efficient, cost-effective approach for primary care providers," in Culligan P, Goldberg R, eds. Urogynecology in Primary Care. Springer-Verlag, London UK, 2007.

Schorge J, et al. eds. William's Gynecology. McGraw-Hill Medical, New York NY, 2008.

Tulikangas P. Chapter 4: "Pathophysiology of incontinence and pelvic floor dysfunction," in Culligan P, Goldberg R, eds. Urogynecology in Primary Care. Springer-Verlag, London UK, 2007.

Whitley N. A Manual of Clinical Obstetrics. JB Lippincott, Philadelphia PA, 1985.

Zimmerman C. Chapter 35: "Surgical correction of defects in pelvic support, A: Pelvic organ prolapse," in Rock J, Jones H, eds. Te Linde's Operative Gynecology, 9th ed. Lippincott, Williams & Wilkins, Philadelphia PA, 2003.

Learning to Recognize Normal Perineal Anatomy

Baden W, Walker T, eds. Chapter 3: The anatomy of uterovaginal support," in their Surgical Repair of Vaginal Defects. JB Lippincott Co., Philadelphia PA, 1992.

Bates B. A Guide to Physical Examination and History Taking, 5th ed. JB Lippincott, Philadelphia PA, 1991.

LeBlond R, et al., eds. Chapter 11: "The female genitalia and reproductive system," in DeGowin's Diagnostic Examination, 9th ed. McGraw Hill Professional, New York NY, 2008.

Varney H, et al. Chapter 56: "Pelvic examination," Varney's Midwifery, 4th ed. Jones & Bartlett, Sudbury MA, 2004.

Functional Disorders of the Urinary Tract

Barr D, et al. "Urinary creatinine concentrations in the US population: implications for urinary biologic monitoring measurements," Environ Health Perspect, 113(2):192-200, Feb, 2005.

Elkins T. "Surgery for the obstetric vesicovaginal fistula: a review of 100 operations in 82 patients," Am J Obstet Gynecol, 170(4):1108-1118, Apr, 1994.

Elkins T, Thompson J. "Lower urinary tract fistulas," in Walters M, Karram M, eds. Urogynecology and Reconstructive Pelvic Surgery. Mosby, St Louis MO, 1999.

Hilton R, Ward A. "Epidemiological and surgical aspects of urogenital fistulae: a review of 25 years' experience in southeast Nigeria," Int Urogynecol J Pelvic Floor Dysfunct, 9(4):189-194, 1998.

Leach G, et al. "L N S C3: a proposed classification system for female urethral diverticula," Neurourol Urodyn, 12(6):523-531, 1993.

Sand P, et al. "Pelvic floor electrical stimulation in the treatment of genuine stress incontinence: a multicenter, placebo-controlled trial," Am J Obstet Gynecol, 173(1):72-79, Jul, 1995.

Waaldijk K. "The (surgical) management of bladder fistula in 775 women in northern Nigeria" (doctoral thesis). University of Utrecht, Utrecht Netherlands, 1989.

ASSESSING PELVIC ORGAN PROLAPSE

Baden W, Walker T, eds. Chapter 2: Fundamentals, symptoms and classification," in their SURGICAL REPAIR OF VAGINAL DEFECTS. JB Lippincott, Philadelphia PA, 1992.

Barber M, et al. "Effect of patient position on clinical evaluation of pelvic organ prolapse," OBSTET GYNECOL, 96(1):18-22, Jul, 2000.

Bent S, Saint S. "The optimal use of diagnostic testing in women with acute uncomplicated cystitis," DIS MON, 49(2):83-98, Feb, 2003.

Bragi R, et al. "Differences in pelvic floor area between African American and European American women," AM J OBSTET GYNECOL, 187(1):111-115, Jul, 2002.

Bump R, et al. "The standardization of terminology of female pelvic organ prolapse and pelvic floor dysfunction," AM J OBSTET GYNECOL, 175(1):10-17, Jul, 1996.

DeLancey J. "Anatomy and biomechanics of genital prolapse," CLIN OBSTET GYNECOL, 36(4):897-909, Dec, 1993.

Garrey M, et al. GYNECOLOGY ILLUSTRATED. Churchill Livingstone, New York NY, 1978.

Hellman L, Pritchard J. WILLIAM'S OBSTETRICS, 14th ed. Appleton, Crofts, New York NY, 1971.

Kolder V, MD. Editing comments, Aug, 1990.

Netter F. ATLAS OF HUMAN ANATOMY, 4th ed. Saunders Elsevier, Philadelphia PA, 2003.

Netter F. THE CIBA COLLECTION OF MEDICAL ILLUSTRATIONS: VOL. 2, REPRODUCTIVE SYSTEM. CIBA Pub, Summit NJ, 1954.

Nichols D, Randall C. "Types of genital prolapse," in Nichols D, Randall C, eds. VAGINAL SURGERY, 3rd ed. Williams & Wilkins, Baltimore MD, 1989.

Singh K, et al. "Three-dimensional magnetic resonance imaging assessment of levator ani morphologic features in different grades of prolapse," AM J OBSTET GYNECOL, 188(4):910-915, Apr, 2003.

Snell R. CLINICAL ANATOMY FOR MEDICAL STUDENTS, 3rd ed. Little, Brown & Co., Boston MA, 1986.

Sorger L, MD. Editing comments, Feb, 1991.

Wexner S, Bartolo D. Chapter 20: "Anterior rectocele," in CONSTIPATION: ETIOLOGY, EVALUATION AND MANAGEMENT. Butterman Heinmann, Oxford UK, 1995.

ANORECTAL DISORDERS AND INCONTINENCE

Fenner D, et al. "Fecal and urinary incontinence after vaginal delivery with anal sphincter disruption in an obstetrics unit in the United States," AM J OBSTET GYNECOL, 189(6):1543-1549 (discussion 1549-1550), Dec, 2003.

Harris R, Speights S. Chapter 19: "Anal incontinence," in Lentz G, ed. UROGYNECOLOGY. Oxford U Press, New York NY, 2000.

Howard D, et al. "Fistula-in-ano after episiotomy," in OBSTET GYNECOL, 93(5, Pt 2);800-802, May, 1999.

Mahony R, et al. "Randomized, clinical trial of bowel confinement vs. laxative use after primary repair of a third-degree obstetric anal sphincter tear," DIS COLON RECTUM, 47(1):12-17, Jan, 2004.

Nygaard I, et al. "Anal incontinence after anal sphincter disruption: a 30-year retrospective cohort study," OBSTET GYNECOL, 89(6):896-901, Jun, 1997.

Owen J, Hauth J. "Episiotomy infection and dehiscence." in Gilstrap L, Faro S., eds. INFECTIONS IN PREGNANCY, Alan R. Liss, New York NY, 1990.

Parks, et al. "A classification of fistula-in-ano," BR J SURG, 63(1):1-12, Jan, 1976.

Power D, et al. "Obstetric anal sphincter injury: how to avoid, how to repair: a literature review," J FAM PRAC, 55(3):193-200, Mar, 2006.

Rogers R, et al. "Obstetric anal sphincter lacerations: an evidence-based approach, Part 1: anatomy and risk factors," FEMALE PATIENT, 27(4):21-24, Apr, 2002.

Rothenberger D, Goldberg S. "The management of rectovaginal fistulae," SURG CLIN N AM, 63(1):61-79, Feb, 1983.

INTIMATE GROOMING, BODY ART AND FEMALE GENITAL SURGERY

NOTE: The natural, healthy genitalia of either sex do not usually require surgical intervention or manipulation. This section includes all types of practices that alter the natural genital anatomy in some way, whether they be imposed upon or chosen by the girl or woman for personal, cultural or medical reasons.

PUBIC AND GENITAL HAIR GROOMING PRACTICES

Pubic hair covers the mons pubis. Genital hair refers to that which covers the labial surfaces that lie between the legs. The evolutionary purpose of pubic and genital hair remains a matter of debate among researchers. Some of the postulated reasons we have this hair include that the hair facilitates dispersal of pheromones to attract the opposite sex, protection of the genitals from friction during sexual activity, provision of warmth for the genitals, protection of the genitals from dirt, and dispersal of excess moisture by trapping a layer of air between the genitals and clothing.

Removal of the pubic hair has been practiced among men and women in some cultures for hundreds of years. In the West, there has been a surge of interest in pubic hair removal since the 1990s. This trend evolved as tiny micro bikinis like the Brazilian bikini became popular among celebrities, prompting them to remove their pubic hair because so much more of the mons is visible in these suits. Trimming, shaping, dying, shaving or permanently removing the pubic and genital hair has since become quite popular among both sexes in the childbearing population in the United States and abroad.

Removal of the pubic hair may be chosen for a variety of reasons, including:

- As a matter of grooming. A shaven pubic area creates a hairless bathing suit line and is considered sexy.
- Many like the smooth feel of their shaven skin, which feels more sensual to them.
- Islamic tradition recommends that pubic and underarm hair be removed. This practice is considered mandatory in some Muslim communities.
- Swimsuit models, lingerie models, pornographic film actors and exotic dancers may be required to shave their pubic hair for professional reasons.
- To meet cultural standards of beauty as many cultures find women with little or no pubic hair more attractive (from a feminist perspective, shaving renders the female body more childlike, accenting her vulnerability).
- Control of the natural moisture in the genital area. Pubic hair, especially when it is thick and full, is believed by hair-removal advocates to provide an ideal environment for bacterial growth.
- Control of genital odor, especially in menstruating women.
- To facilitate sexual activity by rendering the genitals more visible, removing hair as a barrier to access to the genitals and by eliminating the problems of hair in the mouth during oral sex and pulling of the hair during sexual contact.

Counseling pregnant women who are contemplating pubic hair removal

If a woman is already pregnant and expresses a desire to begin removing her pubic hair, discuss with her why she wants to begin at this time. Encourage her to discuss this with her partner. Have her partner present when you explain that shaving used to be a standard of care when prepping women during early labor, but it was found to actually increase the rate of postpartum infection. The shaving being done on women who had never previously shaved, the accompanying inevitable nicks and abrasions from the razor and the routine performance in a hospital (hotbed of pathologic organisms) were all likely contributing factors to this increase in peripartum infection rates.

Nevertheless, when she first starts shaving, her skin will be more sensitive. Her ability to reach her genitals will be increasingly impaired by her enlarging belly. Shaving the pubic area and genitals is widely regarded as a specific skill among those who do it regularly, so much so that many women have pubic hair removed at a salon. The use of improper or careless technique can result in several complications such as pimples, rashes, inflamed hair follicles and ingrown hairs, none of which are pleasant to deal with, pregnant or not. Although she can have her partner do the shaving for her (which I would definitely recommend if she wants to go ahead), it would be better for her (or her partner) to trim her pubic hair and wait to begin shaving until after the birth and after her tissues have returned to their nonpregnant baseline.

If she wants to go ahead and begin shaving before she gives birth, she should be free of any type of infection and otherwise healthy. She should purchase her own shaving equipment that is specifically designed for intimate shaving and clean it after every use. She should plan on not shaving for at least the first 3 weeks after the birth to avoid tiny bits of hair becoming lodged in healing tissues. After she removes the hair, she should wear breathable materials next to genitals because impaired air circulation (synthetic cloth against hairless skin) increases the risk of yoni infection.

Counseling women who come to you who are already removing their genital hair

If a woman comes to you for care who is already in the practice of shaving her pubic hair, there is no particular reason for her to discontinue this practice while she is pregnant unless she is having ongoing problems such as rashes. In that case, continuing to shave during pregnancy, when her immune system is slightly suppressed, will make her more vulnerable to infection. It would be best to resolve any problems and have her trim, rather than shave, her pubic hair, at least until after she gives birth.

Any woman who is grooming her genital hair with products such as waxes, lotions, depilatories or hair dyes, unless they are made of natural ingredients known to be safe, should be warned that these types of products are not recommended for use during pregnancy as their safety for the fetus has not been studied and any product applied to the skin will absorb to a variable extent.

Pubic and genital hair grooming and removal techniques

The process of removing genital hair requires delicate care because the genital area has an uneven surface and thin skin.

Trimming: Trimming the hair is done to reduce its length. This is done as a grooming practice by itself or as a preliminary step when shaving, especially for the first time. It is easily accomplished with a pair of sharp scissors, although it can be tricky to use a sharp tool near the genitals. There are specialized tools available to trim pubic hair without the risk of getting nicked. The Bodworx Longer Hair Body Trimmer is a good tool for this purpose.

Dyeing pubic hair: Many women dye their pubic hair to match their scalp hair. They are often not aware that the dyes can penetrate the skin and that many dyes are quite toxic. There is no product currently on the market that is designed for the purpose of tinting pubic hair.

Women who want to experiment with tinting their hair can use vegetable dyes (available in the baking section of health food stores), henna-based products that are all natural or other natural products that may be available in local health food stores. Dying the pubic hair is not recommended during pregnancy, but if the woman wants to dye it anyway, ask her to avoid shades of red, as coloring the hair red may be confusing when trying to assess the location of bleeding, should that be an issue at the time of birth.

Plucking: Tweezers can be used to remove single hairs. This is obviously a painstaking process that is difficult for a woman to do on herself.

Shaping pubic hair: Sculpting the pubic hair line is a widespread practice. This is often done at a salon. A bikini line cut removes hair from the vulva along the sides and over the mons, resulting in an upside-down triangle pattern. A G-wax removes hair so that a G-string can be worn with no hair showing. The landing-strip cut leaves a central longitudinal rectangle of hair down the center of the labia. Custom designs remove all hair except for a patch centered above the vulva. Shapes can be triangles, arrows, hearts, etc.

Shaving: Shaving removes hair down to the skin and must be repeated frequently, often daily, to maintain effective hair removal. Many women use the same razors that they use on other parts of their bodies to shave their pubic hair, but it is safest to use a razor that is dedicated to the purpose of shaving the pubic and genital area. When the same razor is used to shave all over the body, the risk of developing problems such as ingrown hairs, itching and pubic pimples is greatly increased. There are razors that are specially designed for use in the genital area.

The best tool, however, is an electric pubic shaver, which will reduce the risk of cutting the skin and the other problems associated with shaving with a razor. Pubic shavers usually look like small versions of a man's beard shaver with a rotary foil at the top. The Personal Shaver by Seiko (S-Yard ES1080) is a highly recommended model. Amazon sells it with several accessories (www.amazon.com). Other brands include the Bodworx body shaver and the Body Bare shaver.

Prior to shaving, the hair must first be trimmed very short to enable an electric pubic shaver to work effectively. Since shaving does not remove hair from the root, some may experience ingrown hairs when the hair starts to grow out, especially if special after-shave sprays are not used to prevent the new hair from growing in sideways. Additionally, shaving requires a lot of maintenance because hair grows back in just a couple of days.

Waxing: Waxing the female genitals is relatively easy and is the most common method of regularly removing pubic or genital hair in many communities. "Brazilian" waxing refers to partial genital hair removal, whereas "Hollywood" waxing refers to removal of all the pubic, genital and perianal hair. The main advantage of waxing is that it pulls the hair out at the root, which delays regrowth for 3 to 8 weeks. Regrowth also tends to slow down with repeated waxing. Hair growth can be further slowed with special hair inhibitors to extend the effectiveness of waxing. Although home waxing kits are also available at a fraction of the cost of professional waxing, waxing is quite painful and is usually done in a salon.

Waxing at home: Though painful, many people prefer waxing because it lasts much longer than shaving. Home waxing is ideal for some, and home waxing kits can be purchased at any pharmacy. Bear in mind, however, that the experts at salons work faster, it is easier for them to see what they are doing, and they have the best equipment.

For those who want to try waxing at home, a simple sugar solution can also be used instead of a commercial waxing kit. This cheap and nontoxic formula is a traditional recipe used in Saudi Arabia. You will need:

Olive oil	1 Tbsp. sesame oil
2 cups white sugar	Sauce pan
¼ cup water	Strips of cotton sheet
¼ cup lemon juice	Candy thermometer

1. Coat the surface of a clean counter top or large glass cutting board with olive oil.
2. Place all other ingredients in a stainless steel or glass saucepan, stir to mix and bring to a boil on the stove.
3. Simmer the solution for about 10 minutes or until the sugar reaches approximately 250°F (121°C) (for you candy makers, this is the hard ball stage). This mixture is prone to burning so stir it constantly and watch it carefully.
4. Pour the mixture onto the oiled surface and allow to cool.
5. Once cool but before it sets, lift the sugar, using a spatula if necessary, and form it into a ball.
6. Place it in an airtight container inside the fridge.
7. When ready to use, break off a chunk and heat in microwave until warm and soft (20-30 seconds), so that it becomes pliable in your hands.
8. Smooth a small amount over the hair to be removed.
9. Press a strip of porous fabric firmly over the area.
10. Pull the cotton strip off in the exact opposite direction of hair growth.
11. You can reuse the same cloth strip and sugar by reheating it in the microwave until it fails to pick up more hair.

Depilatories: Hair removal gels, creams, lotions and roll-ons are some of the common types of depilatories. Chemical depilatories are applied to the skin at the location of the unwanted hair and the solution is left for a specified amount of time while it dissolves the hair. These creams work by dissolving the keratin in each hair so it can easily be wiped away. Since the skin also contains keratin, it is vital not to leave a depilatory on too long. Even though there are hair removal creams for the face, pubic region (mons) and legs, there aren't any hair removal creams (as far as I could determine) that claim to be mild enough for the genitalia. In addition, depilatories should not be used during pregnancy.

Permanent removal: Electrolysis and laser treatments are two of the common permanent hair removal solutions. Electrolysis is a tedious process that requires destruction of each hair follicle. Laser treatments use a beam of light to disable an area of hair on your body. These treatments require multiple sessions to completely eradicate hair from the pubic region and cost at least $500 per session.

Shaving tips

Those that choose to shave at home need to know how to do it right, to minimize problems. Advise that the woman choose a time when she is awake, alert and not rushed, especially if she is inexperienced. The genital tissues become more sensitive just before, during and after the peak of the menstrual cycle and during pregnancy. Irritation will be minimized if shaving is postponed until 1 week after a woman finishes bleeding or after pregnancy.

To begin, wash and comb the pubic hair. Trim long pubic hairs down to no more than a ¼ inch stubble with scissors or a hair trimmer. Using scissors takes longer and requires dexterity. A beard trimmer with an adjustable guard can be used to shave pubic hair to a uniform length in no time. A razor should not be used for this purpose. Trimmed wet hair appears shorter once it dries and, because most pubic hair is curly, it will naturally snap back after being trimmed and look even shorter. So just take a little off at a time. Have a large mirror easily available to check progress.

Shaving the genital area is most easily accomplished while in the tub or shower with one leg up and supported on a nonslippery surface. Some women find it easier to reach all of the genital area while seated on an open toilet seat.

Have all your equipment and supplies in easy reach. Do not use a switchblade razor or a disposable razor. If using a safety razor designed to shave pubic hair, use a new blade for each shave.

Regardless of which device is used, shaving can be done either wet or dry. Most sources recommend wet shaving, since soaking the skin makes it softer and easier to shave. Dry hairs often break during shaving. Take a hot bath and gently exfoliate the skin to remove dead cells. If it is inconvenient to take a long, hot shower or bath, place a warm cloth over the genital area for at least three to five minutes. Still, that water makes hair stick to an electric shaver, which is more messy and hard to manage, so the skin and hair can be towel dried after soaking.

A shaving gel or cream can be applied to the mons area, but take care when using anything on the labia themselves, as this skin is very sensitive. Read labels and choose a product intended for pubic shaving if you can find one. If you can't find one, a plain natural oil can be used, such as almond or olive oil. Do not use soap as a shaving cream. Apply a generous amount of lubricant and work it into the skin and hair in a circular motion. Leave it on for two to three minutes. This helps the hairs stand up and allows the blade to cut cleanly, minimizing razor burn.

Always start shaving the genitals from the anal area forward, around the sides and then in front, following the direction of hair growth first. Use one hand to pull the skin taut and the other to slowly shave the hair using long strokes, moving in the direction of hair growth, not against. If using a regular razor, clean it after every stroke to clear away stuck, matted hair on the blades. To shave just inside the labia majora, gently pull and flatten the skin taut with one hand, then slowly and carefully draw the razor across the skin with the other. Shaving against the grain of the hair growth tends to pull the follicles and tear the hairs, leading to more irritation. Therefore, wait until most of the hair is removed and then shave a second time against the grain of hair growth. This produces a clean, close and smooth shave and minimizes skin irritation.

Apply gentle pressure to the shaving head and avoid shaving any one area more than absolutely necessary. Pressing down or shaving over the same area repeatedly does not result in a closer, smoother shave. It does, however, frequently result in razor burns, rashes and bumps that may even turn into ingrown hairs that become infected. After shaving, lightly rub an ice cube over the area to close up open pores, then pat dry and apply a moisturizer.

Complications of pubic and genital hair removal

Cuts, scrapes, razor burn (light abrasions from too many passes of the razor over the same skin) and the like are the usual consequences of hair removal. Chemical burns from depilatories or burns from using wax that is too hot are other possible complications. These problems are handled as you would the same problems in other areas of the body.

Ingrown hairs can also develop as a by-product of hair removal when the hair begins to regrow and curls back or grows sideways under the skin. Usually, pubic hair grows out perfectly from the follicles but when ingrown hairs block the follicles, an inflamed pimple may develop. Like all pimples, they can be painful and itchy and may leave permanent scars.

Shaving the pubic area with a poor quality shaver is the most common cause of ingrown pubic hairs. Ingrown hairs can also develop when hair is broken off under the skin during waxing or tweezing. Other causes of ingrown pubic hair include tight undergarments or pants; dry skin; thick, curly or stiff hair and pubic hair follicles that are clogged with oil or dead skin cells.

There are several simple remedies for ingrown pubic hair. The first method involves applying a hot cloth or hot compress over the ingrown hair. This will help bring circulation to the area to relieve the inflammation and help soften the pubic hair under the skin so that it may rise above the surface on its own. If the ingrown hairs do not surface after a couple of minutes, continue the compress application several times. Should the problem persist, try again in a couple of hours or another day as the pubic hair may not be long enough for you to extract. Whatever happens, do not try to force or squeeze the hair out as this may cause bleeding and permanent scarring. Once a tiny end of the ingrown hair is visible on the surface of the skin, use a pair of sterilized tweezers to pluck the hair. Wash the pubic area, towel dry and apply some antiseptic cream to prevent infections.

Another method of removing an ingrown pubic hair is the use of a hair removal lotion that is certified safe to use on your pubic region by your dermatologist or pharmacist. These creams help to dissolve the ingrown pubic hairs under your skin without causing further skin irritation, but I do not recommend their use during pregnancy.

Once the ingrown hair has been removed, avoid wearing any tight undergarments or pants until all the ingrown hair lesions or other skin problems have completely healed. If a woman tends to develop ingrown pubic hairs just by wearing tight clothes, suggest that she purchase clothes made of softer material or eliminate tight clothing from her wardrobe. Although some people recommend using wax to get rid of the roots of ingrown pubic hairs, this practice may result in additional skin irritation as the wax strips may break open the ingrown hair pimple. Also advise the woman to avoid scrubbing her pubic area with a shower sponge to exfoliate the skin as this may result in additional irritation.

INTIMATE PIERCINGS AND TATTOOS

This chapter offers general information about these practices with a focus on genital piercings and tattoos. The second or later edition of my HOLISTIC MIDWIFERY, VOL. I and VOL. III, has more information on pierced navels and nipples relevant to midwifery practice.

Piercing

Piercing involves perforating the skin to produce a healed tract or fistula. A variety of different types of jewelry or another inert object is then inserted through the wound to hold the edges apart so that it will heal into a tube-shaped tract.

For centuries, women have pierced their ear lobes to facilitate the wearing of jewelry. Beginning in the mid-1990s, body piercing at other sites became popular among young adults in developed countries as a form of body art. As of this writing, between 30 to 50% of young adults ages 18 to 23 have voluntarily undergone some type of piercing at locations other than the ear lobes (Armstrong et al., 2004). Piercing is practiced by both men and women, although women tend to get more general body piercings, perhaps because they are used to wearing jewelry, an inherent component of this practice.

Piercings are usually divided into visible sites (e.g., face or ears) and semivisible sites (e.g., tongue or navel). The arms, tongue, lips, cheek, ear lobes, nose, spine, neck, chest, navel, nipples or genitals may be pierced. Genital and nipple piercings are referred to as "intimate piercings." Each site has its own set of physical complications.

Both sexes engage in genital piercing. Men have more anatomical space for genital piercing and usually wear heavier gauge jewelry. The majority of female genital piercings are located in the labial and clitoral hood areas. Jewelry, usually a captive bead or a straight or curved barbell, is then worn through the tract.

The effect of the piercing depends upon the proper placement of the tract. A practitioner who is inadequately skilled could do permanent nerve damage or sever an artery. Seeking a competent practitioner who has served a genital piercing apprenticeship, who places piercings in anatomically correct locations and who performs swift and smooth procedures are important considerations, especially since piercers are not allowed to administer local anesthetics.

Laws concerning piercing in the US

In the United States, 36 states reviewed their tattooing and body piercing regulations between 1995 and 2005 (Armstrong, 2005). The quality and standardization of legislation concerning body piercing in general varies widely, and as of 2009, no state mentions specific regulations for genital piercings.

Taking a history

Always inquire about piercings when taking a history. When you discover than a woman has piercings, especially at sites other than the earlobes, ask her why she got it (in a nonjudgmental way) and how she takes care of it. Basic education for women with genital piercings should include good hygiene, handwashing and the use of barrier protection during sexual activity. After building that rapport, you will often find yourself serving as a patient advocate against the more subtle and blatant forms of judgmental care that women with genital piercings often encounter in mainstream health care settings.

Reasons for piercings

There are a variety of reasons why women seek genital piercings. Women often consider the choice for some time before becoming pierced. Piercing may be chosen to mark a special event or as a means of overcoming traumatic events, such as divorce, rape or sexual abuse. It may be seen as a way of reclaiming body parts that the person disassociated from at the time of the traumatic event (Caliendo et al., 2005; Meyer, 2000). Women may seek to improve their self-esteem by wearing genital jewelry. Piercing may also be encouraged by a sexual partner. Other reasons include aesthetic appeal, sexual expression, enhancing sexual desire or orgasm pleasure and a feeling of uniqueness. Those who want to control sexual activity might select a form of self-infibulation, wherein the labia majora are pierced and then joined by rings that are hooked together. All of these are examples of women's attempts to set themselves apart. Many pierced women see themselves as risk-takers.

Uniqueness can be exhibited via an increased number of piercings or with piercings placed in an unusual location. For those recovering from a traumatic event, the act of choosing to be pierced is seen as a way of taking control, choosing to be a survivor rather than a victim. In this light, and considering that adult women are making the choice, piercings are viewed as a positive step. More studies are needed to look at the relationship between sexual abuse and genital piercings, particularly the association between a traumatic event and the use of genital piercings to help "reclaim the body" (Stirn, 2003).

Types of female genital piercings

Genital piercings are located according to a woman's individual preference, although certain locations are only suitable for certain types of anatomy and thus are less common. The type and weight of jewelry that any piercing will tolerate depends upon the anatomical site as well as the strength and thickness of the pierced tissue.

Clitoral hood: The large concentration of nerves in the small amount of visible clitoral tissue makes a direct clitoral piercing rare and very painful. Thus, when a woman tells you that her "clit" is pierced, she is usually referring to a hole that has been placed in tissues adjacent to the clitoral shaft or glans. A clitoral hood piercing is most often placed vertically. After placement, the jewelry rests under the hood where it touches the clitoral glans. During arousal, the jewelry stimulates the clitoris as it swells and becomes erect.

Horizontal hood piercings are often illustrated as clitoral hood piercings, but whether they can be done is more dependent on the tissue in the area. Horizontal hood piercings produce a very stimulating response if performed correctly. This piercing may also be done for aesthetic purposes only.

Triangle A: Triangle A piercings are considered by many to be the most stimulating of all genital piercings. They involve inserting jewelry under the clitoral body at the base of the hood. This type of piercing is likely to damage the clitoral root. It requires precision and expert knowledge on the part of the practitioner, who must be able to accurately palpate the clitoral body, which feels like a piece of cord running under the tissue. Stimulation occurs from behind the clitoral body (Anderson et al., 2003).

Labia majora and minora: Stimulation from single or multiple piercings of the labia majora or minora are affected by the changes that take place in labial tissues during sexual arousal and the placement of the piercing. If the labial piercing is near the introitus, the vasocongestion of the labia results in more stimulation for a male partner. If the piercing is located closer to the clitoral area, more pressure may be felt on the clitoral glans, thus increasing the woman's level of sensation.

> **Christina:** The "Christina" is a type of "surface" piercing that is done primarily for aesthetic reasons. It is located where the labia majora join, just below the mons pubis. It does not enhance female sexual response and poses more risk of infection due to the thick, vascular tissue in this area and the difficulty involved in protecting the site during heterosexual intercourse.

> **Fourchette:** A fourchette piercing is a vertical piercing that is usually located in the yoni wall at the most anterior midline region of the fourchette (of the labia minora) at the most anterior region of the perineal body, above the anal opening. It provides stimulation for the male partner during penetration, but does little to stimulate the woman. If a previous clitorotomy has been done, the scar tissue can interfere with the healing of this piercing. Some women report pain during intercourse due to the piercing being pulled into the yoni canal. A fourchette piercing is a set-up for yoni infections due to its close proximity to the anus.

Princess Albertina: This is the rarely performed female version of the "Prince Albert" male piercing (in which jewelry enters the urethra and exits the ventral surface of the penis). In the female version, one end of the piercing is located in the lower portion of the urethra and the other end exits just above or inside the yoni (Halliday, 2005; Pokorney & Berg, 1999). This piercing leaves the woman vulnerable to urinary tract infection and is not recommended.

Piercings and sexual stimulation

Women with genital piercings report a variety of sexual responses. Some are unaware of their piercings and do not experience continual arousal (Miller & Edenholm, 1999), while others report hypersensitivity (Caliendo et al., 2005). Miller and Edenholm found, among women with genital piercings who wear vertical clitoral hood piercings, a strong association with "their desire, frequency of intercourse, and arousal." Piercers report that sexual hypersensitivity is often predominant during the healing phase, as the body is adjusting to the foreign object (the jewelry), and that perceived desensitization is more a return to normal than a true reduction in sensation. They suggest that if clitoral desensitization occurs, changing the type or size of jewelry, or even leaving the piercing site empty for a short time, enhances "resensitization."

Genital piercing in adolescence

Genital piercings are not recommended for those under 18 years of age, even with parental consent, due to the anatomical changes that will occur during the teen years. Physiologically, the tissue is affected by the amount of estrogen in the body. The tissue of the yoni and surrounding area are drier, the labia flatter and the clitoris smaller than they will be once maturity is achieved. According to the Association of Professional Piercers (APP), a reputable piercer will not pierce the genital area of an adolescent.

Care tips and complications of genital piercings

Although the genital region is widely assumed to be one of the most painful locations for body piercing, the pain involved is similar to that of other body piercings, consisting of a quick, sharp, stabbing pain. The thick labia majora are more difficult and uncomfortable to pierce than the thinner labia minora.

After any piercing it is normal to have some bleeding for a few days after the procedure, plus localized swelling, tenderness or bruising (Caliendo et al., 2005). As the tract heals, there may be some discoloration, itching and secretion of a whitish yellow fluid (not pus) that will crust around the jewelry. The tissue may tighten as it heals and the wound contracts. During healing, the open wounds are subject to infection.

Initial healing of the tract occurs from the outside in and can take between six weeks and six months, depending on the site. It can take as long as a year for the tract to fully epithelialize. During this time, movement of the body jewelry within the piercing tract usually poses no problems, but rotating the jewelry deliberately is not recommended as it may disrupt collagen fibroblasts within the tract, prolonging the healing process (Halliday, 2005). Because of the vascular density in the area, genital piercings often heal in as little as 4 to 10 weeks. After healing, there is the potential for induced trauma if tension is placed on inserted jewelry. The fistula can also serve as a reservoir for bacterial debris.

Fresh oral piercings are cared for with 4 to 5 daily mouthwashes using an antibacterial solution. Fresh body piercings should be cared for as outlined by the piercer. Ideally, the site is cleaned twice daily, but if that is impossible, a daily cleansing should take place before bed. Both inadequate and overzealous cleaning will irritate the piercing.

Advise the woman to report warning signs such as heavy yoni bleeding, foul-smelling discharge, fever or flu-like feelings such as chills, problems or pain with urination, and signs of localized infection (such as green, foul-smelling pus; drainage; pain or redness) in or around the piercing. A local infection can be managed by cleaning the site more often and soaking the site in saline. The jewelry is left in place to help the wound drain. If there is no improvement after 2 or 3 days, the woman should report back to you; her piercer may need to be consulted as well.

If she needs a hygiene review, remind the woman to wash her hands prior to cleaning or touching on or near the piercing site. When showering, first wash the rest of the body. On the piercing, use a mild, liquid antibacterial soap (not alcohol, hydrogen peroxide, Betadine or Hibiclens). Work up a lather in the palm and apply it with a fingertip or a clean cotton swab. Gently wash around the sides of the piercing in small circular motions. Rinse well and blot the piercing dry with a disposable paper product. Do not use a towel, because cloth towels can harbor bacteria and catch on piercings, causing injury. If the piercing becomes irritated, the woman can apply a warm saline compress at least once, but preferably twice, daily. Make saline by diluting ¼ tsp of fine-grain, non-iodized sea salt in 1 cup (8 oz) warm water. Soak a clean, chlorine-free paper towel or tampon in the solution, squeeze out the excess and hold the compress to the piercing for 10 to 15 minutes. The piercing can also be soaked in saline by holding a disposable saline-filled paper or plastic cup against the tissue. Always wear clean clothes to bed and change your sheets frequently. (More about caring for oral and other body piercings can be found at [http://safepiercing.org].)

While the tract is healing, sexual activity may continue, but it is recommended that a barrier be used, even during oral sex, to prevent contamination of the site through contact with any type of body fluid. Douching following sex is not recommended, but if the site becomes contaminated with body fluid during sexual activity, clean it promptly. Additionally, if the woman finds sex painful, she should wait longer before resuming regular sexual activity. She should avoid wearing lace or mesh undergarments, which can snag on jewelry, causing discomfort or injury.

Willmott (2001) found that piercings were not associated with an increased incidence of sexually transmitted infections, but more studies are needed to explore whether genital piercings increase this risk.

There are no contraindications to using tampons with genital piercings. If insertion or wearing tampons causes discomfort, allow more time for healing. Be aware that any piercing can be affected by hormonal changes (even ear piercings can become irritated if you're sensitive to body and skin changes). Piercings may exude fluid or be supersensitive during the monthly cycle.

Caring for piercings during pregnancy: Many midwives may have a desire request that anything "foreign" be removed from the areas affected by pregnancy: the nipples, navel and genitals. Nonetheless, women with piercings may be very reluctant to remove their jewelry because of concerns about the piercing tract healing shut, especially in the genital area. Even well-healed genital piercing tracks can shrink, then close quickly, especially those through the clitoral hood and the labia majora. Reinsertion of jewelry can be difficult due to the anatomical closeness of genital structures, requiring the assistance of a piercer and special tools called "insertion tapers" to enlarge the piercing tract to its previous size.

The American Pregnancy Association and the Association of Professional Piercers agree that general body piercings (such as the navel) may be left in during pregnancy as long as the tract is completely healed, is not uncomfortable and does not become distorted as the body changes.

If a piece of piercing jewelry becomes too tight as pregnancy advances, it can be removed by a piercer and replaced with a bendable plastic ring made of polytetrafluoroethylene (PTFE) that is specifically designed for use during pregnancy (see [www.maternity piercings.com]). These rings allow for expansion and greater comfort. Rigid genital jewelry can also be removed and replaced with soft, stretchy material to avoid having the rigid jewelry become a focal point for tears. With labial piercings, it is wise to have all rigid jewelry replaced prior to childbirth, to avoid the possibility of tearing the tissue or trauma to the baby during birth, although clitoral hood jewelry is often left in place. Tearing risk is also of special concern for piercings involving the anus or the urethra. These issues should be discussed with the woman prenatally well before the birth so that she can arrange to have rigid jewelry replaced with space-holding, soft materials prior to the onset of labor.

Piercings and birth: Whether jewelry should be removed at the time of birth is controversial. Some women give birth with genital jewelry in place without any problems (Caliendo et al., 2005). Still, if there is scarring or if tension already on the jewelry that is inserted in a genital piercing appears such that the risk of ripping the piercing tract may be increased, it would be best to avoid this by removing jewelry during the birth. If a surgical delivery is to be performed, it is usually possible to leave traditional genital piercing jewelry in place.

Medical procedures and the need to remove piercing jewelry

While it is important to record the location of any piercings in the medical record, not all medical procedures require the removal of piercing jewelry. Women should be instructed to tell all medical practitioners about their piercings. Take into account the anatomical structures located adjacent to the piercing and the intent of the health care intervention as well as safety and infection concerns. You should always evaluate if the piercing really needs to be removed, or if you would simply prefer that it be removed. If it does require on-the-spot removal, the following can be used as jewelry substitutes: Tygon surgical-grade tubing, nonmetallic sterile intravenous catheter tubing, or soft, clean and thick fishing line (Armstrong et al., 2006b).

Internal yoni examinations can be performed without removing the piercings. If a woman who has a genital piercing has been sexually assaulted, forensic evidence should be collected from the area around the jewelry.

When urinary catheterization is necessary, there is only one uncommon genital piercing (Princess Albertina) that passes through the urethral meatus. A small size urinary catheter could be used to bypass the piercing (Halliday, 2005; Meyer, 2000). If a Foley catheter is to be inserted, extra care must be taken as it is inserted and afterward to keep the perineal area clean.

If the woman requires radiologic studies, simple X-rays are not affected by body piercings. The magnetic fields of an MRI are problematic however, and jewelry attraction and artifacts are possible, meaning metal jewelry must be removed for the procedure. Health care providers must ensure that a woman understands that there is a specific medical or clinical reason for their requesting that she remove her piercing jewelry (DeBoer et al., 2006).

If electrocautery is required, the need to remove genital jewelry depends on the surgical site and the procedure. Just as a wedding band is taped down rather than removed for most surgical procedures, some piercings could also be taped down. The rule is that no electrocautery equipment should physically touch the jewelry (DeBoer et al., 2006).

A woman with piercings should be aware that in the event of an emergency her jewelry may be removed without her consent; the focus will be on her well-being and not the preservation of her piercing tracts.

When jewelry must be removed: Discuss the reasons for removing the jewelry and plan in advance to have a suitable space-holder on hand to keep the tract patent. (It would be a good idea for you to carry space-holders in your birth bag for this purpose.) Planning for temporary jewelry placement to maintain patency even for short procedures (1 to 2 hours) should help to alleviate a woman's fear of tract closure. For example, if it appears that a piercing might tear during birth if the jewelry is left in, replacing the jewelry with a flexible object to maintain patency may suffice to prevent tearing.

Whenever feasible, ask the woman to remove her own piercing jewelry (Meyer, 2000). When a provider must remove genital piercings due to an obstetric or gynecologic emergency, care should be taken to remove the jewelry without further traumatizing the tissue. Extensive skin damage, predisposing the area to the risk of infection, can result when ring or bolt cutters are used to remove the jewelry.

When piercings have been removed, women often seek reinsertion or procure another piercing later (Armstrong et al., 2004).

New piercings during pregnancy

If a woman is contemplating getting pierced while she is pregnant, it would be safest to wait until she has had the baby to avoid the unnecessary risk of complications and infections due to the extra blood volume, increased vascularity (especially in the genital area) and the slight immune suppression of pregnancy (American Pregnancy Assoc., 2008).

If she is intent on getting pierced, advise her to choose piercings located above the neck, although even oral piercings may be problematic for women whose gums become tender during pregnancy (this problem is usually prompted by hormonal changes and exacerbated by nutritional deficiencies). New nipple, genital or navel piercings should be avoided during pregnancy because of the massive changes that these tissues undergo. Any new piercings at this time can produce undesirable results as the tissues return to their nonpregnant normal condition. The gradual stretching of the skin during pregnancy can also make it difficult for new piercings to heal. It is best to go into labor with thoroughly healed piercings in case the jewelry must be removed. Another issue is the introduction of metal jewelry, especially metals that are unfamiliar to the woman's body. New jewelry should be made of surgical-grade metals that the woman knows to be compatible with her body. Women that choose to be pierced during pregnancy should seek a state-licensed piercing studio that is clean and uses sterile equipment. She should inform the piercer that she is pregnant, too, since this may affect how they want to handle the procedure.

Tattoos

Tattoos are another form of decorative body modification that consists of skin markings that permanently alter the pigment for decorative or other reasons. They have been used since time immemorial in numerous cultures. Tattoos may be referred to as "ink," "tats," "art," "pieces," or "work;" and the tattooists as "artists" (Tattoo, 2009).

With the rise of piercings, tattoos have also become very popular with young adults in developed countries, particularly in Europe and the US. A January 2008 Harris Poll (Harris Poll, 2009) estimated that 14% of all US adults have a tattoo. The highest incidence was found among the gay, lesbian and bisexual population (25%) and people living on the West coast (20%). The age group breakdown was as follows: 9% (ages 18–24), 32% (ages 25-29), 25% (ages 30-39), 12% (ages 40-49) and 8% (ages 50-64). Men are just slightly more likely to have a tattoo than women (15% versus 13%).

Tattooing involves the use of a special device for injecting pigment into the skin. Dye disperses throughout a damaged layer of tissue down to the upper dermis, where it activates phagocytes that engulf the pigment particles. During healing, the damaged epidermis flakes away (eliminating surface pigment) while deeper in the skin granulation tissue forms, which is later converted to connective tissue by collagen growth. This mends the upper dermis, where pigment remains trapped within fibroblasts, ultimately concentrating in a layer just below the dermal/epidermal boundary. Its presence there is stable, but in the long term (decades) the pigment tends to migrate deeper into the dermis, accounting for the degraded detail of old tattoos (Tattoo, 2009).

Today, a wide range of dyes and pigments are used in tattoos, from inorganic materials like titanium dioxide and iron oxides to carbon black, azo dyes, and acridine, quinoline, phthalocyanine and naphthol derivatives, dyes made from ash, and other mixtures. As of this writing, the trend for tattoo pigment favors Acrylonitrile butadiene styrene (ABS plastic) as used in Intenze, Millennium and other ABS pigment brands (Tattoo, 2009). The use of plastic-based inks may eventually be proven to be harmful, although ABS is not currently known to pose any particular danger to health.

Tattoos that may be relevant to midwifery care

Breasts: Many women choose to get tattooed on their breasts. However, eventual sagging of the skin in the area will change the way the tattoo looks, particularly for those with large breasts. Most tattoo artists avoid tattooing the nipples, where omission of ink tends not to be so noticeable. Sometimes women seek a tattooed facsimile of a nipple for a breast that has undergone reconstructive surgery involving nipple removal.

Stomach or abdomen: Tattooing the abdomen can be problematic because there is no solid backing to hold the skin down and it is a sensitive area, making the procedure more painful than in some other areas. In addition, abdominal tattoos can change dramatically as a person ages.

Genitals: Genital tattoos are not as painful as one might think, but are nevertheless relatively rare, especially among women. This is primarily because the stretchiness of the skin and the way it moves makes it impossible to create a tattoo image that has a lot of fine detail.

Tattoos and pregnancy

In general, tattoos that are completely healed require no special care during pregnancy and should pose no pregnancy-related problems. However, the changes of pregnancy may very well affect a tattoo. How much so depends upon the quality of the woman's tissue, the location of the tattoo and the way her body responds to pregnancy. Depending on the location, it is possible that the tattoo will stretch and there is no guarantee that it will return to its original shape after the birth. Healing could also be disrupted if a new tattoo is placed over a body region that undergoes lots of stretching. These problems tend to occur mostly with tattoos on the abdomen, although tattoos on the breasts, lower back, the thighs or even the ankles can experience the same types of problems.

A tattoo done on stretched skin can later shrink, becoming dark and shapeless. Women should be particularly wary of getting any tattoo where the shape is important, such as symmetrical tribal designs or Celtic knots. Even simple geometric patterns such as a circle could end up looking like an oval (or worse, an irregular blob). A more forgiving image, such as a cloud scene, is a better bet. Since the entire body undergoes significant fluid changes, even an ankle tattoo can stretch out of shape if a woman experiences swelling during the pregnancy.

Many tattoo artists refuse to tattoo pregnant women. There have been no studies regarding the safety of tattoo ink applied during pregnancy. There is also the slight but very serious risk of contracting a blood-borne disease, especially hepatitis C, during the procedure, even if the tattoo parlor is licenced. Such an infection would massively complicate the pregnancy and pose a serious risk to the fetus, making the option of waiting additionally attractive.

Another possible negative effect of getting tattooed while pregnant is the inherent stress involved, which puts nutritional, physical and psychological stress on the mother and therefore the baby.

The risk of fainting is also a minor concern. It is not uncommon for people who are getting a tattoo to pass out. Anything that puts a woman at risk for falling, losing consciousness or oxygen deprivation such as fainting, is best avoided during pregnancy.

CLITOROTOMY ("EPISIOTOMY")

Note: Review the chapter entitled "Using Surgical Scissors" before studying this one.

A clitorotomy is a surgical incision through the perineal body performed to enlarge the introitus just before the baby emerges. Clitorotomy, when done routinely (as it has been for many decades in the developed world), constitutes one contemporary Western form of ritual female genital mutilation (type IV). For this reason, even though in the West it is a skill that is generally considered essential for midwives to know, it is included in this part of the book, rather than the part entitled "Essential Surgical Skills for Midwives," as a political statement regarding its continued role as a form of ritual mutilation.

Terminology: Why Call It "Clitorotomy" (KLIH-toe-RAH-toe-me)?

Most female genital structures are either an extension of clitoral tissue or involved in its support, protection or function. The yoni and urethra are surrounded by the neurological, cavernous, circulatory and muscular tissue of the clitoris. This makes them clitoral orifices and places an episiotomy in the category of a clitoral incision. Perineal muscles and the perineal sponge embedded within the perineal body (an extension of the clitoral bulbs) are severed when an episiotomy is performed. For all these reasons, the episiotomy (an imprecise term meaning "to cut the external genitals") is more appropriately named "clitorotomy" (to cut the clitoris) and will be referred to as such in this text (Cassidy-Brinn et al., 1984).

Practitioners may be distressed by this term, feeling uneasy about the thought that they are cutting a woman's clitoral tissue. This is exactly what I have in mind. Women may be even more reluctant to allow unnecessary cutting if they realize exactly what is being done. Good. I say, let's call the procedure what it is. If a clitorotomy is necessary, then it should be performed. However, if raising consciousness about what is really being done helps to deter the unnecessary use of this surgical procedure, then my goal in using this term in place of "episiotomy" will have been achieved.

Historical Notes

Clitorotomy first makes an appearance in the literature of obstetrics in 1742 when Fielding Ould, a male midwife, suggested a midline incision to facilitate birth. A little while later, Karl Schuchardt (1893) was the first doctor to report performing an extensive mediolateral clitorotomy to gain better exposure during an operative procedure. Joseph DeLee, however, was the physician who popularized clitorotomy to protect the maternal tissues and the use of forceps to protect the fetal head. During the 1950s and 1960s, the trend gradually moved away from mediolateral to midline incisions in the United States, while mediolateral incisions remained largely the standard of care in Europe. In the US in the

1970s, midwives reentered the field of maternity care in larger numbers and challenged the routine use of clitorotomy, as did the population of childbearing women of that era. During the years that have followed, its routine use has steadily declined. Even so, it is still the most common surgical procedure performed by most obstetricians (Hale & Ling, 2007).

Controversies in Theory

The primary, paradoxical purpose of clitorotomy is to "prevent" injury by inflicting an incision. As with some other forms of female genital mutilation, it has been promoted based on unfounded claims that it offers cosmetic and health advantages and contributes to male sexual pleasure.

The much-touted benefits have included reduction of the time spent pushing, thereby reducing strain placed on the pelvic tissues as well as the stress on the fetus; prevention of severe perineal tears by controlling the direction of laceration, tearing having been believed to be virtually inevitable, especially in first-time mothers; avoidance of anal sphincter injury; substitution of a straight surgical cut for a ragged tear, rendering repair easier for the practitioner; better and more rapid healing; reduction of pain in the postpartum period; prevention of later pelvic floor dysfunction and prolapse and maintenance or even improvement of sexual function. Indications have included these conditions: to better accommodate large babies; to hasten the birth when the baby is believed to be in distress; to enlarge the introitus to allow manual maneuvers during breech births, shoulder dystocia or instrumental deliveries (forceps, vacuum extraction); and to avoid a ragged tear when tearing appears to be inevitable. The benefits of clitorotomy were very much assumed, as no studies that pointed to these presumed advantages were ever done before it came into wide use.

It is true that pushing places strain on the pelvic tissues that can sometimes result in deep tears or avulsions of the internal tissues, including detachment of the origin or insertion points of muscles. Nevertheless, instead of looking for the reasons why this type of damage might be occurring—such as unphysiologic positions for pushing; the use of drugs that unduly relax the tissues; the application of fundal pressure, which was widely used in the era spanning 1910 to 1950, when the promotion of clitorotomy peaked; and the use of instrumental delivery—the solution was to inflict more trauma by cutting the perineum.

It is now acknowledged that routine clitorotomy carries numerous risks. (By routine, I mean performing an incision on every woman who does not give birth before it can be done.) Ironically, many of these risks were long assumed to be reduced by the liberal use of clitorotomy. They include a higher risk of extension with deep tearing; a risk of sphincter disruption, especially when a midline incision is used; greater blood loss; greater risk of infection and fistula formation; and increased postpartum pain. In addition, it is generally not acknowledged that incising the complex vascular sponge embedded in the perineal body may permanently impair sexual functioning. Because most of these complications of routine use have finally been recognized, the number of clitorotomies performed in the US decreased across all ages, races, sources of payment for care and regions of the country from an overall rate of 63.9 per 100 births in 1980 to 39.2 per 100 births in 1998. Nevertheless, when only first-time mothers are considered, nearly all reported rates exceed 65% (Graham et al., 2005).

For some time, it has been understood that muscles do not heal by forming new muscle tissue, but by building other substances, including collagen. This results in the gap filling in with scar tissue, which is weaker, less elastic than undamaged muscle, and prone to reinjury. Since the muscle fibers do not reunite, muscles that were previously of one piece become double-bellied in the area of the scar (Kirk, 2002). Once a muscle is damaged, it can become the source of a great deal of pain. Therefore, it makes no sense to routinely severe perineal muscles, which are so vital to pelvic floor health and function.

In an extensive review of several randomized controlled trials, Carroli and Belizan (2000) and later Carroli and Mignini (2009) found that the risk of having a tear that needs stitches, as well as the risk of anal sphincter damage, is much reduced when clitorotomy is not used routinely. Complications in the healing of the perineum in the first seven days postpartum were also reduced. There was no difference in the rate of severe tearing of the yoni or the perineum and no difference in the amount of postpartum pain, painful intercourse or urinary incontinence. The only advantage afforded by routine clitorotomy seems to be a decrease in what is referred to in the literature as "anterior damage," which would include labial and periurethral lacerations. Both reviews concluded that there was no good evidence to support the routine use of clitorotomy, even in first-time mothers.

At times, I have looked at a perineum and said to myself, "I'm really gambling here by not cutting" because it appeared as though a bad tear was forthcoming (a thought process based on the theory that a directed cut is better than a ragged tear). Afterward, I've generally been glad I refrained, because I've realized that even my tiniest cut would have done more damage than the (sometimes surprisingly) small tear that actually occurred.

Clitorotomies are usually defended by mainstream obstetrics as easier to repair (sometimes true) and better for healing and long-term integrity of the perineal body because they produce straight, clean incisions rather than ragged tears. This hypothesis is based on a general understanding of first-intention healing but there is no research to support this notion when it comes to perineal healing. Tears *can* be very tricky to repair, especially when they involve odd skin tags and detours, but even those clitorotomies that do not extend are almost always deeper and more extensive than the vast majority of spontaneous tears. In the same way that it is difficult to start a rip in the edge of a piece of cloth, a stressed perineum, if it tears at all, will split along the line of least resistance and usually stop thanks to the decussation of muscles fibers in the perineal body. But just snip the edge of the same cloth with a pair of scissors, grasp the edge of the fabric on either side of the snip and pull. This will cause most cloth to tear very easily. In just that same way, a cut starts a line of tissue damage that almost always includes muscle and tends to extend. A spontaneous tear that occurs during pushing in a physiologic (i.e., upright) position will probably not be as extensive and is therefore less likely to do as much damage.

The appropriate use of clitorotomy

Since a tear is usually less extensive and often heals better than a cut, never cut simply to avoid a tear unless you are considering cutting a particularly rigid hymenal ring (which will usually tear anyway) or are faced with some sort of excessive scarring that is refusing to stretch, as would be the case with previous genital alteration in the form of clitoridectomy or infibulation, or a history of sexual abuse, which may not have been disclosed or even recognized in women who have blocked memories of the abuse (see the chapter entitled "Traditional Female Genital Modifications").

Clitorotomies are appropriately performed in instances of acute fetal distress, when you anticipate considerable time from the detection of the distress until birth. When women are informed of the need to birth quickly, however, the knowledge that the baby might be in trouble prompts a surge of catecholamine hormones that helps many mothers push their baby out very fast. Alternatively, a maternal position change or a few contractions without pushing while the mother breathes supplemental oxygen may stabilize the fetal condition. You can gently apply just enough counterpressure against the fetal presenting part with the flat of your palm to take the maximum stress off the perineum between contractions; this will often stabilize fetal heart rate because it relieves some of the pressure on the head. (Do *not* try to push the head back up inside and do *not* try to prevent the birth if it seems inevitable; both can do damage to the baby.) I almost always try these things before making an incision, and one or more of them usually helps, greatly reducing the need to cut due to fetal distress.

Clitorotomy is frequently recommended with anticipated or actual shoulder dystocia. This has always seemed like a waste of valuable time to me. Keep in mind that shoulder dystocia is related to a bony impaction, not one involving soft tissue. Although it may be indicated in some cases, I have never used clitorotomy as part of my shoulder dystocia protocol. Don't be timid about inserting your hands as far as necessary when reaching for those shoulders. Male obstetricians with large hands may be unable to reach far enough into the yoni to deal with certain types of shoulder dystocia without a clitorotomy, but most female birth attendants will not have this problem.

For a while it was thought best to cut a clitorotomy in cases of prematurity to avoid undue pressure on the less-calcified skull of an immature infant. This theory has been refuted with further research (Barrett, 1983). A gentle birth of the baby with the mother in a side-lying position will help relieve pressure on the head. (Ensuring that the baby receives a full cord transfusion after the birth is essential in the care of the preterm baby to avoid brain damage, in part because it keeps the vascular beds in the brain full of blood. See the chapters entitled "The Baby's Journey through Labor to Birth," and "Placenta-to-Newborn Transfusion, Physiologic Closure of the Umbilical Vessels and Severance of the Cord" in HOLISTIC MIDWIFERY, VOL. II, for a complete discussion of normal fetal-to-newborn transition and the role of an intact cord in that process.)

Breech presentation is often considered an indication for clitorotomy. Indeed, it is difficult to cut one after the body is out in the event that you need more room to manipulate the head. Although, as with shoulder dystocia, difficulty with the aftercoming head is usually a bony, not a soft tissue, problem. Ina May Gaskin, a midwife who has much experience with breeches, does not advocate prophylactic clitorotomy. She feels a valid indication is when the scrotum of a frank breech baby is presenting and receiving excessive pressure from prolonged rumping. In this case, relieving the pressure with a small cut will help prevent hematoma formation or more serious scrotal or testicular injury (Gaskin, 1990). Obstetrician Leo Sorger cuts in the very rare cases when descent of the shoulders or head seems to be impeded by soft tissue (Sorger, 1991). He feels that a baby's scrotum can bear a lot of pressure before damage occurs.

Some midwives believe that a clitorotomy is needed to direct damage if a tear seems likely to occur near varicose veins. In fact, you are likely to do far more damage and possibly cut through an unseen vein than to have a vein tear. Blood vessels, even varicosed ones, are fairly elastic, and they will usually remain intact even if the perineum tears. (See other suggestions concerning protecting vulval varicosities in the chapter entitled "Preparing the Perineal Tissues for Birth".)

Rarely, a very rigid perineum resists all attempts to stretch it during fetal descent. Such resistance is usually related to thick scar tissue from a previous tear or cut, but this can happen in a woman with no scar tissue if she has high-tone pelvic floor dysfunction. If such rigidity occurs in an unhealthy woman with poor tissue quality, the result may be a ruptured perineal body through which the baby can pass; sometimes this occurs while the introitus remains intact. Fortunately both of these scenarios are exceedingly rare, but it is good to be aware of such possibilities. If all efforts to facilitate stretching fail, or if a central perineal rupture seems imminent, the only alternative may be to cut the perineum.

Finally, maternal exhaustion is a reason to weigh the merits of a clitorotomy. This must be carefully considered. If the mother is so exhausted that she cannot push any longer and cannot (or will not) rest, eat, and rally, cutting may well get the baby out. But an exhausted mother is more likely to hemorrhage. A woman this exhausted is probably hypoglycemic and dehydrated as well. Do you really want to proceed with this at home? Be sure she has the strength to complete the birth once you cut her. If so and if labor has been long and a cut will save those last 30 minutes of pushing (which may put her over the edge of exhaustion into the danger zone), cutting may be entirely appropriate. It will rarely be necessary, however, if women are free to push in their position of choice.

If you are trying to decide whether to cut, perform a digital exam to make certain that the baby's skull (and not merely a soft enlarging caput), is truly low enough to birth with the aid of a clitorotomy (the biparietal diameter should be fully beneath the pubic bone). A clitorotomy will *not* help if the delay is due to a bony obstruction. You really don't want to have to explain why you have transported a baby with a huge caput and an exhausted, incised, laboring mother to the hospital.

Scars from previous clitorotomies

During prenatal care, inspect existing genital scars and review the chart for any history of discomfort. At the time of birth, if it appears as though a scar may rip, allow it to tear (if it will) and repair it again, rather than cutting to direct any damage. If the perineal muscles or the introitus has been sewn up too tightly (the notorious "husband's stitch" or "lover's knot"), yoni discomfort, particularly on the improperly repaired side of the introitus, is often the chronic result. If so, the tightest points will be eliminated by letting the perineum tear spontaneously. A tear will tell you for sure what was too tight; if you cut, it will be impossible to be certain. Your careful, anatomical, not-too-tight repair will then (very likely) heal much better than the first one. Talk this plan over with your client during prenatal care. At the same time, explain that the faithful performance of prenatal perineal stretching may prevent further damage (in such cases, however, some women may even hope for a tear so the area can be repaired correctly).

Clitorotomies are sometimes necessary when scar tissue from a previous incision is so thick and unyielding that the perineum simply will not stretch. Unyielding tissue may lead to fetal heart rate decelerations secondary to excessive head compression. Whether to cut is always a judgement call, of course, but the need to do so in this case is also rare. The presence of an infibulation often necessitates a clitorotomy, but not invariably. (For full details, see the chapter entitled "Traditional Female Genital Modifications.")

Choosing clitorotomy scissors

A clitorotomy can be cut with any pair of sharp surgical scissors, there are also several styles of scissors have been specially designed for this purpose. Using sharp surgical scissors means an easier and more efficient cut with less tissue trauma. Here is a rundown of what can be used.

Blunt/sharp or blunt/blunt surgical scissors: These basic scissors have blades that are straight from their tips to the finger rings. The tips of the blades may both be rounded or there may be one rounded and one pointed tip. When one end is rounded, it is inserted inside the yoni, since it is less likely to damage the fetal scalp or unintentionally traumatize the maternal tissue. Some companies, such as Snowden-Pencer, make scissors with one finely serrated blade (Diamond-SerEdges), which are ideal for performing a clitorotomy, since serrated surgical scissors are designed to stabilize thick tissue during cutting. Cutting with a serrated edge produces a clean, straight wound that is said to be easier to repair, to promote first intension healing, and to produce minimal scar tissue.

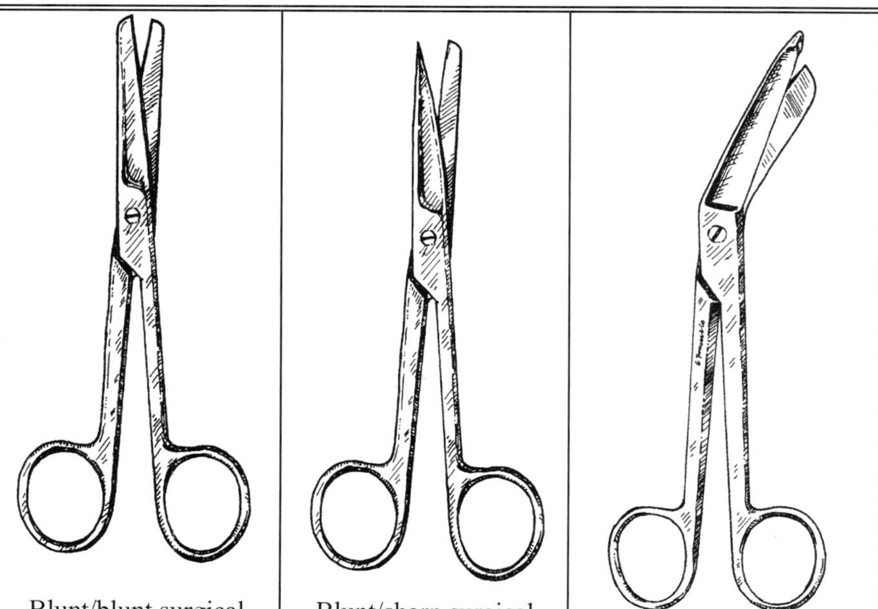

Blunt/blunt surgical scissors | Blunt/sharp surgical scissors | Lister bandage scissors

Right-handed surgical scissors are widely available. Left-handed practitioners can get **Mayo dissecting scissors** that have two small, blunted ends. These are fine, all-purpose surgical scissors entirely suitable for cutting a clitorotomy as well as the other tasks involved in suturing. They are made by V. Mueller (item no. SU1801-001) in a 6.75 inch (171 mm) length and can be special-ordered through Cascade HealthCare Products (www.cascade1.com).

Lister bandage scissors: Lister scissors are constructed so that the blades form a 45° angle to the shaft. This makes for less awkward maneuvering when the scissors are in place in the perineum and you are ready to cut. Hold the scissors blades-down. The outer blade (the one that would go inside the yoni) has a blunt triangular appendage that can be used to help insinuate the blade between the baby's head and the perineum and can be inserted anteriorly when performing an anterior clitorotomy (dividing the closed upper labial tissue) of a woman who has undergone infibulation. The problem with bandage scissors is that they are not designed to cut tissue, so the blades are not as sharp as those of scissors made for that purpose. However, Lister scissors are more readily available in a left-handed design, and this would be very useful for lefties. These are available from the Safety Store on the Internet ([www.safetystore.com], item no. PO16060). These scissors are not designed to cut tissue and do not hold their edge with repeated use, but they may be the best you have access to in a resource-poor setting. I recommend buying a pair and not using them for any other purpose. Once they have been used to cut tissue two or three times, you might want to replace them.

Specialized clitorotomy scissors: The following scissors were designed specifically for use in performing clitorotomies. They are named as they would appear in a surgical instrument catalogue, and sources are given for all of them since they are a harder-to-find item. If you have trouble getting these vendors to sell to you directly, contact any of the midwifery supply businesses that are out there. Cascade HealthCare Products retails for Cardinal Health, where some of these instruments can be obtained.

Barnes (Lawson-Tait) episiotomy scissors: These British-designed scissors feature a gentle angle between the shanks and the blades and a guarded edge on the outer blade similar to the Braun-Stadler scissors. Their most useful unique feature is the finger rings that both point in the same direction to facilitate cutting when the blades are in place. These scissors are 4.85" to 5.5" (125 mm to 140 mm) long. They are available from Downs Surgical in the UK ([www.downs-surgical.co.uk], product code FM-546-01-Q) and from Rocket Medical also in the UK ([www.rocketmedical.com], part no. R20.223).

Braun episiotomy scissors: Braun scissors are the most commonly used type of specialized episiotomy scissors in the United States. Their blades are angled in the manner of a bandage scissors; the outer blade is fat with a rounded outer edge to prevent tissue trauma when it is inserted between the perineum and the fetal scalp. These scissors are more finely constructed and are sharper than bandage scissors since they are intended for surgical use. I could not find them in a left-handed style. These scissors are made by V. Mueller (item no. GL3500) They can be special-ordered through Cascade HealthCare Products (www.1cascade.com).

Braun-Stadler episiotomy scissors: The British version of the Braun, these scissors are of identical design except for their guarded blade, which has a blunted projection along the outer edge, like a fat, blunt knife blade. These scissors are available from Diener Chirurgishe Instrumente (www.diener-gmbh.de) and are listed in their gynecological scissors category (item no. 02-1605.14). They are also available from Rocket Medical in the UK ([www.Rocket Medical.com], part no. R20.225).

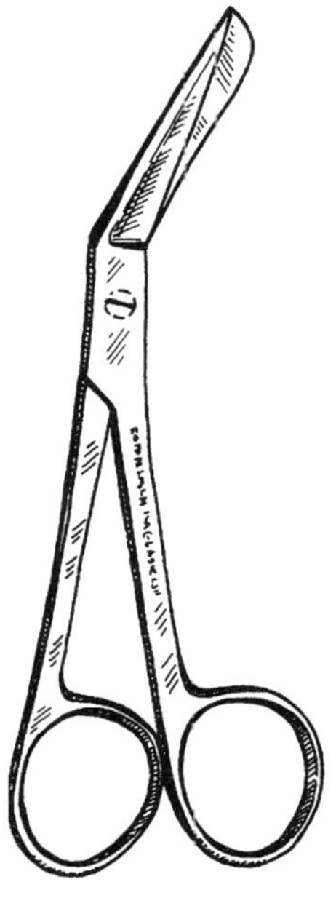

Barnes (Lawson-Tate) scissors

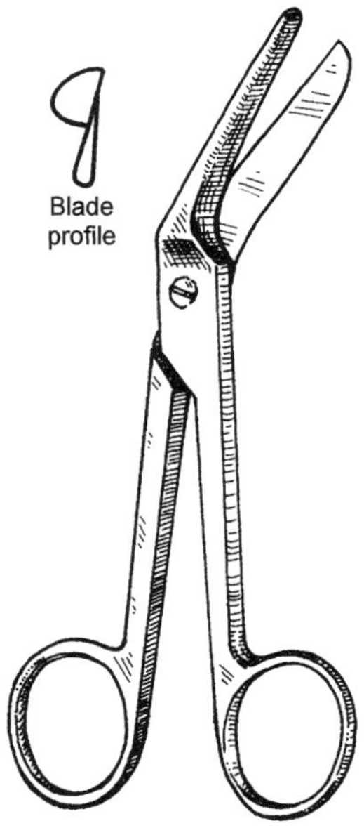

Braun scissors

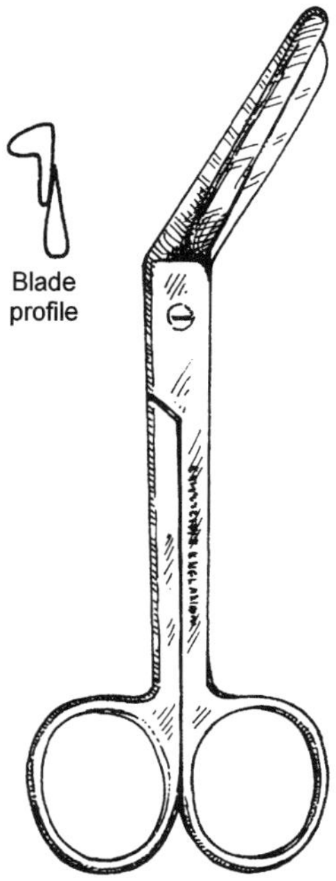

Braun-Stadler scissors

Marbach episiotomy scissors: The blades of Marbach scissors meet the shanks at a 90° angle and are curved to conform to the shape of the baby's head. One blade has a blunt tip to insert between the baby's head and the perineum. These scissors also have strong, serrated edges and are 6" long (152 mm). This design assumes that a long, deep cut will be made, and it may be difficult to produce a more shallow cut with this type of scissors. They are also available from Diener (www.diener-gmbh.de) and are listed as gynecological scissors (item no. 01-1613.15).

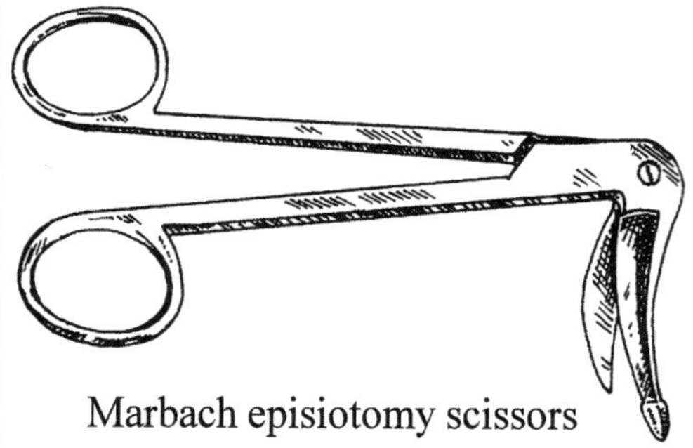

Marbach episiotomy scissors

Schroeder episiotomy scissors: These scissors look like regular blunt/sharp surgical scissors but are specifically designated for making perineal incisions. They are 8.5" (210 mm) in length. This style is made by V. Mueller (item no. GL3480) and is available by special order through Cascade HealthCare Products (www.1cascade.com).

Vant episiotomy scissors: These scissors look just like the Schroeder, except both blades have small rounded (blunt) tips. They are 241 mm long with 76 mm blades and are available through Downs Surgical in the UK (www.downs-surgical.co.uk), item no. FM-561-01-E.

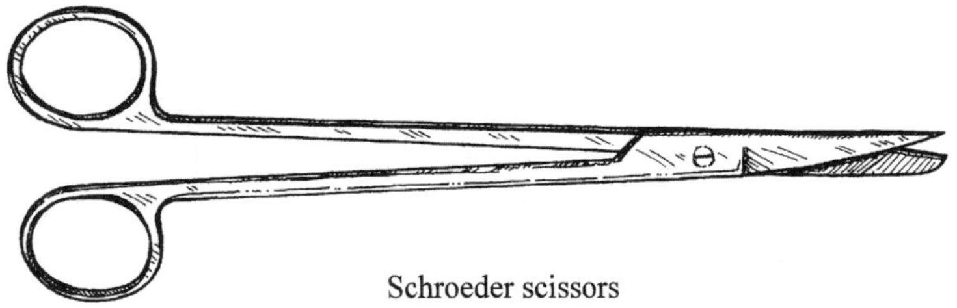

Schroeder scissors

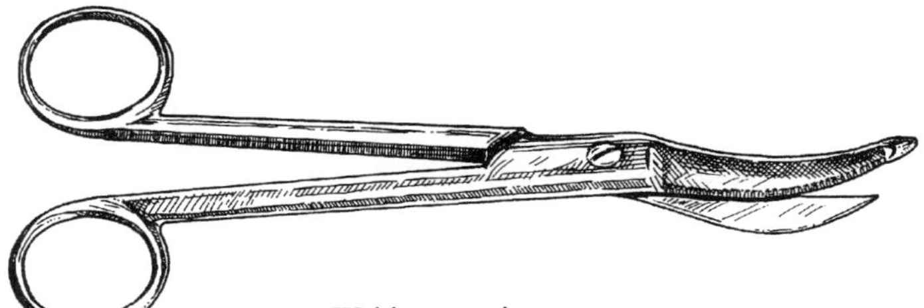

Waldmann scissors

Waldmann episiotomy scissors: The blades of these scissors are similar to those of the Marbach scissors but the shank-to-blades connection is straight. The blades are curved and finely serrated, with a slightly larger inside blade that has a guarded tip. They are 7.75" (197 mm) long. They are made by V. Mueller (item no. GL3510) and are available by special order through Cascade HealthCare Products (www.1cascade.com).

Types of Clitorotomies

The "type" of a clitorotomy performed has to do with the angle of the incision, which is determined by measuring the angle of the incision in relationship to a 0° line drawn down the center of the perineal body (6 o'clock) from the introital midline. There are two primary types of incisions in modern use: the midline and the mediolateral or medio-oblique.

Midline incision

The **midline** or **median clitorotomy** is cut straight down the center of the perineum from the 0° (or 6 o'clock) point, from the introitus toward the anus. Sometimes just releasing the tension with a small cut is all that is needed. Midline incisions are the easiest to perform and the easiest to repair. They are associated with less blood loss, less pain and better anatomic results (O'Leary & O'Leary, 1965; Parker & Brunner, 2003).

Note that midline incisions are unacceptable where the cutting of the perineum is a cultural taboo. Ironically, these same cultures often practice some form of traditional female genital surgery (Chalmers & Omer-Hashi, 2003).

The big downside of midline incisions is that they are also more likely to extend into the anal sphincter. Overall, about 20% of primiparous women who have a midline clitorotomy will have such an extension. Owen and Hauth (1990) found that 9% of primiparous women tear through the sphincter or rectal mucosa with a midline incision, and only 1% had these complications when they were left uncut. Interestingly, multiparous women with a midline cut had fewer third- and fourth-degree extensions that those who received a mediolateral.

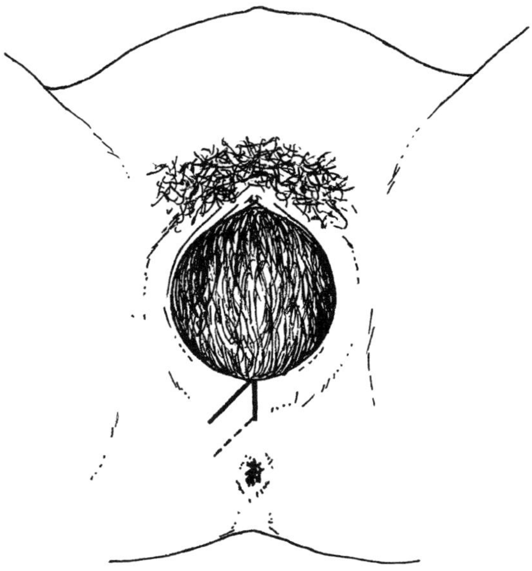

Types of incisions

Darkest solid line–midline
Angled solid line–mediolateral
Darkest line with dashed angled extension–J-shaped

Anorectal extensions are more likely to occur because the incision divides so much of the tissue of the perineum that would otherwise shield the sphincter from close contact with the hard fetal head. Sooklin and colleagues (2007) compared midline and mediolateral clitorotomy and concluded that midline cuts result in a greater number of deep perineal extensions and that such extensions are more likely to occur in women with several risk factors. Observational studies confirm that midline incisions increase the risk of third-degree extension and subsequent anal incontinence.

A median cut may incise the skin, the yoni mucosa, the superficial transverse perineal muscle, the perineal membrane, fibers from the bulbocavernosus muscle or the anal sphincter that cross the midline and the perineal sponge. Deep cuts may involve the puboperinealis portion of the pubovisceral muscle or the urethrovaginal sphincter muscle as well.

A **proctoepisiotomy** is a clitorotomy wherein the anal sphincter is intentionally severed; obviously this is not recommended.

Mediolateral incision

The **mediolateral (angled) clitorotomy** begins at the center of the introitus and is directed to one side or the other at an angle in an attempt to avoid extension into the external anal sphincter.

Appropriate angle of incision: There are many different definitions of the angle and even the shape of this incision. The angles quoted range anywhere from 30 to 90°. Among European hospitals, the angle for a mediolateral cut is most often defined as one of 45°, which would begin at the 6 o'clock point (0°) and be directed midway between the anus and the ischial tuberosity on one side. Others state that the incision should be directed toward one or the other ischial tuberosity, which, depending on maternal pelvic anatomy, can entail an angle as small as 25°. In the US, the recommended angle ranges from "toward the ischial tuberosity" to "at 5 or 7 o'clock" to simply "45°," depending upon the source. Rather than a specific angle, Varney and colleagues (2004) recommend leaving 1 cm between the incision and the anterolateral border of the external anal sphincter, as determined by palpation just prior to cutting but they warn that cutting too far laterally is likely to sever the greater vestibular gland on that side.

The dispute stems from the understanding that the angle of a mediolateral clitorotomy changes significantly from what it was at the time of the incision and where it winds up after the repair (Andrews et al., 2005; Eogan et al., 2006; Kalis et al., 2008a). This occurs because the cut is typically made only after the presenting part is distending the perineum. Stretching distorts the anatomy (especially when women are lying on their back, the safest maternal position for performing a clitorotomy) and irons out the perineal body, thinning and spreading the underlying muscles. Kalis and colleagues (2008a) found that a cut made at an angle of 40° at the point of fetal crowning narrowed to around 20° when the perineum was no longer distended (assessed by measuring the resulting suture line after repair). This means the cut probably sliced through a portion of the (previously dilated) internal and external sphincter muscle after all. Although the before-and-after difference in angles was not as great among women who were cut prior to crowning, it was still significant.

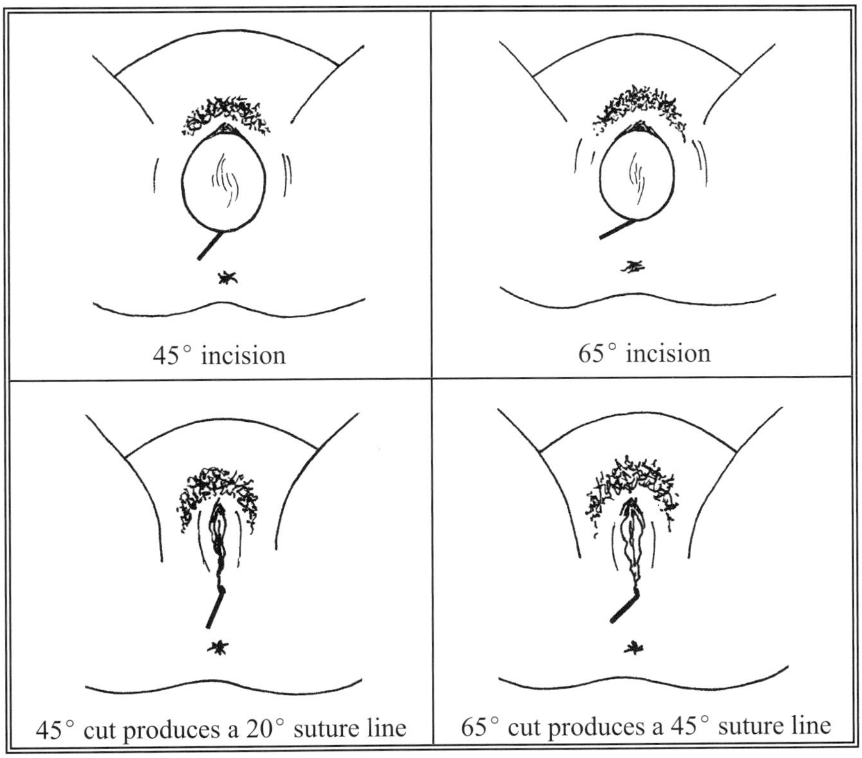

So, the question becomes, if the angle of the incision changes, what angle should be used to define this type of incision: that of the incision itself at the time it is created or that of the resulting suture-line (DeLancey, 2008)? If the incision is to accomplish its goal, it must be made at a wide enough angle to avoid the circumferential parts of the sphincters (although no such cut will always avoid incising the sphincter wing on that side). Thus, in order to create a cut that will result in a suture-line with an angle of 45°, the incision across the fully stretched perineum must be at least 60 to 65° in relation to the perineal midline.

There are also different opinions regarding where the cut should originate. While all the sources I reviewed stated that the joint of the scissor blades should be positioned at the center of the posterior introitus, many drawings that accompany these instructions show the incision originating to one side of the midline. Starting the incision more laterally is not recommended because it will tend to sever even more structures than when it is started in the midline.

Although a mediolateral cut made at a sufficiently lateral angle usually accomplishes the goal of avoiding the main part of the anal sphincter, it also produces more tissue damage as well as a slanted repair that is much more difficult to repair. This incision will cut across the grain of the muscle fibers of the superficial anal sphincter that reach up to blend with those of the bulbocavernosus muscle as well as the puborectalis, facts seldom mentioned in discussions of this type of incision. Sometimes an angled cut extends as far as the thigh muscle (O'Leary & O'Leary, 1965). In spite of these drawbacks, the mediolateral incision is now considered a good alternative because it supposedly spares the anal sphincters when made at an adequately lateral angle.

The problems inherent in the repair of an angled incision make this a questionable choice for midwives unaccustomed to such difficult repairs. In addition, in some studies mediolateral cuts have been associated with poorer pelvic floor function, painful intercourse and more pain in general (Graham & Davies, 2006). DeLancey (2008) pointed out that it has been lauded as protective of the pelvic floor in other studies (Gainey, 1943, 1955; Ranney, 1990), although these studies were done in highly interventive settings on women laboring on their backs, introducing not a few confounding factors. Personally, I have yet to meet a woman who has had a mediolateral clitorotomy with a previous birth who did not suffer from chronic discomfort for at least a year postpartum, frequently winding up with a painful scar for life.

Combination incisions

In the past, some doctors have preferred **"hockey stick"** or **J-shaped clitorotomies**, involving a cut directed straight down and then veering off to the side above the sphincter. Although some European practitioners define this as a mediolateral incision, those that do are in the minority. Theoretically, a J-incision reduces the likelihood of extension into the sphincter and minimizes the excessive damage done by simple mediolateral incisions. It actually offers the worst of both types, frequently extending in both directions and causing long-term postpartum pain (McCutcheon-Rosegg, 1984).

The **Schuchardt incision** (1893) is an angled incision cut deep into one of the posterior yoni sulci and then curved downward and to the side partway around the anus, lateral to the external sphincter. While this incision opens the perineum widely allowing good access for surgical procedures, it cuts through many layers of tissue and is very difficult to repair. None of these combination incisions are recommended for use at the time of birth and have, thankfully, been virtually abandoned by physicians.

Lateral incision

A **lateral incision** involves a nearly horizontal cut that begins at either the 8 or 4 o'clock point (as illustrated in Verspyck et al., 2006). It does not open the introitus very widely, produces profuse bleeding, severs many structures and is very difficult to repair. Needless to say, this is not recommended either (DeLancey, 2008).

Anatomical considerations regarding perineal incisions

While many sources discuss many of the pros and cons of median versus mediolateral incisions, very few focus on the actual structures that are severed with each approach, with the exception of extension into the external anal sphincter. The following chart compares the tissues that may be severed with each technique based on the contemporary understanding of the anatomy of the perineal body.

STRUCTURES DIRECTLY SEVERED DURING CLITOROTOMY	
MIDLINE (WITH NO EXTENSION)	MEDIOLATERAL
Skin and subcutaneous tissue	Skin and subcutaneous tissue
Perineal membrane (narrow midline part; division spreads attached structures)	Perineal membrane (broader lateral banded part; division spreads attached structures)
Superficial transverse perineal m.^	Superficial transverse perineal m.
Bulbocavernosus fibers that cross midline are severed; divides vertical fibers	Bulbocavernosus fascia and m.
	Clitoral bulb (depends on angle* and anatomy)
Urethrovaginal sphincter m.	Urethrovaginal sphincter m. (depends on length)
Perineal sponge	Perineal sponge (depends on angle and anatomy)
	Greater vestibular gland (depends on angle and anatomy)
Puboperinealis m.	Puboperinealis m. (depends on angle and length)
	Puborectalis m. (depends on angle and length)
	Puboanalis m. (depends on angle and length)
Subcutaneous sphincter fibers crossing midline are severed; also divides vertical fibers	Subcutaneous anal sphincter fibers
	Wing of deep anal sphincter (depends on angle, length and anatomy)

^m.=muscle *References to "angle" and "angle and length" pertain to the incision

As you can see, even though a mediolateral cut is intended to result in less damage, it may actually divide a larger number of important perineal structures than a midline incision, although it will generally avoid tearing of the rectal muscosa and will usually preserve the internal anal sphincter.

The two different types of clitorotomies in wide use today have one thing in common: depending upon the angle of the incision, both create damage that is either perpendicular or oblique in relation to the orientation of most of the muscle fibers they sever. Muscles heal best when incisions are made parallel to the direction of their tissue fibers; however, such an incision in the perineal body is not helpful. Because a perineal tear will also sever the muscles perpendicularly or obliquely in relation to the direction of their fibers, the perineal muscle fibers themselves are decussated in the midline because that is the most likely place for a spontaneous tear to occur. Like the crisscrossed threads in fabric, decussation helps stop a tear from extending and thus helps to minimize the impact of any spontaneous damage. This protective feature of the perineal anatomy is undermined when the perineum is cut.

How to cut a clitorotomy

If for any reason you decide an incision is necessary, keep these points in mind:

•Do not cut until you are sure the biparietal diameter is completely beneath the pubic bone and the head is really crowning. If the bony pelvis is too small, a clitorotomy will not help bring the head through the pelvis.

•Do not cut too soon. The perineum should be bulging and the introitus thinned and dilated about 3 cm, with the presenting part right behind it between contractions (not just during contractions). You should expect that the presenting part will emerge during the next two to four contractions (Varney et al., 2004). A premature clitorotomy does not give the tissues a chance to max-imally stretch. Because there is not adequate pressure on the perineum from the presenting part, cutting too soon will be more painful for the mother and will result in more blood loss. It will also be harder to make the incision because the tissue will not be thinned out. Cutting through thicker tissue is likely to result in more extensive muscle damage. On the other hand, cutting too late may result in the tear that you are trying to avoid if the incision is being performed for that reason.

•Do not inject anesthetic in anticipation of needing to do a clitorotomy (exceptions noted in the chapter on "Traditional Female Genital Modifications"). To do so swells the tissue and makes extension more likely. Moreover, Philipson and colleagues (1984) studied 15 mother–baby pairs and found that, when infiltrated into the perineal tissue, local anesthetic reaches maternal plasma in as little as 60 seconds (range: 1 to 12 minutes). Detectable levels also appear in blood samples from the umbilical cord vein at birth. The most consistent correlation with levels involved the length of time between infiltration and birth. Although no drug was detected in neonatal plasma, urinary metabolites of lidocaine were found in neonatal urine up to 48 hours after birth. Even though no signs of lidocaine toxicity were observed in these infants, for women who wish to avoid dosing their fetuses with drugs, this is a serious consideration.

If you wait until the tissue is thinned out sufficiently, the numbing effect of the stretching will eliminate the need for an injection. Besides, most of the time midwives are cutting on the spur of the moment because there is evidence that the baby needs to be born more rapidly. In this setting, the perineum is stretched and time is of the essence. You will not have time to infiltrate the tissue and wait for the anesthetic to take effect. If you are ever in a situation where there is time to inject local anesthetic prior to making the cut, follow the instructions in the chapter entitled "Using Local Anesthetic."

•Have the mother lie down supine with her legs apart. Be sure you have adequate access to her perineum.

•Don sterile gloves. Double-glove your nondominant hand using a nonsterile glove.

•Get your nondominant fingers into place between contractions. Hold your nondominant arm out with your palm toward you and fingers pointed down. Protect the baby by inserting the fingers into the introitus in the midline, between the perineum and the presenting part. It should be almost impossible to insert your fingers into the yoni before making the incision because of pressure from the head, which is why you do it between contractions. If you can insert fingers and scissors easily, you are probably cutting too soon or the presenting part is hung up on the mother's pelvis, in which case widening the perineum will not result in further fetal descent. As you insert your fingers, be sure to push against the posterior yoni wall to smooth out any wrinkles (folds) in the yoni wall that may have formed. Also be sure that fetal scalp or skin is behind your fingers and pressed out of the way. Smoothing the tissues on both sides of your fingers helps minimize the chance of cutting into a fold of tissue, which can either injure the baby's scalp or, if a fold of the yoni wall is severed, can create a buttonhole into the rectal wall. Whenever you cut the perineum, you must check carefully for such damage at the time of yoni inspection and repair (Clark-Collar, 1990).

•Open the scissor blades and insert the blade nearest the perineum into the yoni between your spread fingers. If you are working with scissors that have one blunt, guarded or otherwise specialized blade, place that blade, which is intended to go inside the yoni, between the fingers that are in the yoni. The other blade goes against the perineal skin. Regardless of the angle of the incision you plan to cut, place the joint of the scissor blades at the midline of the posterior fourchette. Be prepared to make the incision as a contraction builds so that the presenting part is pressing against the perineal body. It should be distending the perineum before you cut. Inform the mother of what you are about to do. This warning may prompt her to get the baby out fast. Be prepared to remove the scissors carefully but quickly and put them aside in order to assist the birth if she does.

•Use your nondominant thumb to locate the anal sphincter before you cut; place the tip of your thumb just above the bump of the sphincter.

•Estimate the length of incision needed before making the first cut and adjust the scissors accordingly so that the tip of the external blade is above the sphincter. The length of the cut will double as the introitus stretches (i.e., a 0.27 cm [⅛ inch] cut will open the mouth of the yoni by 0.64 cm [¼ inch]) (Gaskin, 1990). Avoid repeated snipping, as this will leave a more jagged edge. However, it is better to have to extend the incision than to cut too deeply in the first place.

•As you cut, be sure to keep the scissor blades perfectly perpendicular (at right angles) to the plane of the skin surface. This requires a firm grip and a steady hand because healthy tissue will resist the blades. The pressure from the presenting part can easily turn the blades at an angle, especially if the perineum is resisting being cut, as might be the case with tough scar tissue.

•Healthy tissue will be resistant and there may be a slightly gritty feeling as you make the incision.

•**Choose the angle of incision**. If only a little help is needed, cut down the midline.

Varney and associates (2004) recommend the use of mediolateral incisions only when the space needed to get the baby out exceeds the space available between the posterior fourchette and the anterior edge of the anal sphincter muscle.

•**Cutting a midline clitorotomy:** To perform a shallow midline incision, simply snip the center of the perineal skin and yoni mucosa at the 6 o'clock point as the presenting part crowns, making sure you do not deliberately cut into the sphincter. After your initial cut, cut a little further if necessary, taking into account that, once you start cutting, the incision is likely to extend.

Deep cuts that run straight down the perineum involve more complex tissue damage. To minimize this type of damage, it is a common practice to begin by cutting straight down the perineum. If extension is necessary, the scissor tips are directed posteriorly, under-neath the fetal presenting part. The mucosa of the yoni floor is cut (rather than down the perineum) with small bites to avoid cutting too deeply. Theoretically, this redirects any extension of the incision along the mucosa of the yoni rather than down into the perineal body and helps prevent bilateral sulcus tears. To do this, place your nondominant palm down, with your fingers extended into the yoni, spread them wide and then press them down against the yoni floor, placing your finger tips beyond the projected point of extension (i.e., splint the proposed area of incision); then cut along the yoni floor between your fingers. Don't open the scissors blades widely; make a snip, rather than one big chop. Then, reassess the situation (Kolder, 1990; Varney 2004). This technique, however, is not universally supported and some episiotomy scissors are not designed to be used in this manner. I prefer to cut down the perineum rather than back inside, as this seems to produce less deep damage. (I only cut 12 clitorotomies in a little over 500 births [most of these were early in my practice], which may be too few to tell.)

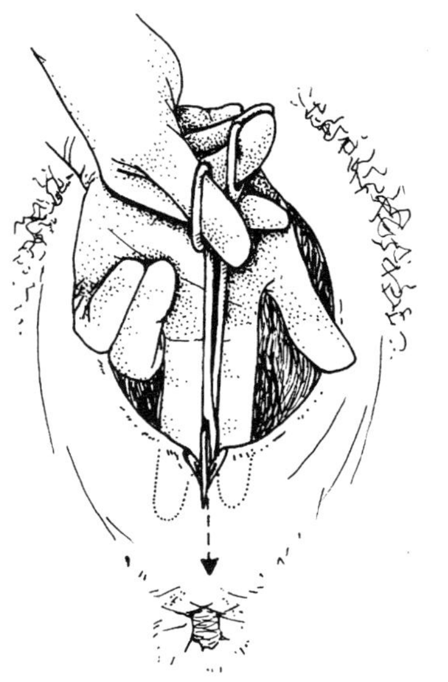

Cutting a midline clitorotomy down the perineum

•**Cutting a mediolateral clitorotomy:** Cut at an angle oblique enough that there is at least 1 cm of tissue between the anal sphincter and the incision. Varney and colleagues (2004) recommend using your nondominant thumb to palpate for the upper edge of the sphincter on the side you will be cutting. DeLancey (2008) recommends an angle of at least 60°. Position the opened joint of the scissor blades in the center of the perineum with the blades directed at the desired angle.

Many authors suggest that the cut be performed on your dominant side: to your left (mother's right) if you are left-handed, and to the your right (mother's left) if you are right-handed. This promotes ease of repair based on handedness, but does not make performing the incision any easier. You can also choose the direction of the incision based on the fetal position, using a cut angled to your right (mother's left) if the baby is LOA, LOP, LSA or RMA and using a cut angled to your left (mother's right) if the baby is ROA, ROP, RSA or LMA. These recommendations are intended to widen and therefore release more tension on the side where the pressure from the descending presenting part is expected to be greatest (i.e., the side of the occiput, the sacrum or the bulk of the head in a face presentation, as the case may be).

- As soon as the incision is completed, leave the scissor blades closed and withdraw them. Hold on to them during the next contraction or place them on a sterile field (an inner wrapper from your surgical gloves will do) in case you need to cut again.
- Withdraw your nondominant hand and have an assistant strip off the top glove, as this glove was used to locate the anal sphincter. Have an assistant ready with a trash receptacle for disposal of this glove.
- After you cut, support beneath the incision to minimize extension.
- If the incision bleeds between contractions, press a dry gauze pad firmly against the incision to prevent excessive blood loss. A cut almost always bleeds more than a tear and an angled cut produces considerably more blood loss than a median cut or tear (Varney et al., 2004).
- If you are cutting because of tough, resistant scar tissue, you may find that, even after making an incision, the perineum does not stretch (or tear for that matter), and you need to lengthen the incision so the baby can be born. If extension is necessary, you will probably have to extend the incision, down the perineum (rather than back along the yoni floor), since that is where the toughest scar tissue will be.

Hymenotomy (HI-men-NOT-toe-me)

The hymenal ring will usually tear during the first term birth. As a rule, this happens easily, but occasionally the tissue is tough and resistant. Some practitioners find that snipping a tough hymen down the center, flush with the yoni wall, will direct the tearing and prevent ragged skin tags with odd, difficult-to-repair deviations. It may also invite a straight tear down the perineum just as a clitorotomy would do. You will have to use your judgment regarding the ethics of cutting prophylactically and the expected helpfulness of a hymenotomy in a particular case. (The two doctors who described this technique to me reported great success at reducing more extensive damage, although the one time I did it the cut did extend slightly.) The hymenal ring itself should not be repaired because it is rich in nerves and will likely be torn again upon

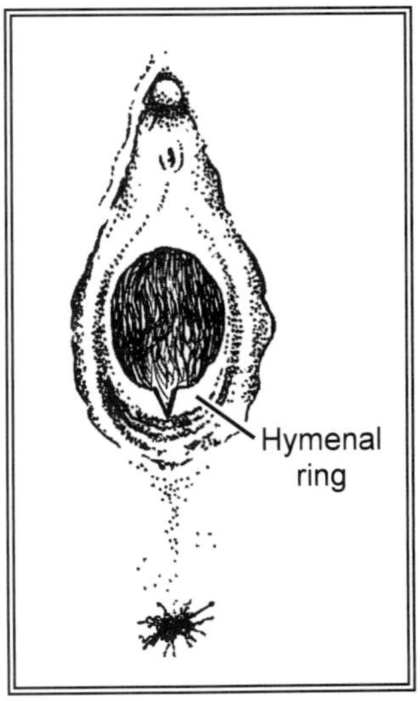

sexual penetration or with the next birth (Kandall, 1990; Kolder, 1990).

Legally Refusing a Medical Intervention

Whether a woman is in your care or someone else's, all women should know the magic—that is, legally binding—phrase to avoid unwanted medical interventions, which is "I refuse to give my consent to __________" or simply "I refuse consent to ________" (fill in the blank). While any other statement can be ignored, practitioners ignore this to their legal peril. Women who wind up in the hospital should know that this is what must be said to stay the hand of any intervening provider and, of course, this phrase can be used wherever care is being provided and must be respected by homebirth practitioners as well.

Female Genital Cosmetic Surgery in Developed Nations

Note: It was difficult to decide in what order to place this chapter. I placed it here because cosmetic surgeries often involve the removal of normal tissues, making it more closely akin to traditional female genital surgeries than to clitorotomy. It should be noted, however, that clitorotomy is often done against a woman's wishes or without her consent or both, while most cosmetic surgeries performed in developed nations are sought out by the woman herself.

The choice to have plastic surgery performed on the genitals and breasts is becoming increasingly common among women in developed nations. Whereas decades ago, upon graduating from high school, well-off young women often got a rhinoplasty ("nose job"), today many young women are also choosing breast augmentation or reduction. This is a worrisome trend because these women have their childbearing years ahead of them and the complications and adverse effects of breast implants can be severe.

Women of various ages are also choosing to have their genitals cosmetically altered with the goal of making them more aesthetically appealing or of enhancing their own or their partner's sexual pleasure. The desire to change normally variant anatomy underscores the continuing need to cultivate a feeling of acceptance and pride in young girls regarding their bodies in all their uniqueness.

Today, genital plastic surgery is as common as other cosmetic procedures, including tummy tucks and breast augmentation. Advocates eagerly point to new advancements and techniques, such as the use of laser devices that typically lessen scarring, pain and recovery time and that are claimed to deliver excellent results. Hype aside, it is important to remember from the detailed review of the delicate and complex pelvic structures in this text, that genital or pelvic surgery is neither simple nor easy. This part of the body is difficult for the most experienced surgeons to restore or enhance, and the likelihood of making a problem worse or having a result fall far short of the goal is a real possibility.

In my opinion, genital surgery should be reserved for cases where it is absolutely necessary for good, medical reasons. The American College of Obstetricians and Gynecologists (ACOG) concurs (2007) and notes that medically indicated surgical procedures may include reversal or repair of female genital cutting and treatment for labial hypertrophy or asymmetrical labial growth secondary to congenital conditions, chronic irritation or excessive androgenic hormones, but that other surgeries have not been proven safe or necessarily even effective and that their long-term sequelae are largely unknown. While choosing a cosmetic procedure does fall into the broad category of female genital mutilation, these are women who are generally of age, freely choosing the procedure, and the procedures are not designed to abnormally narrow the introitus. This makes such surgery a very different practice from crude surgeries designed to narrow the introitus that are performed on young children.

When women still desire genital surgery purely for cosmetic purposes or even when it is needed to correct internal problems, such as prolapse, it would be ideal to wait until after the birth of the their last child so that the repairs are not undone by the stretching of childbirth. There may be some exceptions to this general rule (such as when a condition is greatly debilitating, as would be the case with a large obstetric fistula). A competent urogynecologist can help determine when more immediate surgery is indicated.

Nevertheless, the number of cosmetic procedures on the genitals in each surgical area (labiaplasty, vaginoplasty, and hoodectomy) has been dramatically increasing. In 2005, the American Society of Plastic Surgeons (ASPS) began collecting information on vaginoplasty among their membership (LabiaplastySurgeon.com, 2009). Their data show a growth in these procedures by almost thirty percent (29.9%) since 2006, making it the third most common cosmetic procedure among these practitioners. Moreover, these figures do not include the practitioners that perform the majority of these procedures, which include obstetrician-gynecologists, other cosmetic surgeons and urologists.

Female genital cosmetic surgery (FGCS) is a demanding specialty, and very few surgeons are sufficiently skilled to perform these delicate procedures with good results. Some surgeons, such as urogynecologists and obstetricians, are formally trained in various types of medically indicated female genital surgery. Other practitioners, some of whom are equally competent, especially with cosmetic alternations, are those plastic surgeons, cosmetic surgeons and urologists who have applied themselves to becoming educated and skilled in this specialty. Women should only consider one of these types of surgical specialists who is known to be good at the type of procedure she seeks when having one of these procedures performed.

LabiaplastySurgeon.com was launched around 2003 to address this emerging medical specialty. They offer a roster of physicians from four surgical fields: cosmetic surgeons, obstetrician-gynecologists, urologists and plastic surgeons. The combined knowledge of these practitioners offers women a comprehensive base of information, which they and their partners can use to choose the best surgeon for their needs. According to this web site, they list surgeons from across the country, each of which has been chosen because of their high professional qualifications and credentials in performing such procedures—and their good results. Even so, when choosing a surgeon, I would recommend getting a local referral from a doctor that is known and trusted as well.

This chapter explores different types of genital surgeries that are being sought and what each is intended to do. Any of these surgeries can lead to complications such as infection, adhesions and excessive scarring. Recall that scar tissue is never as flexible or as elastic as undamaged tissue.

Vaginoplasty

The term "vaginoplasty" applies to any surgical procedure intended to treat structural defects of the yoni, to enhance its cosmetic appearance, or to partially or totally construct or reconstruct a yoni. "Vaginoplasty" is a catch-all term used to describe all such surgeries, while the term **neovaginoplasty** refers to procedures involving the partial or total construction or reconstruction of the vulvovaginal complex.

Vaginoplasty involves internal surgery and would almost always be performed under general anesthesia or with the use of spinal anesthesia.

There are several different vaginoplasty techniques. Some involve the use of autologous biological tissue from other parts of the woman's body to construct areas being altered. Tissues may be taken from the oral mucosa, from skin flaps or grafts, from the genital labia, from penile skin or tissue or the scrotal skin (in male-to-female transgender procedures), from the intestinal mucosa and from other parts of the body.

Nonreconstructive vaginoplasty or "vaginal rejuvenation" is usually sought by women who have had multiple childbirths to tighten the tissues and to enhance the sensitivity of the yoni. The restoration of genital tone and appearance is accomplished primarily by removing excess tissue and tightening supportive structures.

The term "designer vagina" refers to an idealized image of female sex organs, which cosmetic surgery strives to achieve. ACOG (2007) warns that this procedure lacks supporting data regarding safety and efficacy. Vaginal rejuvenation surgery can lead to decreased sensory perception in the clitoral glans and over the rest of the genital area, potentially so much so that orgasm can no longer be achieved.

The term "vaginoplasty" has also been applied to several other procedures as well. These are as follows:

- **Hoodectomy:** This technique is the closest female equivalent to male circumcision. Here the clitoral hood is reduced or removed to expose, and thus theoretically heighten sensation in, the clitoral glans.
- **Hymenotomy:** This procedure is a medically necessary surgery wherein an opening is created in a congenitally imperforate hymen to allow for the menses to escape, for sexual penetration and for childbirth.
- **Hymenorrhaphy:** This practice is the medically unnecessary surgical restoration of a ruptured hymen to a "virginal" state.
- **G-spot amplification:** This dubious practice involves injecting collagen into the anterior wall of the yoni in the general region of the G-spot for the purpose of making this area more responsive to stimulation.

Labioplasty

"Labioplasty" refers to the surgical alteration of the labia minora, the labia majora or both. Labioplasty is most often chosen by women who perceive their labia minora as unattractive, usually because they are "too large" (that is, they project beyond the borders of the labia majora) or are irregularly shaped. As recently as 1999, surgeons usually performed labial reduction by simply amputating the protuberant parts and then suturing the edges together. However, this procedure sometimes created a fragile and stiff line of scar tissue as well as eliminating the natural contour and pigmentation of the labia minora. Moreover, other procedural and clinical problems accompany amputation and reduce the likelihood of a favorable outcome. Several years later, surgeons began to use laser surgery and more refined surgical procedures, such as inferior wedge resection and superior pedicle flap reconstruction, techniques associated with fewer complications in the hands of skilled practitioners.

Labioplasty is almost always an outpatient procedure performed under either a local or short-acting general anesthetic. After surgery, women may experience some mild discomfort and a variable amount of swelling, both of which are usually almost resolved after one to two weeks. Recovery times are said to range between three days to two weeks.

Pregnancy and childbirth after female genital cosmetic surgery

Examine the regions that have been repaired and note their appearance in your chart. From 36 weeks until birth, have the woman help her tissues stretch by applying evening primrose, black currant or borage oil to the surgically altered tissues. Regular yoni stretching is also important for these women.

At the time of birth, you can apply more warm oil or straight evening primrose, borage or black currant oil to the tissues to assist with stretching. After the birth, carefully examine the tissues to see what if any damage has occurred.

TRADITIONAL FEMALE GENITAL MODIFICATIONS

Note: Clitorotomy is the predominant form of FGM/C practiced in developed countries today. It is covered in the chapter entitled "Clitorotomy ('Episiotomy')."

This chapter focuses on traditionally dictated cultural practices that permanently alter the female genitals, most of which involve some degree of amputation. These practices are widely regarded as forms of mutilation among nonpracticing cultures. The guiding principles for defining a practice as mutilation include recognizing it as a form of violence against women, as a violation of basic human rights such as the right to health, the rights of children, the right to physical integrity and the right to nondiscrimination on the basis of sex. While the right to culture is also recognized, when a practice conflicts with other, more basic rights, such as the right to physical integrity, the individual rights are considered more fundamental.

International Definitions

In a joint statement, the World Health Organization (WHO), the United Nations Children's Fund (UNICEF) and the United Nations Population Fund (UNFPA) have defined female genital mutilation (FGM) or cutting (FGM/C) as any procedure involving the partial or total removal of the external female genitalia or other injury to the female genital organs for cultural or other nonmedical reasons (Arbour et al., 2008). This is a broad definition, and some things practiced by consenting adults, such as piercing or shaving, fall under its umbrella. By far, however, the most serious practices involve the nonconsensual removal or permanent alteration of the tissues of minor children because these structures can never be restored and their removal typically involves severe physical and emotional trauma followed by acute and chronic health complications.

Terminology

Naming these practices has been a topic of ongoing debate. Health departments, local governments, and the World Health Organization have all been aware of these practices for decades. Efforts to stop FGM/C have been ongoing since the 1940s and escalated dramatically in the 1990s. Local women's groups and midwives in the countries where these practices are prevalent are now campaigning to eliminate them, but there is still much work to do. Thus "mutilation" has been used in most official documents because tissues are removed for no medical reason, as a matter of custom. "Mutilation" accurately describes that these practices permanently alter normal tissues, frequently in ways that pose serious short- and long-term risks. It is considered the best term to use when addressing policymakers.

"Female circumcision" incites less controversy, but it also whitewashes what is really being done, particularly in the United States where "circumcision" is used to refer to male genital mutilation in the form of foreskin removal for cultural reasons, a practice that is still quite prevalent. (In many respects, the "benefits" and "reasons" for male circumcision parallel those put forth to support FGM/C.) The term "excision" is also less offensive and accurately describes those practices that involve removal of tissues. Many foreign terms translate as "female genital cutting," a relatively neutral term that still describes what has been done.

Regardless of which term you prefer, it is always most respectful to find out how each woman from affected communities refers to the practice and use that terminology when you converse with her and her family. Referring to these practices as "mutilation" is not welcomed by most women who have experienced one of these procedures or chosen it for their daughters. Let us remember that Western parents who have chosen male circumcision for their infant sons do not believe they have mutilated or abused him and feel they have acted in his best interest. They are often quite unaware that they have amputated the most sensitive part of his penis and of the negative health consequences of this practice. Likewise, women usually find the term "mutilation" insulting, having never viewed themselves or other women in their communities as mutilated. You must also remember that this practice and its consequences are cultural norms to her and the differences and benefits of not being "done" are likely to be unknown to her (although if she is coming to you in a Western clinical setting, she may be aware that it is not a cultural norm in her new community and be apprehensive as a result).

Types of FGM/C

There are several types and severities of FGM/C. This table introduces and defines the primary categories that these practices fall into:

TYPES OF FEMALE GENITAL MUTILATION (PARTIAL LIST) (ADAPTED FROM HUSTON, 2000)				
PARTS AFFECTED	TISSUES REMOVED & OTHER ASPECTS OF THE PROCEDURE	TERMINOLOGY		WHO TYPE
		COLLOQUIAL	MEDICAL	
Clitoral hood	Hood only	Circumcision	Circumcision, hoodectomy	I
Clitoral glans	Prick or cut glans (no tissue removed)	Sunna	Incision	IV
	Tip of glans	Sunna or Sunna kashfi	Subtotal clitoridectomy	I
	Entire glans	Sunna	Clitoridectomy	I
Clitoral glans, labia minora	Entire glans; scraping of the labia minora, often causing them to fuse during healing	Sunna or Sunna magatia	Clitoridectomy and abrasion of labia minora resulting in labial fusion	IIb
	Glans and labia minora	Excision	Subtotal vulvectomy	IIb
Clitoral glans, labia minora and/or labia majora	Glans, labia minora and often the upper two-thirds of labia majora; raw edges are sutured	Intermediate infibulation	Subtotal vulvectomy and infibulation	IIIb
	As above plus remove entire length of the labia majora with suturing of raw edges	Pharaonic circumcision	Vulvectomy and infibulation	IIIb

Details regarding the four-type, WHO classification system begins on page 267.

Cultural Contexts for the Practice of FGM/C

Origins

The origins of FGM/C are unknown. A variety of theories exist, including that it started in ancient Egypt as a mark of distinction among royalty; mummies have been found with evidence of infibulation. Other theories suggest that it started when black slave women entered ancient Arab societies, or that FGM/C began with the arrival of Islam in some parts of sub-Saharan Africa. Clitoridectomy is believed to have begun in Africa and to have been incorporated as an Islamic cultural practice at the conquest of Egypt in 742 AD. Other evidence points to origins among the Greeks, Romans and Tsarist Russians. Still others think it started in sub-Saharan Africa, before the arrival of Islam, notably among warrior peoples, often as a part of puberty rites. To this day, no one knows for sure how it started or for what reasons.

Regions where FGM/C is currently practiced

In industrialized countries, involuntary FGM/C has primarily taken the form of cutting the routine clitorotomy (WHO classification Type IV). Many other types of FGM/C take a much more severe form as genital structures are removed. In the West until the mid-twentieth century, clitoridectomies (Type I) were carried out to treat a host of "female problems" including masturbation, lesbianism, hysteria and clitoral enlargement (Sheehan, 1981). In addition, a variety of genital cosmetic surgeries, including female circumcision (hoodectomy), have been performed more recently in the West to enhance appearance as well as heighten sexual stimulation (see the chapter entitled "Female Genital Cosmetic Surgery in Developed Nations").

In the developing world, some form of FGM/C is still practiced in 27 countries of Africa and the Middle East. WHO (Arbour et al., 2008) estimates that 100 to 140 million girls and women have already had some form of FGM/C and more than 3 million girls are at risk of being subjected to some type of FGM/C every year (that amounts to almost 6 girls per minute). Slow progress toward eliminating these practices is evident in that older girls and young women in these regions are less likely than older women to have had FGM/C.

Prevalence varies significantly across and within countries. FGM/C is practiced most widely in Africa, but different types of alterations are practiced in other countries as well, although there are as yet no national estimates as to prevalence. Among these ethnic groups are the Daudi Bohra Muslims of northwest India and the Kurdish women of northern Iraq. The list of countries includes Indonesia, Iraq, Israel, Malaysia, Pakistan, Oman, southern Saudi Arabia, Yemen and parts of southeast Asia. In some of these countries, incidence varies greatly depending upon social class. There are also anecdotal reports of FGM/C occurring in several other countries as well, including Colombia, the Democratic Republic of Congo, Peru and Sri Lanka. Countries in which FGM/C is practiced only by migrant populations are not included in the following table (Arbour et al., 2008).

By the year 2000, as many as 228,000 women and girls who had immigrated to the United States had either had FGM/C or were at risk for the practice due to the eagerness of parents to preserve cultural cohesion for their daughters. Twenty-seven percent of those at risk were under 18 years of age, a number that rose by 35% from 1999. Almost 63% of affected women reside in only seven states: California, Maryland, Minnesota, New Jersey, New York, Texas and Virginia. Forty-five percent of these women reside in large metropolitan areas including metropolitan New York City, Washington DC, Baltimore MD, San Francisco, Oakland, San Jose and the Los Angeles-Riverside-Orange County region in California, and St. Paul, MN. Immigrants from Somalia, Sudan, Ethiopia, and other countries have been known to mutilate their small baby girls before entering other countries. Others may arrange through an underground network to have a nonmedical FGM/C performed on their child after they arrive. Others send their daughters back to their native country to have it done.

FGM/C AMONG WOMEN AND GIRLS AGED 15 TO 49					
COUNTRY	PREVALENCE	COMMON TYPES	COUNTRY	PREVALENCE	COMMON TYPES
Benin	13% (2006)•	II	Liberia^	45%	II
Burkina Faso	73% (2006)	II	Mali	91.6% (2001)	I-52%, II-47%
Cameroon	1% (2004)	I & II	Mauritania	71.3% (2001)	I & II
Central African Republic	26% (2005)	1 & II	Niger	2.2% (2006)	II
Chad	44.9% (2004)	II (III in east)	Nigeria	19% (2003)	I & II
Côte d'lvoire	36% (2006)	II	Senegal	28.2% (2005)	II
Djibouti	93.1% (2006)	II & III	Sierra Leone	94% (2006)	II
Egypt*	95.8% (2005)	I-17%; II- 72%; III-9%	Somalia	97.9% (2006)	III
Eritrea	88.7% (2002)	1-64%; II-4%; III-34%	Sudan (northern)*	90% (2000)	1-15%, II-3%, III-82%
Ethiopia	74.3% (2005)	I & II (III border of Sudan & Somalia)	Tanzania, United Republic of	15% (2004-2005)	II & III
Gambia, the	78% (2005-2006)	I & II	Togo	5.8% (2006)	II
Ghana	3.8% (2006)	II	Uganda	0.6% (2006)	1 & II
Guinea	95.6% (2005)	II	Yemen*	22.6% (1997)	
Guinea-Bissau	45% (2006)	I & II	Zambia	1% (2005)	
Kenya	32.2% (2003)	I & II			

•Year data was gathered (when available). *This sample excluded women who had never been married.
^Estimate derived from a variety of local and sub-national studies
(Chart derived from www.childinfo.org/fgmc_tables.php, accessed Aug 25, 2008 and Arbour et al., 2008.)

There is no similar data for Canada, but there are numerous immigrants and refugees residing in Canada that come from regions where FGM/C is practiced. Affected women and at-risk girl children are also living in Australia, New Zealand, France, the United Kingdom and anywhere else where they may travel or immigrate; it is truly an international health care concern as well as a human rights and women's rights issue.

Reasons given for the practice of FGM/C

FGM/C is a male-dictated practice perpetrated by a girl's female relatives. In practicing societies, FGM/C is a manifestation of sex inequality that is deeply entrenched in social, economic and political structures. Like the now-abandoned foot-binding in China and the practice of child marriage, FGM/C represents society's control over women and perpetuates sex roles that are unequal and that harm women. Societies that practice FGM/C are predominantly patriarchal and patrilineal. There is a close link between women's ability to exercise control over their own lives and their belief that the practice should be ended (UNICEF, 2005b).

Where it is widely practiced, it is supported by both men and women, usually without question. Anyone departing from the norm may face condemnation, harassment and ostracism. These punishments are a powerful force and make it very difficult for families to abandon the practice without support from the wider community. Thus, the practices often continue even after their harmfulness is understood because the perceived social benefits are deemed to outweigh the risks (UNICEF, 2005a). When mothers refuse these practices for their daughters, frequently the girls' grandmothers see to it that it is done.

More specific reasons for these practices fall into five broad categories. One or more of the reasons listed may be subscribed to by a specific cultural group.

Psychosexual: Women generally request and perform FGM/C for their daughters because these practices ensure the only culturally acceptable life choice for women: marriage. (Intact Sudanese women are automatically considered prostitutes.) FGM/C reduces or eliminates the sensitive tissues of the outer genitalia, particularly the more superficial parts of the clitoris. Some cultures, recognizing the central importance of the clitoris to female sexual desire, seek to remove it as a means of protecting her from her own sexual nature and save her from temptation and disgrace while preserving her virtue. Excision is also thought to enhance fertility. Many believe that, unless cut off, the clitoris will continue to grow and encourage the girl to become sexually active before marriage. Cultures often believe that FGM/C helps girls mature into women and become full members of the human race.

In these strongly patriarchal cultures, female virginity is an absolute prerequisite to marriage. A virgin bride means that succession rights and inheritance of property cannot be questioned. A small neointroitus demands a higher bride price. Frequently, women are inspected by the man's relatives before they will agree to marriage.

In Egypt and Sudan, female circumcision is thought to increase a man's sexual pleasure during intercourse. Some African tribes believe that the clitoris is the remnant of maleness in women, and the penile foreskin is a remnant of femaleness in men; before a man and woman can come together in marriage, these remnants should be removed.

Some communities attribute awesome powers to female sexuality, holding that a woman's genitalia may blind her birth attendant; that it can cause physical deformity, madness or the death of her infant; or that the clitoris can sting or poison her husband and cause his death.

Sociological: Many cultures use FGM/C as a means of identification with their past ("the ancestors decreed it"), to initiate girls into womanhood and to foster social integration and cohesion. Accompanying ceremonies may be intended to teach the girl her duties as a wife and mother. Traditional practices usually include subjecting girls to powerful social pressure from their peers and family members to undergo the procedure. They are threatened with rejection by the group or their family if they do not follow tradition.

Hygiene and aesthetics: The external genitalia, especially the clitoris, may be considered dirty, unsightly or too large. Removal of these parts is viewed as a sign of maturity, to promote hygiene and to enhance aesthetic appeal. It is believed that FGM/C maintains a woman's physical and mental health.

Religious: FGM/C is primarily a cultural practice that is not mandated by any religion, although it is practiced as such by some fundamentalist groups, including certain groups of Muslims, Falasha Jews of Ethiopia (now living in Israel), some Christian sects (including Catholic, Protestant and Coptic), animists and the followers of many indigenous religions as well as nonbelievers in a variety of regions. Probably the most well-known of these groups is the Muslims. Although many Muslim communities that practice FGM/C do so in the firm belief that it is rooted in Islam, it is not mentioned in the Quŕan or the Hadith, the two primary sacred Islamic texts, and it is not practiced in most Islamic countries. The word "Sunna" is used to describe several forms of FGM/C. This Arabic term is used in Islam and refers to a habitual or customary traditional practice. By applying this term to FGM/C practices, the users incorrectly imply Islamic approval of these practices.

Age when FGM/C is traditionally performed

The age when FGM/C is performed has diverse regional variations, ranging from days-old infants to adolescent girls to adult women, some of whom were not "done" as children who are now requesting the procedure. The traditional practice is usually a component of an initiation into womanhood and is always accompanied by peer pressure.

In most cultures, these operations have traditionally been performed on prepubescent girls. As of this writing, they are being done on much younger children because fathers fear resistance once their daughters enter school, where they may be exposed to Western ideas that condemn the practice. Since the father fears losing the bride price if his daughters aren't "done," he may arrange to have them altered at an earlier age than is traditional in the community. As a result, one of the stated purposes, introduction to adult life, is disappearing. As is true in the West regarding male circumcision, many educated families that have abandoned other traditional and religiously dictated customs may still adhere to FGM/C. The table below, although derived from older data (Shandall et al., 1967) offers an idea of traditional timing.

Age	Country, Region or Tribe (Type When Available)
8 days	Abyssinia
3-6 years	Somaliland (I & II)
5-10 years	Sudan
6-10 years	Egypt
7-10 years	Somaliland (III)
12-13 years	Most other African countries
14-15 years	Introcision–Australia (IV), Bantu peoples–Africa (II & III) ancient Egyptians (II & III)
15+ years	Masai (shortly after marriage), Swahili, Guinea (infibulate after childbirth)

The traditional practice of FGM/C

FGM/C is usually performed by traditional practitioners, generally elderly women specially designated for this task or by traditional midwives who perform FGM/C as a way of making additional money. The role of circumciser elevates a woman's status in her community and assures her a steady income; thus, she has a vested interest in seeing the practice continue.

In many traditional village settings, several girls may participate in an elaborate ceremony during which they receive attention from their relatives and many gifts, although in some Somali groups, no ceremony accompanies the procedure (Hosken, 1993). Typically the girls anticipate a momentous event but usually have no idea what is in store for them. At some point, the girls may be lined up and excised or taken from the group and excised one by one. Pharmaceutical anesthesia is rarely used, although some practitioners attempt to mitigate the pain by such practices as drugging the girl with herbs or alcohol or pouring cold water over the genitals prior to operating. It is frequently a crude procedure performed on struggling, screaming children held down by force in dark huts. The girls are admonished to keep what has been done a secret. Because each community has its own approach regarding the ritual involved and each practitioner varies as to exactly how she alters the anatomy, there are many subtle differences from group to group, and this chapter can only give you a general idea of what to expect.

The instruments used range from single-edged razor blades to broken pieces of glass, knives, stones or fingernails. Instruments may be dull, old or rusty and are often not washed between procedures. Bleeding is staunched and the wound is closed with either catgut or silk suture, thorns or adhesive substances such as homemade herbal poultices, sugar, egg, warm oil, acacia tar, dough, soil or animal dung. Once the bleeding has stopped or the edges of the wound has been approximated by one or more of these means, the girl's movements are often severely restricted until healing takes place.

In urban settings, practices vary according to practitioner. In some countries, health professionals, including Western-trained midwives and physicians, are increasingly performing FGM/C. By 1995, 13% of Egyptian women reported having been circumcised by a doctor. In the same year, 46% of their recently circumcised daughters had been circumcised by a doctor.

Participating health professionals believe that performing FGM/C as a medical procedure with sterile instruments and local anesthesia reduces the pain and physical risks, which is undeniably true. Nevertheless, when resources are limited, care may be as basic as washing the genitals with soap and water or antiseptic and sprinkling penicillin powder on the wound afterwards. They believe medicalization is the first step toward eliminating the practice, and that if they refuse, the family will simply have it performed in the traditional manner. Opponents contend that medicalization only legitimates the practice.

The legal status of FGM/C

Numerous international human rights and health-related organizations have condemned FGM/C as harmful in many ways, and women's rights organizations have become increasingly vocal in their condemnation of these practices. Slowly, countries where FGM/C is prevalent have passed laws prohibiting it, although there are still many regions where traditional FGM/C is practiced that have no such laws. In some places, existing laws would cover the practice, were they enforced. More and more governments in Africa and elsewhere, however, are taking steps to eliminate FGM/C. As of January 2008, 16 African nations had laws banning FGM/C (the date in parentheses indicates the year the law was enacted): Benin (2003), Burkina Faso (1996), Central African Republic (1966), Chad (2003), Côte d'Ivoire (1998), Djibouti (1994), Egypt (Ministerial Decree, 1996, 2007), Eritrea (2007), Ethiopia (2004), Ghana (1994), Guinea (1965, 2000), Kenya (2001), Niger (2003), Senegal (1999), South Africa (2005), Tanzania (1998), Togo (1998) and several states in Nigeria (1999-2000).

Penalties are usually levied against practitioners but may apply to parents and sometimes to both. Sentences may range from a minimum of six months to a maximum of life in prison. Several countries also impose monetary fines. Most have instituted educational and outreach programs to discourage the practice and the use of civil remedies and administrative regulations to prevent it. There have been reports of prosecutions or arrests in cases involving FGM/C in several African countries, including Burkina Faso, Egypt, Ghana, Senegal and Sierra Leone. Nevertheless, where the practice is entrenched, families often find ways to have it done regardless, and in many places the laws against it are not rigorously enforced. In addition, civil unrest and outright war, when and where it occurs, interferes with efforts to eliminate it; communities tend to revert to traditional practices under such circumstances.

In the United States, a federal law criminalizing the practice went into effect in April 1997. The US law makes the practice of FGM/C on a girl under the age of 18 a federal crime, unless the procedure is necessary to protect her health or for medical purposes connected with childbirth. The penalty for violating this law is a fine or imprisonment for up to five years or both. This law specifically exempts cultural beliefs or practices as a defense for conducting FGM/C. Between 1998 and 2006, 16 US states passed their own criminal statutes against FGM/C, all of which vary slightly. They are California, Colorado, Delaware, Illinois, Maryland, Minnesota, Missouri, Nevada, New York, North Dakota, Oregon, Rhode Island, Tennessee, Texas, West Virginia and Wisconsin.

In addition to passing the federal law in 1996, Congress directed the Department of Health and Human Services to determine the populations at risk and to carry out educational outreach to affected communities and medical students. That same year, the Immigration and Naturalization Service (INS) was directed to provide information to immigrants and refugees entering the US from countries where FGM/C is practiced about the adverse health risks and legal consequences of performing the procedure in the United States. Finally in 1997, Congress passed a law requiring US executive directors of international financial institutions to oppose nonhumanitarian loans to countries where FGM/C is practiced and whose governments have not implemented educational programs to prevent it.

Eleven other developed nations that also receive immigrants from regions where FGM/C is practiced have taken similar legal and educational measures. These include Australia (Australian Capital Territory, Northern Territory, New South Wales, South Australia, Tasmania and Victoria [6 of 8 states], 1994-1997), Belgium (2000), Canada (1997), Cyprus (2003), Denmark (2003), Italy (2005), New Zealand (1995), Norway (1995), Spain (2003), Sweden (1982, 1998) and the United Kingdom (1985). France has relied on existing criminal legislation to prosecute both practitioners of FGM/C and parents procuring the service for their daughters. For many more details on legal issues, see the excellent book entitled FEMALE GENITAL MUTILATION: A GUIDE TO LAWS AND POLICIES WORLDWIDE (Rahman & Toubia, 2000) (Reproductive Rights Org., 2008; Womenshealth.gov, 2008).

WHO Categories of Different Forms of FGM/C

Since the 1990s, FGM/C practices have been organized into four broad categories based on the type and extent of the tissues that are affected. The World Health Organization (WHO) (Arbour et al., 2008) has proposed a few subdivisions to allow more specific reference to various practices, but they are not all inclusive because of the many variations of FGM/C practices that exist. Although these definitions are precise, it must be remembered that most of the time this is a very imprecise procedure and more or less of the tissue may be removed than is described here.

Type I (clitoridectomy)

This is defined as partial or total removal of the clitoral glans, the clitoral hood, or both and is often referred to as "clitoridectomy." To distinguish between the major variations of type I, WHO (Arbour et al., 2008) suggests the following subdivisions:

Type Ia: Removal of the clitoral hood only (hoodectomy)

Type Ib: Removal of both the clitoral glans and the hood

Typically the clitoral glans and often a portion of the clitoral body, is grasped between the thumb and index finger, pulled up and away from the pubis and amputated with one stroke of a sharp object. Bleeding is usually stopped by packing the wound with gauze or other substances (such as herbs) and applying a pressure bandage. Western-trained practitioners may ligate the clitoral artery with one or two stitches to stop bleeding.

Although Type Ia is commonly described as removal of the clitoral hood alone, this has not been documented as a traditional practice by most authors, although Shandall and colleagues (1967) list it as such. In some countries, medicalized FGM/C consists of removal of only the hood (Ia) (Thabet & Thabet, 2003), but this appears to be relatively rare (Satti et al., 2006).

Almost all known forms of traditional FGM/C that remove tissue from the clitoral region also cut away some or all of the clitoral glans itself. When type I includes removal of the clitoral glans, sexual sensitivity may be reduced more than in type III when the clitoral glans is left intact beneath the infibulation (Nour et al., 2006). Healing often results in a smooth scar, which can easily be missed during a visual inspection if you are not alert. A variation of type I involves removing only a small part of the clitoral glans. This is referred to as **khifadh circumcision**, and it is done in some Arabic countries and in Egypt.

Type II (excision)

Apart from routine clitorotomy (IV), Type II is the most common form of FGM/C and is estimated to comprise about 80% of all procedures. It is rarely seen in developed countries because those that practice it are typically less well-off, from lower social classes, and not as likely to move from their country of origin. Type II is defined as partial or total removal of the clitoral glans and the labia minora, with or without excision of the labia majora. This is often referred to as "excision," although among French-speaking cultures, the term "excision" is used to refer to all types of FGM/C. To distinguish between the major variations of type II, WHO (Arbour et al., 2008) proposes the following subdivisions:

Type IIa: Removal of the labia minora only

Type IIb: Partial or total removal of the clitoral glans and the labia minora

Type IIc: Partial or total removal of the clitoral glans, the labia minora and the labia majora

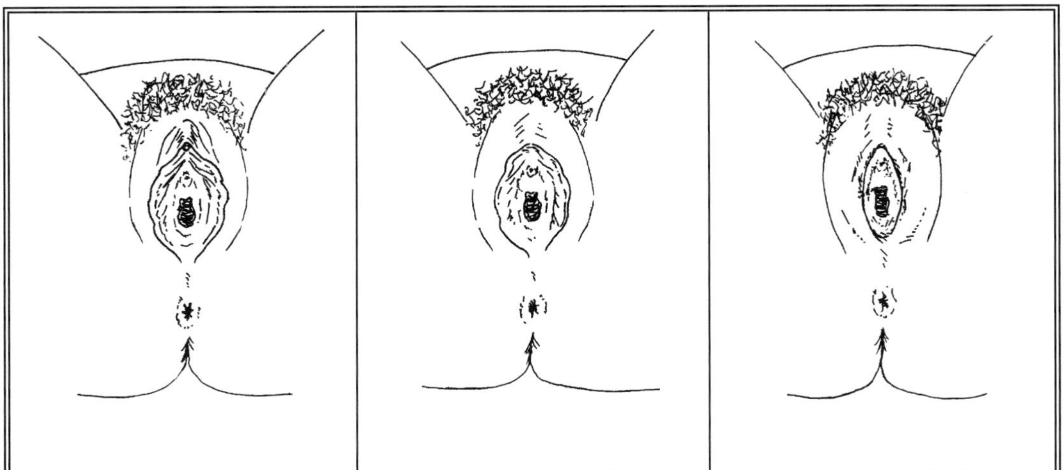

Normal genitalia | Type Ib: Removal of glans and hood | Type IIb: Removal of glans, hood and labia minora

The degree of cutting varies considerably in type II. Commonly the clitoris is grasped as for type I along with the labia minora and both are cut off, often with one stroke. Sometimes, tissue from the labia majora is also removed, and in other cases only the labia minora are cut away, without removal of the clitoral glans. Bleeding is stopped with packing and bandages or by a few circular stitches that may or may not cover the urethra and part of the introitus.

Although no stitching is performed to bring the sides of the two labial stubs together, the raw labial tissues often adhere to each other as they heal, a process known as "sealing." In some parts of Africa, such fusion is accidental; in other areas, it is encouraged. The healed scar does not obstruct the urethra in most cases. However, when the adhesions result in closure of the introitus, the scar mimics a partial infibulation, posing risks similar to those of type III FGM/C and should therefore be categorized as such. What appears to be type II is sometimes a type III procedure that has been defibulated.

Type III (infibulation)

Type III, sometimes called "pharaonic circumcision," is performed in 15 to 20% of all cases of FGM/C. In type III–practicing countries such as Djibouti, Somalia and northern Sudan, the proportion is 80 to 90% across all social classes. Infibulation is practiced on a smaller scale in southern Egypt, Eritrea, Ethiopia, the Gambia, Kenya and Mali, and may also take place in other communities, although the incidence is not known because information is lacking or is still incomplete.

Type III consists of infibulation, a term that derives from the Latin meaning "to clasp or pin." It involves narrowing the introitus by creating a covering seal of scar tissue produced by cutting away the labia minora, the labia majora or both and then joining the remaining edges. New studies have found significant variations in type III, in particular certain cultures make a major distinction between infibulation of the labia minora and of the labia majora (Satti et al., 2006). The most extreme form involves the complete removal of the superficial clitoral structures and the labia minora, together with the inner surface of the labia majora.

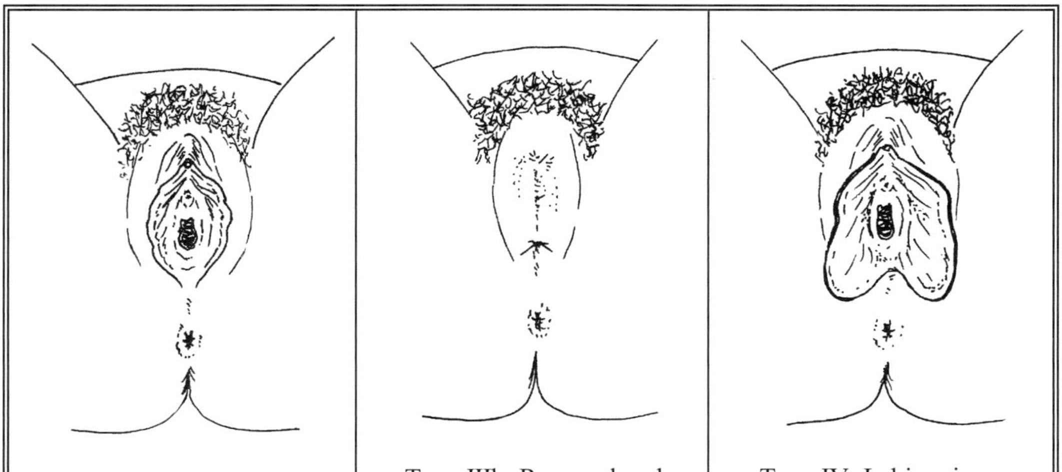

Normal genitalia | Type IIIb: Removal and apposition of labia majora | Type IV: Labia minora elongated

Type III is often, but not invariably, accompanied by partial or total removal of the clitoral glans. Thus, some women retain some (or all) intact clitoral structures or labia minora or both under their covering scar; a very important thing to keep in mind if you are performing a defibulation.

After the tissues are removed, the raw edges of the labia are approximated using one of a variety of techniques such as the application of the adhesive substances mentioned above, the use of suture or thorns to hold the sides together, or both. A small opening is left, often near the posterior end at the level of the introitus to allow the flow of urine and menstrual blood. To prevent closure during healing, the small opening is maintained by placing an object, often a bamboo stick, between the raw edges of tissue. The girl's thighs, knees and ankles are then tied together for two to six weeks while food and fluids are restricted to minimize excretory functions. Typically, bandages are not changed or removed to clean away excrement.

To distinguish between variations in infibulations, WHO (Arbour et al., 2008) suggests the following subdivisions:

Type IIIa: Removal and apposition of the labia minora

Type IIIb: Removal and apposition of the labia majora

The key characteristic of type III is intentional approximation and adhesion of the cut edges of the tissues that are removed, resulting in a functional narrowing of the introitus. Healing results in a tight hood of skin that covers the clitoral area, the urethra and part or most of the introitus, acting as a physical barrier to intercourse. The remaining opening is surrounded by skin and scar tissue and is usually 2 to 3 cm in diameter, but may be as small as the head of a matchstick. Repeated FGM/C appears to be quite frequent among those who practice Type III, usually due to defective healing that resulted in a perforated scar.

In most cases, the introitus itself is not actually narrowed or stitched. One exception is the Western practice of repairing a clitorotomy with a "husband's stitch" or "lover's knot," wherein an extra stitch is placed in the posterior midline of the introitus to "restore virginal tightness." This practice constitutes a very minor, Western variation of infibulation that is fortunately performed far less often than it once was.

If the healed opening is large enough, sexual intercourse can take place after gradual dilation, which may take weeks, months or, in some cases, as long as two years. If the opening is too small to allow for dilation to begin, recutting (defibulation) before intercourse is traditionally undertaken by the husband or one of his female relatives using a sharp knife or a piece of glass. Modern couples may seek the assistance of a Western-trained health care provider for this procedure, although such help is usually sought in secrecy, possibly because it might undermine the social image of the man's virility.

In almost all cases of infibulation, however, and in many cases of sealing after a Type II procedure, defibulation (anterior division of the healed labial scar) must be performed before or during childbirth to allow for birth without tearing the surrounding scar tissue.

Reinfibulation is also a type III procedure to reclose the tissues. It is usually done after a childbirth during which defibulation was necessary. Reclosure is also reportedly done on other occasions. The degree to which the tissues are reclosed varies. If the intention is to recreate a "virginal" appearance, it is often necessary not only to close what has been opened but also to perform further cutting to create fresh raw edges to tighten up the scar. Recent studies have reported that, in some cases, women who were not infibulated prior to childbirth had sutures placed that reduced the size of their introitus after birth. WHO guidelines recommend permanent defibulation to avoid future complications, including suturing the raw edges separately to create a permanent opening and to prevent the formation of adhesions (WHO, 2001a, 2001b).

Type IV (otherwise uncategorized practices)

Type IV includes all other harmful, or potentially harmful, practices that are traditionally performed on the genitalia of girls and women for nonmedical purposes. Most of these practices are less well known and studied than Types I, II and III.

Pricking or **piercing** involves penetrating the genital skin with a sharp object; blood may be let, but no tissue is removed. This has been recommended in some settings in developing regions as a harm-reducing practice to replace more severe forms of FGM/C (Yoder & Mahy, 2001; Njue & Askew, 2004). In developed nations, genital piercing is a type of cosmetic procedure sought by some adult women who then wear jewelry through the healed tract. The jewelry can produce sexually stimulating friction. Tattoos are a variation on genital pricking and are also sought after as a form of body art by some women in developed countries. For details on these practices in developed countries, see the chapter entitled "Intimate Piercings and Tattoos."

Debate as to whether pricking or piercing should be included as a type of FGM/C has been ongoing, both because it is difficult to confirm when it leaves no permanent marks and because it is considered significantly less harmful than most other practices. Others feel that it should be defined as FGM/C to promote documentation of changes from more severe practices and to ensure that it is not used to cover up more extensive procedures. Some women who believe they have undergone pricking have been found to have undergone a wide variety of other procedures, ranging from type I to type III.

Stretching or **elongation** of the clitoral glans, the labia minora or both has been documented in some areas, especially in southern Africa. Generally, prepubescent girls are taught how to stretch their labia over a period of months using products such as oils and herbs. Some cultures elongate the parts even more after giving birth. The elongated labia are intended to enclose the yoni and to enhance both female and male sexual pleasure. Pain and laceration during stretching have been documented, but no long-term consequences are known. The practice has been found mainly in matrilineal societies where women enjoy a relatively high social status. Labial stretching is a form of FGM/C in the sense that there is social pressure on young girls to modify their genitalia and that it produces permanent genital changes (Bagnol & Mariano, 2008; Mwenda, 2006; Tamale, 2006).

Cauterization is a little-known practice that involves the destruction of tissue by burning it with a hot iron. It is used as a remedy for health problems such as bleeding, abscesses, sores, ulcers and wounds as well as for "counterirritation" (to cause pain or irritation in one part of the body in order to relieve pain or inflammation in another). **Circumbustion** as practiced among the Nandi, an eastern Hamite people of northeast Africa, is described as the removal of all the superficial clitoral parts by charring them with a glowing coal held against the tissue with a spoon (Huelsman, 1976).

There are several forms of **cutting** or **incision** that are employed in certain areas. "Gishiri" and "angurya" are local terms used in parts of Nigeria. **Gishiri cuts** are not routinely performed on young girls but are typically made into the yoni wall in cases of obstructed labor. The practice can have serious consequences, including fistula, bleeding and pain. All types of **clitorotomy** also fall in this category and have been discussed in a separate chapter. **Angurya cuts** involve cutting or scraping to remove the hymen and other tissues surrounding the introitus. There is no data on the prevalence or consequences of this practice. Yet another form of cutting is known as **Sunna circumcision** involves multiple, small incisions in the clitoral glans leading to scarification (Huston, 2000). Incision of the genitals of young girls and infants has also been documented (Budiharsana, 2004), as has scraping (Newland, 2006).

Introcision is an aboriginal Australian practice. At puberty a ceremony is held during which a girl's introitus is enlarged by tearing it downward with three fingers bound together with string made from opossum tissue. This is usually performed by an old man trained for the job. It is followed by compulsory intercourse with several young men and sometimes older men to rejuvenate them (Huelsman, 1976).

The **introduction of irritating or harmful substances into the yoni** has been documented in several countries. Generally, adult women use a preparation that may include herbs or other substances on themselves to clean the yoni before or after sexual intercourse or to tighten and strengthen the yoni to enhance their own or their partner's sexual pleasure. The consequences and health risks depend on the substances used, as well as the frequency and methods used. This practice can be defined as a form of FGM, particularly when associated with health risks and high social pressure. The use of irritating feminine hygiene products and routine douching in the developed world can be included in this category.

The wide range of practices included under type IV FGM/C raises a number of questions. It is not always clear which practices should be included. Because of this, it has been generally considered important to maintain a broad definition of FGM/C in order to avoid loopholes that might allow truly harmful practices to continue. Some Western practices, such as cosmetic surgery and hymen repair actually fall under type IV but are legally accepted in many countries and not generally considered to constitute FGM/C. While the result might still be alteration of the genitals and thus technically a mutilation, the free and informed choice of an adult woman to have a procedure performed for specific reasons of her own is a very different matter than imposing cultural pressure on children to have unnecessary, brutally administered surgeries against their will and without their full understanding of possible consequences to their health and well-being.

The lack of clarity concerning type IV practices does not mitigate the urgent need to eliminate the most harmful types of FGM/C that are most prominent and well known—types I, II and III.

Health-Related Consequences of Different Types of FGM/C

Health risks associated with types I, II and III

Immediate risks: The short-term risks of FGM/C are closely related to the type and amount of tissue that is removed. For instance, type I usually includes removal of the clitoral glans and hood (Ib), while type II typically involves removal of both the clitoral glans and the labia minora (IIb) and thus poses greater risks. In type IIa, however, only the labia minora are cut and the clitoral glans is left intact. In these cases certain risks such as hemorrhage may be lower, whereas other risks such as genital infections or scarification may be the same or even greater.

Extreme pain: Cutting nerves and genital tissue causes severe pain, which is compounded when crude instruments are used. Type III FGM/C is an extensive procedure that takes longer that other types to complete (typically 15 to 20 minutes), thus both the pain and the healing is prolonged and intensified accordingly. Since deaths tend to go unreported, mortality statistics are difficult to figure, but are estimated to be as high as 10% for type III.

Proper analgesia is rarely used. Instead, several adults typically hold down the struggling girl during the procedure. This can lead to fractures of the clavicle, femur or humerus, or dislocation of the hip joint. Sometimes, in the midst of the agony, the child bites off her tongue. Even in medical settings where local anaesthetic is available, it is difficult to adequately numb the tissues because the clitoral body and glans are highly vascular with a dense concentration of nerve endings. Multiple painful injections are required and, even then, may not anesthetize the area completely.

Hemorrhage: Blood loss is the most common immediate complication and is frequently life threatening. Clitoral excision severs the dorsal artery of the clitoris, which has a strong flow under high pressure. It can be difficult or impossible to stop the bleeding. Delayed hemorrhage may also occur after the first week if infection causes the clot overlying the artery to slough off. Cutting the labia produces even more damage to blood vessels and may damage the vestibular glands. Acute hemorrhage or protracted bleeding can lead to anemia. The girl may go into shock from loss of blood (hemorrhagic shock) or from severe pain and trauma (neurogenic shock), either of which can be fatal.

Injury to adjacent tissues: The urethra, yoni, perineum and anal area can all be damaged when crude instruments are used; when the operator has limited knowledge of female anatomy, poor eyesight, or a careless technique; when the operation is being performed in poor light or on a writhing victim; or when any combination of these factors are present.

***Damage to the urethra*:** Not only can an injured urethra result in incontinence, but acute urine retention may develop due to swelling and inflammation around the wound, the girl's fear of pain when passing urine or from the injury to the urethra itself. Retention may last for hours or days but is usually reversible. Retention often leads to urinary tract infection.

Infection: It is common for a wound to become infected, usually due to an unhygienic operation; the use of unsterilized instruments; the application of unsterile substances to the wound that provide an excellent growth medium for bacteria; binding of the legs to assist in healing, which prevents wound drainage, or contamination with urine and feces. Infection resulting from faulty healing or an embedded stitch can cause an abscess, which may require surgical drainage. Infections may lead to fever, impaired healing, urinary tract or pelvic infection, tetanus, gangrene, septicemia, anemia or septic shock. Severe infections can be fatal. When the same unwashed instruments are used successively on a series of girls, the risk of transmission of blood-borne diseases increases, although there have been no confirmed cases of such transmission to date.

Impaired healing: Healing may be impaired because of infection, irritation from urine or from rubbing when walking. An underlying condition such as anemia or malnutrition may also have a negative impact. This can lead to a purulent, weeping wound or to a chronically infected ulcer.

Psychological risk: The pain and shock, and the use of physical restraint during the procedure, are reasons why many women describe FGM/C as a traumatic event. Some studies suggest an increased likelihood of fear of sexual intercourse, posttraumatic stress disorder, anxiety, depression and memory loss. The cultural significance of the practice might not protect against these psychological complications. The severity and prevalence of short- and long-term psychological (including psychosexual) trauma may also vary with characteristics other than the physical extent of tissue removal, such as the age and social situation of the girl at the time of the procedure (McCaffrey, 1995).

Long-term health risks of types I, II and III: Numerous long-term risks are posed by types I, II and III, many of which are simply extensions of the short-term risks already described. Type I poses the lowest risk of long-term complications.

Difficulty passing urine: Difficult urination occurs when the urethral opening is damaged or scarred. If the remaining infibulated opening is very small, it can take a woman up to 20 minutes to empty her bladder.

Urinary tract infections: Infection near the urethra can result in ascending urinary tract infections. This is particularly common following type III, when the normal flow of urine is deflected toward the tiny opening in the scar and the tissues under the scar remain constantly wet and susceptible to bacterial growth. **Stasis of urine** resulting from difficulty in micturition can lead to bladder infections, which can spread to the ureters and kidneys. If not treated, kidney stones and other kidney damage may result.

Urinary or fecal incontinence: These conditions can be lifelong and have serious social consequences, including social isolation.

Chronic pain: Pain may develop due to trapped or unprotected nerve endings. A painful neuroma can develop as a result of the entrapment of clitoral nerves in a stitch or in the scar tissue of the healed wound, leading to hypersensitivity and dyspareunia.

Sexual problems: Removal of or damage to highly sensitive genital tissue, especially the superficial clitoral parts, affects sexual sensitivity and can lead to sexual problems such as decreased sexual pleasure.

***Dyspareunia*:** Painful sexual intercourse may develop as a consequence of many forms of FGM/C because of scarring, the reduced size of the introitus and complications such as infection.

***Vaginismus*:** Spasmodic closing of the yoni may result from injury to the vulval area and repeated vigorous sexual intercourse. The introitus closes reflexively, causing considerable pain and soreness.

Calculi: These may form in the yoni or in the space underlying a scar as a result of the accumulation of menstrual blood and urine. This can lead to the formation of an ulcer or a stone that may obstruct the canal.

Fistulas: An open tract may form between the bladder and the yoni (vesicovaginal fistula) or between the rectum and yoni (rectovaginal fistula) as a result of injury to the soft tissues when an infibulation is opened up or when it is resutured as well as during sexual intercourse or obstructed labor.

Reproductive tract infections: Such infections are also common among infibulated women. They are often quite painful and may be accompanied by a discharge. These infections may spread to the uterus, uterine tubes and ovaries and may become chronic.

Infertility: Infertility can result if pelvic infection permanently damages the reproductive organs. A significant factor in the rate of infertility is the anatomical extent of the cutting. Thus, type IIc, which includes cutting the labia majora, is associated with a greater risk of infertility than type IIIa, which entails cutting and infibulation of the labia minora only. Infertility is primarily related to the practices that involve cutting the labia majora as evidence suggests that the more tissue that is removed, the higher the risk for infection.

Cysts: These are common problems associated with all types of FGM. They occur most frequently after infibulation. Implantation dermoid (inclusion) cysts are formed when a fold of skin becomes embedded in the scar. A sebaceous cyst may form due to blockage of a sebaceous gland duct. These cysts range in size from quite small to the size of a tennis ball or even a grapefruit. Cysts occasionally become infected. They may be extremely painful and may inhibit sexual activity.

Difficult childbirth: Problems during childbirth are common, particularly following severe forms of FGM/C. These are discussed in detail beginning on page 290.

Occlusion: Occlusion of the introitus or the urethra or both may occur due to a sealed type II or a type III, due to keloid scarring or due to stenosis. Any of these may result in slow and painful menstruation or urination or both. Retention of the menstrual flow (hematocolpos) may present with a bluish bulging membrane at the introitus that can prevent penetrative sex. It can also cause distension of the abdomen that, together with the lack of menstrual flow, may give rise to suspicions of pregnancy, with potentially serious social consequences. Dribbling of urine is common among infibulated women, probably due both to difficulties in emptying the bladder and to stagnation of urine beneath the scar tissue. Hygiene is often impaired as it can be difficult or impossible to adequately cleanse the area underlying the scar, where secretions, urine, semen and menstrual blood accumulate.

Repeated defibulation and reinfibulation: Additional complications are related to the need to repeat such procedures later in life for a variety of reasons. Defibulation that is accomplished after marriage either surgically or during penetrative sex makes intercourse painful for the woman during the first few weeks after sexual initiation. The male partner can also experience pain as he attempts to penetrate the tiny opening.

Health risks associated with type IV

With the exception of Western forms of genital piercing and clitorotomy, there is little known about the specific health risks of other type IV practices.

Caring for Women Who Have Undergone FGM/C Types I, II or III

The following general guidelines apply whether a woman is pregnant or not.

Educate yourself

When working with women from high-risk regions, you need to be aware that any given woman may have undergone FGM/C. It is important not to make any assumptions about this, however, even if she is from a country where it is practiced widely. Treat each woman and her situation individually. If you are unfamiliar with her cultural background, educate yourself so that you can be sensitive and respectful regarding her cultural beliefs, values and attitudes. Also work to ensure that your own values and attitudes do not interfere with the care you provide.

Many women from FGM/C-practicing countries are afraid that Western care providers will not know how to care for them and will impose unnecessary interventions. Familiarize yourself with the topic in general and what her genitals may look like by studying images in textbooks and on the Internet and talking to other midwives that have direct experience working with such women. It is of utmost importance that you refrain from displaying shock or disgust when she explains what happened and when you examine her and that you know enough to avoid asking inappropriate or embarrassing questions. It is also vitally important to use culturally acceptable, neutral terminology that is familiar to the woman when referring to FGM/C.

Get family permission to help her

Many cultures that incorporate FGM/C dictate that the woman must have permission from a male family member before she can receive any medical care. Therefore, it is important to gain the trust and respect of her male partner or other relatives who may accompany her to appointments. If relevant, obtain special consent in advance from a male relative or her husband before performing a physical exam, preferably at the visit prior to the one when the exam is to be performed. Her family members may prevent her from being examined or treated by male care providers. Be aware of this and be prepared to advocate for her if transport is necessary. Other women may accept a male provider, feeling that the role of the physician is neutral. They may see him as more qualified to assume the role of doctor, although female nurses, midwives and interpreters are always preferred. Once again, individualization of care is vital.

Arrange for an interpreter, if appropriate

If an interpreter is needed, she should be acceptable to the woman and should also be impartial, otherwise there is the risk that her own beliefs and values will bias the interpretation of what is being said.

Taking the history

It is important to establish a trusting relationship with all your clients. This means showing empathy and creating a rapport with each woman. It also means maintaining confidentiality while being respectful and patient as the woman explores whether it is safe to open up to you. Successful history taking will depend largely on your interpersonal communication skills. Women who have undergone FGM/C typically seek care for reasons other than FGM/C. You must always address her health problems as she presents them.

Greet the woman in a manner consistent with her cultural norms. Invite her to sit comfortably near and facing you. Introduce yourself, and address her by name. If a partner or relative has accompanied her, greet them and let them know what you intend to do.

Make it clear with your body language and the way you are sitting that you are ready to listen to her concerns and that she should feel free to share anything she wishes with you. Paraphrase what she says from time to time to check that you have heard her correctly and to avoid misunderstanding.

Begin by asking general questions, such as: "How are you?" "How is your family?" and "Do you have any information you would like to share with me?" When she is relaxed and seems ready to talk about more personal matters, begin your history with questions about her general health, illnesses, etc. When you feel the time is right, start asking about any previous pregnancies and births.

Tactfully inquire about any operations she may have had, including any genital operations. If she reports such operations, ask her if she would like to share any information about it with you. Reassure her that you are familiar with her cultural practices and that it is not a barrier to her getting services. If she starts crying, be patient and offer support. Let her express her feelings and give you the information she wants to share. Then, if appropriate at this point, tactfully ask the woman specific questions about her experiences of urination, menstruation, pelvic pain, any swellings and, if relevant, sexual intercourse (you may have to ask again if she reports no problems and the introitus or urethra appears scarred during your exam). *Remember, to her FGM/C is the norm; she may have numerous urogynecological or anorectal problems that she does not associate with her surgery.*

Affected women may be very slow to share information about their condition, so be patient and do not try to drag information out of her. If the woman is not forthcoming, plan on working on trust and communication during future visits.

Once you have established that a woman believes she has undergone FGM/C, this information and the subsequent clinical examination should be handled with professionalism and discretion. The type of FGM/C she believes to have been performed and any complications as reported by the woman should be noted in her chart or as required by the policy of the health institution where you work.

Physical exam: Always begin a physical exam by doing things that do not involve significant disrobing and are not sexually charged, such as examination of the head and neck and taking her blood pressure. Save breast and pelvic exams until she is comfortable with your touching her, possibly at another visit.

It is always a good idea to examine, at some point, the genitalia of a woman who reports FGM/C, as some women who believe themselves to have had FGM/C are actually found to be intact when examined; likewise others may have much more extensive FGM/C than they realize. Either way, it is very important that you know, in advance, exactly what you may need to deal with at the time of birth. Schedule this appointment when you know you will have plenty of time to go through it in an unhurried manner and time to help the woman process the exam afterward, if necessary.

Genital examination can be very embarrassing for these women. If you are working in a clinic, you should warn the other practitioners in advance that you are planning on examining a woman with possible FGM/C to ensure her uninterrupted privacy during the exam.

If you want another practitioner to be present during the exam, arrange for this in advance and explain to the woman why you want another person present. Have the person there at the beginning of the visit so that the woman can meet her. Prearrange that the person leave the room for some reason so that you can ask the woman if she still feels comfortable having this person present during the exam; if not, examine the woman privately. The woman has the right to refuse, and this must be respected. Emphasize that her care is not conditional on her consent to allow others to attend the examination.

It is paramount that a woman feel confident that she is in safe hands, will not be judged and will never be made an object of curiosity or put on display. Women have reported that one of their most traumatic experiences was a pelvic exam by a care provider unfamiliar with FGM/C during which they were found to be excised and the health provider called in the rest of the staff to look at their "mutilated" genitals.

Prior to the exam, explain what you plan to do slowly and completely; make sure she has understood you (language may be a barrier) and answer any questions she may have. Get her consent to proceed and reaffirm her consent as you go through each portion of the exam. In some practicing cultures, women are taught not to express their fears or pain. Therefore, give the woman permission to tell you how your exam feels and encourage her to express her needs throughout her care. Offer to show her what you are finding using a mirror, but be aware that looking at her genitals, especially in the presence of someone else, may be completely outside her cultural comfort zone. If she is not ready to be examined, postpone the procedure until the next visit or until she is comfortable.

Once you have her consent, prepare to examine her. Leave the room so she can disrobe below the waist. Ask her to lie down on the examination surface with her legs apart and flexed. Provide her with a drape and ask her to cover herself from the waist down until you are ready to perform the exam. Remember that women from many of these cultures are very modest, much more so than many Western women; she should remain as covered as possible during the exam. Always be aware of and respect the woman's reactions.

Arrange a good light source. Wash your hands thoroughly and don gloves. With her permission, lift the covering to expose her genitalia. Visually inspect the external genitalia to identify the type of FGM/C and to check for ulcers, infection, abscesses or swelling. Considering the wide variety of normal variation that occurs in natural genitalia, be sure to look carefully: scarring may only appear as an exceptionally smooth area.

If you find it necessary to palpate her, look her in the eye as you explain to her what you want to do and why before you proceed. If you cannot tell by looking, it is important to assess whether the superficial clitoral structures are present. If they are, they can probably be palpated through the scar. Begin at the upper border of the symphysis and check for the clitoral body by placing your finger in the midline and rocking it side to side, your fingertip should "fall off" the sides of the clitoral body if it is present (try this on yourself and sister students when you practice pelvic exams). Palpate along the body to the tip to try to determine if the clitoral glans is still present. You may need to perform this exam through thick scar tissue and, due to nerve and tissue damage, this exam may be painful, so be sure to follow the woman's lead and stop if she is in pain or becomes distressed.

Most of the time there is no need to introduce fingers into the yoni, as most problems will be obvious during visual inspection of the external genitalia. If it is necessary, explain to the woman why you feel you need to perform a digital exam. Once you have her permission to continue, first slowly try to introduce the tip of your well-lubricated index finger, then introduce the whole finger if the introitus allows. If there is room for more than one finger, introduce the second finger very slowly and observe the woman's reaction, as this may cause pain. For infibulated women, the introitus may be very tight and may not admit even a fingertip. In such cases, you should not attempt to introduce any fingers.

If the use of a speculum seems necessary and possible, try a pediatric speculum first. A bimanual exam may be done using a single finger within the yoni and palpating the uterus and ovaries via a rectal exam. If bimanual examination is difficult, ultrasound may be helpful in determining if the pelvic organs are normal (Lightfoot-Klein & Shaw, 1991).

After completing the procedure, thank the woman for her cooperation. In cases where you have introduced fingers into the yoni, look for abnormal yoni discharge before taking off your gloves. Assist the woman into a sitting position and leave the room until she is fully clothed. Invite her to sit comfortably while you record your findings and discuss them with her. Drawing a sketch of the appearance of the vulva in your records may help to avoid unnecessary examinations in future.

Dealing with physical complications of FGM/C in the clinical setting

Midwives in developed countries will primarily be dealing with adult women who have a healed wound and may present with numerous long-term complications. Midwives in all countries, but more likely midwives in developing countries, may at times be presented with a child that has recently undergone a procedure and is now having complications that have frightened the parents to the point that they are seeking your care for her. Should this occur, it is important that you welcome them and make them feel safe.

Must you report FGM/C to authorities? In regions where laws exist against these practices, there may be an overarching duty of providers to report suspected instances of child abuse. Nevertheless, because the parents intended to benefit, not harm, their child and because the risk of additional harm after FGM/C is usually nonexistent, reporting a procedure that has already occurred may not be warranted (again, compare it to Western parents' choosing to circumcise their sons). If there are other still unaffected girls in the family, however, and the provider learns of the intention to perpetrate the practice on these girls, reporting may be warranted under state law to protect these children. Plus parents are not liable if the procedure took place outside the US, and many parents have their girls done before moving. For those known to have been in the US for a longer time, the procedure may have taken place during a trip abroad. Unjustified reporting can be extremely detrimental to the well-being of the family. Once trust has been established, explain the local laws to the parents and discourage the future practice of FGM/C (Toubia, 2000).

Dealing with short-term physical complications

Managing short-term physical complications varies depending on what is going on and may range from simple support to counseling to emergency interventions. Here are some notes on dealing with immediate and short-term complications.

General care: In each instance you will administer an analgesic so that your care does not increase the pain. Then clean a fresh wound, inspect it for the extent of damage, bleeding and signs of infection, prescribe antibiotics as appropriate and advise keeping the wound dry during healing. Arrange follow-up visits to continue to monitor healing.

Bleeding: Inspect the wound and staunch the bleeding by packing it with sterile gauze; advise keeping the wound dry and recheck the girl in a few days.

Assess the seriousness of the bleeding and how much has been lost (remember that a child has a much smaller blood volume than an adult). Administer IV fluids, monitor vital signs and transfer her immediately to a hospital for blood transfusion if necessary. If blood transfusion is not available, transfer her to a tertiary-level facility immediately. It may be the policy of health institutions to prescribe Vitamin K, especially in bleeding babies. If so, take action as required by the policy.

A traditional compound (i.e., one containing ash, herbs, soil or cow dung), which can lead to tetanus or other infections, may have been applied to the wound. Therefore, a tetanus vaccine and antibiotics may be recommended in accordance with national guidelines.

Severe pain and injury to tissues: The management of pain associated with FGM/C is the same as under any other circumstances. If routine measures do not relieve the pain, or the girl is in shock, refer the parents or the woman for medical attention.

Shock: Treat the girl for shock by elevating the legs, and keeping her warm. If she is having difficulty breathing, administer oxygen and be prepared to resuscitate. Give IV fluids to replace lost fluid. Check vital signs every 15 minutes. If the woman or child's condition does not improve, refer her for medical attention. (See HOLISTIC MIDWIFERY, VOL. II, for a detailed discussion of hemorrhagic shock.)

Infection and septicemia: First, look for signs of infection and anything that might be contributing to the infection, such as obstruction of urine. Obtain a specimen of yoni discharge with a swab and obtain a urine sample to perform cultures and sensitivity. Any obstructions should be removed. Arrange a follow-up visit within 36 hours and again in seven days to assess progress. If infection persists or seems severe to begin with, refer the client for medical evaluation.

Urine retention: If the girl is unable to pass urine because of pain and fear, give her strong analgesics and use techniques to encourage her to pass urine, such as turning on a water tap. If retention is due to infibulation, offer defibulation counseling to herself and her partner if she is an adult; discuss it with both her and her guardian if she is a child. If retention is due to an injured urethra, refer her to a urogynecologist.

Urinary catheterization when the meatus is covered with scar tissue: If a woman who has not been defibulated requires catheterization, you may need to insert your finger under the scar and retract it gently to locate the urethral meatus before you can insert the catheter (Lightfoot-Klein & Shaw, 1991).

Anemia: Anemia may develop due to blood loss or infection, especially from malaria, particularly in children. Assess the severity of the anemia and send blood for hemoglobin, hematocrit, red cell count, ABO typing and, if appropriate, malaria testing. If a simple iron-deficiency anemia is found and is mild, give folic acid, iron tablets and advice regarding a nutritious, iron-rich diet. In cases of malaria, treat appropriately. If the anemia is severe or a hereditary anemia is discovered, refer the client for medical evaluation.

Dealing with long-term physical complications

Midwives in developed countries are more likely to encounter adult women with these types of problems, many of which may present at any time, including in pregnancy. For women who have had type III FGM/C, many of their problems stem from a tight introital opening. For these women, defibulation is frequently the best remedy. A complete discussion of defibulation begins on page 285.

Scarring: Keloid scar tissue may form that obstructs the introitus. Inspect the genitalia for the presence and size of the keloid tissue. Removal is complicated because removing keloids usually results in the formation of more. If the keloid is small, advise the woman to leave it alone and reassure her that it will not cause harm. If the keloid is large, is causing difficulties during intercourse, is likely to obstruct fetal descent, or is psychologically distressing to the woman, refer her to a specialist experienced in removing keloid scars. Pregnant women with large keloids may require surgical delivery if the scar obstructs the introitus and cannot be removed before term.

Stenosis of the introitus is handled by gradually dilating it with increasingly larger objects (such as dildos) or by manual stretching, depending upon the tightness of the stenosis and the elasticity of the scar.

Cysts: Dermoid (or inclusion) and sebaceous cysts are common complications of all forms of FGM/C. Inspect the genitals to assess for the presence, location and size of cysts. Small noninfected cysts may be left alone after counseling the woman that it is harmless. Alternatively, you can refer her to have them removed under local or regional anaesthesia. However, before interfering with a small cyst, it is important to determine if corrective surgery might result in further damage and scarring of remaining sensitive tissue or blood vessels, as might be the case if the cyst overlies clitoral parts. If such a risk exists, inform the woman so she can choose whether to proceed with removal.

If the cyst is large or infected, refer the woman for excision or marsupialization (cutting the anterior cyst wall and forming a pouch to allow drainage), either of which are usually performed under general anesthesia.

Clitoral neuroma: Clitoral nerve tissue may become trapped in fibrous scar tissue following clitoridectomy. This can result in extremely sharp pain over the fibrous swelling during intercourse; even friction from underpants may be enough to cause pain. A neuroma cannot usually be seen, but can be detected by carefully touching the area around the clitoral scar with a delicate object, such as a cotton swab, and asking the woman if she feels any pain. Under general anesthetic, the neuroma feels like a small pebble underlying the mucosa. If the symptoms are mild, advise the woman to wear loose pants and give her an analgesic (for example, lidocaine cream) to apply to the area.

If symptoms are severe, refer the woman for surgical excision of the neuroma. This is not commonly required, and the woman should be carefully counseled before such a step is taken. The symptoms may be psychological, the result of the trauma of excision or the fear of sexual intercourse.

Vulval abscesses: An abscess may develop as a result of deep infection, faulty healing or an embedded stitch. Inspect the site to assess the extent of the problem. Apply an analgesic ointment to relieve pain. Then palpate to determine the extent of the swelling. Small vulval abscesses can be treated with antibiotics, herbal or saline sitz baths and vulval hygiene. Large abscesses may require surgical intervention, which may involve incision and drainage of the abscess under general anesthesia, or administration of antibiotics as indicated by swab culture. If an abscess does not clear up during a pregnancy, the woman may need to have a hospital birth. Monitor the abscess closely.

Urinary tract infection (UTI): Urinary tract infections are common among women who have undergone type III FGM. This can be due to obstruction of the urine in infibulated women or the presence of urinary stones or previous injury to the urethra. Inspect the vulva carefully to establish the cause of infection. If infibulation appears to be the cause, counsel the woman or parent on the need to open up the infibulation. Perform a urine analysis to identify what organism is involved and treat the UTI. Advise the patient to drink plenty of water. If UTI is recurrent, refer the client for medical evaluation.

Chronic pelvic infection: This condition may be the result of obstructed yoni secretions due to occlusion of the introitus, the presence of yoni stones or stenosis. Take a yoni swab for culture and sensitivity. Give antibiotics that are appropriate and available locally, e.g. tetracycline (500mg every 6 hours for 10 days) or doxycycline (100 mg twice daily for 10 days). If the infection is fungal, metronidazole (Flagyl) may be prescribed. If the woman has a husband or partner, treat him for the infection as well. If the woman has type III FGM, counsel her on the benefits of opening the infibulation. If symptoms persist or if the cause of the infection is due to an obstruction because of stones or due to injury, refer her to a urogynecologist.

Infertility: Infertility is often a consequence of severe pelvic infection and may occur in nulliparous women (primary) or after the birth of one or more children (secondary). In rare cases it is due to failure of penile penetration because of a very tight introitus. Take a history and inspect the genitalia to identify the problem. If infertility is the result of failure to penetrate, counsel the woman and her partner on the benefits of defibulation. Otherwise, refer her to a gynecologist for specialist care.

Fistulas and incontinence: Vesicovaginal (VVF) or rectovaginal (RVF) fistulas resulting in incontinence may have their origin in injury to the external urethral meatus or injury due to obstructed labor. Assess the child or woman to identify the cause of incontinence and the type of FGM/C. Confirm the presence, level and the severity of any fistula. (See the chapters entitled "Functional Disorders of the Urinary Tract" and "Anorectal Disorders and Incontinence.")

In cases of stress incontinence, counsel the client and start pelvic floor exercises to strengthen the muscles, or refer her to a urologist for further evaluation and treatment. Women with a fistula must be referred for specialist repair. If infection is present, she should by treated with pharmaceuticals as appropriate.

Yoni obstruction: Partial or total obstruction of the yoni may occur because of infibulation, stenosis or a hematoma, any of which may be accompanied by hematocolpos. Unmarried girls may be suspected of being pregnant because of the amenorrhea and swelling of the abdomen. Sometimes, young girls are punished for this condition. Assess the woman to identify the problem and type of FGM/C. If she has been infibulated, counsel on the need for opening up. If the woman has hematocolpos, stones or stenosis, refer her for surgical intervention under general anesthetic. In cases of yoni stenosis, surgical intervention may involve dilation.

Menstrual disorders: Many excised women report severe dysmenorrhea with or without menstrual irregularity. One possible cause is an increase in pelvic congestion due to infection or other unknown conditions; anxiety over the state of the genitals, sexuality or fertility is another. Try to establish the cause of dysmenorrhea by taking a history and performing a clinical exam. Find out how she feels and support her in dealing with the situation. Consider giving antispasmodic drugs to relieve pain. If dysmenorrhea is due to the accumulation of menstrual flow as a result of infibulation, counsel her regarding the need for opening up the scar. If the condition is severe, refer her to a urogynecologist for further evaluation.

Ulcers: Vulval ulcers may develop when urea crystals become trapped under the scar tissue. Counsel the woman on the need for opening up her infibulation, and advise her that her vulva should be kept open thereafter. If she decides to proceed, once she is defibulated, apply antibiotics to the ulcer with or without 1% hydrocortisone cream to stimulate healing. Also give her healing herbs such as comfrey to use in sitz baths; this can be suggested if she declines defibulation as well. If the ulcer fails to heal, refer the woman for surgical excision of the tough fibrous walls of the sore.

Psychosocial and sexual problems

Women who have had FGM/C can all be expected to have some sort of psychosocial impact from the procedure. FGM/C can affect self-confidence and self-esteem and cause problems in relationships; these would mostly be classified as psychosocial or sexual problems. In some instances girls and women from FGM/C-practicing communities seek care for physical problems for which no sign can be found when they are examined. Their complaints are, in fact, "psychosomatic"; that is, they are psychological problems that the woman experiences or unconsciously disguises as physical discomfort. Anxiety about their genitals or about sexual relationships may manifest themselves this way. Often the girl or woman is unaware that her symptoms are rooted in psychological anxieties.

Counseling should never be hurried. If either of you is pressed for time, it may be better to make an appointment for another mutually convenient time. When the client has opened up to you, ask her about her eating and sleeping patterns and her menstrual patterns and sexual relationships in a very tactful manner, as these questions may embarrass her and result in communication breakdown. Use "open-ended" questions—i.e., questions that require more than a simple "yes" or "no" answer and that do not suggest an answer in the wording—and thus offer the woman the chance to explain things in some detail. Use observation skills continuously to pick up nonverbal cues, and tell the woman what you have observed to give her the chance to tell you more about the situation. Listen carefully and empathetically. Use all your senses to try to understand her cultural context. It may not be easy the first time you meet her, but arrange for subsequent visits to explore more. Assess the woman's intellectual status and her ability to understand information and to comprehend her situation. Refer women who are severely disturbed for more specialized care.

Psychosocial and sexual problems are identified by first taking her reports of a physical problem seriously and examining her to assess for yourself. If there is no physical evidence of a problem, talk to her more about her feelings and the symptoms (it could be that a physical problem exists that you cannot detect during an external exam).

Sometimes a woman is aware that her symptoms are not the real cause of her problems, but she is too shy to discuss them directly and seeks care for physical complaints in the hope that her health care provider will be able to read between the lines. It is not easy for these women to discuss sexual problems. Moreover, in areas where FGM/C is practiced, sex is often a taboo topic; she may not even have a sufficient vocabulary to express herself to you, especially if your first languages differ. It is essential for the midwife to pick up nonverbal cues of psychosocial problems, by observing body language and listening carefully to the tone of voice, which may give more meaning to what the woman is telling you and what she may be feeling.

Empathize with the woman as she describes a disturbing experience. Explain to her how you can help. Advise her that there are various ways of conducting sexual relationships; teach her appropriate techniques by which both she and her partner may be aroused. If she wants her partner to be involved in the discussion, invite him or her to join you at the next appointment.

FGM/C does not necessarily prevent a woman from reaching orgasm or enjoying sex. Therefore sexual problems may be due to fear of pain rather than a physical cause. However, if sexual intercourse is not possible as a result of infibulation or extensive scarring, the issue of opening up the tight introitus should be addressed. Assist the woman and her partner, when appropriate, to make an informed decision on the steps to be taken to solve the problem. Assist them to act on their decision by giving advice on how to proceed. Set up an appointment for another counseling or follow-up session to prepare for the next step. If the problem persists, refer them to a specialist.

Prenatal care for women who have had FGM/C

This section focuses on special considerations for pregnancy, building on what has already been covered. Regardless of the type of FGM/C that was done, these women require particularly sensitive and culturally competent maternity care. Many women from developing countries approach pregnancy and birth with a great fear of dying.

Caring for women with type I, II and IV FGM during pregnancy: When types I, II or IV FGM have not resulted in any particular complications, the woman will not require any special treatment during pregnancy other than softening the scar tissue and yoni stretching.

Reassure her that she is not at high risk because of her condition and invite her to ask any questions about her excision or any other issues relating to her pregnancy. Find time to counsel her about sexual issues and to give her support. During prenatal visits, ask the woman if she needs any special help but do not ask about her excision unless she wants to discuss it. Pregnancy provides a good opportunity to educate and inform women regarding basic health, normal and excised genitals, childbirth and postnatal care.

Types I, II and IV FGM/C can produce severe vulval and yoni adhesions, scarring and stenosis that may resist stretching, obstruct childbirth or interfere with necessary internal exams. In the event of miscarriage, passage of the conceptus may be obstructed. Urinary tract or pelvic infections can cause pain and interfere with the normal progress of the pregnancy. Dermoid cysts and keloids may cause discomfort and perhaps obstruction during birth.

Caring for women with type III FGM during pregnancy: Visually inspect the genitals to confirm type III FGM or a sealed type II. Where these practices are common, the vulval area should be inspected early in prenatal care as a matter of routine.

As a general rule, if the urethral meatus is visible (i.e., if there is no covering scar tissue from the meatus downward), or if two fingers can be introduced through the scar opening and into the introitus without discomfort, the scar tissue is unlikely to cause major problems at the time of birth. Women whose introital opening is 1 cm or less in diameter are at greater risk for major perineal tearing during birth; defibulation prior to term is recommended. If the woman has been pregnant before, her previous experiences during labor will indicate whether she is likely to have problems this time.

Preparing the tissues for birth: Taking evening primrose oil (or another linoleic acid–rich oil) internally and massaging it into the scar tissue on a daily basis during the last six weeks of pregnancy will go a long way toward helping the tissues stretch and not tear at the time of birth.

Defibulation: Among those who have a sealed type II or a type III FGM, defibulation may be called for at any time in a woman's life to relieve symptoms. However, midwives will almost always be called upon to consider defibulating a woman in relation to a pregnancy. If this has not been done prior to conception, it may be necessary to allow for a normal birth.

It is never illegal to perform a medically indicated defibulation with a woman's informed permission. In the US, reinfibulation is also allowed on women over the age of 18, although you can refuse to do it. Make clear your professional limits from the beginning of your discussion. You may need to remind her of them later as well.

***Indications for defibulation*:** Opening up an infibulation is indicated for the following conditions: urinary retention (common in children); recurrent urinary tract and kidney infections; severe genital tract infection (especially when treatment has not been successful); severe menstrual problems; difficulty with penetration during sexual intercourse; incomplete miscarriage or abortion; the medical termination of pregnancy; normal childbirth (opening ≤ 1 cm in diameter); the prevention of massive perineal tearing at the time of birth; the diagnosis and treatment of diseases requiring manual or speculum examination; certain contraceptive methods for family planning and certain religious or purification purposes in traditional settings. That being said, there are several midwives who have attended infibulated women that I have heard from who report that, with care and attention to the perineum at the time of birth, these women often stretch without lots of tearing, especially those that are multiparas.

Some women who have been educated about their genital function may request defibulation or surgical reconstruction of her genitals in the hope of regaining sexual sensitivity. While this does happen sometimes, in other cases it does not. It is important to be very clear that you *cannot* guarantee what the outcome of surgery will be, especially as far as sexual function is concerned.

***Counseling women regarding defibulation*:** There are many situations when permanently opening an infibulation is the best and safest option for a woman. Nevertheless, the woman must be thoroughly informed and counseled and must come to her own decision to go ahead with it. Sometimes a woman may be ambivalent about being opened up; that is, she may want it but be fearful of the consequences. Counseling should aim to help her reach an informed decision about which she is confident. Make it clear to the woman (and others as appropriate) that your recommendations are based on a careful consideration of her individual health and well-being. If the family refuses to give consent for a minor or an adult woman to be opened up, providing them a written statement of medical necessity and answering their questions thoroughly may help to alleviate their concerns.

During counseling, include the partner and arrange to speak with him (or her) in at least one separate session as well. Give the woman factual information about the effects of type III FGM on the anatomy and physiology of the reproductive system, on pregnancy and birth, and on associated complications. Explain how her genitals will look and feel afterward, emphasizing the difference between natural and infibulated genitalia, including changes in urination, menstrual flow, genital moisture and sexual activity. Explain that she can expect increased postoperative sensitivity in the vulval area that was previously covered by the scar for at least 2 to 4 weeks following the procedure and that it may last for a while. Inform her of the legal status of FGM/C in her country of residence and in her native country, if relevant.

If she is currently pregnant, also discuss the benefits of opening up her infibulation for her general health prior to birth. Explain that, once she is opened up, it may be possible for her to give birth over an intact perineum. Opening the scar during pregnancy has advantages besides preparing for delivery. It means that clean samples of urine can be obtained and that yoni infections, premature rupture of membranes and other events can be more easily investigated should they occur. Pregnant women whose infibulation is so tight that it will not permit normal birth and who refuse to be defibulated either prior to or during pregnancy should be informed that defibulation may be required at the time of birth, when it is more dangerous for the mother. It is unlikely that any woman will refuse entirely as it is culturally accepted that defibulation is necessary to allow for birth.

Give the woman (and her partner) complete and clear information about the defibulation procedure and make sure she has understood. Inform her that the scar will be cut in the midline and then the sides will be sutured separately, not resutured together to recreate a small opening.

Several sessions may be needed to prepare the woman and her family psychologically for the procedure. Instruct her regarding the importance of vulval hygiene and the need to keep her vulva clean and dry during healing. Discuss pain relief options. Advise the woman and her husband or partner regarding when it will be safe to resume sexual activity (generally 4 to 6 weeks after the procedure). Information about these discussions should be clearly recorded in the prenatal records.

***Timing defibulation in pregnancy*:** Defibulation should be performed during the second trimester between the 20th and 28th weeks of pregnancy to allow time for the sides of the wound to heal before term.

It is recommended to avoid defibulation during the first trimester because there is a higher risk of miscarriage at that time. If the woman happens to have a miscarriage after she is defibulated, she may blame it on the surgery, and word may spread to her community that defibulation may threaten a healthy pregnancy. Such a situation might make it more difficult to convince other women of the benefit of performing the surgery prior to term.

***How to perform a defibulation*:** Defibulation can be performed when a fully informed woman is ready for it to take place.

***Gather your supplies and equipment*:** Gather together antiseptic swabs, a pair of straight scissors, a dilator (if you have one), two hemostats, sterile gauze, sterile gloves, a 5 mL (cc) syringe and needles, local anesthetic, suture, stitch scissors, needle holder, lubricant, sterile towels, antiseptic solution, a receptacle for used instruments and antiseptic hand washing solution.

***Prepare the mother*:** Prepare the mother as for an internal exam. Review again what you have already discussed with her about the opening up. Emphasize that the main reason for the problems she has suffered is the infibulation and that opening the infibulation will help to relieve many of these problems. Talk to her about having a support person with her and ensure total privacy in the procedure room. Defibulation may trigger flashbacks of the original event; warn her of this possibility and help her breath through the procedure as you talk through each step.

***Administer local anesthetic*:** Wash your hands, don sterile gloves, expose the genitalia and clean the perineal area with antiseptic swabs. Introduce an index finger, a closed forceps or a metal cervical dilator slowly and gently into the opening and work the tip underneath the skin to lift the scar tissue. Infiltrate 2 to 3 mL (cc) of local anesthetic into the midline area where the cut will be made along the scar and to either side of the scar. Palpate over the region where the clitoral body and glans should be to determine if these structures underlie the scar and take care not to inject anesthetic into these structures.

***Defibulation procedure*:** With your finger or a dilator inserted into the opening in the scar, introduce the tips of the scissor blades pointed toward the symphysis pubis, between the anterior side of the finger or instrument and the overlying tissue to avoid injury to underlying and adjacent tissues (or to the baby, if the procedure is done during labor).

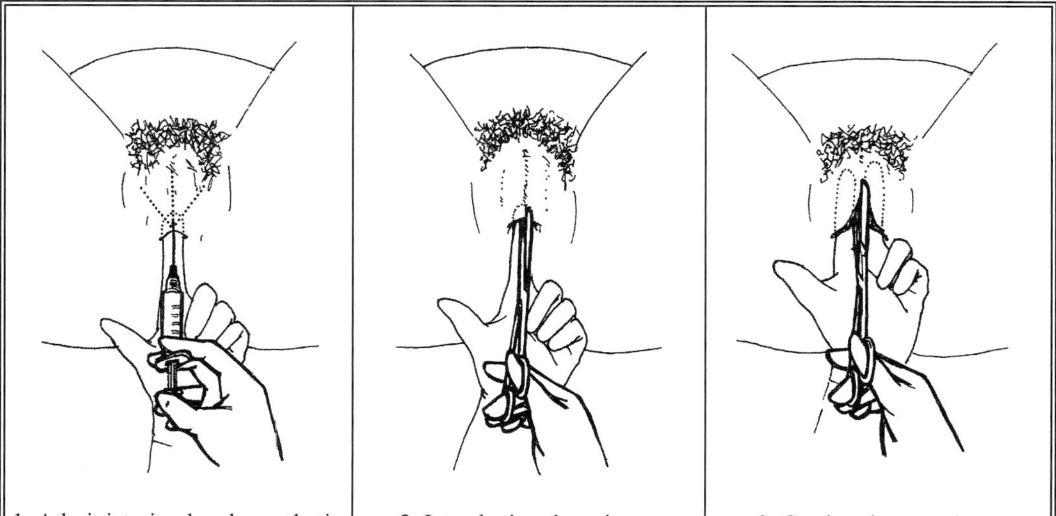

1. Administering local anesthetic | 2. Introducing the scissors | 3. Cutting the scar tissue

If the introitus is too tight to admit your finger, cut just far enough up the midline so that you can remove the instrument, insert a finger or fingers up to the anterior apex of the flap and then continue the incision. You may need an assistant to help you manage the instruments. This way, your fingers can help guide the incision and will help you avoid cutting into any underlying labial or clitoral tissues that remain. Before you begin to cut the tissue, be sure that your finger directly underlies the scar and that any remaining labia minora are not bunched up between your finger and the underside of the scar.

Insert the tips of the scissors (Fig. 2), making sure your finger stays between the blade and the underlying tissue. If using an instrument instead of a finger to elevate the infibulation, open it slightly and slip the tips of the scissors between the ends of the elevating instrument. Make an incision toward the pubic bone in the midline. Divide the tissue enough so that you can insert two fingers to guide your cut until you reveal the meatus; then stop. Cut exactly along the midline of the scar towards the symphysis pubis until the urethral meatus is exposed. It is common with type III to find structures beneath the scar that are still intact such as the clitoral body, the glans, the labia minora or all three.

Do not separate the scar above the level of the urethra because you may cut into clitoral blood vessels, which can result in bleeding that is very difficult to control. An incision about 5 to 7 cm long in the direction of the urethra is usually appropriate.

In most cases, there is little bleeding from the relatively avascular scar tissue. Even so, if you are doing this during labor, it is wise not to do it too early, as more blood may be lost than is really necessary. Wait until the presenting part is starting to distend the tissues, but not so long as to risk the possibility of excessive tearing from the pressure.

Suture the raw edges of each side to prevent the tissue from resealing and to avoid infection (Fig. 5). Use either 3-0 chromic gut or 4-0 synthetic. Small, shallow interrupted stitches or continuous basting stitches can be used. Use continuous stitches whenever the scar tissue allows it because they secure hemostasis better, respond better to swelling, lessen the likelihood that a sinus tract will form and will probably be more comfortable as they involve far fewer knots.

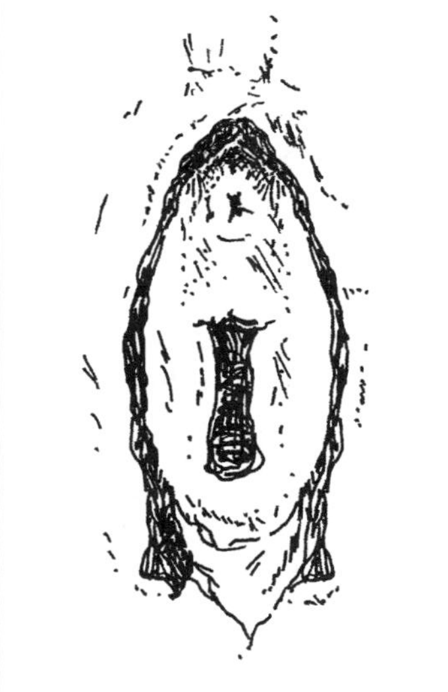

4. Close-up of opened infibulation with raw edges on either side

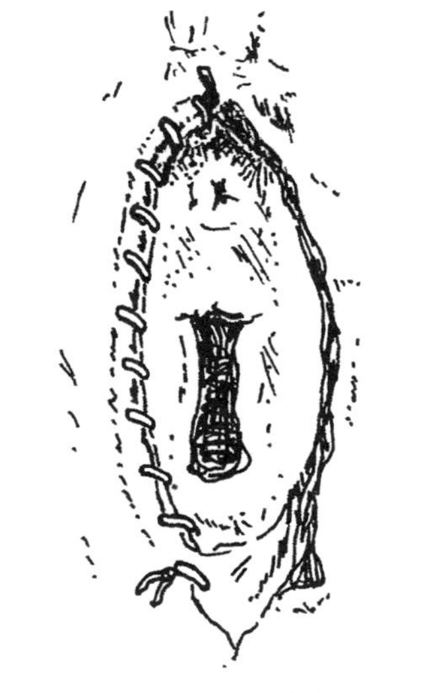

5. Close-up of partial repair using continuous stitches

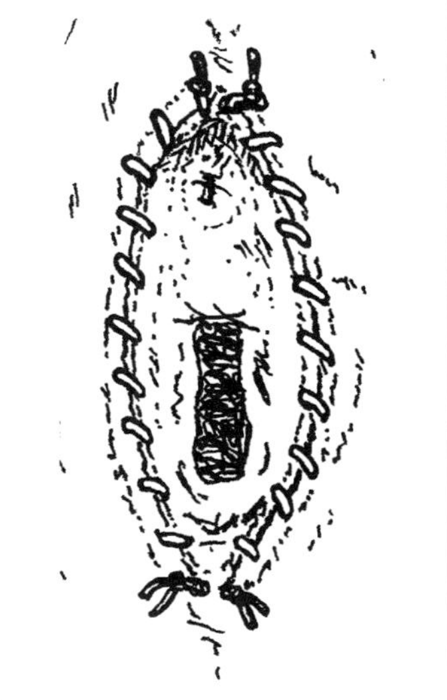

6. Completed repair

Postoperative care: Analgesia should be prescribed following the procedure. Postoperative pain restimulates the pain of the initial FGM/C and may reinforce negative ideas about being opened up. Antibiotics may also be prescribed depending on the situation.

Reassure the woman that sensitivity tends to dissipate, but it can take a while. She will also get used to the feeling of wet genitals. Suggest that she takes sitz baths (warm water containing salt or herbs or both) three times a day followed by gently drying the area and applying a soothing cream (Lansinoh Lanolin or calendula cream can be used if synthetic suture was used) for the first 1 to 2 weeks. Advise her on the importance of personal hygiene.

Advise the woman and her husband when to resume sexual intercourse. Typically they should wait 4 to 6 weeks. This may require counseling over several sessions. Advice and culturally appropriate counseling regarding sexual matters require great sensitivity, and should be carefully tailored to the needs of the woman and her family.

Make a follow-up appointment to monitor healing and to deal with any issues that may arise concerning her genitals or sexual relationship. Home visits are an ideal time to discuss these things with the woman and her family; they will need further support and counseling in order to cope successfully with the many changes following the defibulation.

Male partners in particular need psychosexual counseling to help them understand and accept sexual changes and to ensure they do not try to persuade the woman to be reinfibulated. When women must be referred to community services for follow-up, the midwife who performed the procedure must provide clear information to the health care provider who will be responsible for follow-up to ensure there is no lapse in support.

Caring for affected women during labor or birth

In most cases, a woman at term will have received at least some antenatal care. However, there will be some who have not had any care, and their first contact with a health care provider will be when they call or arrive in labor on the doorstep of the birthing center or hospital. Whatever the circumstances, assure the woman that her condition will be managed and that the care providers are ready to offer any service she needs. The following pointers are specific to labor.

Although, as previously mentioned, some infibulated women do stretch adequately, the greatest risk during labor is obstructed fetal descent due to scar tissue. Knowing if defibulation will be necessary requires attentive midwifery care. Should an infibulated woman with a resistant scar find herself in unattended labor, she and her baby may die as a result of being unable to give birth without having someone there to open her scar. A surgical delivery may be necessary if a tight infibulation has not been opened up during pregnancy and labor is allowed to become obstructed. Possible effects on the newborn include fetal asphyxia due to prolonged labor or neonatal brain damage due to obstructed labor, birth injuries due to difficult delivery, or death as a result of delivery complications.

Assessment during labor: Take a history of labor and perform a physical examination as you would for any woman. Examine the genitalia to assess the tightness of the introitus, and whether it will allow for normal delivery or not. If the introitus is tight, explain to the woman the problems associated with having a tight opening at the time of birth. Also perform an abdominal examination and auscultate the fetal heart. Palpate the bladder (also ensure that the bladder is emptied regularly).

Monitoring the progress of labor: If the situation allows, labor can be assessed using external parameters such as contractions, descent and fetal heart rate patterns. Observe the woman closely and monitor her vital signs hourly. Give clear and simple information to the client about what to expect during delivery. Note all these observations in her record.

If there is a problem during labor that absolutely requires an internal exam but the introitus is so tight that an internal exam is impossible, the scar can be opened along the midline. Explain the situation to the mother and follow the procedure as outlined on pages 287.

Management of a tight introitus in women with types I, II and IV FGM/C during labor: When FGM has caused introital stenosis and inelasticity of the perineum, there may be a need for a clitorotomy. Generally speaking, women with type I FGM/C are able to deliver normally without any intervention unless there is extensive scarring. Usually a tight introitus will have been identified during the first phase of labor, and the woman informed of the possible eventual need for a clitorotomy at that time. If, however, the woman has arrived for care when she is pushing, explain to her that you may need to increase the size of the opening by performing a clitorotomy and inform her of when and how this will be done (as already described, this should be at the height of a contraction, using clitorotomy scissors).

Management of women with type III or a sealed type II FGM during labor: In cases where the infibulation has not been opened during pregnancy and the woman is in early labor, she should receive a crash course in the circumstances that may require defibulation. Explain the physical changes involved and that it will be repaired open, not reclosed.

Inspect the introitus to assess whether it is going to be able to stretch sufficiently to allow for birth. Assess the opening by slowly and carefully trying to introduce one finger into the yoni to measure the tightness of the introitus. If this is successful, try to move the finger upward and downward and left to right. If there is space for a second finger, insert it too. Then try to spread the two fingers and check for resistance. If it is impossible to introduce one finger, or even the tip of a finger, the introitus is extremely tight: equivalent to type III FGM. If you can introduce a finger but cannot stretch the opening because of resistant scar tissue, it will be necessary to open up the introitus via defibulation or a clitorotomy.

If defibulation is needed, explain the situation to the mother and follow the procedure as outlined on page 287. When indicated, the vulva should be opened up during pushing at the height of a contraction to minimize pain, taking care not to cause injury to the baby or structures underlying the scar. Once the upper scar tissue has been divided, assess the condition of the perineum as you would for any other birth: she may not need any more cutting to get the baby out.

In some cases, where the scar has caused extensive inelasticity of the skin around the yoni, a clitorotomy may be needed in addition to defibulation. Usually after cutting you assist the baby to emerge slowly. After the birth of the baby and the placenta, and after the immediate needs of the mother and baby have been attended to, the cut edges of the scar and any other injuries must be sutured. If there is no time to discuss the procedure in detail with the woman—if, for example, she arrives and birth is imminent—make sure everything is discussed with her afterward. It is probably best to go over everything the following day, when the woman should be counseled about the procedure and the importance of not being resutured to reduce the size of the opening.

Immediate postpartum care

Immediately after the birth of the placenta and a suitable time has passed for bonding, the mother should be assessed and tears should be repaired as you would do for any woman (see HOLISTIC MIDWIFERY, VOL. II). Check for lacerations and hemorrhage from deep tears or injury to blood vessels. Suture tears or incisions immediately if they are bleeding excessively. Tears may involve the urethra and bladder anteriorly and rectum posteriorly.

In cases of type III FGM when an existing infibulation has obstructed labor, it is vital that the woman and her baby be thoroughly assessed after delivery.

Care of affected women in the days and weeks following birth

At the visits following the birth assess the mother's genitalia for bleeding, signs of infection and proper healing. Also assess the mother's psychological and emotional state.

Women with type I, II and IV FGM with no birth-related complications should be advised like any other woman. Assure her that you are available to answer questions about her own care, that of the baby or concerns about sexual matters.

Women with type III FGM/C who needed to be defibulated at the time of birth will need additional information, counseling and support to help them adapt to the changes they can expect and to discourage them from seeking reinfibulation after discharge from your care. Discuss with her the feeling of wetness and increased sensitivity in her opened vulva, which she might not have experienced before. Advise her to wear loose underwear to reduce discomfort caused by friction.

Complications may include wound infection, which may lead to delayed onset bleeding, repair breakdown or even septicemia. Urine retention may develop if the repair was not done correctly. Injury to adjacent tissues due to tears that you missed at the time of birth, that were improperly repaired or that break down may result in incontinence of urine or feces, fistulas or sexual problems.

When a woman requests reinfibulation

Women who have been defibulated may request that they be resutured after they give birth or after the complication that prompted defibulation has cleared up. You can express sincere concern regarding this decision as to the success of such a repair—avascular scar tissue is likely to heal suboptimally and is more prone to infection—and the long-term impact on her health and well-being (if defibulation was done to help clear up a condition, it could easily return after reinfibulation is performed) (Rosenberg et al., 2009). However, she should not be made to feel badly that she wants to be reinfibulated. In countries where there are laws against reinfibulation, it is relatively simple to deal with the situation, since the midwife can honestly state that the law forbids her to resuture. However, in countries where there are no such laws or where the law does not prohibit reinfibulation of adults, as is the case in the US for women 18 and older, a request for resuturing can cause a real dilemma for the care provider. In such situations the midwife should follow her own practice protocols or the guidelines of the health facility where she works. Whatever the legal status of FGM and resuturing, counseling and education are extremely important, and every effort should be made to discourage the practice of reinfibulation. If the woman insists on reinfibulation after thorough counseling and you decide to do it for her, discuss leaving the scar open enough to allow exposure of the introitus and preferably the urethra.

Keep in mind that even if the woman chooses not to be reinfibulated, this decision may place her in danger at home from a partner or family members that believe she has been corrupted by your influence or that of the dominant culture. This may result in her family forbidding her from seeking further care. Therefore it is vital to engage her family members in decisions of this type.

Counseling women regarding their daughters and FGM/C

A women with any type of FGM/C who gives birth to a baby girl should be counseled about the physical and legal consequences of allowing her daughter to be excised. The husband and other family members who may be influential in decisions about FGM/C, especially her mother and mother-in-law, should be counseled as well. Explain the local laws to them in as nonjudgmental a fashion as possible. In countries where the practice is clearly illegal, you can point out that she has chosen to come to a culture where this practice is not used and needs to respect those laws. If she is in a Western country where male circumcision is permitted, she may be confused as to why this practice is not illegal, when female excision is. You can explain that amputation of the male foreskin is a matter of great controversy, and still not viewed by some as being as harmful, as is true of female excision in her culture.

Contraceptive use in women who have had FGM/C

The only obstacle to contraceptive use occurs with those types that require insertion (intrauterine devices and barrier methods such as the diaphragm, the female condom, spermicides and the cervical cap) in women whose introitus is narrowed. To the extent that the introitus can be restored to a more normal dimension, any method that is acceptable to the woman may be used.

(Daly, 1978; Hosken, 1994; Saadawi, 1982; Shaw, 1985; Toubia, 2000)

References and Further Reading on Intimate Grooming, Body Art and Female Genital Surgery

References Used in Multiple Chapters

Chalmers B, Omer-Hashi K. Female Genital Mutilation and Obstetric Care. Trafford Pub., Victoria BC, Canada, 2003.

Rodriguez S. "Rethinking the history of female circumcision and clitoridectomy: American medicine and female sexuality in the late nineteenth century," J Hist Med Allied Sci, 63(3):323-347, Jul, 2008.

Pubic and Genital Hair Grooming Practices

Bodworx International. "Tip list for shaving your vagina hair-removal," www.hair-removal-shaver.com/shaving-tip-vagina.html, accessed Oct 28, 2008a.

Bodworx International. "Why should I shave my pubic hairs?" www.hair-removal-shaver.com/should-i-shave-my-pubic-hairs.html, Mar 12, 2008, accessed Oct 28, 2008b.

Bodworx International. "You can learn to trim pubic hair like a pro," www.hair-removal-shaver.com/trim-pubic-hair.html, accessed Oct 28, 2008c.

Carr K. "Pubic hair removal solutions: is anal hair naturally normal for men than women," www.buzzle.com/articles/pubic-hair-removal-solutions-is-anal-hair-naturally-normal-for-men-than-women.html, Sep 1, 2008, accessed Oct 28, 2008.

Jones M. "Pubic hair shaving tips," www.buzzle.com/articles/pubic-hair-shaving-tips.html, Mar 12, 2008, accessed Oct 28, 2008.

Williams N. "How do I get rid of ingrown hairs in pubic region?" www.buzzle.com/articles/how-do-i-get-rid-of-ingrown-hairs-in-pubic-region.html, May 24, 2007, accessed Oct 28, 2008a.

Williams N. HairRemovalHaven.com, www.HairRemovalHaven.com, Jun 2, 2007, accessed Oct 28, 2008b.

Williams N. "How to select the right solution for the removal of pubic hair," www.buzzle.com/articles/how-to-select-the-right-solution-for-the-removal-of-pubic-hair.html, Jun 14, 2007, accessed Oct 28, 2008c.

Williams N. "Hair removal for genitals: how to choose the right solution," www.buzzle.com/articles/hair-removal-for-genitals-how-to-choose-the-right-solution.html, Jul 11, 2007, accessed Oct 28, 2008d.

Intimate Piercings and Tattoos

American Pregnancy Association. "Body piercing during pregnancy," www.Americanpregnancy.org/pregnancyhealth/bodypiercingduring.htm, 2007, accessed Sep 11, 2008.

Anderson W, et al. "The urologist's guide to genital piercing," BJU Int, 91(3):245-251, Feb, 2003.

Armstrong, M. "Tattooing, body piercing, and permanent cosmetics: a historical and current view of state regulations, with continuing concern," J Environ Health, 67(8):38-43, Apr, 2005.

Armstrong M, et al. "Genital piercings: what is known and what people with genital piercings tell us," Urologic Nursing, 26(3):173-179, Jun, 2006a.

Armstrong M, et al. "Pregnancy, lactation, and nipple piercings," AHWONN Lifelines, 10(3):212-217, Jun-Jul, 2006b.

Armstrong M, et al. "Toward building a composite of college student influences with body art," Issues in Compr Pediatr Nurs, 27(4):277-285, Oct-Dec, 2004.

Caliendo C, et al. "Self-reported characteristics of women and men with intimate body piercings," J Advanced Nursing, 49(5):474-484, Mar, 2005.

Carroll S, et al. "Tattoos and body piercings as indicators of adolescent risk-taking behaviors," Pediatrics, 109(6):1021-1027, Jun, 2002. (Comment in Pediatr 111[5, Pt 1]:1126, May, 2003; author reply, 1126.)

DeBoer D, et al. "Managing body jewelry in emergency situations: misconceptions, patient care and removal techniques," J Emerg Nurs, 32(2):159-164, Apr, 2006.

Earth's Magic, Inc. "Will having a tattoo affect my pregnancy?" http://tinyurl.com/m4uwsn. Accessed Sep 17, 2008.

Halliday K. "Body piercing: issues and challenges for nurses," J Forensic Nurs, 1(2):47-56, Sum, 2005.

Harris Poll. "Three in ten Americans with a tattoo say having one make them feel sexier,"No. 15, http://www.tinyurl.com/2dp911, Feb 12, 2008. Accessed Aug 25, 2009.

Meyer, D. "Body piercing: old traditions creating new challenges," J Emerg Nurs, 26(6): 612-614, Dec, 2000.

Miller L, Edenholm M. "Genital piercing to enhance sexual satisfaction," Obstet Gynecol, 93(5, Pt 2):837, May, 1999.

Pokorney C. Berg R. Body Art: A Comprehensive Guidebook and Model Code. National Environmental Health Association, Denver CO, 1999.

Stirn A. "Body piercing: medical consequences and psychological motivations," Lancet, 361(9364):1205-1215, Apr 5, 2003. (Comment in Lancet , 361(9376):2250, Jun 28, 2003).

Teshima-Miller L. "rec.arts.bodyart ___*Frequently asked questions (FAQ)," Usenet rec.arts.bodyart, www.faqs.org/faqs/bodyart/1997. Accessed Sep 17, 2008.

Willmott F. "Body piercing: lifestyle indicator or fashion accessory?" Int J STD AIDS, 12(6):358-360, Jun, 2001.

Wikipedia contributors. "Tattoo." Wikipedia, the Free Encyclopedia, http://en.wikipedia.org/wiki/Tattoo, last updated and accessed Aug 25, 2009.

Young C, Armstrong M. "What nurses need to know when caring for women with genital piercings," Nurs Womens Health, 12(2):129-138, Apr-May, 2008.

Clitorotomy ("Episiotomy")

Anderson M. "Principles of wound healing in the repair of the episiotomy" (unpublished paper), Hawthorne NY, 1975.

Andrews V, et al. "Occult anal sphincter injuries—myth or reality?" Br J Obstet Gynaecol, 113(2):195-200, Feb, 2006.

Andrews V, et al. "Are mediolateral episiotomies actually mediolateral?" Br J Obstet Gynaecol, 112(8):1156-1158, Aug, 2005.

Banta D, Thacher S. "The risks and benefits of episiotomy," Women & Health, 7(3-4):165, Fall-Win, 1982.

Barrett J, et al. "The effect of type of delivery on neonatal outcome in singleton infants of birth weight of 1000 g or less," JAMA, 250(5):625-629, Aug 5, 1983.

Carroli G, Belizan J. "Episiotomy for vaginal birth," Cochrane Database Syst Rev. (2):CD000081, 2000.

Carroli G, Mignini L. "Episiotomy for vaginal birth," Cochrane Database Syst Rev. (1):CD000081, Jan 21, 2009.

Cassidy-Brinn G, et al. Woman-Centered Pregnancy and Birth. Cleis Press, Pittsburgh PA, 1984.

Chaliha C. "Anal function: effect of pregnancy and delivery," Am J Obstet Gynecol, 185(2):427-432, Aug, 2001.

Chalmers I. Effective Care during Pregnancy and Birth, Vol 2: Childbirth. Oxford U Press, New York NY, 1989.

Childbirth Graphics. Slides: "The effect of giving birth on the muscles of the pelvic floor and episiotomy anatomy," Childbirth Graphics, Rochester NY, 1987.

Clark-Collar T, CNM. Editing comments, Spr, 1990.

DeLancey J. "Episiotomy: what's the angle?" Int J Gynaecol Obstet 103(1):3-4, Oct, 2008.

DeLancey J, et al. "Internal and external anal sphincter anatomy as it relates to midline obstetric lacerations," Obstet Gynecol, 90(6):924-927, Dec, 1997.

Downer C, et al., eds. A New View of a Woman's Body: A Fully Illustrated Guide by the Federation of Feminist Women's Health Centers. Feminist Health Press, Los Angeles CA, 1991.

Eogan M, et al. "Does the angle of episiotomy affect the incidence of anal sphincter injury?" Br J Obstet Gynaecol, 113:190-194, 2006.

Fenner D, et al. "Fecal and urinary incontinence after vaginal delivery with anal sphincter disruption in an obstetrics unit in the United States," Am J Obstet Gynecol, 189(6):1543-1549 (Discussion, 1549-1550), Dec, 2003.

Formato LS. "Routine episiotomy: is it always necessary?" J. Nurse-Midwifery, 30(3): 144-148, May-Jun, 1985.

Fornell EU, et al. "Obstetric anal sphincter injury ten years after: subjective and objective long term effects," Br J Obstet Gynaecol, 112(3):312-316, Mar, 2005.

Fritsch H, et al. "Anal sphincter complex: reinterpreted morphology and its clinical relevance," DIS COLON RECTUM, 45(2):188-194, Feb, 2002.
Frudinger A, et al. "Changes in anal anatomy following vaginal delivery revealed by anal endosonography," BR J OBSTET GYNECOL,106(3):233-237, Mar, 1999.
Fynes M, et al. Chapter 4: "Childbirth and pelvic floor injury," in Pemberton J, et al., eds. THE PELVIC FLOOR: ITS FUNCTION AND DISORDERS, WB Saunders, London UK, 2002.
Gainey H. "Postpartum observation of pelvic tissue damage: further studies," AM J OBSTET GYNECOL, 70(4):800-807, Oct, 1955.
Gainey H. "Postpartum observation of pelvic tissue damage," AM J OBSTET GYNECOL, 45:457-466, 1943.
Gaskin IM. Informal video presentation on breech births, MANA conference, Kansas City MO, Nov, 1990.
Gibb D. Chapter 5: "Operative obstetrics," in Maxwell D, ed. SURGICAL TECHNIQUES IN OBSTETRICS AND GYNECOLOGY. Churchill Livingstone, New York NY, 2004.
Goldberg R. Chapter 3: "Effects of pregnancy and childbirth on the pelvic floor," in Culligan P, Goldberg R, eds. UROGYNECOLOGY IN PRIMARY CARE. Springer-Verlag, London UK, 2007.
Graham I. EPISIOTOMY: CHALLENGING OBSTETRIC INTERVENTIONS. Blackwell Press, Oxford UK, 1997.
Graham I, Davies C. Chapter 5: "Episiotomy: the unkindest cut that persists," in Henderson C, Bick D, eds. PERINEAL CARE: AN INTERNATIONAL ISSUE. MA Healthcare Ltd., London UK, 2006.
Graham I, et al. "Episiotomy rates around the world: an update," BIRTH, 32(3):219-223, Sep, 2005.
Hale R, Ling F. EPISIOTOMY: PROCEDURE AND REPAIR TECHNIQUES. American College of Obstetricians and Gynecologists, Washington DC, 2007.
Hartmann K, et al. "Outcomes of routine episiotomy: a systematic review," JAMA, 293(17):2141-2148, May 4, 2005.
Henderson C, Bick D, eds. PERINEAL CARE: AN INTERNATIONAL ISSUE. Quay Books, London UK, 2005.
Kalis V, et al. "The incision angle before and after repair of mediolateral episiotomy," INT J GYNAECOL OBSTET 103(1):5-8, Oct, 2008a.
Kalis V, et al. "One Europe . . . how many definitions of mediolateral episiotomy," www.ics office.org/publications/2007/pdf/0274.pdf, accessed Mar 7, 2008b.
Kalis V, et al. "The perineal body length and injury at delivery" (article in Czech), CESKA GYNEKOL, 70(5): 355-361, Sep, 2005.
Kandall C, MD. Conversation regarding cutting the hymen to reduce ragged tearing, Apr 9, 1990.
Kirk R. BASIC SURGICAL TECHNIQUES, 5th ed. Churchill Livingstone, London UK, 2002.
Kitzinger S. "Episiotomy," MOTHERING, (55):62-65, Apr-May-Jun, 1990.
Kitzinger S, Simpkin P, eds. EPISIOTOMY AND THE SECOND STAGE OF LABOR. Pennypress, Seattle WA, 1984.
Kolder V, MD. Editing comments, 1990.
Kudish B, et al. "Operative vaginal delivery and midline episiotomy: a bad combination for the perineum," AM J OBSTET GYNECOL,195(3):749-754, 2006.
Lieberman A. "Must you have an episiotomy?" AMERICAN BABY, 30, 35, Feb, 1989.
Mahony R, et al. "Internal anal sphincter defect influences continence outcome following obstetric anal sphincter injury," AM J OBSTET GYNECOL, www.ajog.org, 217.el-217.e5, Mar, 2007, accessed Mar 2007.
McCutcheon-Rosegg S. NATURAL CHILDBIRTH THE BRADLEY WAY. Penguin, New York NY, 1984.
Nager CW, Helliwell JP. "Episiotomy increases perineal laceration length in primiparous women," AM J OBSTET GYNECOL,185(2):444-450, Aug, 2001.
Nisbet M, Brown R. PERINEAL REPAIR. Davis and Geck, Cyanamid Australia, 1992.
Nygaard I, et al. "Anal incontinence after anal sphincter disruption: a 30-year retrospective cohort study," OBSTET GYNECOL, 89(6):896-901, Jun, 1997.
OGCCU, Clinical Guidelines: Section B: 5.9.4.4. "Infiltration of the perineum and cutting an episiotomy," revised ed. King Edward Memorial Hospital, Perth Western Australia, Apr, 2005.
O'Leary JL, O'Leary JA. "The complete episiotomy: analysis of 1224 complete lacerations, sphincter-otomies, and episiproctotomies," OBSTET GYENCOL, 25(2):235-240, Feb, 1965.
Ould F. TREATISE OF MIDWIFERY IN THREE PARTS. Facsimile reprint. Gryphon Editions, Classics in Obstetrics and Gynecology Library, New York NY [1742] 1990.
Owen J, Hauth J. "Episiotomy infection and dehiscence." in Gilstrap L, Faro S, eds. INFECTIONS IN PREGNANCY. Alan R. Liss, New York NY, 1990.

Parker L, Brunner J. Chapter 32: "Gynecologic surgery for obstetric patients," in Rock J, Jones H, eds. TE LINDE'S OPERATIVE GYNECOLOGY, 9th ed. Lippincott, Williams & Wilkins, Philadelphia PA, 2003.
Perinatal Education programme, Skills workshop 9: "Performing and repairing an episiotomy," Perinatal Education Trust, South Africa, Jan 2006, www.gfmer.ch/PEP/pdf-MCM-2006/MCM_SW-9-2006.pdf, Aug 31, 2007.
Peyton V. Chapter 20: "Episiotomy and Obstetrics Tears," in Lynge C, et al., eds. 20 COMMON PROBLEMS: SURGICAL PROBLEMS AND PROCEDURES IN PRIMARY CARE. McGraw-Hill Pro., New York, NY, 2001.
Philipson E, et al. "Maternal, fetal, and neonatal lidocaine levels following local perineal infiltration," AM J OBSTET GYNECOL, 149(4):403-407, Jun 15, 1984.
Ranney B. "Decreasing numbers of patients for vaginal hysterectomy and plasty," SD J MED, 43(7)7-12, Jul, 1990.
Robinson P, Beattie P. "Perineal anatomy and episiotomy," N Z MED J, 115(1150):144, Mar 22, 2002.
Rogers R, et al. "Obstetric anal sphincter lacerations: an evidence-based approach, Part 1: anatomy and risk factors," FEMALE PATIENT, 27(4):21-24, Apr, 2002.
Sartore A, et al. "The effects of mediolateral episiotomy on pelvic floor function after vaginal delivery," OBSTET GYNECOL, 103(4):669-673, Apr, 2004.
Schuchardt K. "Eine neue Methode der Gebärmutterexstirpation" (article in German), CENTRALBL F CHIR, 20:1121-1126, 1893.
Shafik A, et al. "A novel concept for the surgical anatomy of the perineal body," DIS COLON RECTUM, 50(12):2120-2125, Dec, 2007a.
Shafik A, et al. "Physioanatomical relationship of the external anal sphincter to the bulbocavernosus muscle in the female," INT UROGYNECOL J, 18(8):851-856, Aug, 2007b.
Shafik A, et al. "Surgical anatomy of the perineal muscles and their role in perineal disorders," ANAT SCI INTERNAT, 80(3):167-171, Sep, 2005.
Shiono P, et al. "Midline episiotomies: more harm than good?" OBSTET GYNECOL, 75(5):765-770, May, 1990.
Shute W. "Episiotomy: a physiologic appraisal and a new painless technic," 14:467-472, Oct, 1959.
Sooklim R, et al. "The outcomes of midline versus medio-lateral episiotomy," REPROD HEALTH, 4:10, Oct 29, 2007.
Sorger L, MD. Editing comments, Feb, 1991.
Stepán J, et al. "How exact is the performance of mediolateral episiotomy?" (article in Czech), CESKA GYNEKOL, 72(6):381-385, Dec, 2007.
Sultan AH. "Obstetric perineal injury and anal incontinence," CLINICAL RISK, 5:193-196, 1999.
Thacker S. "Midline versus mediolateral episiotomies," BMJ, 320(7250):1615-1616, Jun 17, 2000.
Thorpe JM, et al. "Selected use of midline episiotomy: effect on perineal trauma," OBSTET GYNECOL, 70(2): 260-262, Aug, 1987.
Varney H, et al. Chapter 79: "Cutting an episiotomy and repairing episiotomies and lacerations," VARNEY'S MIDWIFERY, 4th ed. Jones & Bartlett, Sudbury MA, 2004.
Verspyck E, et al. "Episiotomy techniques" (article in French), J GYNECOL OBSTET BIOL REPROD (PARIS), 35 (Suppl. 1):1S40-1S51, Feb, 2006.
Viswanathan M, et al. THE USE OF EPISIOTOMY IN OBSTETRICAL CARE: A SYSTEMATIC REVIEW. Evidence Report/Technology Assessment No. 112. (Prepared by the RTI-UNC Evidence-Based Practice Center, under Contract No. 290-02-0016.) AHRQ Publication No. 05-E009-2. Agency for Healthcare Research and Quality, Rockville MD, May, 2005.
Way S. "Social construction of episiotomy," J CLIN NURS, 7(2):113-117, Mar, 1998.
Wheeless C. "Guest editorial: ten steps to avoid fecal incontinence secondary to fourth-degree obstetrical tear," OBSTET GYNECOL SUR, 53(3):131-132, 1998.

Female Genital Cosmetic Surgery in Developed Nations

ABC News. "Demand for 'designer vagina' Surgery Rising in UK," May 25, 2007.
American College of Obstetrics and Gynecology (ACOG). Committee Opinion No. 378: "Vaginal 'rejuvenation' and cosmetic vaginal procedures," OBSTET GYNECOL, 110(3):737-738, Sep, 2007.

Cosmetic Surgery. "Cosmetic surgery of the female genitalia," www.cosmeticsurgery2.com/cs-female1.htm. Accessed Mar 17, 2009.

LabiaplastySurgeon.com. www.labiaplastysurgeon.com/, accessed Mar 17, 2009.

Maas S, et al. "Functional and aesthetic labia minora reduction," PLASTIC RECONSTRUCTIVE SURG, 105(4):1453-1456, Apr, 2000.

Munhoz A, et al. "Aesthetic labia minora reduction with inferior wedge resection and superior pedicle flap reconstruction," PLASTIC RECONSTRUCTIVE SURG, 118(5):1237- 1247, Oct, 2006.

Ollivier D. "Designer vaginas," www.salon.com, Nov 14, 2000.

Wikipedia contributors. "Vaginoplasty." WIKIPEDIA, THE FREE ENCYCLOPEDIA, http://en.wikipedia.org/w/index.php?title=Vaginoplasty&oldid=277796242, accessed Mar 17, 2009.

Women's Health News. "Vaginal 'rejuvenation' not safe or necessary," http://womenshealthnews.wordpress.com/2007/08/31/vaginal-rejuvenation-not-proven-safe-or-necessary/, accessed Mar 17, 2009.

TRADITIONAL FEMALE GENITAL MODIFICATIONS

Arbour L, et al., eds. ELIMINATING FEMALE GENITAL MUTILATION: AN INTERAGENCY STATEMENT UNAIDS, UNDP, UNECA, UNESCO, UNFPA, UNHCHR, UNHCR, UNICEF, UNIFEM, WHO. World Health Organization, Geneva Switzerland, 2008.

Bagnol B, Mariano E. "Elongation of the labia minora and use of vaginal products to enhance eroticism: can these practices be considered FGM?" FJEM, 3(2):43-53, 2008.

Banks E, et al. "Female genital mutilation and obstetric outcome: WHO collaborative prospective study in six African countries," LANCET, 367(9525):1835-1841, Jun 3, 2006.

Barber G, ed. FEMALE GENITAL MUTILATION: AN RCN EDUCATIONAL RESOURCE FOR NURSING AND MIDWIFERY STAFF. Royal College of Nursing, London, UK, 2006.

Budiharsana M. FEMALE CIRCUMCISION IN INDONESIA: EXTENT, IMPLICATIONS AND POSSIBLE INTERVENTIONS TO UPHOLD WOMEN'S HEALTH RIGHTS. Population Council, Jakarta Indonesia, 2004.

Daly M. GYN/ECOLOGY: THE METAETHICS OF RADICAL FEMINISM. Beacon Press, Boston MA, 1978.

Daniels S, midwife. Conversation regarding clitoridectomy, MANA conference, El Paso, TX, 1991.

Hosken F. THE HOSKEN REPORT: GENITAL AND SEXUAL MUTILATION OF FEMALES, 4th ed. Women's International Network News, Lexington MA, 1993.

Hosken F. "Female genital mutilation," WOMAN OF POWER, 18:42-45, Fall, 1990.

Huelsman B. Chapter 10: "An anthropological view of clitoral and other female genital mutilations," in Lowry TP, Lowry TS. THE CLITORIS. Warren Green, St. Louis MO, 1976.

Huston P. FEMALE GENITAL MUTILATION AND HEALTH CARE: CURRENT SITUATION AND LEGAL STATUS, RECOMMENDATIONS TO IMPROVE THE HEALTH CARE OF AFFECTED WOMEN. Women's Health Bureau, Health Canada, Winnipeg MB Canada, Fall, 2000.

International Confederation of Midwives. "Position statement: female genital mutilation," The Hague, The Netherlands, adopted at Counsel meeting, Brisbane Australia, Jun, 2005.

Jenkins G, Nanayakkara S. "Female genital mutilation," O & G MAG, 10(2):29-32, Win, 2008.

Lightfoot-Klein H, Shaw E. "Special needs of ritually circumcised women patients," JOGNN, 20(2):102-107, Mar-Apr, 1991.

Lovel H, et al. A systematic review of the health complications of female genital mutilation including sequelae in childbirth," World Health Organization, Geneva Switzerland, 2000.

McCaffrey M. "Female genital mutilation: consequences for reproductive and sexual health," SEX MARITAL THER, 10(2):189-200, Apr, 1995.

Momoh C, O'Donnell S. Position paper no. 21: "Female genital mutilation (female circumcision)," Royal College of Midwives, London UK, Jun, 1998.

Mwenda KK. "Labia elongation under African customary law: a violation of women's rights?" INTERNAT J HUMAN RIGHTS, 10:341-357, 2006.

Newland L. "Female circumcision: Muslim identities and zero tolerance policies in rural West Java," WOMEN'S STUDIES INTERNATIONAL FORUM, 29:394-404, 2006.

Njue C, Askew I. "Medicalization of female genital cutting among the Abagusii in Nyanza Province, Kenya," Population Council Frontiers in Reproductive Health, Washington DC, 2004.

Nour NM, et al. "Defibulation to treat female genital cutting. Effect on symptoms and sexual function," OBSTET GYNECOL, 108(1):55-60, Jul, 2006.

Rahman A, Toubia N. FEMALE GENITAL MUTILATION: A GUIDE TO LAWS AND POLICIES WORLDWIDE. Zed Books, New York NY, 2000.

Reproductive Rights Organization. "Fact sheet: female genital mutilation (FGM): legal prohibitions worldwide," www.reproductiverights.org/pdf/pub_fac_fgm_1.08.pdf, accessed Sep 6, 2008.

Rosenberg L, et al. "When cultures collide: female genital cutting and US obstetric practice," OBSTET GYN, 113(4):931-934, Apr, 2009.

Saadawi N, El. THE HIDDEN FACE OF EVE: WOMEN IN THE ARAB WORLD. Beacon Press, Boston MA, 1982.

Satti A, et al. "Prevalence and determinants of the practice of genital mutilation of girls in Khartoum, Sudan," ANNALS OF TROP PAEDIATR, 26(4):303-310, Dec, 2006.

Shandall A, et al. "Circumcision and infibulation of females: a general consideration of the problem and a clinical study of the complications in Sudanese women," SUDAN MED J, 5(4):178-212, 1967.

Shaw E. "Female circumcision: what kind of maternity care do circumcised women need and can US caregivers provide it?" AM J NURS, 85(6):685-687, Jun, 1985.

Sheehan E. "Victorian clitoridectomy: Isaac Baker Brown and his harmless operative procedure," MED ANTHROPOL NEWSL, 12(4):9-15, Aug, 1981.

Tamale S. "Eroticism, sensuality and 'women's secrets' among the Baganda," INSTITUTE OF DEVELOPMENT STUDIES BULLETIN, 37:89-97, 2006.

Thabet SM, Thabet AS. "Defective sexuality and female circumcision: the cause and the possible management," J OBSTET GYNAECOL RES, 29(1):12-19, Feb, 2003.

Toubia N. CARING FOR WOMEN WITH CIRCUMCISION: A TECHNICAL MANUAL FOR HEALTH CARE PROVIDERS. Rainbow Publications, New York NY, 2000.

Toubia N, Sharief EH. "Female genital mutilation: have we made progress?" INTERNATIONAL J GYNECOL OBSTET, 82:251-261, 2003.

UNICEF. "Female genital mutilation/female genital cutting: a statistical report," UNICEF, New York NY, 2005a.

UNICEF. "Changing a harmful social convention: female genital mutilation/cutting," INNOCENTI DIGEST, UNICEF, Florence Italy, 2005b.

Walker A, Parmar P. WARRIOR MARKS: FEMALE GENITAL MUTILATION AND THE SEXUAL BINDING OF WOMEN. Harcourt Brace & Co., San Diego CA, 1996.

Womenshealth.gov. "Female genital cutting," www.womenshealth.gov. Accessed Sep 6, 2008.

World Health Organization. ELIMINATING FEMALE GENITAL MUTILATION: AN INTERAGENCY APPROACH. WHO Press, Geneva, Switzerland, 2008.

World Health Organization. FEMALE GENITAL MUTILATION: INTEGRATING THE PREVENTION AND THE MANAGEMENT OF THE HEALTH COMPLICATIONS INTO THE CURRICULA OF NURSING AND MIDWIFERY, A TEACHER'S GUIDE. World Health Organization, Geneva Switzerland, WHO/RHR/01.16, 2001a.

World Health Organization. FEMALE GENITAL MUTILATION: INTEGRATING THE PREVENTION AND THE MANAGEMENT OF THE HEALTH COMPLICATIONS INTO THE CURRICULA OF NURSING AND MIDWIFERY, A STUDENT'S MANUAL. World Health Organization, Geneva Switzerland, WHO/RHR/01.17, 2001b.

World Health Organization. FEMALE GENITAL MUTILATION: THE PREVENTION AND THE MANAGEMENT OF THE HEALTH COMPLICATIONS, POLICY GUIDELINES FOR NURSES AND MIDWIVES. World Health Organization. Geneva Switzerland, WHO/RHR/01.18, 2001c.

World Health Organization. FEMALE GENITAL MUTILATION: A JOINT WHO/UNICEF/UNFPA STATEMENT. World Health Organization, Office of Pub., Geneva Switzerland, 1997.

Yoder P, Khan S. "Numbers of women circumcised in Africa: the production of a total," DHS Working Papers series, Marco International, Calverton MD, Mar, 2008.

Yoder P, Mahy M. "Female genital cutting in Guinea: qualitative and quantitative research strategies," (DHS Analytical Studies No 5), Macro International Inc., Calverton MD, 2001.

NOTES:

SURGICAL TOOLS, EQUIPMENT AND RELATED SUPPLIES

SELECTING SUTURING TOOLS, RELATED SUPPLIES AND EQUIPMENT

The Importance of Quality Tools

Even though you may be a student currently, I strongly encourage you to invest in the best equipment you can possibly afford. Buying cheap equipment is false economy. If you buy high-quality needle holders and scissors from the start, the stainless will be fine enough to minimize rusting, the hinges will work better, and the total construction will be more precise. Plus, you won't wind up having to replace poorer-quality equipment, which will eventually result in your spending what you might have spent on one good instrument in the first place.

Your needle holder, suture scissors and cord scissors should be the very best quality, since they are probably your most-used pieces of equipment. A good needle holder will probably be your most expensive instrument. A cheap needle holder will not hold needles with great reliability, a shortcoming that is especially irritating when you are just beginning to learn. Students, feeling a better piece of equipment is an unjustified expense since they aren't "really using it yet," often make the misguided cheaper choice. Midwives who anticipate suturing only occasionally will often purchase cheaper needle holders too. I urge you not to make this mistake. Students will learn faster and with less frustration when using good tools. Also, the less you suture, the more crucial it is to have a needle holder that will perform reliability. With infrequently used instruments, such as Allis clamps and ring forceps, you can get by with equipment of lesser quality; if properly maintained, it last a very long time.

Left-Hand–Dominant Equipment

Surgical instruments are typically designed for those who are right-hand dominant. A few instruments, such as tweezer-type forceps, are designed for use by either hand with equal grace. Cutting with right-handed scissors, however, may be especially problematic if you are left-handed. Left-handed scissors were more widely manufactured years ago, but casting dies wore out, manufacturers were disinclined to make new dies and mass production largely fell by the wayside. As of this writing, it appears that the availability of left-handed instruments has improved somewhat, although they are still not available in all styles of instruments.

In the United States, V. Mueller and Snowden-Pencer (both part of CardinalHealth, [www.cardinal.com]) offer some styles of high-quality needle holders and a few scissors for left-handed persons. Although left-handed instruments tend to be expensive, they are well worth the money if you can afford them. One of these fine tools, properly cared for, should last throughout your career. Call Cascade HealthCare Products to special order these instruments. Details regarding left-handed instruments are given in the descriptions that follow. Otherwise, lefties are just going to have to learn to use right-handed instruments.

Surgical Instruments for Suturing

Now let's demystify the tools used for suturing and related activities. Some are important, while others are nice to have but not essential. If you look at an instrument catalogue, hundreds of tools may be listed, all named after a doctor or procedure but with hardly any information about their intended use. This text will fill in some of those gaps. Once you have an idea of what you want, go window-shopping at a surgical supply store (if there is a large one in your area), examine another midwife's instruments, peruse catalogues or have a sales representative show a group of midwives some basic instruments in different styles and sizes to get an idea of what will work best for you before you invest.

Even the least expensive surgical instruments are, relatively speaking, well-made tools. They require the skilled work of an instrument craftsperson. The production of a single instrument can take up to six weeks. The cheapest instruments are usually made in Pakistan. Most of them have a mirror finish and are intended to be disposable or semi-disposable. Surgical-grade instruments are also made in Pakistan as well as Germany, Malaysia, Hungary, the United States and Poland. They typically have a matte or satin finish and are usually backed with a lifetime warranty. High-quality tools are marked with the company name, part number and country of origin. New instruments have a flawless feel, although hinges may feel stiff at first.

Needle holders (drivers)

Needle holders have specialized jaws that can be locked together. The jaws of most needle holders have crisscrossed serrations on each inner surface, and some also have a small oblong cut-out. Both features enable them to hold a needle very securely. Between the finger holes, a locking mechanism called a **ratchet** clamps the jaws together to maintain a secure grip on the needle without any effort from you. Hemostats are not designed to hold a needle and make a poor substitute; don't aggravate yourself by trying to learn with one.

Ordinary stainless steel is a poor choice for jaw material because the needles are harder than it is and the teeth wear quickly; for this reason the jaws are usually made of specially processed metal. Snowden-Pencer, V. Mueller and Miltex (Carb-N-Sert), among others, have some needle holders with tungsten carbide inserts made from prehardened metal. Tungsten carbide jaws have sharp, precise serrations that hold the needle without slipping and are distinguished by gold-plated shanks and finger rings. These carbide inserts can be replaced if worn out, but a midwife in a small practice should never have to go to this expense as these fine instruments should last a lifetime. Miltex and others chamfer, or bevel, the edges of these super-hard jaws to prevent them from accidently severing suture material when it comes in contact with the edges. Expect to pay at least $125 to $150 (US) for one of these fine-quality needle holders. You won't regret it.

Miltex also offers a less-expensive line of needle holders with Ceram-A-Grip® jaws, a technology originally developed for the aerospace industry. This unique, extremely durable ceramic material improves the gripping power of the instrument. It is fused to the stainless steel jaws of the needle holder. These premium needle holders outperform standard stainless steel patterns and provide many of the same benefits of a tungsten carbide insert, but at a lower cost. Their finger rings are green.

Needle holders come in various sizes to match the size of the needles being used. The styles mentioned here are suitable for use with the needles typically employed for perineal repair.

Olsen Hegar needle holders have a combination jaw that incorporates a small pair of scissors. Designed for surgery requiring many interrupted stitches, they are a poor choice for perineal repair because it usually requires continuous stitches, and a combined scissor–needle holder increases the likelihood of accidently cutting the wrong segment of the strand (especially when you are first learning).

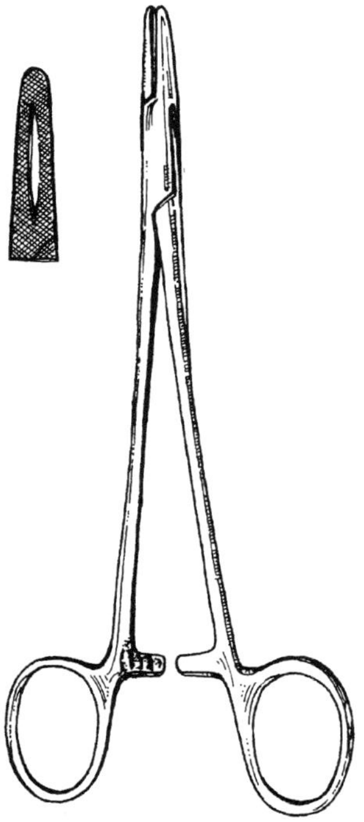

Mayo-Hegar needle holder

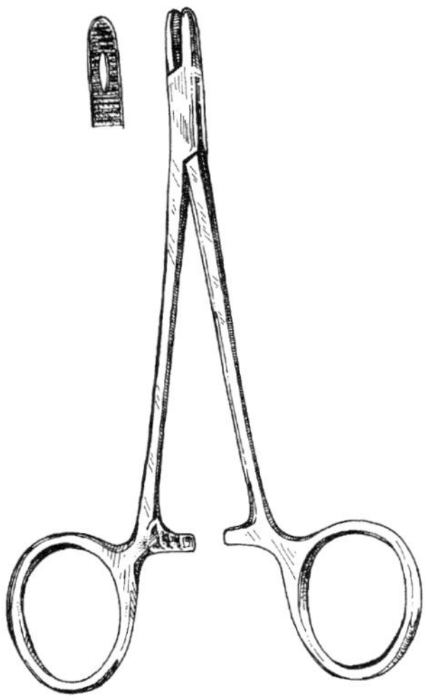

Derf needle holder

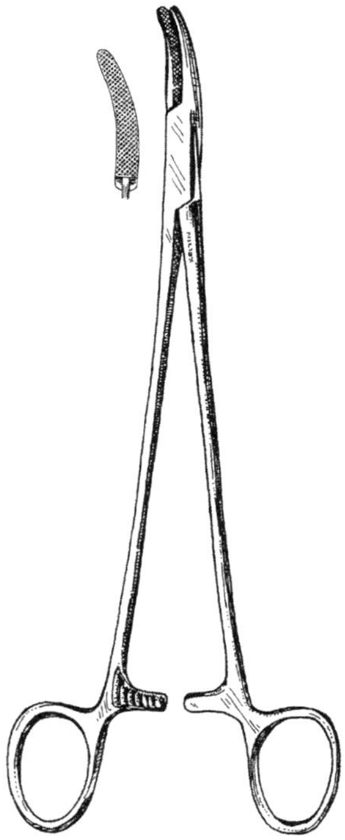

Heaney needle holder

A 6 to 8 inch long **Mayo-Hegar** style is a good, all-purpose needle holder. Longer instruments are designed primarily for other types of surgical applications and will get in your way during perineal repair. Instruments that are too short, however, will make maneuvering in deep or tight spaces awkward. Mayo-Hegar needle holders with serrated jaws are available from V. Mueller and Snowden-Pencer in left-handed models.

The **Baumgartner** is a smaller version of the Mayo-Hegar and is an ideal second needle holder when using finer needles during labial repairs. The **Derf** is an even more delicate tool and makes another good choice for fine work. A 5" **Halsey** with serrated jaws is available from V. Mueller and Snowden-Pencer in a left-handed model (CardinalHealth Cat. No. OP7513-001) and is very similar to the Derf and Baumgartner needle holders.

Some repairs require putting the needle in the jaws at an angle, as is the case when suturing in the bottom of a deep wound. A good-quality needle holder with tungsten carbide jaws will usually hold a needle at an angle without slipping. The **Heaney needle holder**, however, has curved jaws that allow you to place the needle in the jaws perpendicular to the shaft, which is the most stable way to grip the needle, thus making it easier to perform some types of repairs that require inserting the needle into the tissue at an odd angle.

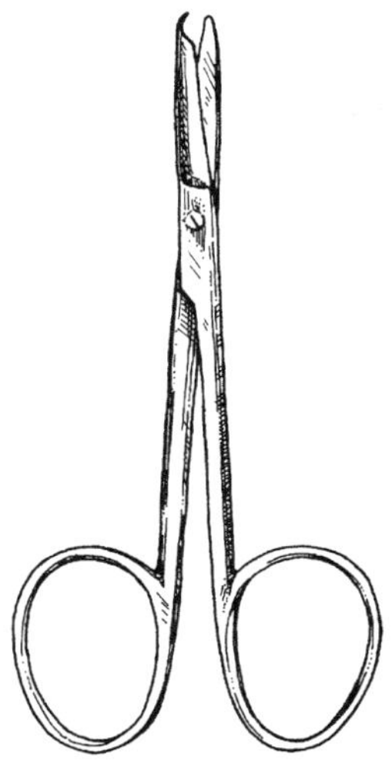

Spencer delicate stitch scissors

Stitch scissors

If you can afford it, also invest in a pair of stitch (hook) scissors that have one blade with a C-shaped cut-out (called a "notched blade") to help isolate and hold a single strand in place so it can be cut.

Spencer delicate stitch scissors are an excellent size. Alternately, you might prefer to use scissors with angled blades, which allow better visualization for cutting in tight places. I could not find left-handed stitch scissors available anywhere.

Operating (OR) scissors (nurse's scissor; straight bladed suture scissor): These scissors come in several styles. **Sharp/blunt scissors** have a sharp-tipped point on one blade and a rounded tip on the other. **Blunt/blunt scissors** have two straight blades with rounded tips. Either can be used to cut a clitorotomy. Blunt ends help avoid inadvertent tissue damage when the midwife cannot see both tips. They can also be used for trimming skin tags, opening inclusion cysts or cutting treads during suturing.

Most scissors are made entirely of stainless steel and cut by a crushing action. Micro grind or Supercut™ (Miltex) scissors have a top blade that is razor sharp and a lower blade that has a very finely serrated edge to grip the tissue while the top blade slices through it. This feature is identified by black shanks and finger rings. These scissors are super sharp when new but lose their edge rapidly and must be sharpened frequently (three to four times yearly in hospital settings). Some scissors have a tungsten carbide cutting-edge inserts welded or vacuum-brazed to the blades. These super-hard inserts stay sharper longer, but cannot be replaced once they have been worn down. Such scissors are designated by gold plating on the rings and shanks.

Extremely sharp scissors will cut through tissue so easily it can pose the risk of cutting too deeply, so be careful. They should never be used to cut the umbilical cord because using a duller blade with a crushing action promotes hemostasis. A pair of good-quality scissors with regular cutting blades is adequate for most midwifery applications.

Left-handed midwives can obtain **Mayo dissecting scissors** (CardinalHealth Cat. No. SU1801-001) from V. Mueller Instruments. These scissors have blunt/blunt blades and are suitable for trimming suture, removing skin tags and performing the rare clitorotomy. For less expensive alternatives, check out offerings through hairdresser supply houses and left-handed specialty stores on the web. Any pair of small, well-made stainless steel (the best choice) or chrome (if you can't find anything else) scissors could be used to trim suture. You might have to replace them more often, but they won't be nearly as expensive as left-handed surgical scissors. (See, for example [www.anythingleft-handed.co.uk] and [www.heim erdingercultlery. com]).

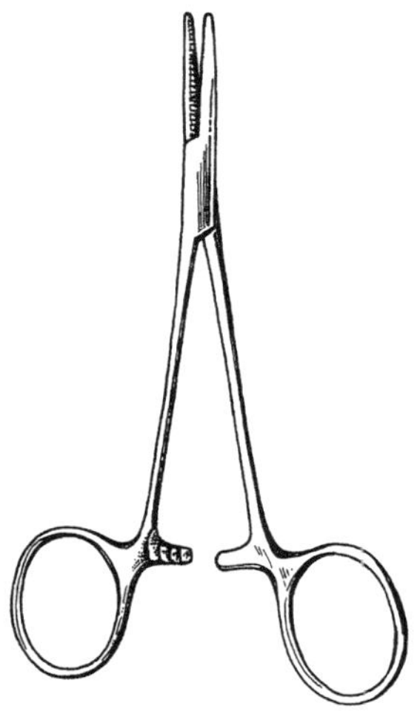
Halsted mosquito forceps

Hemostats: These clamps have long, flat, serrated jaws and a ratchet between the finger holes and come in many different styles. The relatively small **Halsted mosquito forceps** or any similar style without teeth at the tip can be used to clamp off a bleeding blood vessel as you prepare to ligate it. Some sort of hemostat is also needed for third- and fourth-degree repairs (you'll need four). Don't buy them too short or the rings will get in your way during repairs; you want them to be at least 5" long.

Thumb forceps (dressing forceps/ tissue forceps)

Tweezer-style forceps are often generically referred to as "thumb forceps" because of the way they are manipulated. These types of forceps, used as an extension of your nondominant hand, keep your fingers away from the needle and thereby allow you to avoid puncture injuries. These nonlocking clamps are available in a variety of styles.

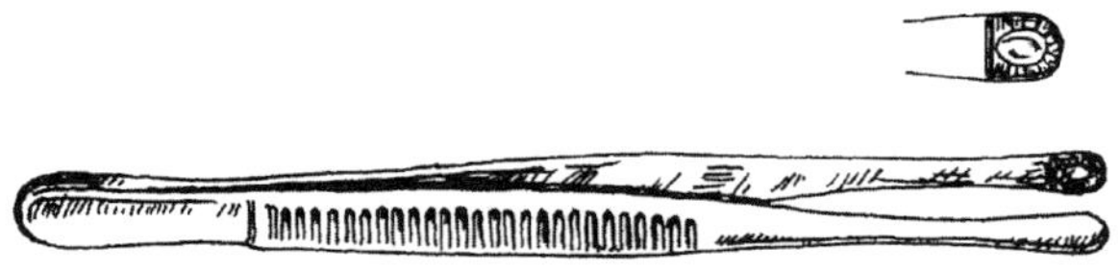
Russian forceps

Tissue forceps (sometimes called **thumb forceps with teeth**) are designed to manipulate tissue. They come in many models, which may have smooth tips, crosshatched tips or serrated tips. They may also have tiny projections, often called "mouse's teeth" at the tips. Common arrangements of teeth are 1×2 (two teeth on one side that interlock with a single tooth on the other), 7×7 and 9×9.

Counterintuitively, teeth will damage tissue less than a smooth surface because you can maintain a grip while applying less overall pressure (Wikipedia contributors, 2009). Tiny interlocking teeth can grasp very tiny skin tags to facilitate their removal. Forceps with smooth or crosshatched ends and no teeth are intended for manipulating gauze, suture, needles and similar items. They can be used to hold the tip of the needle halfway through a stitch as you reposition your needle holder to retrieve the needle. A regular hemostat or a second, smaller needle holder can be used this way too, but are more likely to damage the needle.

Dressing forceps (intended primarily to manipulate materials such as gauze) have blunt ends and serrated jaws. Examples include Adson, Brown-Adson multitoothed, Cushing, Russian and Standard pattern.

Either standard tissue forceps or Adson tissue forceps with 1×2 teeth or Potts-Smith dressing forceps with serrated jaws for fine work are appropriate for midwifery applications. **Russian tissue forceps** are another good, all-purpose choice for midwives. Although they are designed for use in tissue, they have broader serrated jaws than most similar instruments and can also grip a needle firmly. A 5" to 7" length is a good size. (See the chapter entitled "Using Thumb [Tissue or Dressing] Forceps" for details.)

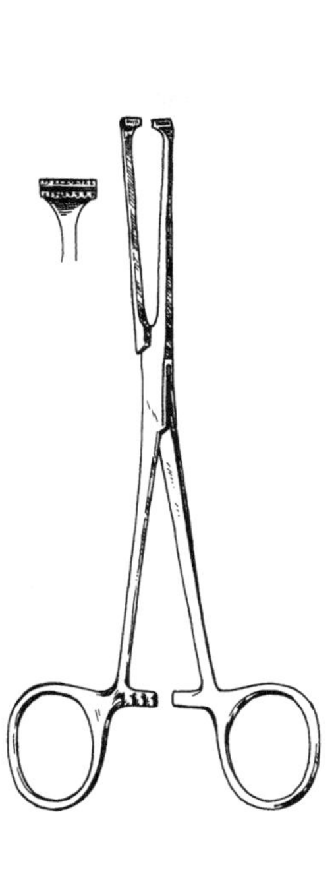

Allis clamps

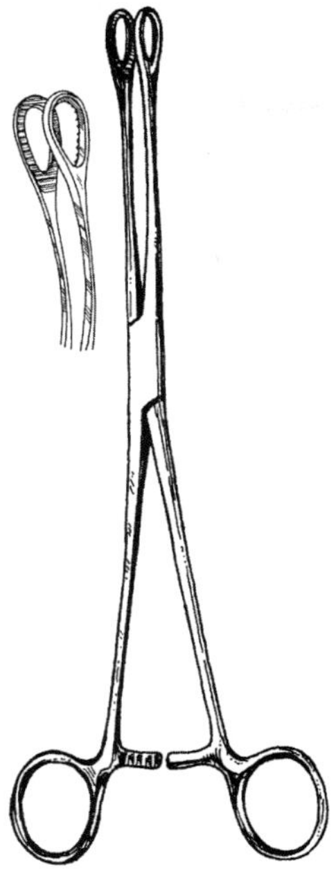

Foerster sponge-holding forceps

Allis clamps

You'll need two specialized hemostats called "Allis clamps" if you ever plan to tackle repairing anal sphincters. These are also good for grabbing and holding small skin tags away from the rest of the tissue before removing them and can be used for cervical examination as well. They have blunt teeth on each blade to assist in holding tissue and a ratchet between the finger rings. Clamps with four teeth on one blade and five on the other are good for our purposes. Wider blades may not work well in very small spaces.

Sponge-holding (ring) forceps

Foerster sponge-holding forceps have serrated jaws; open, oval ends; and a ratchet between the finger rings. The ends may be straight or curved. They are used to pull down the cervix for examination and repair, to clamp off a bleeding cervix and to aid visualization during examination of the posterior yoni (see the chapter entitled "Examining the Perineum after Birth"). Get two forceps of medium length (7 to 9 inches long) and keep one with your birth instruments. They also come in very handy for grasping and removing trailing placental membranes without tearing. To make remembering easy, I will use the term "ring forceps" when referring to this instrument.

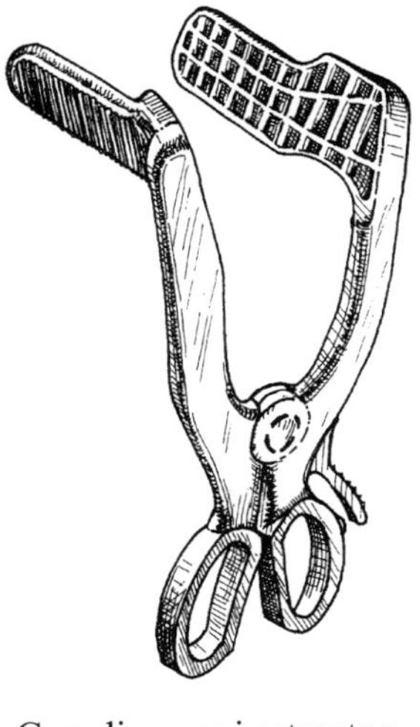

Guardian yoni retractor

Yoni retractor

A retractor is a surgical device designed to hold tissues apart so that the surgeon can gain access to deeper structures. Most perineal repairs can be completed without a retractor. When you need one, however, it can really make the repair much easier to perform. Although there are many styles of stainless steel retractors that can be used for perineal repair, the best choice for a midwife who works independently to use is the **Guardian vaginal retractor** (Cooper Surgical, 2005). This is a sterile, single-use, latex-free, plastic retractor that has a hinged blade with finger rings, a blunt blade on each side and a locking mechanism. The plastic is warm to the touch and lightweight. The proximal ends of the blades are concavely curved, and the distal blade ends are set at a divergent angle, maximizing exposure. This feature, plus the textured outer surfaces of the blades, minimizes slippage once the device is in place. To effectively retract the tissues, it is usually inserted like a speculum, only sideways, allowing adequate visibility and access to the complete circumference of the yoni, the perineum and the cervix. Once in place with the handle in the 6 o'clock position, the blades are parted, which opens the yoni by pushing back the walls on either side, fully exposing the ceiling, the lower sulcus groves and the floor of the yoni. These are the areas where tears occur most frequently, although the retractor can be oriented in any direction necessary to accomplish the repair.

Use of a retractor lessens the likelihood of a needlestick accident because you can see what you are doing better and you are not trying to retract the tissues with your fingers. It also facilitates tissue-layer approximation, and best of all, it leaves both hands free to do the suturing. It is exceptionally well suited for clitorotomy and perineal repair in the home or birth-center setting. This product retails for around $26.00 each or $135 for a box of six.

A stainless steel lateral vaginal retractor is available from Gynex (www.gynex.com). It works the same way as the plastic one but can be sterilized for reuse. It comes in three blade lengths: medium (55 mm), large (about 72 mm) and extra long (100 mm).

Disposable suture kits: In the UK, where bovine spongiform encephalopathy was first recognized and where a number of cases of the human version of this disease (new variant CJD) have occurred among persons of childbearing age, midwives are now using single-use disposable suture equipment for all perineal repair (Gifford, 2010). This is because the suspected agent of infection, prion protein, is very difficult to destroy. A number of UK vendors have one-time-use sterile instrument packs for suturing; be sure to check to see exactly what is included with the pack. Among them are Nu-Care Products, UK www.nu-careproducts.co.uk and www.medisave.co.uk. Both have sterile instrument packs of various types. These kits are relatively inexpensive. Having one on hand for back-up in case you don't have time to process instruments between births is a good idea. They are not great quality, but will work fine for a single use.

Suturing Supplies: Needles and Thread

Wound healing is a natural and spontaneous process. However, sometimes tissue is disrupted to the point that it cannot heal naturally without complications, such as possible disfigurement or loss of function. In such cases, it will heal best when dead tissue and foreign bodies are removed, any infection treated and the sides of the wound held together until the healing process restores the tissue's ability to withstand normal stresses and stay together without artificial support. When artificial support is called for, skilled use of suture materials with specially designed needles provides accurate and secure wound closure.

There are many types of surgical threads and needles, and several ways these materials are packaged for surgery. Be sure the suture material and needle you plan to use are appropriate for your purposes. This chapter includes many suggestions to help you in your selection process.

Suture material

The surgical thread used for repairs is commonly called "suture." Choice of suture material is predicated upon the biological interaction of the materials and the tissues to be repaired as well as the movement of the part of the body that is injured. The suture must be strong enough to the hold edges of the wound together artificially until they have healed enough to stay together on their own. The material must also be somewhat stretchy to accommodate tissue changes, such as swelling and shrinkage, that are inherent in the healing process. Like any other foreign object, suture material produces an immune response, invites infection and must be broken down in the body. Only the minimal amount that is required for the job should be used.

Minimum Standards for Knot Tensile Strength for USP sizes of Suture			
Type of material	**2-0**	**3-0**	**4-0**
Chromic gut	5.7 lb	3.9 lb	2.4 lb
Absorbable synthetic	6.2 lb	3.9 lb	2.4 lb
Actual Vicryl knot	7.9 lb	5.0 lb	3.2 lb

(Ethicon, 1985)

Characteristics of suture materials: Suture materials have a variety of qualities, the combination of which make them suitable for certain types of repairs. The strength of the suture strand is of primary importance. **Tensile strength** is the amount of tension or pulling, expressed in pounds or kilograms, that a strand can withstand before it snaps in two. This characteristic is assessed by dividing the force required to break a strand by its cross-sectional area. **Knot tensile strength** is the most critical factor because the knot is the weakest link in a suture strand. The US Pharmacopeia (USP) defines knot tensile strength as the force required to break a strand when applied to the free ends after it has been tied, using a surgeon's knot, around a quarter-inch rubber tubing. The European Pharmacopeia (EP) measures knot tensile strength after a creating half of a square knot (a single throw knot). The suture's tensile strength should not exceed the tensile strength of the tissue to be repaired but should ideally be at least as strong as normal tissue through which it is placed. After it is placed, **breaking strength retention (BSR)** measures the tensile strength retained by the strand over time. A strand with a knot tensile strength of 20 lbs that has 50% BSR at 1 week has a tensile strength of 10 lbs at that point (Chu et al., 1996).

Extensibility refers to the stretchiness of the suture. Familiarity with a material's extensibility helps one know when a knot is snug. Ideally the material is stretchy enough to allow for normal edema and returns to its original length as edema resolves. This property is known as **load elongation**. The material should stretch immediately when slightly stressed, but no more than that so it can continue to keep the wound edges closed; this characteristic is known as a **resistance to creep** (Edlich & Long, 2005). **Tissue drag** denotes the strand's resistance to passing through tissue; lower drag minimizes trauma.

Of all the qualities of suture, **hand** is the most subtle. It refers to the firmness of the strand, the feel of the suture during use, the smoothness with which it passes through tissue and the way in which knots can be set and snugged down (Ethicon, 2005a).

Sizing: The diameter of a strand is denoted by different calibers or gauges (weights or thicknesses of the strand) in either USP or EP (metric) sizes. The USP uses two different

SIZE EQUIVALENCES FOR ABSORBABLE SUTURES				
United States Pharmacopeia (USP)		Metric--European Pharmacopeia (EP)	Suture Diameter (mm)*	
Organic	Synthetic	Organic & Synthetic	Min.	Max.
1-0	**1**	4	0.40	0.49
2-0	**1-0**	**3**	0.30	0.39
3-0	**2-0**	**2.5**	0.25	0.29
4-0	**3-0**	**2**	0.20	0.24
5-0	**4-0**	**1.5**	0.15	0.19

*Minimum and maximum size standards in mm–millimeters. The USP & EP adhere to the same diameter standards. (Chu, 1997)

size standards: one for catgut and one for synthetic materials. Size is designated by a number assigned to each gauge. Smaller sizes are numbered from 11-0 or 11/0 (the smallest) to 0 (or 1-0) (for example, 3-0 is shorthand for three zeros or 000). From 1-0, strand diameter increases from 1 to 6. The EP size standard is the same for all materials and uses a numeric code that directly relates to the size of the strand expressed in tenths of a millimeter.

Strand diameters vary slightly among various materials. A given size in a gut suture is always slightly larger than the same size in a synthetic material. The sizes most frequently used in perineal repair are listed in the table above, with those most often used in bold.

Size has a direct bearing on a strand's tensile strength. The finer the strand, the less tension it will tolerate, and thicker strands have higher tensile strength. Nonetheless, thickness does not significantly influence breakdown time (i.e., 2-0 dissolves at about the same rate as 4-0).

The rule is, use the finest strand that corresponds to the strength of the tissues in which it will be placed. This minimizes trauma as the sutures pass through tissues and ensures that the smallest possible mass of foreign material is left in the body to dissolve. For most birth-related repairs, you can use either 3-0 chromic gut or 2-0 synthetic (EP size 2.5). This is a good all-purpose size suited to a variety of below-the-skin tissues. Use 4-0 synthetic (EP size 1.5) for fine labial, clitoral, periurethral or rectal mucosa repair and 2-0 chromic or 1-0 synthetic (EP size 3) to repair the deep perineal muscles, the cervix, the lateral yoni walls and the anal sphincters. Alternatively, Peyton (2001) suggests using 3-0 or 4-0 chromic gut for rectal mucosa repairs, reasoning that chromic gut is absorbed more quickly, thereby reducing the risk that a rectovaginal fistula will develop. The trade-off is that chromic prompts a greater inflammatory reaction, presenting yet another risk for fistula formation.

Types of materials: Suture materials are classified according to the origin of the strand material (organic or synthetic), the time it takes for the strand to break down in the tissues (absorbable or nonabsorbable) and the structure of the material (monofilament [essentially one strand] or multifilament [several thin strands that are braided together]).

There are two primary manufacturers of sutures in the US. Ethicon (a division of Johnson & Johnson) and Syneture (a division of Covidien). (Syneture suture was formerly sold under the brand name Davis & Geck or D&G.)

Nonabsorbable materials, such as cotton, steel and silk, retain their tensile strength for much longer than 60 days, and undissolved particles remain in the tissue. An eyed needle of the appropriate size and weight and silk suture make good, relatively inexpensive practice materials. However, nonabsorbable suture should not be used for perineal repair because its use is associated with significant pain and a higher rate of wound breakdown. It also must be removed once healing is complete.

When healing is expected to be relatively quick, as is the case with perineal tissue, choose a material that will lose its tensile strength at about the same rate that the damaged tissue will regain strength and that will be absorbed so that no foreign material remains in the tissue after healing is complete. **Absorbable sutures** are designed to gradually break down in tissue within a predictable period of time and are preferred for use in areas where wound contamination cannot always be prevented. In addition, perineal tissues tend to heal well and usually do not require continued artificial support (Anderson, 1975).

For all kinds of suture, loss of tensile strength and the rate of absorption are separate phenomena. One material may lose tensile strength quickly and be absorbed slowly while another may maintain tensile strength throughout healing and then absorb rapidly. These factors are influenced by the material used, the body chemistry of the individual, and the characteristics of the wound.

Absorbable organic material: Natural-fiber materials are the most economical type of absorbable suture and are commonly used for repairing birth-related damage. Organic suture is made from purified connective tissue consisting primarily of collagen that is taken from either the submucosal layer or the serosal layer of bovine (cattle) small intestines or from the submucosal fibrous layer of ovine (sheep) intestines. (Gut suture is no longer sold in the United Kingdom and other parts of Europe due to regulatory changes prompted by concerns regarding spreading bovine spongiform encephalopathy [mad cow disease].) This material is commonly referred to as "catgut." Although suture has never been made from the gut of cats, this term is probably a transliteration of "kit," an old word for a fiddle. "Kit" was likely derived from the Greek word *kithara*, meaning a lyre, harp, or lute. These instruments were strung with material made from sheep gut (Haubrich, 1984).

After harvest, the connective tissue is processed by slicing it into long ribbons that are chemically treated to render them useful as suture material. **Plain gut** is simply tanned with dilute aldehyde (a form of formaldehyde) to increase its strength and resistance to enzyme action in the tissues. It maintains its tensile strength for only seven to 10 days, produces more tissue reaction than does chromic gut and is completely dissolved after 70 days. For all these reasons, plain gut is inappropriate to use for perineal repair.

Chromic gut is plain gut that has been treated with chromium trioxide, a process that significantly increases its resistance to absorption in tissue. Producing less tissue reaction than the plain variety, it is the best organic choice for perineal repair (Anderson, 1975). Chromic gut is available in different degrees of strength. Any standard or full-strength strand can be used; this suture is simply labeled "chromic gut." Material designated as "mild" or "medium" chromic does not retain its tensile strength long enough for use in perineal repair.

After gut ribbons are treated, two or more are twisted together to produce strands of the desired thickness. Even though more than one ribbon is used in processing, the ribbons are fused into a single strand that is classified as a monofilament material. Unfortunately, combining several ribbons in this way produces a strand that is somewhat more prone to fraying during knot tying than a synthetic monofilament alternative. The strand is dried and polished to a uniform thickness to eliminate high and low spots (minimizing the tendency to fray) and finally sterilized and packaged in a dilute (<50%) isopropanol alcohol solution that acts as a preservative and prevents the strand from drying out and becoming stiff. Natural gut material is a yellowish tan color. Ethicon also makes gut with blue dye.

Because using gut suture introduces a foreign animal tissue into human tissue and because it requires lysosomal enzymatic action to break it down, it produces marked white blood cell response (i.e., inflammation) in comparison to synthetic materials. Gut also has a lot of **strand** or **package memory**, a term that refers to a material's tendency to retain kinks or bends from its packaged posture instead of lying flat, even after it is gently stretched out. This relative lack of flexibility means that learning to tie secure knots with it takes practice.

***Absorption characteristics of organic suture*:** Salthouse and colleagues (1969) found that gut reabsorption occurs due to sequential attacks by lysosomal enzymes. All stages of the healing process prompt the production of enzymes that act on any foreign material and attempt to break it down. Absorbable gut suture is designed to breakdown in the presence of these enzymes by a process, known as **proteolysis (PRO-tee-OHL-ih-sis)**, that is similar to normal digestion. In most types of tissue, this process is started by acid phosphatase, with leucine amino-peptidase playing a more important role as absorption progresses. Collagenase may contribute to the enzymatic degradation of collagen sutures.

The dissolution of absorbable natural-fiber suture begins with a reduction in tensile strength followed by a loss of mass as the material starts to dissolve. Generally speaking, chromic gut retains 34% of its original tensile strength after about 10 to 14 days, with some measurable strength remaining for up to 21 days. Dissolution is usually complete after 90 days. In practice, however, the time it takes for gut's tensile strength to diminish and for total absorption to occur varies widely, the rate depending upon the tissue in which it is placed and the enzymatic response of the individual. In my experience with perineal repair, chromic gut's tensile strength is significantly reduced by a week to 10 days, and it is usually broken down completely by six to eight weeks. If infection is present, gut suture has a tendency to break down more rapidly, which is an advantage of using an organic material. Suture that remains in an infected wound provides a hiding place for bacteria.

Absorbable synthetic material: There are many types of synthetic materials, some of which are well suited for perineal repair. They come in single or braided multifilament strands.

***Synthetic monofilament suture*:** To achieve a happy balance between the advantages of a synthetic material and the benefits of gut, Syneture (www.syneture.com) has developed synthetic monofilaments that strive to mimic chromic gut. Synthetic products produce less tissue reaction than does gut suture and are less allergenic as well. Whenever organic fiber suture comes into contact with body fluids, especially blood, it tends to get sticky; this is less of a problem when synthetic monofilaments are used.

Caprosyn (Syneture) is a synthetic gut substitute. This uncoated suture is made from Polyglytone 6211™, a synthetic polyester that consists of glycolide, caprolactone, trimethylene carbonate and lactide. Although wound approximation using Caprosyn is the same as for chromic when it is initially placed, its tensile strength, compared to chromic, falls at a faster rate, meaning the tensile strength of Caprosyn becomes weaker than the same size strand of chromic gut would do over the same period of time.

Biosyn (Syneture) is an uncoated monofilament synthetic made from glycolide, trimethylene carbonate and dioxanone. Compared to Caprosyn, it lasts longer in tissue and maintains its tensile strength longer, qualities that make it an ideal choice for anal sphincter repair.

Both undyed Caprosyn and Biosyn look like clear fishing line, so they are very difficult to see in tissue. For this reason, I recommend using either of these materials dyed (both are available with violet dye). As with chromic gut, these monofilament synthetics also have a high degree of strand memory, making maintaining appropriate tension on a partially tied knot somewhat more challenging.

Monocryl (Ethicon) is a monofilament suture composed of Poliglecaprone 25™, a copolymer of glycolide and epsilon-caprolactone. This material is Ethicon's closest match to Caprosyn. Monocryl, however, only provides 10 to 14 days of wound support while taking much longer than Caprosyn to absorb (91 to 119 days), the worst of both worlds. Monocryl can be used for perineal repairs when prolonged support is not required and there is no other material available but, the monofilament materials Caprosyn or Biosyn made by Syneture are better suited for most birth-related repairs.

PDS II (Ethicon) is composed of polydioxanone and comes clear or with violet dye. **Maxon (Syneture)**, the nearest equivalent product from Syneture, is made of polglyconate, a copolymer of glycolic acid and trimethylene carbonate. Both products dissolve more slowly and retain some tensile strength for more than six weeks, plus their monofilament structure minimizes the chance of infection. These properties make them the recommended materials for repair of the external anal sphincter but inappropriate for other obstetric repairs. Products that offer such extended support also carry risks such as prolonged irritation and knot extrusion to the skin surface, which can cause pain or even infection.

***<u>Synthetic multifilament suture</u>*:** A variety of multifilament synthetic sutures have also been developed. These products are made of polyglycolic acid, which is inherently rigid. To overcome this inflexibility, the material is extruded in thin ribbons that are braided together, which creates a very pliable strand. Multifilament strands retain their tensile strength longer than chromic. Their tensile strength for matched calibers is greater than gut, and knot security is maintained for a few weeks longer. Their absorption rate varies somewhat, depending upon the product, but is always much slower than chromic.

Vicryl (Ethicon) is made of Polyglactin 910™, a copolymer made from lactide and glycolide acids, both of which are natural carbohydrate derivatives. Vicryl is said to completely absorb in 56 to 90 days but, in most cases, it is gone by 56 days.

Syneture produces several multifilament synthetics, of which **Polysorb** is the most similar to Vicryl. It is composed of Lactomer™, a polyester made of glycolide and lactide. Faulkner and colleagues (1981) found knotted Polysorb to be stronger and easier to tie than Vicryl.

Dexon (Syneture) is made from a polyglycolic acid similar to that used in Vicryl. Dexon is totally absorbed after 60 to 90 days. It can be used in perineal repair, but Polysorb is the better choice, as it has a shorter absorption time.

***Rapidly absorbing multifilament synthetic*:** To eliminate some of the disadvantages of other multifilament materials, Ethicon developed **Vicryl Rapide**, a braided polyglactin suture irradiated to alter its molecular structure to achieve a faster absorption rate. It has a tensile strength that is initially greater than chromic gut, although reduction of its tensile strength occurs more rapidly than with chromic gut, and sutures begin to fall out after seven to 10 days. It is totally absorbed after about 42 days, 66% faster than coated Vicryl. This fast dissolution rate means that suture remnants should not require removal later, after healing takes place. Vicryl Rapide is suitable for repair of lacerations sustained by healthy women who have a history of healing well. Syneture offers no similar product.

Antibacterial multifilament synthetic suture: To address the issue of braided suture harboring infectious organisms, Ethicon introduced **Vicryl Plus Antibacterial suture**. This is plain coated Vicryl that has been impregnated with the antibacterial agent Igracare MP (generic name, triclosan). Vicryl Plus is available in 0, 2-0 and 3-0 sizes swaged to a CT-1 needle. This suture handles and behaves exactly like plain coated Vicryl.

Triclosan has been shown to inhibit colonization of the suture by *Staphylococcus aureus*, *Staphylococcus epidermidis*, Methicillin resistant *S. aureus* (MRSA) and Methicillin resistant *S. epidermidis* (MRSE). All of these microorganisms have proven links to surgical-site infections. Animal studies have demonstrated that antibacterial suture inhibits bacterial colonization of the treated strand after direct in vivo challenges using these bacteria.

Ethicon uses the same antibiotic in **Monocryl Plus** and **PDS Plus**. These products are effective against the organisms listed above as well as *Escherichia coli* and *Klebsiella pneumoniae* (Johnson & Johnson, 2008).

The use of antibacterial suture only adds to the already overwhelming use of antibiotics. In women already known to have an intrauterine infection, however, and therefore having pathogen-laden lochia, the use of an antibacterial suture may be a reasonable precaution, particularly when the woman's immune system is weakened due to malnutrition, infection or other illness or when anal structures need repair.

***Coating*:** Synthetic multifilament suture also comes coated or uncoated. Coating is a special treatment to make the surface of the suture smoother, thus enhancing its passage through tissue, lessening the stickiness factor (multifilament materials tend to get stickier than monofilament synthetics during use) and making knot tying and repositioning easier. Coating also reduces (but does not eliminate) **capillarity**, whereby fluid and bacteria travel into the spaces between the braided ribbons of multifilament sutures. Thus, coating may minimize the tendency of braided synthetic ribbons to harbor bacteria to some degree. Coating materials vary between manufacturers:

- **Ethicon** uses a lactide, glycolide and calcium stearate coating that produces an adherent, nonflaking, waxlike lubricant comprising 2% to 5% of the strand's overall weight. Vicryl is not available uncoated.
- **Syneture** uses a "II" (Dexon II) designation for its Polycaprolate coating, a glycolide and epsilon caprolactone copolymer that comprises approximately 1% of the strand's overall weight. Do not use uncoated Dexon (marked "S"[smooth]).

These are considered water-insoluble coatings that have chemical constituents similar to the suture material and are broken down over time with the material by hydrolysis.

Coated multifilament synthetics are more pliable and have less memory than chromic material (i.e., it does not recoil to its original shape as much, a quality which contributes to initial knot security), but its smooth surface tends to encourage knots to slip over time, so more throws are required to create a secure knot. Midwives also report that these materials tangle more than chromic gut.

Uncoated braided synthetics are not recommended for perineal repair; they are significantly harder to handle, and knots are harder to tie and often impossible to reposition or tighten once begun. (More details regarding the different types of synthetic sutures are included in the chapters entitled "Tying Surgical Knots" and "Perineal Infections.")

***Dyes*:** Vicryl comes with or without purple dye, and Dexon comes with or with-out green dye or in a bicolor of woven green and beige. Undyed multifilament products are light beige. Although dye is supposed to make it easer to see, I find undyed beige multifilament suture to be very visible in the repair. Using undyed material means one less chemical for the mother's body to have to disperse. When the undyed material looks like fishing line, however, dye may be useful, as is true for monofilament synthetic materials.

***Absorption characteristics of synthetic suture*:** Synthetic sutures, be they monofilament or multifilament, elicit a minimal acute inflammatory tissue reaction, followed by gradual encapsulation of the suture strand by fibrous connective tissue. Progressive loss of tensile strength comes next. Eventual absorption occurs via **hydrolysis (hi-DROHL-ih-sis)**, that is, dissolution via contact with water in the body. Once the strand has been broken down into its constituent parts, it is eventually absorbed and metabolized by the body.

The breakdown time for various synthetic sutures is only somewhat influenced by an individual's body chemistry; since the fibers are broken down by hydrolysis rather than proteolysis, their breakdown is less subject to individual variation than is the case with chromic gut. Hydrolysis occurs most readily in an alkaline environment. The acidic environment of the healthy yoni helps the suture material maintain its integrity well beyond the minimum time needed to ensure proper closure (Sanz, 1987).

The longer staying power of most synthetic materials keeps the wound edges together longer and thus minimizes the risk of wound dehiscence (separation of the edges), a real advantage in tissues that heal more slowly or receive more stress. This benefit makes synthetics an excellent choice for repair of the labia, rectal mucosa and anal sphincters. Carefully sutured perineal wounds, on the contrary, are usually healed closed within two weeks by primary intension; at that point they no longer require artificial support. A disadvantage of synthetic material is that fragments remaining in the tissue long after healing is complete can cause local irritation and require removal. Another problem is that braided strands can harbor bacteria, which can lead to, or exacerbate, an infection. In addition, unlike chromic gut, infection does not hasten the absorption of synthetic sutures, and some think it actually delays it (see the chapter entitled "Perineal Infections" for more details). Despite these drawbacks, there are birth practitioners who use synthetic multifilament exclusively.

***Choosing a synthetic suture*:** Either Vicryl Rapide or Polysorb are good choices for basic repair in healthy, well-nourished women who have superficial tears that will not require prolonged support. I do not recommend either product for unhealthy women; difficult repairs; or labial, muscle, rectal mucosa, or anal sphincter repair. Whenever greater tensile strength is needed for a longer period of time—which I have found helpful in performing labial and periurethral repairs—Biosyn, Vicryl, or Dexon II are your materials of choice. Reserve Biosyn for women that you expect to require prolonged wound support as it has the longest absorption profile of these materials. For maximum wound support, use PDS II or Maxon (generally only recommended for anal sphincter repair).

In my opinion, absorbable synthetic suture is the only appropriate material for anal sphincter repair. Although some providers do use chromic gut for this purpose, the proper synthetic has more staying power and increases the chances of a successful repair. Plus, there is no point in running the risk of a suture reaction and dehiscence in an area where adequate healing is so critical. Synthetic suture may also be used for rectal mucosa repair. However, since this tissue heals rapidly, some use 3-0 or 4-0 chromic gut with equal success.

Summary of suture types: This table reviews materials midwives typically use.

SUTURE MATERIAL	INITIAL TENSILE STRENGTH*	DEGREE OF KNOT TENSILE STRENGTH RETAINED DURING BREAKDOWN		EFFECTIVE WOUND SUPPORT	TOTAL ABSORPTION TIME
Chromic gut	8.0 lbs (2-0)	34% by 2 weeks (varies widely)	None by 3 weeks (varies widely)	10 to 14 days (varies widely)	Within 90 days (varies widely)
Coated Vicryl	13 lbs	Minimal loss 1st 7 days, 65% by 2 weeks	40% by 3 weeks	21 days	56 to 70 days
Vicryl Rapide	9.9 lbs	50% by 5 days	None by 12 days	About 10 days	Within 42 days
PDS II	11.5 lbs (plain 2-0 PDS)	70% at 2 weeks	25% at 6 weeks	35 to 42 days	180 days or more
Monocryl	No data available	50 to 60% by 7 days 20 to 30% by 12 days	None by 3 weeks	10 to 14 days	180-210 days
Dexon II	12.4 lbs	Minimal in 1st 7 days, 65% by 2 weeks	35% by 3 weeks	21 days	60 to 90 days
Polysorb (Vicryl alternative)	15.6 lbs	80% by 2 weeks	30% by 3 weeks	21 days	56 to 70 days
Biosyn	No data available	75% by 2 weeks	40% by 3 weeks	21 days	90 to 110 days
Caprosyn (gut alternative)	No data available	50 to 60% at 5 days	20-30% by 10 days	About 10 days	Within 56 days
Maxon	12.6 lbs (2-0)	80% at 7 days	25% at 6 weeks	35 to 42 days	210 + days

*Tensile strength varies with the diameter of the strand. Values give only an idea of the relative strength of each product prior to tying and are usually tested on 2-0 but I could not confirm that for every type of product.

Packaging: Most sutures are individually packaged in double envelopes. The suture strand itself is wrapped around a paper or plastic holder to prevent tangling and allow easy removal of the needle and strand by the surgeon. This holder is contained in a sterile foil packet that is sealed inside an outer envelope with a clear window through which to view the foil packet, which shows the size and type of suture and needle it contains.

Most tears can be completed with a single packet of 27 or 30 inch (68 to 75 cm) suture. Longer strands tangle more easily and can be unwieldy to use. Long strands also mean dragging more suture through the woman's tissues, with chromic gut being particularly vulnerable to fraying when exposed to too much friction. Longer strands are also more costly. Reserve the use of long strands for extensive tears needing a lot of suture.

Needles

The selection of the proper needle is as important as the choice of suture material. Since the only purpose of the needle is to weave the suture material in and out of the tissue, it should be designed to do so easily while producing as little tissue trauma as possible.

Characteristics of surgical needles: Today's surgical needles are made of high-quality stainless steel especially developed to minimize the harboring of microorganisms while maximizing several important characteristics. **Strength** is determined by how well a needle resists deformation during repeated passes through tissue. The **surgical yield strength** refers to the amount of angular deformation or bending the needle can withstand before becoming permanently bent. **Ductility** refers to the needle's resistance to breaking when subjected to a given amount of bending under pressure or **load**. Needles are designed to be flexible enough so that they bend somewhat before they break. **Sharpness** refers to the precision of the point and is especially important when repairing delicate tissue or skin, because a sharp needle will produce the least scar tissue. Sharpness is determined by the angle of the point as well as the taper ratio of the needle tip. Surgical needles are given a micro-thin coating of lubricants and are otherwise treated to allow smooth passage through tissue with very little resistance.

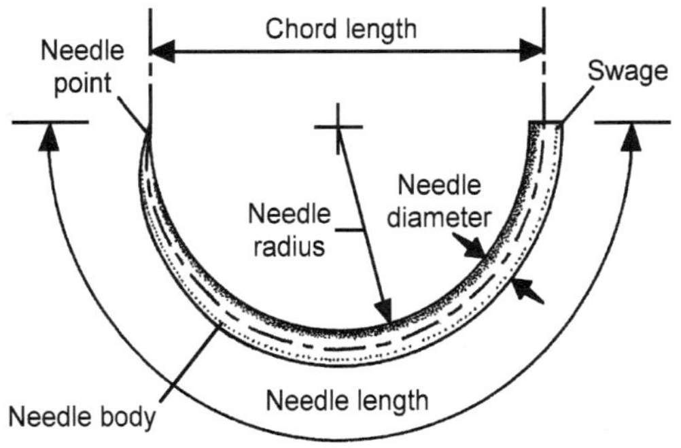

Parts of a half-circle needle

The parts of a suture needle: The **chord length** is the straight-line distance between the needle tip and the swaged tip; for a half-circle needle, this would be its diameter if the curve of the needle were continued to complete a full circle. **Needle length** measures the curve of the shaft from the needle tip to the swaged end. The **radius** is the distance from the center of the circle to the needle wire if the curve of the needle were continued to complete a full circle. Needle **diameter** denotes the gauge or thickness of the needle wire. The **body** or **shaft** of the needle is the portion of the wire that extends from the swaged end to the point where the wire begins to taper as it nears the tip. The needle's **point** enters the tissue first. It includes the entire tip, from the end to where the wire widens to merge with the maximum cross-section of the body.

Attachment of the needle and suture: For most applications, one end of the sterile suture strand is permanently inserted or swaged into the hollow end of a single-use needle. The swaged end of the needle is often flattened slightly to enhance its ability to remain securely positioned in the needle holder. The diameter of the needle should match that of the strand to which it is swaged as closely as possible. Swaged suture is easier to use than a threaded needle because it does not become unthreaded and eliminates the additional bulk of a threaded needle, leaving a smaller hole in the tissue. Suture also comes double swaged—i.e., with a needle on each end—a handy arrangement when you have a very large tear requiring two different types of needles (fortunately, a rare occurrence). Be sure not to get swaged suture with detachable needles, which is designed for easy needle removal during surgery requiring many interrupted stitches; such suture is inappropriate for perineal repair.

Sizes and types of needles: Surgical needles are made in different diameters in a variety of straight and curved shapes. Those used for perineal repair are all half-circle needles, which allow you to take a deep bite in a small space and then easily locate the point as it exits the tissue. Using more widely curved needles in a small space tends to produce stitches that are too wide and may also hamper your ability to maneuver.

Students are often surprised to learn that relatively large needles are recommended for most birth-related repair. A 36.4 or 37 mm size needle is ideal for most internal repair and for closure of the outer perineum. Believe me, needles much smaller than this size easily get lost in the tissue, an anxiety-producing experience for everyone concerned. Very shallow perineal repairs can be performed with a somewhat smaller needle. A very fine needle can be used for labial and rectal mucosa repair.

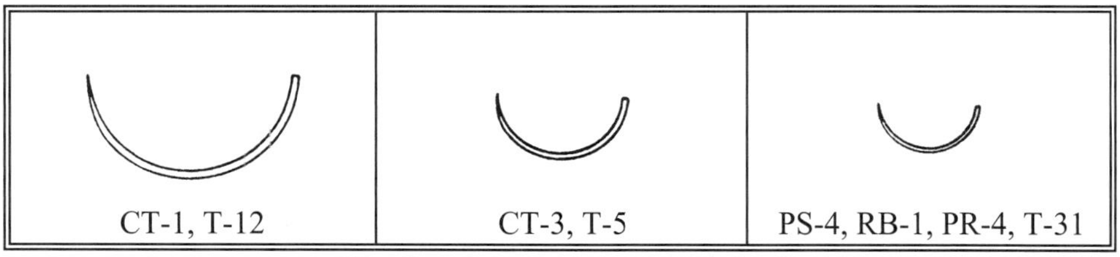

(Needles shown are the actual size.)

***Needle points*:** There are also a variety of styles of needle points with smooth or cutting tips.

A **taper point needle** is ideal for most perineal repair. Its smooth, rounded body and sharp point spreads tissue without slicing it. This combination minimizes trauma to delicate mucosa, with the needle point often rolling by blood vessels rather than puncturing or cutting into them, and minimizes other accidents such as the severing of sutures already in place. If a woman has a history of poor nutrition or is currently unhealthy, use only taper point needles for her repair.

Blunt taper point needles (Ethiguard™ [Ethicon] and Protect•Point™ [Syneture]) are available to help reduce the number of needlestick accidents. These needles have a tapered tip with a rounded, blunt point that can dissect friable tissue but require considerably more pressure to penetrate most tissues than do conventional needles. Ethicon's Ethiguard needles are ribbed along the shaft and the body is flattened.

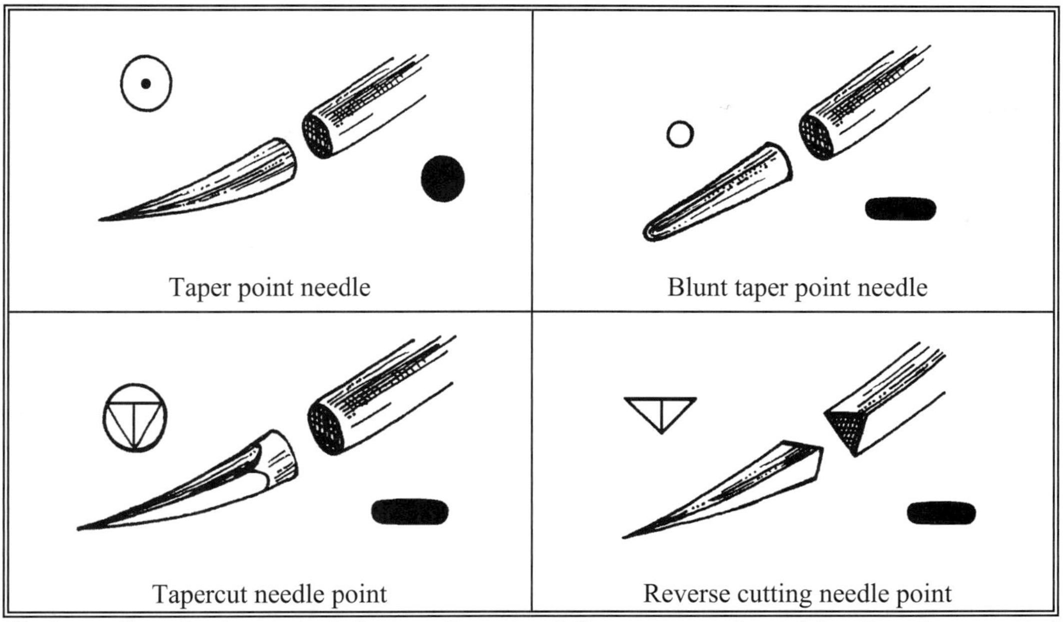

(Each needle point image includes, on the upper left, a cross-section of the tip, a large central drawing of the point profile, and, on the lower right, a cross-section of the needle body.)

Mornar and Perlow (2008) surveyed obstetric providers and found that many were satisfied with the performance of blunt-tipped needles for perineal repair, although when using a minimal amount of anesthetic, a blunt tip is likely to cause more pain. Blunt-tipped needles, however, may be the best choice for women with unhealthy, friable tissue, as this point is likely to pass easily through their tissues, especially when repairing mucosa. Don't use a blunt tip when repairs require penetration of the tough skin surface, as may be necessary during labial repairs. The variety of appropriately sized sutures swaged to blunt-tipped needles is limited.

Cutting needles: A **tapercut (trocar) point** combines a sharp taper point with a reverse cutting tip. Three sharp cutting edges extend about 1/32" from the tip, where they blend into a round taper body. This point is designed to cut through old scars while still making a very small hole and is generally the best cutting needle to use in this highly vascular tissue. A tapered body passes smoothly, minimizing the danger of cutting into the surrounding tissue.

Unfortunately, tapercut needles are not available in all the needle–suture combinations that are best suited to perineal repair. Therefore, reverse cutting needles can be used as an alternative in some cases (see the tables that follow for recommended products). There are several types of cutting needles that are designed to penetrate skin cleanly, thus minimizing scarring. These needles have one or more sharp edges along a portion of the wire that slice, rather than puncture, the tissue. They cut through blood vessels more easily as well and their use results in more bleeding.

Reverse cutting needles are the only type appropriate for repairing the skin or tough scar tissue. The first third of the needle wire is triangularly shaped; the remaining two-thirds of the wire is flattened, with rounded corners. The apex of the triangular portion forms a cutting edge that runs along the outer (convex) curve of the shaft. It produces an incision on the far (inferior) side of the needle's path, leaving a flat wall of tissue on the near (superior) side of the needle's path. This arrangement maximizes penetration of tough tissue while minimizing tissue trauma when the suture strand is manipulated during knot tying.

Recommendations: suture materials for specific types of tears

A list of properly sized, swaged suture in the two most popular brands follows. All multi-filament synthetics listed are undyed and coated. All monofilament synthetics are dyed violet unless otherwise noted. The most desirable suture–needle combinations are not always available: substitutes have been suggested when possible.

General repair of the yoni mucosa and perineum: For most repairs, use 3-0 chromic gut or Vicryl Rapide on a taper point half-circle needle (lengths are rounded off).

Brand	Code	Needle: Code, Point (Length)	Suture Material	Suture Length
Ethicon	810H	CT-1 Taper (36.4 mm)	3-0 Chromic gut	27" (68.5 cm)
Ethicon	922H	CT-1 Taper (36.4 mm)	3-0 Chromic gut	36" (91 cm)
Ethicon	942H	V-34 Tapercut (36.4 mm)	3-0 Chromic gut	36" (91 cm)
Ethicon	J259H	CT-1 Taper (36.4 mm)	2-0 Coated Vicryl (undyed)	27" (68.5 cm)
Ethicon	J945H	CT-1 Taper (36.4 mm)	2-0 Coated Vicryl (undyed)	36" (91 cm)
Ethicon	J917H	V-34 Tapercut (36.4 mm)	2-0 Coated Vicryl (undyed)	36" (91 cm)
Ethicon	JB945	CTB-1 Blunt taper (36.4 mm)	2-0 Coated Vicryl (undyed)	36" (91 cm)
Ethicon	VR945	CT-1 Taper (36.4 mm)	2-0 Vicryl Rapide (undyed)	36" (91 cm)
Ethicon	VR917	V-34 Tapercut (36.4)	2-0 Vicryl Rapide (undyed)	36" (91 cm)
Syneture	CG-810	GS-21 Taper (37 mm)	3-0 Chromic gut	30" (76 cm)
Syneture	CG-922	GS-21 Taper (37 mm)	3-0 Chromic gut	36" (91 cm)
Syneture	CG-962	KV-34 Tapercut (37 mm)	3-0 Chromic gut	36" (91 cm)
Syneture	9266-51	GS-21 Taper (37 mm)	2-0 Dexon II (undyed)	30" (76 cm)
Syneture	9268-51	GS-21 Taper (37 mm)	2-0 Dexon II (undyed)	36" (91 cm)
Syneture	9253-51	KV-30 Tapercut (27 mm)	2-0 Dexon II (undyed)	36" (91 cm)
Syneture	9042-51	BGS-21 Blunt taper (37 mm)	2-0 Dexon II (undyed)	36" (91 cm)
Syneture	CL-811	GS-21 Taper (37 mm)	2-0 Polysorb (violet)	30" (76 cm)
Syneture	CL-923	GS-21 Taper (37 mm)	2-0 Polysorb (violet)	36" (91 cm)
Syneture	CL-943	KV-34 Tapercut (37 mm)	2-0 Polysorb (violet)	36" (91 cm)
Syneture	CLT-953	BTP-1 Blunt taper (37 mm)	2-0 Polysorb (undyed)	36" (91 cm)
Syneture	CM–811	GS-21 Taper (37 mm)	2-0 Biosyn (violet)	36" (91 cm)
Syneture	CMT-811	BTP-1 Blunt taper (37 mm)	2-0 Biosyn (violet)	36" (91 cm)
Syneture	CC-843	GS-21 Taper (37 mm)	2-0 Caprosyn (violet)	30" (76 cm)
Syneture	CC-953	GS-21 Taper (37 mm)	2-0 Caprosyn (violet)	36" (91 cm)
Syneture	CC-1945-G	KV-34 Tapercut (37 mm)	2-0 Caprosyn (undyed)	36" (91 cm)

Shallow repairs near the skin edge of the perineum: When the skin of the perineum is to be repaired, use a tapercut or taper point needle swaged to one of the suture materials in the following table. The Ethicon CT-2 and SH taper needles are the same size, but the SH needle has a smaller diameter and should only be used to repair unscarred tissue because it might bend as you try to drive it through tough scar tissue.

Brand	Code	Needle: Code, Point (Length)	Suture Material (Color)	Suture Length
Ethicon	882H	CT-2 Taper (26 mm)	3-0 Chromic gut	27" (68.5 cm)
Ethicon	G172H	SH Taper (26 mm)	3-0 Chromic gut	27" (68.5 cm)
Ethicon	J269H	CT-2 Taper (26 mm)	2-0 Coated Vicryl (undyed)	27" (68.5 cm)
Ethicon	J416H	SH Taper (26 mm)	3-0 Coated Vicryl (undyed)	27" (68.5 cm)
Ethicon	VR417	SH Taper (26 mm)	2-0 Vicryl Rapide (undyed)	27" (68.5 cm)
Syneture	9232-51	V-20 Taper (26 mm)	2-0 Dexon II (undyed)	30" (76 cm)
Syneture	GG-122	V-20 Taper (26 mm)	3-0 Chromic gut	30" (76 cm)
Syneture	GM-323	V-20 Taper (26 mm)	2-0 Polysorb (violet)	30" (76 cm)
Syneture	GM-123	V-20 Taper (26 mm)	2-0 Biosyn (violet)	30" (76 cm)
Syneture	GC-323	V-20 Taper (26 mm)	2-0 Caprosyn (violet)	30" (76 cm)

Anal sphincter repair: The next table lists synthetics suitable for internal and external anal sphincter repair and both chromic and synthetic materials that can be used to place a deep layer of stitches in the yoni. Never use a cutting needle of any kind to repair the sphincters.

Brand	Code	Needle: Code, Point (Length)	Suture Material	Suture Length
Ethicon	J260H	CT-1 Taper (36.4 mm)	1-0 Coated Vicryl (undyed)	27" (68.5 cm)
Ethicon	J946H	CT-1 Taper (36.4 mm)	1-0 Coated Vicryl (undyed)	36" (91 cm)
Ethicon	JB260	CTB-1 Blunt taper (36.4 mm)	1-0 Coated Vicryl (undyed)	27" (68.5 cm)
Ethicon	JB946	CTB-1 Blunt taper (36.4 mm)	1-0 Coated Vicryl (undyed)	36" (91 cm)
Ethicon	VR945	CT-1 Taper (36.4 mm)	2-0 Vicryl Rapide (undyed)	36" (91 cm)
Ethicon	Z339H	CT-1 Taper (36.4 mm)	2-0 PDS II (violet)	27" (68.5 cm)
Syneture	CG811	GS-21 Taper (37 mm)	2-0 Chromic gut	30" (76 cm)
Syneture	9266-61	GS-21 Taper (37 mm)	1-0 Dexon II (undyed)	30" (76 cm)
Syneture	9042-61	BGS-21 Blunt taper (37 mm)	1-0 Dexon II (bi-color)	36" (91 cm)
Syneture	CL-954	GS-21 Taper (37 mm)	1-0 Polysorb (undyed)	36" (91 mm)
Syneture	CLT-955	BTP-1 Blunt taper (37 mm)	1-0 Polysorb (undyed)	36" (91 cm)
Syneture	CM-812	GS-21 Taper (37 mm)	1-0 Biosyn (violet)	30" (76 cm)
Syneture	CM-924	GS-21 Taper (37 mm)	1-0 Biosyn (violet)	36" (91 cm)
Syneture	CMT-812	BTP-1 Blunt taper (37 mm)	1-0 Biosyn (violet)	30" (76 cm)
Syneture	CC-844	GS-21 Taper (37 mm)	1-0 Caprosyn (violet)	30" (76 cm)
Syneture	CC-824	GS-21 Taper (37 mm)	1-0 Caprosyn (violet)	36" (91 cm)
Syneture	6267-51	GS-21 Taper (37 mm)	2-0 Maxon (green)	30" (76 cm)

Fine labial, skin tag or rectal mucosa repair: The following materials are suggested for labial and skin tag repair; use either a taper, tapercut or reverse cutting plastic surgery point (designated PS or P). Use only a taper point needle for rectal mucosa repair.

Brand	Code	Needle: Code, Point (Length)	Suture Material	Suture Length
Ethicon	J507G	PS-4 Reverse cut (16 mm)	4-0 Coated Vicryl (undyed)	18" (46 cm)
Ethicon	J241H	RB-1 Taper (17 mm)	4-0 Coated Vicryl (undyed)	27" (68.5 cm)
Ethicon	VR214	RB-1 Taper (17 mm)	4-0 Vicryl Rapide (undyed)	27" (68.5 cm)
Syneture	9728-31	P-24 Reverse cut (17 mm)	4-0 Dexon II (undyed)	18" (45 cm)
Syneture	9106-31	CV-23 Taper (17 mm)	4-0 Dexon II (undyed)	30" 76 cm)
Syneture	GL-884	CV-22 Taper (13 mm)^	4-0 Polysorb (undyed)*	30" (76 cm)
Syneture	UL-215	CV-23 Taper (17 mm)	3-0 Polysorb (undyed)*	30" (76 cm)
Syneture	UC-214	CV-23 Taper (17 mm)	4-0 Caprosyn (violet)	30" (76 cm)

^4-0 Polysorb not available swaged to a CV-23 taper needle. Polysorb not available in any size swaged to a small tapercut needle.

*4-0 Polysorb is not available with dye in packets appropriate for perineal repair.

Antibacterial sutures: Use Vicryl Plus when the risk of infection is significantly increased.

Brand	Code	Needle: Code, Point (Length)	Suture Material	Suture Length
Ethicon	VCP258H	CT-1 Taper (36.4 mm)	3-0 Vicryl Plus (undyed)	27" (68.5 cm)
Ethicon	VCP259H	CT-1 Taper (36.4 mm)	2-0 Vicryl Plus (undyed)	27" (68.5 cm)
Ethicon	VCP260H	CT-1 Taper (36.4 mm)	1-0 Vicryl Plus (undyed)	27" (68.5 cm)
Ethicon	VCP944H	CT-1 Taper (36.4 mm)	3-0 Vicryl Plus (undyed)	36" (91 cm)
Ethicon	VCP945H	CT-1 Taper (36.4 mm)	2-0 Vicryl Plus (undyed)	36" (91 cm)
Ethicon	VCP840D	CT-1 Taper (36.4 mm)	1-0 Vicryl Plus (undyed)	36" (91 cm)
Ethicon	VCP232H	CT-2 Taper (26.01 mm)	3-0 Vicryl Plus (undyed)	27" (68.5 cm)
Ethicon	VCP269H	CT-2 Taper (26.01 mm)	2-0 Vicryl Plus (undyed)	27" (68.5 cm)
Ethicon	VCP218H	SH-1 Taper (21.82 mm)	4-0 Vicryl Plus (undyed)	27" (68.5 cm)
Ethicon	VCP214H	RB-1 Taper (17.45 mm)	4-0 Vicryl Plus (undyed)	27" (68.5 cm)
Ethicon	VCPB944H	CTB-1 Blunt taper (36.4 mm)	3-0 Vicryl Plus (undyed)	36" (91 cm)
Ethicon	VCPB945H	CTB-1 Blunt taper (36.4 mm)	2-0 Vicryl Plus (undyed)	36" (70 mm)
Ethicon	VCPB946H	CTB-1 Blunt taper (36.4 mm)	1-0 Vicryl Plus (undyed)	36" (70 mm)
Ethicon	VCP916H	V-34 Tapercut (36.4 mm)	3-0 Vicryl Plus (undyed)	36" (91 cm)
Ethicon	VCP917H	V-34 Tapercut (36.4 mm)	2-0 Vicryl Plus (undyed)	36" (91 cm)
Ethicon	VCP518H	V-34 Tapercut (36.4 mm)	1-0 Vicryl Plus (violet)	36" (91 cm)
Ethicon	PDP339H	CT-1 Taper (36.4 mm))	2-0 PDS II Plus (violet)	27" (68.5 cm)

(Anderson & Romfh, 1980; Chalmers, 1989; Davis, 2004; DeLancey, 1987; Ethicon, 1985, 1994a, 1994b, 2009; Lin & Long, 1999, 2005; Sanz, 1987; Syneture, 2007; Syneture online catalogue [www.syneture.com], 2008; Varney et al., 2004)

Other concerns regarding suture materials:

Care and storage of suture materials: All suture materials should be stored in a cool, dry place away from heat sources and moisture. Damaged packages should be discarded. Expiration dates should be checked periodically, especially if certain types of suture are used infrequently. When you receive an order, record the types of suture, number of packets of each and their expiration dates in your pharmaceutical record book before you store them.

Cost: Suture is very expensive. Synthetic is about twice as expensive (or more) as its chromic gut equivalent. Have plenty of what you will use most frequently on hand, and purchase just two or three packets of sizes you will need only rarely. This way, you'll be properly equipped without investing a small fortune.

Tissue Adhesives

Synthetic tissue adhesives have been used for many years in Europe, Canada, the Middle East and Asia. In 1998, the FDA approved their use in the United States. Homebirth midwives, many of whom want to offer their clients as many options as possible, have clients who refuse suturing, have an aversion to suturing or who have limited access to suture materials due to legal constraints, have expressed a great deal of interest in tissue adhesives as an alternative to needles and thread.

Tissue adhesive is in a class of glues that adhere when they contact basic substances such as water or blood to form a strong bond. These adhesives are in the same family as cyanoacrylate household adhesives such as Super Glue. Over-the-counter cyanoacrylate glues contain methyl alcohol because it is inexpensive. It cures by a chemical reaction called **polymerization**, which produces heat. Methyl alcohol has a pronounced heating action when it contacts tissue and may even produce burns if the glue contacts a large enough area of tissue. Rapid curing may also lead to tissue necrosis. Midwives generally do not observe such reactions because minimal amounts are being used for perineal repair. Nevertheless, with their greater toxic potential, over-the-counter products are inappropriate for use in human tissue (Quinn & Kissick, 1994).

The medical-grade products currently available contain either butyl, isobutyl, or octyl esters. They are bacteriostatic and painless to apply when used as directed, produce minimal thermal reaction when applied to dry skin and break down in tissue. They are essentially inert once dry. Butyl products are rigid when dry but provide a strong bond. Octyl products are more flexible when dry but produce a weaker bond. Originally popular were *n*-butylcyanoacrylate formulas, such as Histo-Acryl Blue, a combination of adhesive with blue dye. Histo-Acryl Blue is now only used for short, straight wounds, however, because in 1998, a new, more versatile compound, octylcyanoacrylate (Dermabond), was introduced.

Dermabond has many advantages over the previous formulas. It contains a plasticizer that makes it flexible and thus useful for irregular or moving surfaces, as well as having bactericide properties and a higher breaking strength. The repaired wound requires manual support for only 30 to 60 seconds while the adhesive dries. While wounds so repaired are at greater risk for breaking open immediately after closure, after seven days there is no difference when compared to sutured wounds. The glue peels away after healing.

Packaged in sterile, plastic-covered glass vials, Dermabond can be stored at room temperature. The vial comes with either a rounded or chisel-shaped applicator tip. The chisel shape allows easier application of adhesive to many wounds without the need to apply undue pressure, which can invert the wound edges. This adhesive is available in two viscosities, with the higher viscosity formula less prone to dripping. The high-viscosity, chisel-tipped applicator is probably the best one to use for perineal repair.

Dermabond is intended for closing fresh lacerations in tissues under low tension with clean, even edges that come together easily and without gaps. There should be little to no oozing of blood, and the lacerations should be in an area where adhesive runoff can be controlled or avoided. While Dermabond is used to close many wounds that would ordinarily be repaired with sutures, its use is contraindicated on mucous membranes, hairy areas, weight-bearing areas or areas that undergo stress, all of which are characteristics of the perineal area. Tissue adhesive alone is not suitable for repair of any sort of deep wound as it cannot be used to glue together the raw sides of the wound; it is only intended to bridge across a wound and to be applied to intact skin on either side of a wound. Thus, perineal lacerations with characteristics that might make them suitable candidates for closure with tissue adhesive (were its use not in every other way contraindicated for such wounds) can probably be left to heal without any artificial closure. The exception is shallow but irritating labial tears, which might respond well to closure with tissue adhesive if the region were not so moist and the tissue so nearly like mucous membrane (Trott, 2005). For details on how midwives and obstetrical providers have used tissue adhesive for perineal repair, see the chapter entitled "Alternative Closure Techniques."

Sea vegetables: In the never-ending effort to reduce the trauma that women experience at birth and to eliminate the need to suture, some midwives have experimented with using pieces of sea vegetables as an organic form of tissue adhesive (Gilpin-Blake & Elliott, 2001). Given a choice between seaweed and synthetic adhesives, sea vegetables are the far less toxic alternative and are easy to obtain at most health food stores. Nori is sold in sheets and kelp leaves are sold in large pieces, making them especially good for this purpose. Many midwives, however, report that sea vegetables do not work well for this purpose (Scholles, 2009). See the chapter entitled "Alternative Closure Techniques" for details about how seaweed has been used by midwives

Additional Tools, Supplies and Equipment to Have on Hand

Medical exam and surgical gloves

There are basically two kinds of medical gloves. Nonsterile Exam gloves are sold singly in boxes. They used to perform nonsterile procedures, such as internal exams when the membranes are intact or the newborn exam. Surgical gloves are sterile, more precisely sized, sold in pairs, fit better and are more expensive than exam gloves. Some midwives include at least one pair of properly sized sterile gloves in a custom birthing kit; then clients pay for gloves. Surgical gloves are used for any type of precision work that requires sterility, which may include manual removal of the placenta and suturing.

Medical gloves are usually made of natural or synthetic rubber latex. With the prevalence of latex protein allergies among hospital personnel, however, synthetic nonlatex materials (e.g., vinyl, nitrile and neoprene [polymers and copolymers of chloroprene]) are widely available as well. The reported barrier integrity of gloves varies with the type and quality of material, intensity of use, length of time used, manufacturer, when tested (before or after use) and the method used to detect glove leaks. Generally, defects turn up in vinyl gloves more frequently than in latex gloves, the difference in defect frequency being greatest after use. Even so, intact vinyl gloves provide protection comparable to that of latex gloves. Limited studies indicate that nitrile gloves have leakage rates similar to latex gloves. Some gloves are designed to minimize puncture wounds during suturing, but this is accomplished by increasing the material's thickness, which reduces tactile sensitivity.

It is also important to decide the length cuff you need for the glove. Generally, the length of the glove depends on the level of splash protection needed or the depth of immersion in a solution (or during an exam). For maximum protection of the hand, wrist and forearm, measure from the tip of the middle finger to the desired length along your arm so that you can discuss the lengths available from your distributor. Unfortunately, well-fitted medical gloves do not come in lots of different lengths (Measure your hands, 2009).

Sterile gloves are sometimes sold powdered, which makes them easier to put on, but some people are allergic to the talc inside some powdered gloves. Talc allergies can be addressed by using talc-free gloves. Even if one does not have an allergy, talc exposure is best avoided as it is irritating to the respiratory tissues; this is particularly true for babies. Alternative materials for powdering include cornstarch (now available in many products, although a significant number of people are also allergic to corn), tapioca starch, potato starch, or arrowroot powder. I do not recommend do-it-yourself powdering because the powder can easily become contaminated.

Exam Glove Size	Surgical Glove size	
XS (Extra small)	5.5 to 7"	14 cm
S (Small)	6 to 8"	15 cm
M (Medium)	6.5 to 9"	16 to 17 cm
L (Large)	7.5 to 10"	19 to 20 cm
XL (Extra large)	8.5 to 11"	21 to 28 cm

Measure your hand to get a general idea of your glove size. The most commonly recommended method involves measuring around your palm at the level of the knuckles (widest point). Wrap the tape around your hand, make a fist, and measure. The other method calls for using a ruler or a flexible tape measure to measure from the base of your palm (where the hand joins the wrist) to the tip of the middle finger. The number of inches (or cm) equals your numerical glove size. Surgical gloves usually come in 12 to 15 inch (305 to 381 mm) lengths in whole and half sizes ranging from 5.5 to 12. Glove size varies among brands, so you will then need to try on different kinds of gloves to find the best fit. A properly fitted glove provides maximum protection. Gloves that are too big can impair dexterity; gloves that are too small can cause hand fatigue (Davis, 2008).

For example, if your hand measures 7 inches, you would wear a medium sized exam glove or a size 6.5 to 9 (16 or 17 cm) surgical glove. If your hand measures over 7 inches you may need to use the next size up, but this will depend upon the brand. Store gloves in a cool, dry place. While there are currently no FDA-required expiration dates for gloves, after two years of proper storage, the gloves should be carefully inspected to make sure they are continuing to provide adequate barrier protection. More about gloves can be found beginning on page 442.

Light

A bright, glare-free light is essential. There are many small, high-intensity flashlights or desk lamps on the market that serve the purpose well. A miner-style hat can be used, although it may be a nuisance as you attempt to maneuver. There are also many smaller bright head lamps, intended for hiking and camping, that attach around the head with an elastic strap. One of these would work well and can be gotten at any good outdoor gear shop such as REI. Ask your clients to have a good flashlight on hand as a backup.

Assistant

Enlist someone to help you, either your apprentice or someone else at the birth. I once had this role filled by a two-year-old who wasn't allowed to be at the birth because his mother felt unsure of his response; he held the light more unflinchingly than some nonmidwife adults! Because it's a good idea to keep someone with the mother for emotional support, don't count on the mother's partner to assist you.

The assistant's job is to hold the light and (if older than two) hand you supplies, hold tissue open, assist in maintaining asepsis, etc., and, if an apprentice, to learn.

Sterile gauze squares

These are used to clean the torn area and blot up blood as you work. Four × four inches is a good, all-purpose size. Facial tissue or toilet paper can substitute in a pinch, but it must be used carefully as it tends to shred. Gauze can also be used to form a tampon to keep lochial discharge at bay, which will improve visibility and make repair easier.

Urinary catheters

These are needed if you must drain the bladder or if a tear has occurred in or near the urethra. If periurethral tears are very close to or through the urethra and require repair, inserting a catheter can help prevent accidental closure of the urethral lumen. A straight, #10 French size is small enough to minimize the trauma of insertion but large enough to act as a landmark. A balloon catheter is not needed but can be used if that is all you have.

An appropriate set-up for examination and repair

It is difficult for a woman to assume many labor positions if the bed is too soft, and it is very difficult to perform a proper exam or to sew somebody up with her bottom sinking into the bed. You need good visibility, easy access to the perineum and the ability to assume a position that affords you some degree of comfort as well. Don't short-change this last requirement; if you are miserably uncomfortable, you will be distracted and it will be harder to do a good job. Assess furniture that can be used during suturing when you do your prenatal home visit. Check the bed for firmness. Have a board placed under the mattress (or put the mattress on the floor) if necessary. Two chairs with seats of the same height can be used to support the mother's feet for a perineal exam or repair. For an extensive repair, you could have the woman lay on a dining table with her bottom at the edge and with chairs to support her feet (Kolder, 1990). This assumes that there is a suitably sturdy table available; in many cases, there is not.

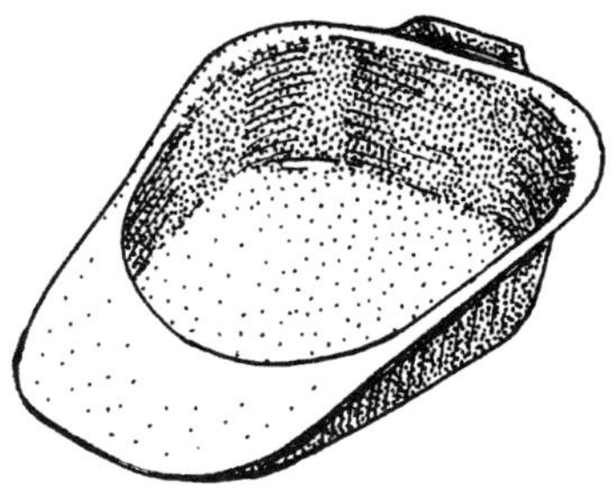

Fracture pan

Devices to elevate the woman's bottom during examination and repair: While a firm bed does help, performing complex repairs at home without benefit of an exam table with stirrups can be challenging, to say the least. The simplest and cheapest way to remedy this situation is to place a large book in a plastic bag and insert this underneath the woman's sacrum. Books and the like are not contoured, however, and can become uncomfortable during lengthy repairs.

An inverted placenta pan or a fracture pan in a plastic bag can also be placed beneath the mother to elevate her bottom for repair. The bottom of the fracture pan is tapered; place the narrow end under the woman's sacrum.

Cookie sheet or tray

Metal cookie sheets make excellent portable instrument trays. Cover one with an underpad or clean towel taped around the bottom of the tray. Most clients have a cookie sheet or a metal serving tray, so you don't necessarily have to carry one. If you purchase a tray, be sure it is does not have a nonstick or painted surface that will wear and peel, as you will be washing it often.

Crock pot

A crock pot makes a handy, portable warmer for compress water. If a woman doesn't have a crock pot, she can almost always borrow one. It works much better than trips back and forth from the kitchen with boiling hot water throughout the pushing phase of labor. Any such heating device should be cleaned thoroughly prior to use and put through a dishwasher if possible.

Local anesthetic

Any of the "-caine" drugs can be used locally. Spray anesthetic made with a "-caine" drug in a 10% concentration is available from various supply houses and is, by far, the best thing to use. Plain lidocaine, Xylocaine or Novocain 1% or 2% are the most popular injectable types. They all come in multi-use vials. (For more details see the chapter entitled "Using Local Anesthetic.")

Sharps container

A special container designed to receive sharp objects used in medical settings should be obtained to dispose of suture needles, syringes, blood tubes and any other waste that could potentially cause a puncture wound. If you have employees that are exposed to bodily fluids, check with your local health department or OSHA office for proper protection and disposal procedures. If you are working in an area where no such container is available, use a plastic bottle with a cap and tape a label over the side with "SHARPS CONTAINER" written in red ink and dispose of sharps in it.

Biohazard bags

If you are required to deal with a medical waste management company, you will need specially marked biohazard bags for all your disposable medical waste.

Crochet hook

A very small stainless steel crochet hook can be used to help remove stitches. Thumb forceps with a fine tip and tiny teeth can also be used for this purpose.

Scalpel

You could use a scalpel to make a tiny slice to remove a subcuticular synthetic stitch that is causing irritation. You will need a handle and a compatible no. 11 blade, which looks like the blade on an X-acto knife: an elongated triangle sharpened on the hypotenuse edge. This is a real extra, however, which you can easily do without.

Syringes and hypodermic needles

You can use either glass or disposable syringes, although glass syringes are increasingly harder to find. Disposable ones are easy to use, and you don't have to worry about contamination. Syringes come in all sizes. A 10 cc syringe with a 1½ inch needle is usually recommended. If you use anesthetic sparingly, a 3 cc. syringe with a 1 inch needle will be plenty big enough. If you have access to an autoclave and disposable syringes are hard to get where you practice, it may be worth getting some glass syringes to use with disposable needles. Disposable syringes contain a tiny bit of silicone as a lubricant for the plunger. The only way to avoid such additives is to use glass syringes.

A 22 to 25 gauge, 1 inch needle will do in most cases. (Gauge refers to the size of the lumen of the needle; the larger the number, the smaller the size.) Do not use reusable needles. Disposable ones are sterile and always sharp.

If you are using anesthetic that is packaged in vials, you may need to go back into your vial for more solution. It is a good idea to carry extra individually wrapped needles for this purpose. If you work with any solutions sold in individual ampules, you will also need filter needles to use when you remove the solution from the ampule. These filter needles keep shards of glass out of the fluid you will inject. Once the fluid is withdrawn from the vial, the filter needle is removed and replaced with a regular needle that is used for injection.

Peri-Rule

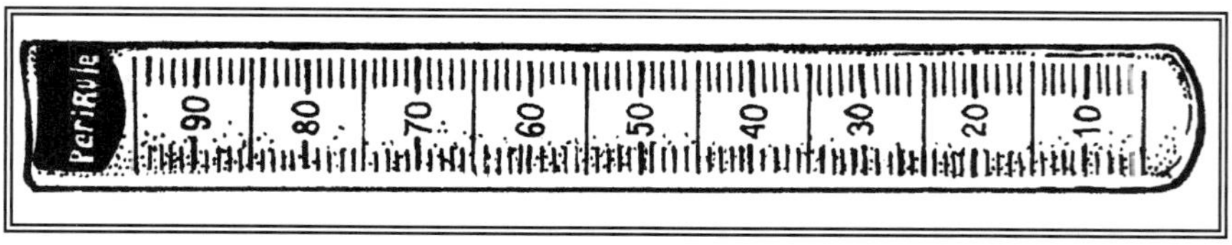

In response to the suture versus let-it-heal-on-its-own debate, midwives in the United Kingdom felt that a more objective way to measure tears would be useful. They noted that there was no system for classifying the actual size of a tear, other than the subjective opinion of the care provider who attended the birth. Reliance on professional judgement for the assessment of size is simply guesswork, however. How big, exactly, is a "small tear"?

The Peri- Rule™ is the first practical, validated tool for the reliable measurement and objective assessment of the depth of first- and second-degree perineal tears. It consists of a single-use ruler constructed of soft, medical-grade plastic with rounded edges, so that it can be painlessly inserted into a tear. It has a millimeter scale molded into the plastic on one side that leaves the surface almost completely smooth. It is 105 mm long, 10 mm wide and 4 mm thick. It also comes with a paper form to record your findings.

The Peri-rule is not sold sterile but can be cleaned and autoclaved at 273.2°F (134°C) for three minutes or boiled for twenty minutes or more without any shrinkage, distortion or flaking of the scale. Baking the ruler is not recommended as it does warp the scale.

There are numerous benefits of having an objective way of assessing tear depth. It enables improved data gathering of the rate and severity of tearing and better correlation of these data with outcomes; it also helps individual practitioners better assess the tears that are occurring among women in their care and the tearing rates when different birthing practices are employed. Objective measurement assists in teaching clinical skills. As of this printing, the Peri-Rule is not sold in the US but can be ordered from the UK. (See the website at www.wound-assessment.co.uk or www.peri-rule.bham.ac.uk for more information.)

Midwives who do not want to invest in Peri-Rules can scratch marks on one of the outer sides of the end of their thumb forceps in at least 5 mm increments to create a way to approximate this measurement. The problem with this approach is that the scratches damage the instrument and create a place for particulate matter and bacteria to hide. Therefore, particular attention must be paid to cleaning these marks thoroughly before sterilizing the instrument. Marked instruments should be checked carefully to make sure that the end that is marked remains intact with no cracks or other signs of damage. Even if you do not want to measure tears, a single mark at 1.25 cm can help you assess the need for two layers of stitches in deep tears. How to measure a tear with a Peri-Rule is explained in the chapter entitled "Assessing the Degree of Damage and the Need for Repair."

Herbs

Hemostatic (HE-mow-static) herbs arrest bleeding, and astringent herbs constrict tissue. Both can be useful during suturing to help stop bleeding so that repair can proceed. A water-based infusion for topical use or a grain alcohol–based tincture to be given orally can be made from any of the following: witch hazel bark, bayberry bark, or white oak bark. Commercially prepared calendula solution can also be used to sooth tissue and arrest bleeding. Look for a product that does not contain alcohol.

A water-based infusion of one of the astringent herbs listed above could be prepared during labor. An infusion will not only help with bleeding from tears but will be very soothing to hemorrhoids as well. Commercially prepared liquid extracts of any of these herbs in a nonalcohol base are a good alternative to alcohol-based solutions. You could also prepare a decoction and preserve it with a few drops of tincture of benzoin.

Because tinctures contain grain alcohol, they should not be used topically if it can be avoided. If an infusion is not available, place the amount of tincture you will use in a small quantity of boiling water; allow the alcohol to burn off for a few minutes before using, then soak a clean gauze square and press it into the tear.

Valerian, skullcap, Motherwort or other nonnarcotic nervine tinctures can be given orally for their calming effects. Rescue Remedy is the Bach flower remedy for crisis and can be safely given for any type of trauma. Herbs used for a postpartum herbal bath are discussed in the chapter entitled "Postpartum Care and Comfort Measures." Also see the chapter entitled "Herbal Medicine" in the Appendices.

75% silver nitrate/25% potassium nitrate swabs or applicator sticks

These can be ordered through any drug store if you can get a prescription. They can be used to cauterize sensitive spots or raw areas that are not healing well. See the chapter entitled "Examining Tears and Repairs in the Weeks Postpartum."

Sterile water-based lubricant (such as Astroglide or K-Y)

Lubricant may be necessary to perform exams in labor, but after the birth the lochia will provide plenty of lubrication most of the time. Some practitioners lubricate suture to ease pulling it through tissue. A water-based lubricant applied to chromic gut will not do any harm, as it does not break down by hydrolysis, but such solutions should not be used on synthetic sutures. Lubricating suture is not recommended by manufacturers, who have tried to take care of this issue by coating multifilament strands and by producing monofilament strands. Oil causes suture to deteriorate and should never be used for this purpose.

Povidone iodine (Betadine) solution and scrub

This is used by some practitioners to lubricate suture. It can also be used to wash hands and wipe down surfaces. Some midwives use a diluted solution to gently clean the perineal area before repair, but this is not necessary to prevent infection. (I prefer using saline solution or an herbal solution that also promotes healing.) Povidone iodine solution in gel (or sterile water-based lubricant such as K-Y) can be used to lubricate the tip of a urinary catheter. Some people are highly allergic to iodine, so you must ask before it is used. As general rules, do not combine alcohol and iodine, and do not use one after the other because burns may result. Iodine stains can be removed by soaking cloth articles in a strong solution of Borax laundry booster for several days. Iodine solution should not be used to clean metal instruments as it will promote pitting of the metal, which can eventually lead to rusting.

Hydrogen peroxide (70%)

Have a bottle of regular drug store peroxide on hand or, better yet, include it in the items list for your homebirth clients so they have it on hand. It is great for getting blood out of fabrics and has limited uses as a wound irrigant.

Items and products used to clean and sterilize instruments

The basis of the ability to safely administer injections, treat wounds and perform surgery is a group of procedures known as **aseptic** or **sterile technique**. The difference drawn between these two by some authors is subtle. When referring to equipment preparation, **asepsis** is defined as the complete absence of living microorganisms brought about by physical means such as autoclaving or gamma radiation. When not merely used as a synonym for "aseptic," **sterile** may also refer to the absence of living microorganisms when this state has been produced using chemical disinfectants.

A fundamental aspect of good surgical technique is beginning with absolutely clean and sterile instruments. It is important to maintain your instruments in top shape by using products specifically designed for this purpose.

Gloves for cleaning: It is a good idea to wear disposable exam gloves during cleaning to protect yourself. Disposing of the gloves eliminates worry about cross-contamination when you go to clean the instruments used at another birth.

Sterilization device: An autoclave can be used to sterilize steel equipment as well as glass and, in some units, cloth by applying extreme heat, steam and pressure to the articles placed in the sterilization chamber. Air is removed to create a vacuum, then superheated steam is applied. There are several types of autoclaves in use. Among these, the ones most relevant to midwifery practice are as follows.

Gravity displacement (downward displacement): In these units a heating element is submerged in a pool of water, which, when heated, produces steam. As steam is lighter than air, it forces the air in the sterilization chamber downward and out through a drain hole. Once the temperature in the sterilization chamber is sufficient, the drain hole is closed automatically and the sterilization process begins. This type can be used on liquids and instruments.

Autoclaves tend to be very expensive, yet pressure sterilizers that use steam heat are available and less costly than a traditional autoclave. These devices are similar to a pressure-cooker and can be obtained in either electric or nonelectric models. The nonelectric ones can be used on any stove top. The electric version costs about $700.00 from Cascade HealthCare Products and would be a good investment if you can afford it. These gravity displacement sterilizers reach 259°F (126.2°C).

Positive pressure displacement is an improvement upon the design of a downward displacement unit. Steam is created in a second, separate chamber and held until the proper amount to displace all of the air in the sterilization chamber is accumulated. The steam is then released into the sterilization chamber in a pressurized blast, forcing the air out through the drain hole and starting the sterilization process. This process a more accurately displaces the air than does downward displacement.

Finally, the porous load sterilizer is primarily intended to process porous items such as dressings, gowns and other textiles. In addition, they are capable of sterilizing medical and surgical equipment wrapped in porous materials, such as lint-free cloth, but they cannot be used to sterilize liquids.

Autoclaves are also classified as either type "N" or type "B". "N" autoclaves are suitable for sterilizing solid, unwrapped instruments. Type "B" autoclaves can be used on both wrapped and hollow instruments, which means a piece of equipment can be sterilized with no further handling now for use later.

Ultrasonic cleaning device: Most instrument manufacturers recommend ultrasound as the most effective way to clean surgical instruments, particularly those with hinges, box locks and other moving parts. Despite this advice, purchasing an ultrasonic device will be prohibitively expensive for all but the largest practices and is not very well suited to schlepping to births.

Cleaning brushes: Instrument cleaning brushes are available for all types of instruments. Midwives need a general-purpose toothbrush-style brush with nylon bristles to clean surgical instruments. A brush with stainless steel bristles is ideal for cleaning box locks, needle holder jaws and other hard-to-clean parts. A properly designed metal bristle instrument brush will *not* harm the surface of the metal but should never be used on coated instruments. Brass-bristled brushes should never be used on stainless steel instruments because mixing metals is not recommended. Spectrum makes soft-bristled stainless steel brushes that tests have shown do not damage the surface of matte- and satin-finished metal instruments.

Sterilization tape: This surgical masking tape has stripes that indicate sterility by changing color after a certain period of being exposed to a certain temperature. Using it on paper instrument wrappers can help you monitor sterility in home ovens and let you know if a wrapped packet has been previously sterilized. Unfortunately, the adhesive stains cloth. You will not need this tape if you use self adhesive sterilizing envelopes.

Instrument tongs: Any type of stainless steel tongs will do to remove loose instruments from a sterilization device. Do not get ones that have plastic-coated finger rings, as the coating may harbor bacteria. Modern autoclaves have trays from which the pouched instruments can be removed by hand or have a means of hanging the paper packages on a rack, eliminating the need for tongs.

Instrument cleaning agent: Instrument cleaning solution can be used to remove biological debris before sterilization. Although many midwives use povidone iodine for this purpose, it is not a suitable instrument cleansing agent. An ideal instrument detergent is low-sudsing and a good wetting agent while having a neutral pH (6.5 to 8, 7 is ideal), which protects the chromium oxide coating of fine-quality stainless steel. Solutions that are either too acid or too alkaline will damage the metal, eventually leading to pitting and breakage. Solutions that are too acidic will also cause tungsten carbide inserts on needle holders and scissors to loosen. Solutions that are overly alkaline will dissolve tungsten particles and cause premature wear. Spectrum (www.spectrumsurgical.com) and Miltex (www.miltex.com) make excellent cleaning products.

Instrument lubricating agent: An instrument lubricating agent is used to coat stainless steel instruments after cleaning and before sterilization. It helps prevent rusting and reduces wear and tear. Dilute concentrated agents with distilled water whenever possible; if no distilled water is available, used filtered water. Miltex offers a spray bottle for use with their Instrument Milk. Filling it in advance eliminates the need to dilute solutions at births. It can easily be carried in your birth bag in the event that you need to process instruments quickly.

This table summarizes the products offered by Miltex and Spectrum for instrument cleaning and lubrication.

Product (M-Miltex; S-Spectrum)	Ref No.	Use
Instrument Prep Enzyme Foam, 24 oz spray (M)	3-760	Holding and presoak
Spectra-Moist, 32 oz spray (S)	SS6	
EZ-Zyme All Purpose Cleaner, 32-3/4 oz packets (M)	3-750	Holding and presoak; soak cleaning ultrasonic cleaning; manual cleaning laundry presoak
Spectra-Soap, 1 gallon concentrate (S)	SS2	
Spray Lube, 8 oz spray bottle (M)	3-700	Prior to autoclaving or other heat sterilization
Spectra-Lube, 32 oz spray bottle (S)	SS3	
Surgical Instrument Cleaner, 8 oz spray bottle (M)	3-720	Soak cleaning; ultrasonic cleaning manual cleaning
Spectra-Sonic 1 gallon of concentrate (S)	SS1	
Surgical Instrument Stain Remover, 3 oz jar (M)	3-740	Stain removal
Spectra-Scrub powder, 3 oz jar (S)	SS7	
Nylon-bristled instrument cleaning brush (M)	3-1000	Manual cleaning
Nylon-bristled brush, 7" length (S)	45-303N	
Stainless steel-bristled instrument cleaning brush	3-1001	
Stainless-steel-bristled brush, 7" length (S)	45-303SS	

Cold sterilization solution: Specially formulated cold solutions are available for sterilizing instruments. Most chemical/cold sterilization solutions, however, render instruments sterile only after ten hours of immersion. Because of the prolonged time required, cold sterilization may not be the best choice for a busy practice. In addition, this prolonged chemical action can be more detrimental to the instruments than the usual 20 minute autoclave cycle. Furthermore, it is not recommended to sterilize instruments with tungsten carbide insert jaws by using chemical/cold sterilization solutions, which may deteriorate the instrument's jaw. If the instruments need to be "disinfected" only, a chemical/cold sterilization soak is acceptable, as disinfection will take approximately 10 minutes or so. Always check the manufacturers' specifications for the exact time recommended (Miltex, 2008).

Sterilization pouches: Medi-Plus makes instrument pouches with one clear plastic side so you can see what they contain. They have an indicator on the bag that changes color when sterilization has occurred. They can be used in any steam-pressure sterilization technique to package several instruments in a set. If used in an oven, they must be placed on a clean baking/cooling rack and then on an oven shelf with a pan of boiling water placed below them; these pouches must not heated above 200°F (93.5°C) in an oven or they will melt.

Individual paper or plastic pouches can be used to sterilize individual instruments by placing one instrument in each pouch. Make sure the pouch is wide enough for instruments with ratchet locks to be sterilized in an open (unlocked) position. If wrapping instruments in a cloth, make sure it does not contain detergent residue, which can stain instruments.

Care, Cleaning and Sterilization of Surgical Instruments

High-quality equipment lasts longer, but no instrument will tolerate abuse. Most surgical instruments are made of so-called stainless steel, which is, in most respects, an ideal material as it resists rust, takes a fine point and retains a keen edge. Better–quality instruments are often treated with a layer of chromium oxides that helps the steel resist damage. It is, however, important to keep in mind that stainless steel is only stain resistant and can stain or rust.

The following tips will help all your instruments last longer:

- Handle all instruments gently, as the finely crafted, precision tools that they are.
- Use designated surgical instruments only for their intended purpose.
- During cleaning, handle each instrument individually whenever possible.
- Avoid bouncing, dropping or tossing instruments; place them where you want them.
- Avoid weighing instruments down by placing heavier equipment on top of them.
- Protect the tips by never placing an instrument down tip-first and avoid placing other instruments over the tips.
- Contact with blood (because it contains iron) and saline are both corrosive and among the most common causes of deterioration of stainless steel. Once you are completely done using an instrument, open the ratchet or hinge and place it in a holding area until you are ready to clean it. To prevent blood from drying on your instruments, saturate a towel in tap water and lay it over them. A spray-on instrument moisturizer may also be used, but that costs money and a wet towel does the job.
- Wash and dry soiled instruments as soon as possible after use.
- If you wish to put identifying marks on your instruments, do not use a vibrating or impact marking device. If you do mark them, mark the shanks rather than the area near or on the box lock or hinge. This will decrease the likelihood of early hinge fracture.

Cleaning

All instruments, even brand new ones, should be cleaned before sterilization to remove biological and industrial debris. If an instrument is not thoroughly cleaned, it cannot be considered sterile because residual biological material that remains stuck may remain infectious and, even if not, offers a medium for microbial growth.

Used instruments should be cleaned and dried as soon as possible. Avoid soaking in water and never soak them in saline, laundry stain removers, chorine bleach, Lysol or any other solution not specifically formulated for cleaning surgical instruments. The only exception to this rule is when prion contamination is suspected (see page 452 for more on this topic). If you must use household soap, use the mildest dishwashing liquid available that is designed for handwashing dishes, or use liquid Dreft or Fairy soap. Do not use anything with abrasives in it.

Wear gloves throughout cleaning. Disposable exam gloves are fine for this purpose. To begin cleaning, scrub each instrument with a nylon-bristled brush (a soft-bristled toothbrush dedicated to this purpose works well). A piece of gauze or a sponge can also be used. Open all joints completely and scrub them from all sides.

Rinse each instrument well and recheck all joints, teeth and serrated surfaces for dried blood or other biological debris. If a nylon brush does not remove all visible debris, use a brush with stainless steel bristles that is intended for cleaning matte- or satin-finish surgical instruments (do not use to clean mirror-finish instruments). Metal bristles can remove baked-on debris in needle holder or hemostatic jaws as well as stains that nylon bristles cannot remove.

Thoroughly rinse each cleaned instrument for at least 30 seconds in distilled water if you have it or filtered water or tap water if you don't. Move jointed instruments through their full range of motion under running water to ensure that all debris has been removed. Reinspect for debris and if the instrument is clean, dry it thoroughly with a clean towel and then check each one for damage, as described beginning on page 336.

Once that is done, open all ratchets and part scissor blades. Hold each instrument up by one ring over a clean towel, several thicknesses of newspaper, or a clean trash bag and apply a 30 to 60 second spray of a nonsilicone, water-soluble surgical- instrument lubricant to condition the joints and leave a film that deters corrosion and preserves cutting edges; never use industrial oils or lubricants. Alternatively, place the open instruments on a clean towel and spray each side. After spraying, open and close the hinges a couple of times to work the lubricant into all the crevices. Allow the instruments to air dry for a few moments. You could lay them on a small, clean cake rack or hang them from a finger ring on a chopstick dedicated to this purpose. Good cleaning and lubricating practices will eliminate many possible problems with instrument wear. If you are not using a lubricant, the instruments can be prepared for sterilization after thorough cleaning.

When finished, be sure to remove debris from your cleaning tools, use a disinfectant or let soak in bleach for 1 hour, rinse again. These tools should then be sterilized separately from your surgical tools in boiling water or, preferably, an autoclave or pressure cooker.

Preventing and dealing with rust

While stainless steel can rust, most of what appears to be rust is actually blood or tissue, which can harden into a yellowish brown crust. This should be removed with good cleaning or a soft toothbrush. If blood and tissue debris are allowed to remain on an instrument during sterilization, after a while corrosion will develop in the contaminated areas.

New instruments usually have some residual magnetization from the manufacturing process in their lock boxes, serrations and ratchets that will gradually diminish over time. New instruments are therefore more vulnerable to rusting because this residual magnetism attracts tiny metal fragments to the surface and holds them there. Some older instruments were made of chromium-plated iron; when the plating flakes off, the iron underneath it will start to rust. Sometimes the screws of instruments are made from a different material than the instrument itself, which can result in the rusting of the screw or the surrounding metal. A humid environment or steam cleaning may be contributory factors to the development of rust. Another source of particles could be a metal screw that is part of an autoclave.

In order to prevent rust formation, iron instruments or rusty instruments should not be sterilized in the same autoclave as stainless steel instruments. When parts containing iron are sterilized in an autoclave, rust particles might remain inside the autoclave and precipitate on stainless steel instruments during a subsequent sterilization. This is why it is important to remove rust from an instrument as soon as possible and before it is sterilized. Never sterilize home-crafted instruments that are not made out of good-quality stainless steel together with your better-made stainless steel instruments.

Rusting weakens metal and can lead to a tension rupture at the joint in an instrument with a lock box, especially if rusted instruments are autoclaved with the ratchet engaged in its tightest position. To avoid such damage, make sure that all locking instruments are left un-engaged and slight open during sterilization.

There are two ways to remove rust. One is to scrub it gently with a soft, metal-bristled brush designed for use with instruments; if you can get the rust off with a brush, great. The other method is to soak the instrument in Coca-Cola. This is the only solution that I am recommending that is not intended to be used for surgical instruments; I do so because it is readily available and will remove some of the rust and will soften the rest of it so that it is easy to remove. The two methods can also be combined in stubborn cases.

Coca-Cola contains an acid that helps dissolve rust but that can also damage metal. Pour some Coca-Cola in a bowl and add the rusty instrument, add more Coke so that the instrument is submerged. Set a timer to ensure that you remove the instrument within 30 minutes and then clean it immediately. Thoroughly wash and rinse the cleaned instrument to remove all rust and any Coca-Cola residue (Haddad & Worst, 1999).

Checking your instruments for wear and damage

While midwifery instruments do not get the same kind of use they would get in a hospital setting, they can still be damaged. After thoroughly cleaning and rinsing, check to be sure that each instrument is undamaged and in good working order. This is an excellent job for your assistant. Each type of instrument has different areas of weakness that need to be examined frequently.

If you find damage or wear discontinue use, especially if the damage may compromise the function of the instrument or there is a risk of a piece breaking off during use. If it is a high-quality instrument, contact the manufacturer for replacement. If it is not, replace it, preferably with a higher-quality instrument.

Welded instruments: Carefully examine any parts that are welded together and any area where an instrument shaft changes shape, as these areas are particularly vulnerable to cracking.

Scissors: Open the blades widely and look along the edges of the blades to ensure that they are smooth, free of nicks, bent areas and burrs. Check to be sure scissor edges are sharp. Make sure the tips of the blades are present and either sharp (if pointed) or properly rounded (if blunt). Close the blades and check to see if the tips of the blades meet precisely, with no offsetting at the ends. Look along tungsten carbide inserts for pitting and cracks.

The cutting action should be smooth when opening and closing the rings. Scissors become dull at the tips first, their weakest area. To test cutting, open the blades three-quarters of the way and close them to the tip. All scissors used in tissue should be able to cut through four layers of gauze to the tip. Fine or delicate scissors should cut cleanly through a surgical glove. Medium-sized scissors should cut through a single layer of stocking or cast netting or two layers of gauze; large or utility scissors should cut through a double layer of stocking or plaster-cast netting. Stitch scissors should cleanly cut through all types of dissolvable suture without chewing or snagging and through an exam glove without pinching. Check both sides of a screwed or otherwise hinged area for cracks.

Needle holders: Inspect to make sure tungsten carbide inserts are present and free of pitting or cracks. Check the serrations on the jaws for wear (smoothing of serrations), cracks and missing portions. A new serrated jaw will have an even cross-hatched pattern over the entire surface of the tungsten carbide insert. Inspect both sides of the neck (located at the base of each jaw) and the box lock (the hinged area located between the neck and the shanks) for cracks and baked-on blood. The shanks should be straight and the ratchet action should be precise and smooth as you open and close the rings. When the ratchet is fully engaged to its last tooth, the edges of the jaws should meet evenly. Minimally, a needle holder should hold a needle so that is cannot be turned easily when the handle is clamped to the second ratchet tooth. A good needle holder will usually hold the needle firmly when engaged to the first tooth of the ratchet.

All other hinged instruments: Check all hinged instruments to see that they work properly and have no play in them when wiggled up and down and back and forth with your fingers in the rings; be sure the tips of the jaws are aligned. Examine the box lock for cracks.

All instruments with ratchets: Open the ratchet and check for worn or broken teeth.

Hemostats: The ratchets of hemostatic instruments are designed to remain engaged on any of their teeth. Open and close the hemostat. The action should be smooth. Then engage the ratchet on each tooth. It should hold without coming undone. To test whether the ratchet is "sprung," set it on the first tooth. Now hold the instrument by the jaws and tap the flat side of the rings softly and evenly on a flat surface. If the hemostat does not remain engaged on the first ratchet tooth or if the ratchet comes undone while tapping, it needs to be repaired or replaced. To test tension in a hemostatic instrument, close the rings until the jaws touch, leaving the ratchet unengaged; there should be a space of 1/16 to 1/8 of an inch between the first ratchet tooth of each shank.

Make sure the jaws meet with no overlap and that the tip ends meet exactly. Check the box lock and serrations in the jaws for blood and debris and cracks.

For hemostats with teeth, such as Allis forceps, the jaw teeth should interlock precisely. For ring forceps, the oval tips should match exactly, and the serrations of the jaws should be intact and free of debris.

Tissue, dressing and thumb forceps: The amount of pressure required to open and close these types of forceps changes with use. There should be no clicking or sticking when testing the tension required to press the tip ends together. Inspect the tips to ensure that they meet exactly. Serrated tips should be free of debris. Look for cracks, especially at the joined end. If the forceps has toothed tips, be sure the teeth are all present and that they fit together exactly. Examine them carefully for breaks or cracks, using a magnifying glass if necessary. If the forceps have a pin stop between the levers, make sure it is not broken, cracked or gone.

Metal retractor or yoni speculum: Check the blades, especially the tips, for bends, prongs, sharp edges or burrs. If a retractor has a release lever, it should spring back into place and open and close smoothly. Disassemble specula and check for debris and cracks, especially in or around the screw. Ensure that all parts are present, rust-free and in good working order.

Testing old instruments for plating defects: Let's say you inherited a set of old instruments from a relative. Very old instruments often have a metal finish that will eventually start to flake off. To test a finish, don exam gloves. Hold the instrument over a white surface and rub it vigorously between your palms; look for metal flakes. Once flaking begins, the instrument should not be used again because these flakes can come off during use and contaminate the site of repair.

Rust versus stains: A stain is a surface deposit, while rust is a more rare but serious condition, that occurs due to penetrating damage to the metal. A stain can be removed, but rust leaves permanent pitting in the metal. Most areas that are discolored orange or brown may appear to be rusted but are really only stained. Rub a pencil eraser over the discolored area. If the spot comes off completely, it is a stain; if not, it is rust. If a pit mark is revealed beneath the stain, it has been caused by corrosion and will eventually become rusty.

The chart on the following pages gives some common types of instrument damage, why they occur and how to remedy the situation.

PROBLEM	LIKELY CAUSE	SOLUTION
Dark or light spots	Water droplets condensing and evaporating slowly during air drying allows minerals from the water to deposit on the metal, especially sodium, calcium and magnesium.	Apply an instrument stain remover. Follow autoclave instructions exactly; leave door closed until all stream has escaped. Check for a leaky autoclave gasket or valve. Wash towels and wraps with a neutral pH detergent. Allow instruments to dry thoroughly before storing them.
	Instrument wrappers or towels may contain detergent residue.	Check towel with litmus paper for alkaline (>8 pH) detergent residue. Wash them with less soap, double rinse or both to remove all detergent.
Rust-colored film	Foreign matter inside plumbing pipes, water softeners.	Use distilled or demineralized water for cleaning and sterilizing.
Bluish stains	Prolonged use of cold sterilizing solution causes it to become corrosive.	Change sterilizing solution frequently. Use distilled water and a rust- inhibiting lubricant.
Brownish or orange stains	Perform the eraser test. If stain rubs off and no pitting exists, the problem is most likely from detergent residue on towels or the use of a high-alkaline (>8 pH) detergent, such as chlorhexidine, that left a phosphate surface deposit.	Change to neutral-pH detergent made to clean instruments. Check pH of towels with litmus paper to look for alkaline (>8 pH) detergent residues. Rinse instruments thoroughly in warm running water for at least 30 seconds after cleaning.
	Use of products containing polyphosphates, which have a copper-solubilizing action on parts of the sterilizer, causing a layer of copper to be deposited on the instruments by electrolytic action.	Use a stain remover on both the instruments and the autoclave. If problem persists, use distilled or demineralized water in the autoclave, especially if the local water supply is high in iron or other minerals. Experiment with another cleaning agent, measure accurately and be sure the autoclave fills with cold water before use.
	Could also be from: dried or baked-on blood, iodine or Betadine residue, cold sterilization solution, soaking in saline	Clean thoroughly and avoid contact with non-indicated cleaning agents as much as possible.
Dark brown or black stains w/pitting	Exposure to an acidic substance such as: low-pH (<6 pH) detergent residues on instrument surface or from towels, other chemical compounds used for “cold soaking,” bleach, dried blood	Follow all recommendations as above. If pitting remains, send instrument back to manufacturer for evaluation.
Blue-black or blue-green stain	Reverse plating may occur when different metals are cleaned together using ultrasound (for example, stainless steel with chrome). Exposure to saline, blood, potassium chloride, bleach.	Separate instruments made of different metals during cleaning and sterilizing. Avoid contact with inappropriate cleaning agents.
Purplish-black stains	Exposure to ammonia, amine chemicals, blood, potassium chloride and many other compounds or a high-pH detergent	Avoid using detergents with chloride bases or with a pH range above 8.5.

PROBLEM	LIKELY CAUSE	SOLUTION
Rust or corrosion	Imperfect chrome plating on instruments may result in the release of carbon particles from the improperly plated areas. These particles deposit on the plated parts, resulting in rust.	Separate instruments made from different materials during cleaning & sterilizing. Avoid purchasing chrome-plated instruments when possible.
	Inappropriate cleaning agents	If you must use a contraindicated soap, always rinse with distilled or deionized water, especially if the water is "hard" (high in mineral content).
	Use of water containing iron.	
	Detergent residue in cloth instrument wrappers	Rinse and dry cloth instrument wrappers thoroughly before use.
	Dried blood mimics rust; if baked on, cracks may form, especially near box locks.	Clean promptly and dry thoroughly. Preheat the autoclave and don't rush drying time, just crack the door.
Bluish-gray w/possible pits	Improper preparation of cold sterilization solutions	Follow solution manufacturer's instructions carefully, especially temperature and soak times. Use distilled or demineralized water, change solution per manufacturer's instructions.
Rainbow or multicolored stains	Excessive heat caused by a local "hot spot" during sterilization; this can compromise the tensile strength of the metal	Check your autoclave for proper temperature.
Black stains	Exposure to ammonia.	Do not use ammonia on instruments.
Cracked box locks	Blood and debris buildup that is allowed dry and that is not thoroughly removed.	Thorough cleaning with ratchets open before blood dries.

(Miltex instrument stain table, 2007)

Packaging instruments for sterilization

It is nice to package your most used instruments and your seldom-used instruments as sets in separate pouches (for example, you could separate your birth instruments and your suturing instruments into two sets). Open the finger rings of scissors slightly. Unlock all clamping instruments and sterilize them in an open position. Instruments locked during heat sterilization can experience cracked hinges or other problems because of heat expansion. Place heavy instruments on the bottom of the pile (when two layers are required). In addition, when using sterilization wrappers, instruments should be placed in them with the tips pointing in the same direction, with the finger rings nearest the opening of the pouch (or near the door of the autoclave or uppermost if using a pressure cooker with no wrappers). This way, you can reach in to a grasp an instrument without touching the tips.

When wrapping instruments in cloth, use one piece of cloth to enclose the instruments in an inner packet and a second piece of cloth as a dust cover.

Sterilization procedures

Since birth is not a sterile event, the primary purpose of sterilizing birth instruments is to avoid cross-contamination from one woman to another. Cleaning and sterilization beforehand allows you to go to each birth with instruments that have been throughly decontaminated from the previous birth.

"Sterile" is an absolute term that means no living organisms have survived. To "disinfect" refers to something that has been basically cleaned, but some organisms may have survived (Miltex, 2007b). The chain of resistance to destruction (from most to least hardy) is: prions (malformed protein particles that are very difficult to destroy. Prions are thought to cause transmittable spongiform encephalopathy), spores, mycobacteria (e.g., tuberculosis), non-enveloped (entero) viruses (e.g., polio), fungi (e.g., yeast), vegetative bacteria (e.g., staph), lipid (enveloped) viruses such as hepatitis and HIV, and syphilis. (If allowed to air dry, syphilis dies almost immediately once outside the body.) For more about each of these infectious agents refer to UNDERSTANDING DIAGNOSTIC TESTS. For information on prions go to www.midwiferybooks.com and check for updates to the text if you have the 7th edition or earlier.

Sterilization device: If you have access to an autoclave or an electric steam-pressure sterilizer, great. Follow the directions that are included with it exactly; some of the suggestions given below for other types of sterilization methods may be helpful as well. If you are using an autoclave, add distilled or filtered water whenever possible.

When using most portable tabletop autoclaves or other steam-based heaters, avoid overloading the chamber because an air pocket may form that inhibits steam penetration. At the end of the autoclave cycle and before the drying cycle, you may need to unlock the door and open it no more than a crack, about 1/4" (6.4 mm). Then run the dry cycle for the period recommended by the autoclave manufacturer. If the autoclave door is fully opened before the drying cycle, cold room air will rush into the chamber causing condensation on the instruments that may result in water stains or cause moisture to condense on the packs, leaving them wet.

Make sure autoclave filters and chambers are cleaned as recommended by the manufacturer. A Surgical Instrument Stain Remover (3-740) is effective in removing stains and cleaning the autoclave chamber. If you have any unusual staining on your instruments after sterilization, obtain Miltex's Instrument Care video tape (Item no. 3-810) or contact a Miltex or Spectrum representative (Miltex, 2007b) for tips on how to avoid this in the future.

Home oven: If you do not have a sterilization device, you can sterilize your instruments in an oven set to 320°F (160°C). This should kill all microorganisms and their pathogenic by-products but may actually preserve prions (see page 452). You should carry an oven temperature gauge in your birth bag, since oven temperatures frequently vary. Because of such variations, preheat the oven to 350°F (180°C) for 20 minutes before placing your instruments in it. The extra time and heat helps compensate for temperature irregularities of individual ovens. This is more than enough time and heat to kill spores. Be sure to check the oven thermometer before you put the instruments in and then at intervals during the sterilization process.

Wrap your cleaned instruments in three layers of white cloth (you can buy a cotton sheet and make at least two sets of square, hemmed wrappers used only for this purpose). When the oven is up to temperature, place the wrapped instruments in a clean paper bag and put them in a clean pan in the center of the preheated oven on the upper shelf. Put a separate pan of water on the lower oven shelf to minimize scorching of your wrapper. Sterilize the instruments for two hours.

Pressure cooker: You can also use a home pressure cooker if there is time for the packets to dry after processing. Pressure cooking is not ideal if you expect to be called to another birth within eight hours, as there is no time to allow the packets to air dry before you have to leave for the next birth. Time considerations also make this method a poor choice for sterilizing while doing immediate care after the birth because you will still have a packet of wet instruments by the time you are ready to go home.

To proceed, place a vegetable steamer in the bottom of the cooker. Fill the cooker with water so that it almost reaches the bottom of the steamer base. Place cleaned instruments in a disposable sterilization pouch or wrap them in new aluminum foil and set them in the steamer. Place your instrument tongs in the pot outside the packet, handle up, so they can be used to lift the packet from the cooker. If you have neither foil nor sterilization pouches, simply place the cleaned instruments in the cooker.

Secure the lid, position the jiggler and raise the pressure to maximum (regular rocking motion of the jiggler). Now adjust the heat so the jiggler maintains a steady rocking motion, and cook for a minimum of 25 minutes. Then turn off the heat. Remove the pot from the burner if you're using an electric stove.

When the pressure has reduced, remove the instrument packet, or if not already in a packet, use the tongs to move each instrument from the pressure cooker directly to clean cloth instrument wrappers (Hobbs, 1990). Cover the instruments with a second wrapper immediately. After sterilization and placement in clean wrappers, if the instruments are damp, they should be allowed to air dry before handling. Once completely dry, place instruments in more dry, clean cloth wrappers or in disposable sterilization pouches.

Boiling water: If you have no other choice, you can boil your instruments in enough water to cover them for a minimum of 25 minutes. This will kill most microorganisms but will not deactivate prions. Remove them from the water as for pressure cooking and place them in instrument wrappers. Don't make boiling them a habit, as it will ruin your tools and does not destroy all pathologic agents.

Handling sterilized instruments

Handle the cool instruments with sterile gloves. If placing them into sterilization pouches have an assistant hold the pouch open while you transfer the instruments to the pouch. The surface that the cloth wrappers rest on should have been disinfected, dry, and in a place of minimal activity that is at least waist high, since moisture and air currents, dust or dirt from talking and moving about may interfere with maintaining sterility.

Storing your sterilized instruments

Once sterilized and completely dry, the wrapped instruments can be placed in a new sealable plastic bag and then put away in your birth bag until you are ready to use them at the next birth. One week is the usual time limit to consider something sterile. However, if the instrument packs are not opened and are kept clean and dry, and you are not in a hospital or other high risk setting with prevalent resistant or highly contagious pathogens, such as the tropics, it is perfectly safe to forego additional sterilization between births unless the instruments sit around for longer than, say, 30 days or unless their wrappers become damaged, damp or soiled. (Block, 1983; Codman, 1987; E Davis, 2004; Hobbs, 1990; Williams, [n.d., ca. 1985).

Humid climates: To avoid the growth of organisms as well as the development of rust, instruments must be stored dry. In hot, highly humid climates surgical instruments, microscopes, slitlamps, ophthalmoscopes and lenses should all be protected from moisture and fungal contamination. This can be accomplished by using a monsoon box. To make a box, rig up a small light fixture fitted with a small 5 to 15 watt incandescent light bulb inside a closed cabinet or in a wooden box that is large enough to hold the articles you want to keep dry. The warm air inside the box has a lower relative humidity than the air in the ambient room environment, and this will help keep your instruments dry.

Another way to protect instruments like ophthalmoscopes is to place a small bag of silica gel, or other dehydrating chemical, inside the case with the instrument. If a desiccant product is not available, a small bag of dry rice can be used to absorb water from the humid air (Haddad & Worst, 1999).

References and Further Reading on Surgical Tools, Equipment and Related Supplies

References Used in Multiple Chapters

Anderson R, Romfh R. Technique in the Use of Surgical Tools. Appleton Century-Crofts, New York NY, 1980.

Davis E. Heart & Hands: A Midwife's Guide to Pregnancy & Birth, 4th ed. Celestial Arts, Berkeley CA, 2004.

Salthouse T, et al. "Relationship of cellular enzyme activity to catgut and collagen suture absorption," Surg Gynecol Obstet, 129(4):691-696, 1969.

Trott A. Wounds and Lacerations: Emergency Care and Closure, 3rd ed. Elsevier Mosby, Philadelphia PA, 2005.

Selecting Suturing Tools, Related Supplies and Equipment

Adoni A, Anteby E. "The use of Histoacryl for episiotomy repair," Br J Obtet Gynaecol, 98(5):476-478, May, 1991.

Anderson M. "Principles of wound healing in the repair of the episiotomy" (unpublished paper), Hawthorne NY, 1975.

Bowen M, Selinger M. "Episiotomy closure comparing enbucrilate tissue adhesive with conventional sutures," Int J Gynaecol Obstet, 78(3):201-205, Sep, 2002.

CardinalHealth catalogue. Allegiance Surgical Instruments. www.cardinal.com, McGaw Park IL, 2006.

Cascade HealthCare Products. Product Catalogue, www.1cascade.com, accessed Oct, 2008.

Chalmers I. Effective Care during Pregnancy and Birth, Vol. 2: Childbirth. Oxford U Press, New York NY, 1989.

Chu C. Chapter 4: "Classification and general characteristics of suture materials," in Chu C, et al., eds. Wound Closure Biomaterials and Devices. CRC Press, Boca Raton FL, 1996.

Cooper Surgical, Inc. "Guardian Vaginal Retractor" (product brochure). Cooper Surgical, Inc., Trumbull CT, revised Apr 2005.

Coulthard P, et al. "Tissue adhesives for closure of surgical wounds," Cochrane Database Syst Rev, (2):CD004287, 2004.

Davis D. "Choosing and using the right surgical glove" Workhorse Pub., www.cardinal.com/mps/brands/gloves/selection/surgglove.asp, 2001, accessed on Oct 14, 2008.

DeLancey J. Basic Exercises: Surgical Technique. Davis-Geck, Wayne NJ, 1987.

Dineros-Fernandez A, et al. "CAPROSYN, another major advance in synthetic monofilament absorbable suture," J Long-Term Effects Med Implants, 14(5):359-368, 2004.

Dunn D. Wound Closure Manual. Ethicon, Inc. Johnson & Johnson Co., Somerville NJ, 2008.

Edlich R, Long W. Syneture Surgical Knot Tying Manual. US Surgical/Tyco Healthcare, Norwalk CT, 2005.

Ethicon, Inc. Ethicon Product Catalogue. Johnson & Johnson Co., Somerville NJ, updated Feb 16, 2009.

Ethicon, Inc. Knot Tying Manual. Johnson & Johnson Co., Somerville NJ, 2005a.

Ethicon, Inc. Synthetic Absorbable Sutures (product brochure). Johnson & Johnson Co., Somerville NJ, 2005b.

Ethicon, Inc. Advanced Wound Closure (product brochure). Johnson & Johnson Co., Somerville NJ, 2005c.

Ethicon, Inc. Wound Closure Manual. Johnson & Johnson Co., Somerville NJ, 1999.

Ethicon, Inc. Vicryl RAPIDE (product brochure). Johnson & Johnson Co., Somerville NJ, 1995.

Ethicon, Inc. Wound Closure Manual. Johnson & Johnson Co., Somerville NJ, 1994a.

Ethicon, Inc. Ethicon Product Catalogue. Johnson & Johnson Co., Somerville NJ, Aug 1, 1994b.

Ethicon, Inc. Wound Closure Manual. Johnson & Johnson Co., Somerville NJ, 1985.

Ethicon, Inc. Suture Use Manual: Use and Handling of Sutures and Needles. Ethicon Inc., Somerville NJ, 1977.

Faulkner B, et al. "Biomechanical performance of a braided absorbable suture," SURG GYNECOL OBSTET, 153:497-507, 1981.

Gifford, KA. Personal conversation, May, 2010.

Gilpin-Blake D, Elliott S. "A natural alternative to suturing," MIDWIFERY TODAY, (60):32, Win, 2001.

Greenberg JA, et al. "Randomized comparison of chromic versus fast-absorbing polyglactin 910 for postpartum perineal repair," OBSTET GYNECOL, 103(6):1308-1313, Jun, 2004.

Gynex.com. www.gynex.com, accessed Feb, 2008.

Harris T. "Suitable suture material for perineal repair," BRIT J MIDWIFERY, 9(11):678-681, Nov 1, 2001.

Haubrich W. MEDICAL MEANINGS: A GLOSSARY OF WORD ORIGINS, 2nd ed. Harcourt Brace Javanovich, San Diego CA, 1984.

Johnson & Johnson Co. "Essential prescribing information: Monocryl Plus Antibacterial suture," www.jnjgateway.com/home.jhtml?loc=USENG&page=viewContent&contentId=09008b9881159515&parentId=09008b9880609524, accessed Feb, 2008.

Jueneman F. "Stick it to um," INDUSTRIAL RESEARCH DEV, 19, Aug, 1981.

Kaye D. "Clinical sterilizers: an overview," www.articlealley.com/article_60215_17.html, Jun 6, 2006, accessed Jun 7, 2010.

Kettle C. "Pregnancy and childbirth. Perineal care: Repairing first- and second-degree tears, absorbable sutures in first- and second-degree tears," BMJ CLINICAL EVIDENCE, 9:1571- 1583, 2003.

Kettle C. "Suture materials used for perineal repair following childbirth," BRIT J MIDWIFERY, 6(12):760, Dec 3, 1998.

Kettle C, Johanson RB. "Absorbable synthetic versus catgut suture material for perineal repair," COCHRANE DATABASE SYST REV, (2):CD000006, 2000.

Kettle C, et al. "Continuous versus interrupted perineal repair with standard or rapidly absorbed sutures after spontaneous vaginal birth: a randomized controlled trial," LANCET, 359(9325): 2217-2223, Jun 29, 2002.

Kolder V, MD. Editing comments, Aug, 1990.

Leroux N, Emmanuel B. "Impact of chromic catgut versus polyglactin 910 versus fast-absorbing polyglactin 910 sutures for perineal repair: a randomized, controlled trial," AM J OBSTET GYNECOL, 194(6):1585-1590, Jun, 2006.

Lin K, Long W. "Revolutionary advances in skin stapling and tissue adhesives," US Surgical/Tyco Healthcare, Norwalk CT, Jan, 2006.

Lin K, Long W. SCIENTIFIC BASIS FOR THE SELECTION OF SURGICAL NEEDLES AND SUTURES. US Surgical/Tyco Healthcare, Norwalk CT, Mar, 2005.

Lin K, Long W. SCIENTIFIC BASIS FOR THE SELECTION OF SURGICAL NEEDLES AND SUTURES. US Surgical/Tyco Healthcare, Norwalk CT, 1999.

Mainstone A. "Sutures, surgical needles and perineal trauma," BRIT J MIDWIFERY, 12(12):771-776, Dec 2, 2004.

"Measure your hands," http://www.therapygloves.com/measurehands.html. Accessed Dec 17, 2009.

Miltex.com. www.miltex.com, accessed Feb, 2008.

Miltex, Inc. MILTEX SURGICAL INSTRUMENTS. Miltex Instrument Co., Inc., New York NY, 1986.

Mornar S, Perlow J. "Blunt suture needle use in laceration and episiotomy repair at vaginal delivery," AM J OBSTET GYNECOL, 198(5):e14-15, May, 2008.

Peri-Rule.com. www.peri-rule.bham.ac.uk, accessed Dec, 2008.

Quinn J, Kissick J. "Tissue adhesives for laceration repair during sporting events," CLIN J SPORT MED, 4(4): 245-248, 1994.

Rocket Medical. INSTRUMENTS FOR GYNAECOLOGY (product catalogue). Watford, UK, www.rocketmedical.com, accessed Oct, 2008.

Sanz L. "Wound management matching materials and methods for best results," CONTEMP OB/GYN, 30(5): 86-114, Nov, 1987.

Scholles H. Personal communication, 2009.

Snowden-Pencer, Inc. DIAMOND-LINE INSTRUMENT CATALOGUE. Feb, 1990.

Spectrum Surgical Instruments. www.spectrumsurgical.com, accessed on Feb, 2008.

Syneture. SYNETURE PRODUCT CATALOGUE, 2007. United States Surgical, Norwalk CT, 2007.

Syneture. INDERMIL TISSUE ADHESIVE, (product brochure). United States Surgical, Norwalk CT, 2006.

Syneture. SYNETURE FAMILY OF MONOFILIMENT SYNTHETIC ABSORBABLE SUTURES, (product brochure). United States Surgical, Norwalk CT, 2005.

Szarmach R, et al. "An innovative surgical suture and needle evaluation and selection program," J LONG-TERM EFFECTS MED IMPLANT, 12(4):211-229, 2002.

Timesco. GYNAECOLOGIC AND OBSTETRIC INSTRUMENTS CATALOGUE. Timesco, London UK, (www.timesco-surgery.co.uk), accessed Nov, 2008.

Tyco Healthcare. "Polysorb coated, braided synthetic absorbable sutures," (package insert), United States Surgical, Syneture, Gosport UK, Mar, 2006.

Varney H, et al. Chapter 79: "Cutting an episiotomy and repairing episiotomies and lacerations," in their VARNEY'S MIDWIFERY, 4th ed. Jones & Bartlett, Sudbury MA, 2004.

von Fraunhofer J, Chu C. Chapter 3: "Surgical Needles," in Chu C, et al., eds. WOUND CLOSURE BIOMATERIALS AND DEVICES. CRC Press, Boca Raton FL, 1996.

Wark G. "Types of autoclaves," www.ehow.com/about_5031514_typ3es-autoclaves.html, accessed Jun 6, 2010.

Wikipedia contributors. "Forceps." WIKIPEDIA, THE FREE ENCYCLOPEDIA, http://en.wikipedia.org/wiki/Forceps, accessed Jan 28, 2009.

Wound Assessment. www.wound-assessment.co.uk, accessed Feb 2008.

Zederfeldt B, Hunt T. WOUND CLOSURE: MATERIALS AND TECHNIQUES. Davis & Geck, Wayne NJ, 1990.

CARE, CLEANING AND STERILIZATION OF SURGICAL INSTRUMENTS

Association of Operating Room Nurses (AORN). "Recommended practices for the care and cleaning of surgical instruments and powered equipment. Association of Operating Room Nurses," AORN J, 65(1):124-128, Jan, 1997.

Block S, ed. DISINFECTION, STERILIZATION AND PRESERVATION, 3rd ed. Lea & Febiger, Philadelphia PA, 1983.

Codman & Shurtleff, Inc. THE CARE AND HANDLING OF INSTRUMENTS. Johnson & Johnson, Randolph MA, 1987.

Haddad D, Worst J. STANDARD OPERATING PROCEDURE MANUAL FOR: MAINTENANCE OF MICROSURGICAL INSTRUMENTS, REPAIR OF MICROSURGICAL INSTRUMENTS. Fred Hollow Foundation Inc., Randwick Australia, Apr, 1999. (Available in PDF at (http://tinyurl.com/haddadworst99), accessed Feb 12, 2008.)

Hobbs V, Midwife. Editing comments, 1990.

Miltex. "Instrument stains," www.miltex.com, accessed Nov, 2007a.

Miltex. "Recommended steps in cleaning, sterilization and maintenance of surgical instruments," www.miltex.com, accessed Nov, 2007b.

Schultz R. INSPECTING SURGICAL INSTRUMENTS: AN ILLUSTRATED GUIDE. Spectrum, Stow OH, 2005.

Spectrum. INSTRUMENT PROCESSING ESSENTIALS: SURGICAL INSTRUMENTS, REPAIRS, INSTRUMENT ACCESSORIES, 7th ed. (product catalogue). Spectrum Surgical Instruments, Stow OH, 2004.

Williams V. "Sterile (?) techniques and home birth," unpublished paper, (n.d., ca. 1985).

BASIC SURGICAL PRINCIPLES

How Wounds Heal

Understanding how materials used to bring the edges of a wound together or how leaving a wound to heal on its own may affect the tissue requires a basic understanding of how wounds heal. A **wound** is defined as any type of tissue injury, especially when caused by physical means and when it involves the interruption of the continuity of the tissue. Tissue damage activates defense processes to restore the tissue's integrity and strength and results in natural and spontaneous healing.

Ideally, every injury would be repaired by regeneration of the same type of tissue that was destroyed. In reality, only the epidermis and the mucosal tissues heal by regeneration. Other tissues, such as muscle, fat, fascia, blood vessels, etc., heal by laying down collagen, a white protein that, in this case, becomes **scar tissue**.

Normal healing

This description is largely based on Myers (2008) unless otherwise noted. Healing begins immediately upon injury. It occurs in four phases that partially overlap. These phases are hemostasis, inflammation or preparative, proliferative and maturation. Each of these phases is an important part of normal healing. If a phase is either too short or too prolonged, healing will be impaired.

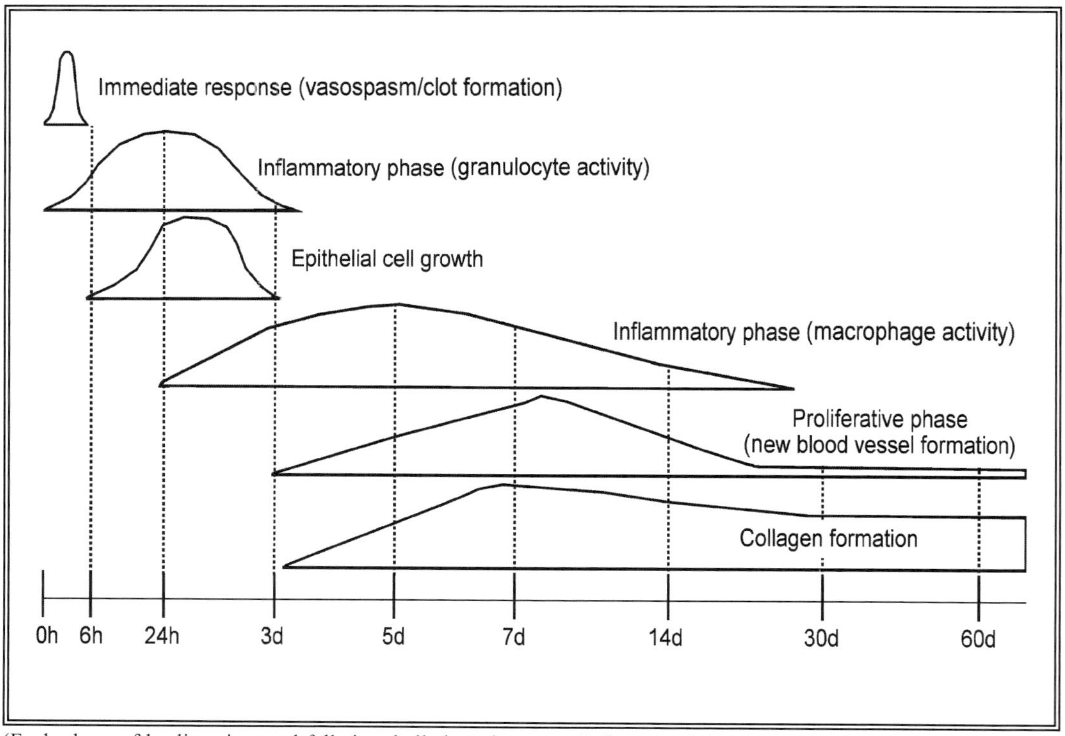

(Each phase of healing rises and falls in a bell-shaped curve. Collagen activity tapers slightly at about 24 days but remains quite high beyond 60 days.)

The first thing that happens after injury is bleeding, which triggers **hemostasis**. Damage to surface tissue leads to constriction of superficial blood vessels for about 10 minutes. Platelets begin to accumulate in the damaged blood vessels along the edges of the wound. The clotting cascade is activated and, within minutes, the wound begins to fill with coagulated hemostatic agents. In surface wounds, coagulated blood and other agents enter the wound, where they gradually dry to form a scab.

As hemostasis is occurring, the **inflammation** or **preparative phase** begins and lasts through the first three to seven days of healing. This healthy response involves both vascular and cellular activities that remove debris and prevent infection. It also signals cells needed for repair and healing to come to the site of the injury.

As fluid containing plasma proteins, red and white blood cells, and clotting agents fills the wound, mast cells degranulate. This releases inflammatory mediators such as prostaglandins and histamine, which prompt local undamaged blood vessels to dilate. The complement system is activated, attracting granulocytes to the wound, followed shortly by lymphocytes. During the first 12 to 24 hours, neutrophils (a type of granulocyte) peak. The white cells work together to remove debris (a process called débridement [de-BREED-ment]) and bacteria from the damaged tissues. After about 24 to 48 hours, monocytes enter the wound in large numbers and by day 5 are the predominant type of WBC. They also work to destroy cellular debris, consume bacteria, and stimulate new vessel formation, as well as releasing healing regulators such as growth factors and prostaglandins and prompting fibroblasts to release collagen. These processes are aided by immunoglobulins that mix with the other wound exudates.

The white cells produce inflammation within a few hours that lasts three to seven days and causes localized swelling (tumor), pain (dolor), warmth (calor), redness (rubor) and decreased function (functio laesa) around the wound (words in parentheses are the Latin terms). At first the wound oozes sanguinous (blood-rich) fluid that changes to a clear or pale yellow fluid called "serous exudate." As this fluid mixes with proteins and white blood cells, it forms a pale yellow to cream-colored layer over the surface of the wound. If this layer becomes quite thick, it is called "slough," which is yellow to tan in color and has a stringy or mucinous texture. During this period, the wound's tissue tensile strength is low.

After two to four days the **proliferative phase** begins, when neovascularization, that is, new vessel and tissue growth, takes place, usually becoming most active by day 7. It starts with fibroblast cells traveling via the general circulation to the wound surfaces. Fibroblasts rapidly divide and begin to produce new collagen fibrils by day 2. These tissue-building cells adhere to and hold the wound surfaces together by forming a collagen matrix in the wound known as "granulation tissue," which contains myofibroblasts. Peak synthesis occurs between days 5 and 7, and the wound has its greatest collagen mass by 3 weeks. Collagen protein is a primary component of connective tissues. New collagen is gelatinous and is laid down randomly in an amorphous pattern that has little tensile strength.

With time, collagen fibers crosslink as they remodel into an organized basket-weave pattern. For this to proceed without the formation of too much collagen, lysis takes place, breaking down old or damaged collagen that is cleared from the site by macrophage cells so that new collagen can replace it. The balance between synthesis and lysis results in a period about 7 to 10 days after injury when the healing wound is most vulnerable to dehiscing (breaking open) or becoming infected.

Eventually, enough mature collagen is laid down to allow the wound to withstand normal activity without separating. How long this takes varies according to the tissues that are injured and the stress placed on them. Skin and fascia are the strongest tissues but regain tensile strength slowly during healing. Mucosa is weaker but heals much more rapidly. In wounds that heal by primary intension (types of healing intension are explained later in this chapter), proliferation occurs in a few days. The proliferative phase begins rapidly and then slows, with the major repairs ending around the 14th day.

As connective tissue reknits, lymphocyte channels are also restored, blood vessels form buds (which appear as tiny red dots), granulation tissue develops, and capillary beds are temporarily established to nourish the healing tissue. Tiny blood vessels begin to bridge the wound surfaces forming loops that are surrounded by actively growing fibroblasts, causing the red dots to connect. At this point, the healing surfaces of the wound become pink and rosy and finally a bright, beefy red as the vascular bed is established, an appearance referred to as **granulation**. This thick vascular bed brings nutrients and oxygen to the healing site. Granulation tissue is most visible in open wounds that heal by secondary intention. Vascularity decreases by day 21, with continued regression as the wound matures.

Other damaged tissues are also replaced during the proliferative phase. Within 12 to 72 hours of the injury, epithelial cells from the basal layer of the epidermis begin to undergo functional changes that facilitate migration of intact cells from the wound edges over the surface of the wound. They travel over the damaged dermis and under the clot. Epithelial cells move in a sheet of cells or by "leap-frogging" over viable tissue, giving the wound a pink appearance. They can only move across moist granulation tissue (a dry wound or a scab impedes this process). Keeping wounds moist speeds healing, thus the moist environment of the perineum supports the healing process. The cells advance from the edges toward the center of the wound, where they meet. Continued replication reestablishes the normal skin layers over the months following the injury.

The wound regains only 5% of its original strength by two weeks and only 35% of its original strength by one month post injury. It takes several months for a wound to achieve its fully healed tensile strength. The final appearance of any scarring will not be evident for six months to a year or more.

Wound contraction also occurs during the proliferative phase as fibroblasts are transformed into myofibroblasts. When the collagen matrix is sufficiently firm, cell-exerted force squeezes out growth factor. Once the growth factor is available, the fibroblast expresses the contractile proteins, sticks more firmly to the matrix and starts to contract, pulling the matrix tightly together. This process liberates yet more growth factor that in turn stimulates other fibroblasts to become contractile. The mechanical nature of this process ensures that contraction only occurs when the matrix is "ready" (Wipff et al., 2007). Myofibroblasts have properties similar to smooth muscle cells and fibroblasts and are the primary facilitator of wound contraction. As myofibroblasts mature and cross over themselves, they shrink, pulling the edges together, reducing the size of the opening in the tissue and resulting in a smaller wound that requires less scar tissue to heal.

Linear wounds contract faster than square or rectangular wounds and round wounds contract the least efficiently. Wounds that penetrate below the skin level contract the most. Wound contraction can lead to excessive scarring in some areas of the body, such as the neck and face. Surgical wounds that close by primary intension have minimal contractile response because perfect alignment of the wound edges reduces the amount of collagen needed as well as the amount of epithelial migration required to close the wound.

The **maturation** or **remodeling phase** occurs as collagen deposition is completed. It begins around the 20th day, although timing varies, and it lasts until the wound structure becomes solidified by the formation of scar tissue and tensile strength is increased, which can take up to 18 months and sometimes longer. During this phase, the vascularity of the wound gradually decreases as the strength of the healed wound rises.

At this point, scar tissue begins to form. A **scar** is an area of fibrous tissue that replaces normal tissue after an injury. It has fewer blood vessels and may lack sensory neurons, hair and skin glands. The amount of scar tissue that forms depends upon the amount of granulation tissue that developed during the proliferative phase. The pink-red color of the newly formed scar fades so that it more closely matches the surrounding skin. It also lies flatter to the skin surface over time as the collagen fibers reorganize and remodel. Torn muscle fibers do not reunite as they heal: they are connected by intervening fibrosis, and thus a tear that occurs perpendicular to the orientation of the muscle fibers results in a double-bellied muscle once it heals (Kirk, 2002).

The forces that pull the edges of a wound apart will remain a factor after the sutures have dissolved or have been removed. Significant collagen synthesis continues from 5 to 42 days postoperatively. After that, any additional gain in tensile strength will be due to remodeling, or cross-linking, of collagen fibers rather than to collagen synthesis. The amount of collagen that ultimately forms creates the final scar. Tensile strength continues to increase up to one to two years post injury. Previously wounded tissue is never as strong or as elastic as it was before injury. A recovery of 80% of the original tensile strength is considered excellent.

The healing potential of the yoni and perineal region: The yoni and rectal mucosa and other soft tissues of the genitals are forgiving and usually heal well. This is because the environment is ideally arranged to optimize healing: the area is constantly moist; the mucosa heals rapidly and without scars; the vascularity of the area speeds the resolution of swelling and the transport of tissue nutrients and waste products; and the tissues are held naturally in approximation when the legs are together, reducing strain on the tissues and any sutures that are placed. The mildly acidic (3.8 to 4.2) pH of the yoni also helps, because it tends to inhibit bacterial growth and thus infections of the perineal area are uncommon.

Impaired healing

A variety of things can go wrong in the healing process. These problems are more likely to occur in malnourished individuals, as well as those taking steroid medications, those with diabetes and those with immune disorders. Proper healing can only occur in living tissues, so the presence of necrotic tissues can impair healing and breed infection.

On one hand, when the **inflammatory phase** is impaired or absent, reflected by decreased or absent signs and symptoms, wound healing will be prolonged. An inflammatory response can be encouraged using débridement or electrotherapeutic stimulation and lavage techniques. On the other hand, chronic inflammation impairs healing because it prevents new tissue from forming. Such inflammation can be caused by a foreign object in the wound, by repeated mechanical trauma or by the use of cytotoxic agents.

Hypogranulation results when the wound cannot build enough granulation tissue to fill the wound cavity, as might occur in a large, deep, unsutured wound. This lack of adequate granulation in turn impairs epithelial migration, resulting in skin cells lining the sides of the wound cavity rather than bridging the gap; this can create a skin-lined fistula or blind pocket. A perimeter of scar tissue around the wound edge can also impair epithelial cell migration. Therapies aim to protect and enhance the granulation process. Wiping the edges of the wound or lightly filling the hole with a suitable material may decrease the risk of premature epithelization. Serial débridement can also help form healthy granulation tissue by restimulating inflammation.

The opposite problem, **hypergranulation**, is more likely to occur in young, healthy women of childbearing age. This involves continued growth of granulation tissue after the wound defect is filled, resulting in a mound of tissue (proud flesh) that projects above the surface of the surrounding skin. Hypergranulation also impairs epithelization because the skin cells have trouble climbing up the mound and sometimes produce a rolled edge instead.

Excessive granulation can be prevented by protecting the wound from trauma such as inappropriate whirlpool use. Once hypergranulation develops it will often regress, at least somewhat, on its own. If it is bothersome and does not regress, it can be resolved in three ways: apply pressure to reduce the oxygen supply to the cells, which helps to slow the overgrowth; cauterize it by applying silver nitrate to the mounded tissue (see pages 571, 595 for how to do so) or surgically remove the tissue.

Hypertropic scars result when there is an overproduction of immature collagen during the proliferative and maturation phases. This produces red, raised, fibrous lesions within the boundaries of the wound. Such scars develop more readily in wounds that cross lines of tension in the skin or in large or infected wounds with prolonged inflammation. Dark-skinned persons are at greater risk for hypertropic scarring. Applying compression, as well as massage, steroids or surgery can be used to alter the scar.

Keloid scarring also occurs when the secretion of immature collagen exceeds the necessary minimum but results in a bulkier scar. It is more likely to occur in those with dark pigmentation or in wounds that overlie areas of increased tissue tension. Keloid scars extend beyond the original edges of the wound and rarely regress on their own. They are more likely to form when there is trauma to the healing wound. These scars present as nodular masses of collagen randomly arranged in swirls or clusters.

Contracture is the abnormal shortening of a wound to the point of deforming underlying structures. It usually occurs when wounds, especially burns, cross a joint.

Dehiscence occurs when healing or healed wound edges separate due to insufficient collagen formation or inadequate tensile strength. Although dehiscence is usually associated with infection, the wound edges probably separate prior to the onset of any infection. Once dehiscence occurs, the wound is treated if infected, protected from stress and usually left open to heal.

Wound healing patterns

First intention healing (primary closure) occurs when a wound heals by primary union. The edges of the wound lie against each other, either naturally or because they are sutured, leaving virtually no dead space (**dead spaces** are areas in the wound where the damaged surfaces remain separated, either naturally or because of inadequate suturing). The wound edges are clean (or cleansed) so that they are free of foreign material and cellular debris, greatly reducing the inflammatory phase. There is little to no tissue loss or devitalization. Healing occurs by regeneration and resurfacing of the tissue, although the actual rate and pattern of healing differs depending upon the tissue involved. There is minimal edema, no local infection and no serous discharge. The proliferation phase primarily consists of reepithelialization and may begin as soon as 24 hours after closure of a surgical incision. Healing occurs quickly with no separation of the wound edges. The proximity of the edges means that the body does not have to work as hard to fill the gap between the sides of the wound with a large area of granulation tissue. This decreases the distance that new blood vessels and keratinocytes must traverse and minimizes bacterial invasion. Wound contraction is minimal and occurs quickly. There is very little scarring because minimal tissue building is needed to close the gap. Paper cuts and other small cutaneous wounds typically heal by primary closure.

Second intention healing (**secondary closure**) occurs when healing involves the formation of granulation tissue containing fibroblasts and the wound closes by contraction, with the secondary growth of epithelium. When wounds are too extensive for the edges to lie against each other without support and are not repaired, disrupted healing is the result. Leaving wounds unsutured is desirable when a contaminated wound cannot be thoroughly cleaned before suturing, as it leaves the wound open for additional cleansing or débridement and thus lessens the chance of infection. Second intention healing can also occur in a sutured wound in the presence of an infection, an allergic reaction, excessive trauma, tissue loss (leaving a larger gap that must be filled), imprecise reconstruction of the tissues or anything else that may disrupt healing. (Keep in mind that the excessive use of injected local anesthetic swells the tissue and may result in a big gap the next day due to misjudging how tight to make the stitches.) Such disruptions produce further tissue destruction and suppress healing to a certain extent.

In secondary closure, healing is a more complex and prolonged process, in which the inflammatory phase is often pronounced and in which wound contraction plays a more important role. These wounds heal from the inside out. Granulation tissue forms in the sides of the wound, closing the wound cavity as the tissue contracts. Epithelization and granulation must be sufficient to fill in the gap between the surfaces of the wound, prolonging the healing time and creating a bigger, more contracted and sunken scar; the larger and deeper the wound, the longer this will take. Excessive granulation tissue may form and bulge from the wound's surface, necessitating removal to allow epithelization to occur. Secondary healing produces tissues that may be less functional and more sensitive to thermal or mechanical injury (such as soaking in too hot water or abrading the wound).

Third intention healing (**delayed primary closure** or **tertiary intention healing**) takes place when a wound that does not involve significant tissue loss or devitalization has not been sutured (sometimes done intentionally in the hospital to allow drainage when infection is present) or when a repair has completely broken down (dehisced [de-HISSED]) due to gross infection, a severe suture reaction or excessively tight stitches.

The wound is cleaned and left open. Sterile, fine-mesh gauze, which may first be soaked in warmed sterile saline, is inserted in the wound and changed twice daily. This allows the tissues to remain exposed to air and to begin the healing process by developing new circulatory tissue and resistance to infection. The wound is cleansed and observed for several days. The wound may or may not require débridement, which involves taking off a layer of surface tissue, often by scraping, to remove debris or necrotic tissue. Whether this is done depends upon the condition of the tissue and the judgement of the practitioner. Débriding creates a new wound, resulting in a deeper and wider wound and thus more scarring.

After four to five days of observation, if there is no evidence of infection and red granulation tissue is present, the wound is sutured. This timing is based on the low incidence of infection when closure is postponed for at least 96 hours. If these prerequisites are not met, the wound is left open to heal by secondary intention.

When the wound is sutured, the tissue layers must be accurately matched and securely stitched. After closure, the wound gains strength rapidly. In a few days its strength is equivalent to that of a wound that was closed initially, and later may be even stronger than a wound that heals by primary intention. This mode of healing does not necessarily produce excessive scarring and cosmetic results are usually good.

(Chapter based on Boyle, 2006; Ethicon, 2005; Sanz, 1987; Stotts, 1990; Zederfeldt & Hunt, 1990)

Practical Principles of Surgical Repair

Note: Study the preceding chapter before launching into this one.

The primary purpose of wound repair is to hold the sides of the damaged tissue together so they are next to each other, increasing the likelihood of healing by primary intention. Correct repair of a wound helps stop bleeding, minimizes infection and closes all pockets so that no dead spaces remain. In perineal body repair, an open space left below a sutured area may heal as is (apart) and weaken pelvic support. Suturing promotes tissue integrity by supplying artificial support during healing, and it helps preserve cosmetic appearance by minimizing the amount of scar tissue that must form to fill the wound. Suturing restores and supports the anatomical alignment of the tissues during the healing process. Tissue is less likely to heal well when a woman is not in good health, and more artificial help is needed to promote tissue integrity.

The following principles enhance the uncomplicated healing of sutured tissues:

- Provide adequate hemostasis (i.e., stop bleeding) before repair.
- Ensure that the wound is free of contamination before closure. If clots or other debris are sewn into the wound, they will promote excessive inflammation and provide a medium for bacterial growth.
- Avoid removing tissue unless absolutely necessary. Removal of tissue, such as skin tags, leaves a wider gap and requires the formation of more scar tissue to heal.
- Use appropriate suture material. The ideal suture material would hold the tissue together long enough for the edges to heal so they remain together once it dissolves or is removed. It would offer adequate knot security, produce minimal tissue reaction, maintain adequate tensile strength, be flexible and pliable, be nonallergenic, not promote infection and absorb at a predictable rate. The appropriate material will vary depending upon the location of the injury. The perfect material has not yet been developed.
- Avoid using threadable needles, which cause more tissue trauma.
- Use taper point needles whenever possible. In the perineal area, cutting needles do more damage. Reserve them for excessively scarred tissue or skin repair only.
- Use local anesthetic sparingly. Doing so enhances accurate approximation and proper healing. Topical anesthetic provides adequate pain relief for most women while eliminating artificial swelling resulting from injections. Excessive injected anesthetic causes increased tissue swelling and more postpartum pain, while making approximating tissue more difficult due to distortion. Excessive swelling impairs healing because it interferes with circulation to the wound.
- Aim for a quality repair rather than getting it done quickly; haste invites mistakes. The way to shorten the time repairs take is to become proficient with basic techniques and to eliminate wasted motions, not to simply work faster (DeLancey, 1987).
- Place stitches so that they provide maximal tissue support while remaining loose enough to allow good circulation. This produces a stronger repair than when the stitches are too tight. Tight suturing impairs circulation, resulting in poor

oxygenation and thus increasing the likelihood of poor healing, dehiscence and infection.

- Precisely approximate wound edges. Edges should touch but not roll together (invert) and should be accurately joined to meet their original other half or side.
- Place stitches that are at least as deep as they are wide. This makes maximum use of the size of needle chosen, helps prevent rolled edges during knot tying and guards against poor tissue alignment.
- Avoid excessive layering of sutures, which leads to more pain and poor healing. This is especially true of deeper layers as well as when the areas of pressure produced by stitches overlap, which further impairs circulation and oxygenation. At the same time, you want to achieve adequate closure to the depth of the wound to eliminate dead space. Dead space is created when wound edges are not brought together to begin with, when they separate, or when air becomes trapped below the tissue surface. Such spaces result in a weaker repair. Moreover, serum or blood can collect there, predisposing the wound to infection.
- Avoid placing sutures through the external skin surface.
  - It tends to encourage bacterial growth.
  - The inflammatory response to the foreign suture material may lead to excessive scarring. This is particularly true of chromic gut materials.
  - It provides a pathway along which skin cells can migrate during healing and form a pinhole-sized blind pocket in the skin surface or even a fistula.
- If stitched at all, ideally the skin should be closed with a subcuticular stitch, especially in cases of large, ragged labial or skin tears. This will enhance healing and significantly reduce postpartum discomfort. (Ethicon, 2005; Fleming, 1990; Sanz, 1987; Varney et al., 2004)

Biological response to suture materials

The introduction of any foreign material produces a tissue reaction. The acute response to suture material is usually mild (lasting about three days), with an increase in white blood cell response, especially neutrophils, resulting in a slightly increased inflammatory reaction. The neutrophils are then replaced by other blood cells (monocytes, plasma cells and lymphocytes). The acute response will be more pronounced if complicated by infection, allergic reaction or trauma.

References and Further Reading on Basic Surgical Principles

References Used in Multiple Chapters

Elkin M, et al. NURSING INTERVENTIONS AND CLINICAL SKILLS, 2nd ed. Mosby. St Louis MO, 2000.

Ethicon, Inc. ADVANCED WOUND CLOSURE (product brochure). Johnson & Johnson, Somerville NJ, 2005.

Fleming N. "Can the suturing method make a difference in postpartum perineal pain?" J NURSE-MIDWIFERY, 35(1):19-25, Jan-Feb, 1990.

Sanz L. "Wound management: Matching materials and methods for best results," CONTEMP OB/GYN, 30(5):86-114, Nov, 1987.

Sherris D, Kern E. ESSENTIAL SURGICAL SKILLS, 2nd ed. Saunders, Philadelphia PA, 2004.

Sutton J. LET BIRTH BE BORN AGAIN: REDISCOVERING AND RECLAIMING OUR MIDWIFERY HERITAGE. Birth Concepts UK, Middlesex UK, 2001.

Timby B. CLINICAL NURSING PROCEDURES, JB Lippincott, Philadelphia PA, 1989.

Varney H, et al. Chapter 79: "Cutting an episiotomy and repairing episiotomies and lacerations," VARNEY'S MIDWIFERY, 4th ed. Jones & Bartlett, Sudbury MA, 2004.

How Wounds Heal

Anderson M. "Principles of wound healing in the repair of the episiotomy" (unpublished paper), Hawthorne NY, 1975.

Baxter H. Chapter 3: "Surgical wounds and their care," in Maxwell D, ed. SURGICAL TECHNIQUES IN OBSTETRICS AND GYNECOLOGY. Churchill Livingstone, New York NY, 2004.

Body in Balance. "How muscles heal." www.bodyinbalance.com/muscular_injury_muscularpain.htm, accessed Aug 11, 2008.

Boyle M. WOUND HEALING IN MIDWIFERY. Radcliffe Pub, Oxford UK, 2006.

Cascade HealhCare Products. On-Line catalogue, www.1cascade.com, accessed Nov, 2008.

Dunn D. WOUND CLOSURE MANUAL. Ethicon, Inc., Johnson & Johnson Co., Somerville, NJ, 2008.

Kettle C. Chapter 4: "The management of perineal trauma," in Henderson C, Bick D, eds. PERINEAL CARE: AN INTERNATIONAL ISSUE. Quay Books, London UK, 2005.

Kirk R. BASIC SURGICAL TECHNIQUES, 5th ed. Churchill Livingstone, London UK, 2002.

Montgomery RD. "Healing of muscle, ligaments, and tendons," SEMIN VET MED SURG (SMALL ANIM), 4(4):304-311, Nov, 1989.

Myers B. WOUND MANAGEMENT: PRINCIPLES AND PRACTICE, 2nd ed. Pearson, Upper Saddle River NJ, 2008.

Salthouse T, et al. "Relationship of cellular enzyme activity to catgut and collagen suture absorption," SURG GYNECOL OBSTET, 129(4):691-696, 1969.

Stotts N. "Seeing RED and YELLOW and BLACK: the three-color concept of wound care," NURSING90, 20(2):59-61, Feb, 1990.

Trott A. WOUNDS AND LACERATIONS: EMERGENCY CARE AND CLOSURE, 3rd ed. Elsevier Mosby, Philadelphia PA, 2005.

Wipff PJ, et al. "Myofibroblast contraction activates latent TGF-beta1 from the extracellular matrix," J CELL BIOLOGY, 179(6):1311-1323, Dec 17, 2007.

Woodward S. WOUND HEALING. Davis-Geck, America Cyanamid Co., Wayne NJ, 1988.

Zederfeldt B, Hunt T. WOUND CLOSURE: MATERIALS AND TECHNIQUES. Davis & Geck, Wayne NJ, 1990.

Principles of Surgical Repair

DeLancey J. BASIC EXERCISES: SURGICAL TECHNIQUE. Davis-Geck, Wayne NJ, 1987.

NOTES:

ESSENTIAL SURGICAL SKILLS FOR MIDWIVES

TYING SURGICAL KNOTS

Surgical knots are used to tie off a single stitch or to anchor a series of continuous or running stitches. Good knot-tying technique is essential to the integrity of your repair. While it is true that you can perform perineal repair using only square knots, each type of knot has its pros and cons, so variations on the square knot as well as the Aberdeen knot are covered in this chapter. Tying well-executed knots needs to become second nature to you. Practice!

Anatomy of a tied stitch

A tied stitch has two parts: the loop and the knot. The suture that passes through the tissue (the woman's side) is called the **loop**. A **knot** closes the loop, holding the ends of the strand, and therefore the torn tissue, together. A knot consists of two or more **throws** (discussed below) that are snugged down to close the loop around the divided tissue. The **ears**, or ends, of the strand are trimmed long enough to allow them to slip slightly without coming untied.

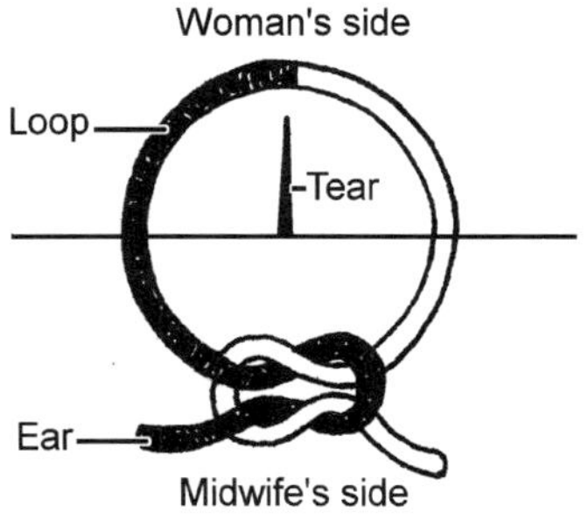

Parts of a knot

The midwife's side of the stitch is the tied part. When considering a simple, interrupted stitch, the segment of the strand that exits the tissue after the loop is created is often referred to as the **fixed end** because it is attached to the needle; I will call this the **needle end**; it is shown in black. The other end of the strand that remains is called the **free end** because, in a simple interrupted (or single) stitch, that end is left sticking out of the tissue with nothing attached; it is shown in white.

A **throw** is the weaving of the two segments together. A **single-wrapped throw** (a wrap is called a **turn** in some sources) is formed by winding one segment around the other one-half (180°) to a full turn or revolution (360°). A **double-wrapped throw** is formed when the free segment is wound around the other twice or two full turns (720°).

After wrapping, the throw is slowly advanced, or **run down**, and snugged against the tissue to bring the wound edges together and keep them approximated. The effort required to advance a throw is called **knot rundown force**. The force required varies among suture materials; some allow rundown and readjustment of knot tension after rundown more easily than others. When the first throw is being snugged down, the amount of tension needed to bring the wound edges together without strangling the tissue is assessed, and the tension is readjusted if necessary. After the first throw is in place, more throws are created until the knot is secure. **Knot configuration** is the number of throws needed to complete a knot.

Knot shorthand: An international code may be used to describe surgical square and granny knots. The number of wraps in each throw is designated by an Arabic numeral. Parallel throws (as in a square knot) are designated by an " = " sign. Crossed throws (as in a granny knot) are designated by an ×. Thus, a square knot formed by using two single parallel throws is coded 1=1. A knot made with two crossed throws is coded 1×1. A slip knot is designated with an S (for example, a single-wrap, double-throw slip granny knot is coded like this: S×S).

Knot integrity

A knot is always the weakest link in a suture loop. The force required to break a knot is always less than that required to break an untied strand of the same material. This is due to the bending, creasing, friction and tension required to form a knot, all of which weaken the strand. The relationship between the tensile strength of an unknotted strand and a knotted strand of the same material is called **knot efficiency** and is expressed as a percentage (the % of knot efficiency = tensile strength of knotted suture ÷ tensile strength of unknotted suture). The amount of force required to break a knotted strand is influenced by the type of knot used, the strand material, the diameter of the strand and the tissue in which it is placed. Once in place, absorbable materials display a progressive decrease in knot-breaking strength. As the suture breaks down in the tissue, it weakens and the knot tends to weaken faster because of the stress to which it has already been subjected during tying.

To a point, knot security is enhanced as the number of throws increases. An ideal configuration uses enough throws to form a secure knot that will fail by breaking rather than by unraveling. The ideal number of throws varies for each type of suture. Once the ideal configuration has been created, however, additional throws do not enhance knot security because they weaken the strand too much, increasing the risk that the knot will break; thus, too many throws only create a bulky knot and provide additional hiding places for bacteria.

Some additional points to keep in mind are as follows:

- Choose the simplest knot for the task and the suture material.
- Nontension ties are used in soft and delicate tissues and to ligate blood vessels and are thus appropriate for most birth-related repairs. Here, the initial throw is snugged down flat to keep it tight, without tugging on the ends. The ends must remain loose, or the throw will loosen by the time the rest of the knot is completed.
- Ideally, the suture material and the knot used allow each completed throw to be easily advanced to the wound edges. During rundown, equal, constant and adequate tension is slowly applied, in opposite directions, to each end of the suture. By applying about 80% of the breaking strength of the knotted material, you avoid breaking the strand while creating a knot that is unlikely to slip. Uniform tension creates a more secure knot; too little tension results in a knot that tends to slip. Jerking the suture or running down a knot too rapidly weakens the strand and produces less secure throws that are more likely to loosen over time.
- Strive to tie a tight knot over a loose loop. Each loop must be tight enough to bring the wound edges together while remaining loose enough to allow for swelling and subsequent tissue shrinkage as edema resolves. Poorly tied stitches will often unravel and those that are tied too tightly may even break if the pressure in edematous tissue encompassed by the loop rises above capillary pressure. Impaired capillary blood flow and a fall in oxygen levels may lead to cell death, with loss of tissue strength and an increased risk of wound dehiscence, infection or necrosis. Overly tight sutures may also cut through healthy tissues. (Unhealthy tissues may shred, however, even when stitches are appropriately tight.) Even when no such clinically obvious problems arise, tight stitches do not make a repair more secure, will not restore an already lax pelvic floor, may cause a repair to heal

unanatomically tight and will, at the very least, be more uncomfortable.

- Avoid pulling the strand back and forth in the tissue (seesawing) or unnecessarily rubbing the segments together during rundown as either can cause unnecessary tissue trauma and weaken the strand, especially when using gut materials.
- Avoid pulling on the loop during rundown, as this may tear or avulse the tissue.
- Be sure the first throw is properly placed and snugged down before beginning the second throw. At first you will need to check the knot both visually and by touch. With more experience, you may be able to check by touch alone.
- Each knot introduces additional foreign material for the body to break down. Place as few knots with as few throws as possible to minimize tissue irritation.
- All knots slip to some degree. How much slippage occurs depends upon the suture material, moisture and knot type as well as how well the knot is tied and whether the ears are left long enough to compensate for tissue changes. Ears should be trimmed straight across the strand to a length of approximately 3 to 5 mm, at the most. If the ears are too short, the knot may unravel; if they are too long, they will poke and irritate the tissue. Some practitioners cut the ears of a knot left above the tissue surface, as may occur with a labial repair, nearly flush with the knot to avoid poking. When you plan to trim ears very short, an extra throw should be placed beforehand, but it is best to always leave a short ear as an extra precaution.
- A poorly tied knot may reduce the strength of the strand by over 50% (Kirk, 2002).
- Don't leave suture that has been clamped or otherwise damaged in the tissue or the knot, as such insults weaken the strand. (Edlich & Long, 2008; Sanz, 1987; Varney et al., 2004; Zederfeldt & Hunt, 1990; Zikria, 1981)

Suture materials and knot tying

Each suture material requires a specific knot configuration. Chromic gut is somewhat rough; its knot security is considered to be very good to only fair (depending on the source), and its stiffness makes it more awkward to manipulate. In contrast, synthetic monofilament sutures are similar to fishing line, which manipulates easily but the resulting knots also tend to slip after they are tied. Most monofilament synthetics also have more memory than do multifilament synthetics, which have very little. Thus, monofilament synthetics are more difficult to snug down. As a rule, synthetic multifilament sutures are generally easier to handle and to tie than monofilament sutures because they behave more like sewing thread. The braided and twisted construction of multifilament materials provides a high coefficient of friction and, according to the manufacturers, the knots tend to remain snug after they are laid down (although, independent sources report only fair to good knot–security for these products [von Fraunhofer & Chu, 1996]). This also means that the knot is hard to reposition once in place; using coated suture tends to mitigate this tendency to a degree (Ethicon, 2005). More details about how to tie different suture materials can be found on page 383.

Handedness of the tie

When a wound is aligned with your spine (vertically or longitudinally oriented) and the needle holder is manipulated with your dominant hand, the needle passes through the tissue from your dominant to your nondominant side (i.e., from right to left if you are right-handed and from left to right if you are left-handed). After the suture is in place, the needle end of the strand will have moved to your nondominant side and the free end of the strand will remain on your dominant side. When one end of the strand is fixed (to the needle in this case) and a hand tie is used, surgeon's typically use the nondominant hand to pinch and push the free end through the loop as each throw is wrapped. Confusingly, however, surgeons refer to the hand *opposite* the one wrapping the free end when designating whether a tie is right-handed or left-handed. (The opposite hand will usually be the dominant one manipulating the needle holder, but, it is also possible, for example, for a right-handed surgeon to manipulate the free end with her dominant hand and thus tie "left-handed.") With an instrument tie, the dominant hand uses the needle holder to place the stitch *and* to pull the free end through the loop. Thus, the hand that pulls the free end through the loop, in this case the dominant hand, still denotes the handedness of the tie. In all cases, the free end is wrapped because this avoids having to disengage the needle from the holder and prevents having to pass a swagged needle through the knot loop, an awkward process that greatly increases the risk of needlestick injuries.

All the illustrations in this chapter depict **right-handed ties** and assume a stitch has been taken, thus the needle (black) end is shown on the left. Other knot–tying manuals usually show bicolored cord as well but the handedness of ties is not always explained. Use the rules outlined above to determine the handedness of ties depicted across a vertical incision. If tying is demonstrated across a horizontal incision (or two horizontal layers), the stitch can be formed either forehand (starting with the palm toward the tissue, the needle passes toward oneself, from the far [or upper] side to the near [or lower] side of the wound) or backhand (starting with the palm up, the needle passes away from oneself, from the near [or lower] side to the far [or upper] side of the wound). The segment being manipulated is still the free end, and the hand opposite the one doing the wrapping still determines the handedness of the tie.

Practicing Knot Tying

Practice materials

To learn the basic mechanics of knot construction start by tying to a fat, round object, such as the finger ring of a coffee mug, to get the idea of making a loop in your head, plus a fat object spreads the knot out as it is tied so you can better see how it is constructed. It is also helpful to have on hand a small (4" square) board with a hook attached in the center it to practice hand and instrument ties, although you can use the mug handle for all your practice and it will always be easy to see the knot configuration. Tie the ends of two 10 inch pieces of cotton cord together. Color one side with an indelible marker to represent the needle end; the white half represents the free end. Or, obtain heavy cord in white and a color (or a light color [for white] and another darker color) and sew them together at one end.

Square knot

The **flat square** or **reef knot** is the most commonly used surgical knot. Depending upon the suture material, it can be up to 10 times stronger than a granny knot (DeLancey, 1987). Ancient peoples ascribed magical powers to this knotting technique.

Place the mug on a table, in front of you. Pass the cord through the handle, with the lighter segment on your dominant side. This positioning mimics that used during suturing when the knot will usually need to be made by stretching the segments away from the loop toward you (i.e., you will be tying knots on the near-side of the loop, rather than above it). Numbers in parentheses in the following text correspond to the drawings on the next page.

A square knot is formed with two throws, also called "half-hitches." First, the loop is placed through the tissue (a vertical tear is shown because the majority of your knots will be tied over a longitudinally oriented wound). The first throw is started by crossing the segments (1), thus closing the loop. In a surgical knot, the free end of the strand is always wrapped around the colored (needle) end (2). The ends of each segment are now on opposite sides from where they started out (3).

After completing (3), the first throw is run down or tightened by steadily applying *equal and opposing tension to each segment at the level of the tissue surface* (4), thus completing the first half-hitch. Equalizing tension during rundown ensures that each segment makes a half turn around the other. The application of unequal tension results in a slip knot by causing the segment to which less tension is applied to wrap completely around the other, more tense and therefore straighter segment.

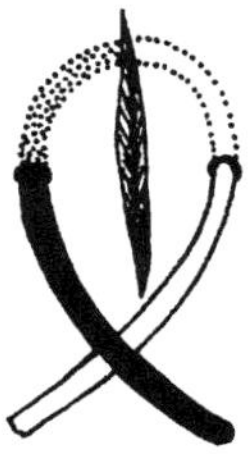	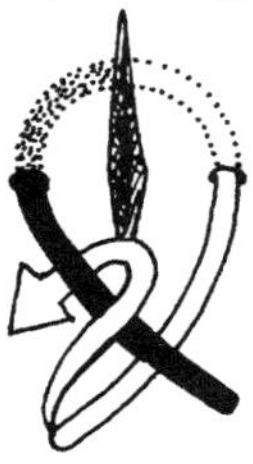	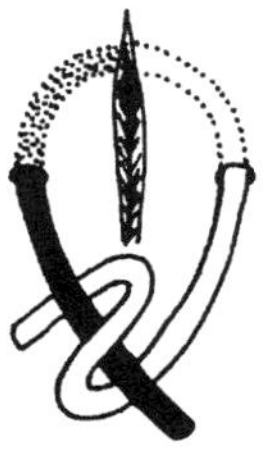	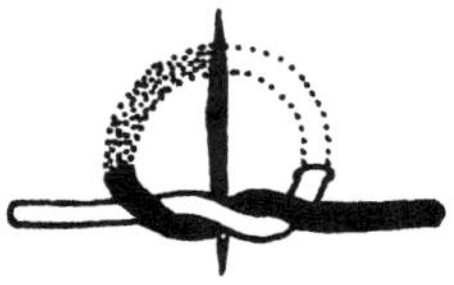
1. Cross the colored segment over the white to create a loop.	2. Wrap the white segment toward you, over and around the colored segment.	3. So it looks like this.	4. Tighten by pulling segments in opposite directions.
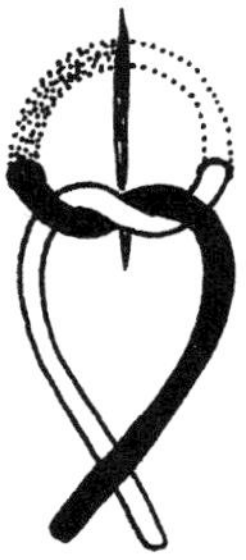	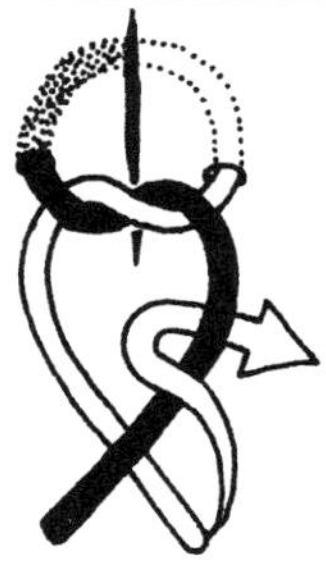	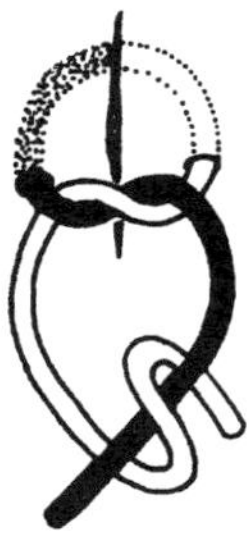	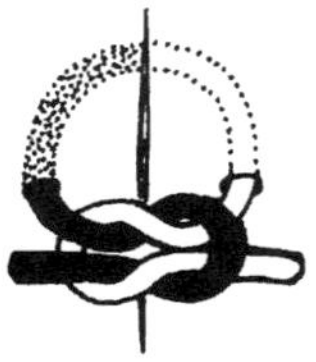
5. Begin a second throw by crossing the colored segment over the white.	6. Wrap the white segment toward you, over and around the colored segment.	7. So it looks like this.	8. Tighten by pulling segments in opposite directions.

During rundown, the knot must be snugged into place directly over the wound, not off to one side, at an angle. Pulling straight out to either side of the loop at the level of the tissue transfers all the tension to the knot and also avoids unnecessary tension on the tissue. Examine the completed half-hitch throw (4) and note that the segments are now reversed, with the colored segment now to the right in this example.

A square knot is distinguished by the way the segments are crossed for the second throw and the direction that one segment is wrapped around the other; the crossing and wrapping is alternated with each throw. For example, if the first throw begins with the left segment crossed over the right and the free (white) end is wrapped around the needle (colored) end in a toward-you, over and around direction for the first throw (as illustrated on the last page in steps 1, 2, 3 and 4), the second throw must start with the right segment crossed over the left. The white end *must* then be wrapped around the colored end in the same manner but, because the segments were crossed as in step 5, it is wrapped in the opposite direction (as illustrated in 5, 6 and 7 above; compare steps and 2 and 6). Another way of saying this is that the knot is tied by crossing the left segment over the right to form the first throw and the right segment over the left to form the second throw (or vise versa). In a simple square knot, it does not matter in which direction one segment is crossed or directed in the first throw, as long as the direction is reversed for the second. In a surgical knot, you want to make sure that the free end is always the one being wrapped (as illustrated here). A square knot is constructed using a minimum of two throws that exhibit this mirror-image (so called because the steps are reversed), or "parallel," construction.

The formation of a double-throw square knot can be confirmed by checking for parallel construction, wherein two parts of the needle (colored) segment pass under one side of the knot and two parts of the free (white) segment pass over the other side of the knot (alternating the direction of each throw results in the segments lying parallel with each other; see arrows in the drawing below). The ends of the strand should also lie almost parallel with the segment that forms the loop. To begin learning to tie a square knot, practice using the simple technique illustrated on the previous page. After tying each knot, confirm that it is a square knot by examining its configuration.

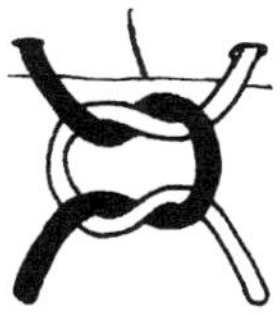	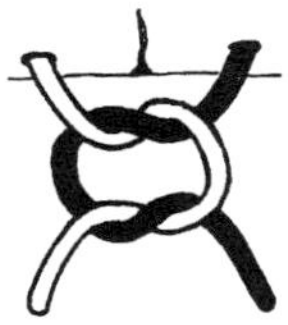	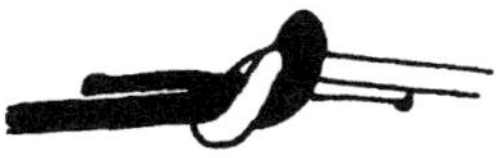
Square knot with two single-wrapped throws: one side	Square knot: the other side	Looking down on the knot to confirm that the ends lie parallel with the loop

<u>Similar types of knots that should be avoided</u>: There are a few variations on this knot that can cause problems if they are used instead of a classic square knot.

Granny knot: I will now explain granny knots, so you can tell the difference. If you are easily confused by subtle differences, you may want to skip to "friction knots" at the bottom of page 367 and just focus on getting the square knot in your head.

A granny knot is a pseudo–square knot with identical, or crossed, construction. The first half-hitch is formed in the same manner as for a square knot, as illustrated in steps 1, 2, 3 and

4 below. For the second half-hitch, the movements are repeated: the segment that is now to your nondominant side is also crossed in front of the segment that is now to your dominant side and emerges in front of the dominant-side segment. Thus, a granny knot is formed by crossing and then passing the end that winds up on the nondominant side of the loop in the same direction for each throw (right over left, right over left, or vise versa).

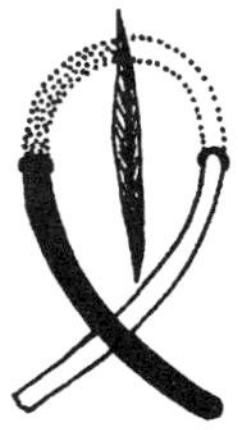	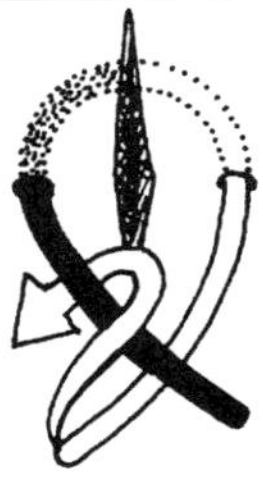	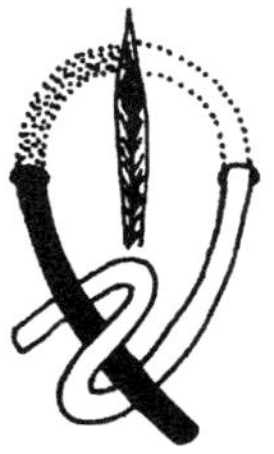	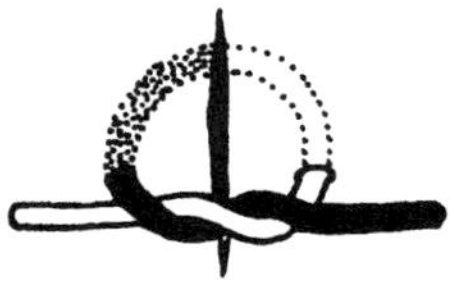
1. Cross the colored segment over the white to create a loop.	2. Wrap white segment toward you, over and around colored segment.	3. So it looks like this.	4. Tighten by pulling segments in opposite directions.
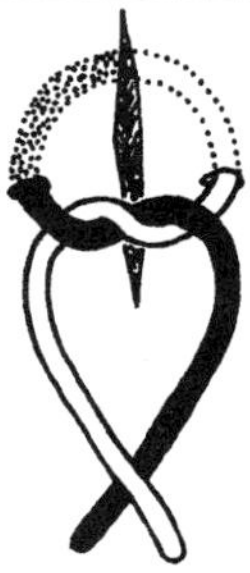	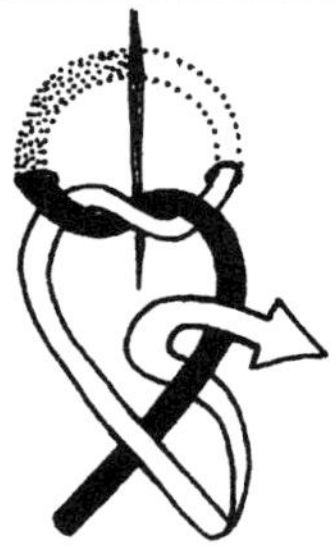	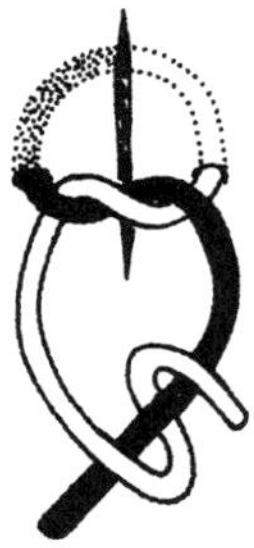	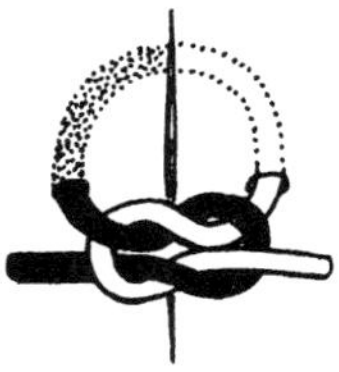
5. Begin a second throw by crossing the white segment over the colored.	6. Wrap the white segment away from you, over and around the colored segment.	7. So it looks like this.	8. Tighten by pulling segments in opposite directions.

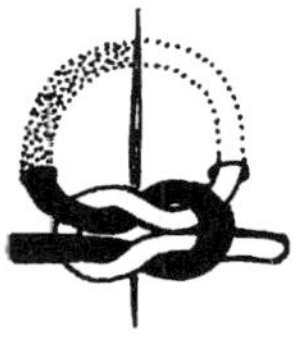	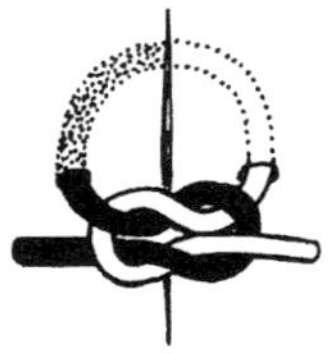
Square knot	Granny knot
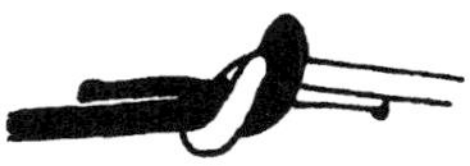	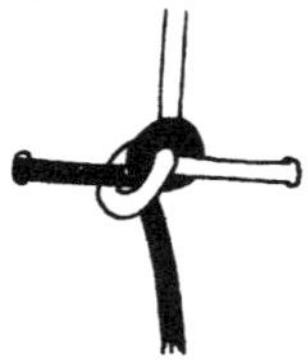
Looking down to see that the ends of the segments are parallel with the loop	Looking down to see that the ends of the segments are at right-angles to the loop

The formation of a granny knot is confirmed when the colored segment passes under and over one side of the knot and the white segment passes under and over the other side and when the ends of the segments project at right angles to the loop (study the two illustrations on the preceding page).

Study and compare the following drawings carefully to see how the segments are crossed and wrapped in each type of knot to create the second throw.

SECOND THROW–SQUARE KNOT			
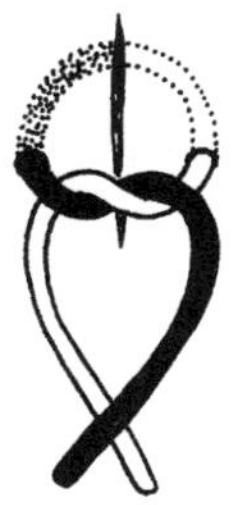 5. Begin a second throw by crossing the colored segment over the white.	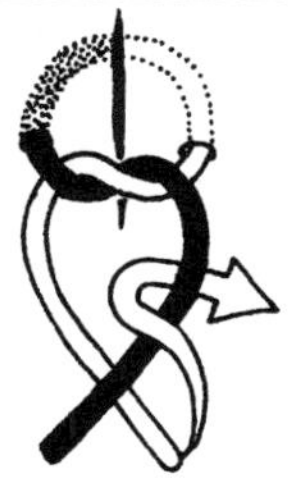 6. Wrap the white segment toward you, over and around the colored segment.	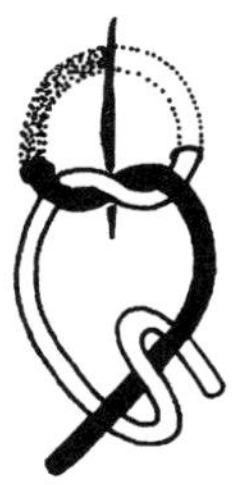 7. So it looks like this.	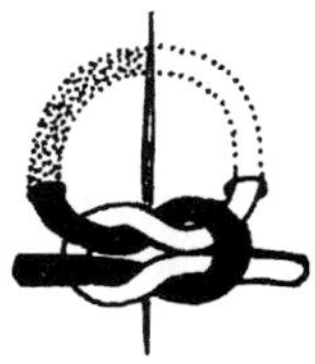 8. Tighten by pulling segments in opposite directions.
SECOND THROW–GRANNY KNOT			
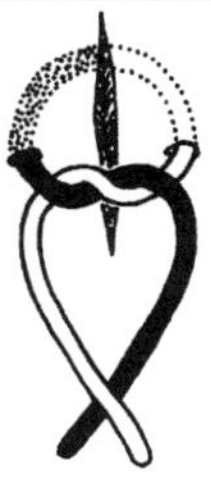 5. Begin a second throw by crossing the white segment over the colored.	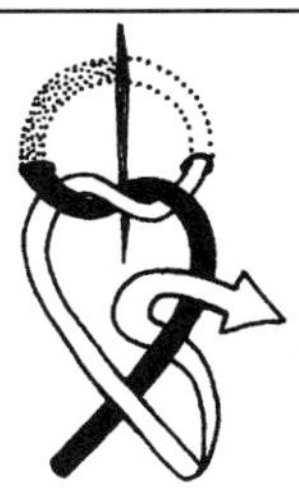 6. Wrap the white segment away from you, over and around the colored segment.	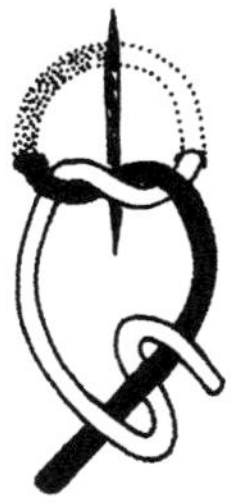 7. So it looks like this.	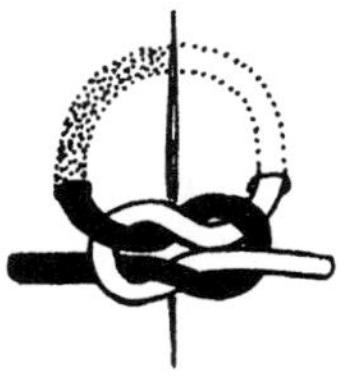 8. Tighten by pulling segments in opposite directions.

Surgeon's friction knots: It is also important to understand what creates a friction knot and why they can be problematic in the types of repairs midwives typically perform. A **surgeon's (friction** or **tension) knot** is a square knot made using one double-wrap throw followed by a single-wrap throw (2=1). Double wrapping the first throw increases the friction on the segments thus temporarily "locking" them, which helps to keep the first throw in place, holding the wound edges together long enough to complete the second throw.

Double–wrapping cannot be relied upon by itself, however, because any tension from the woman's side will cause the throw to slip. A double-wrapped throw is also much more difficult to properly position initially and to readjust later if it is not tied appropriately tight in the first place. Because of the additional friction double-wrapping creates, the strand is more likely to break than slip if an attempt is made to readjust this type of knot.

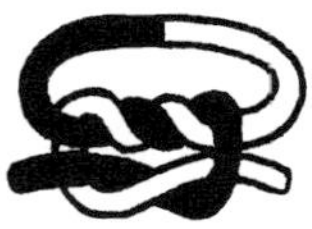	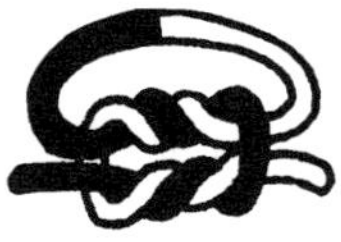	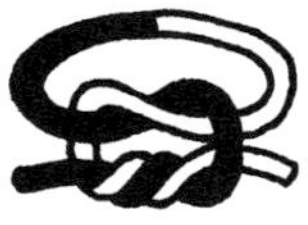
Surgeon's knot	Double-double surgeon's knot	Reversed surgeon's knot

A **double-double surgeon's knot** has two double-wrapped throws (2=2). A single-wrap followed by a double-wrapped throw (1=2) is called a **reversed surgeon's knot**.

Wound orientation and tying square knots: The direction in which the wrapped segments are pulled during rundown is determined by the orientation of the wound and the suture loop. The suture loop is usually at a 90° angle to the orientation of the wound. It is easiest to form a secure square knot when the knot overlies a tear or incision that runs perpendicular to the spine of the practitioner (that is, side-to-side across the tissue), because the suture loops will be vertically oriented. This makes it easy to apply equal tension to each segment in a horizontal plane in relation to the tissue surface, parallel with the orientation of the loop as the knot is snugged down. This always allows the hands to separate as they pull in opposite directions away from the wound, leaving the knot visible at all times.

In contrast, midwives work with tears that almost always are longitudinal or nearly so in relation to their spine (that is, running up and down in the tissue) and that are frequently in small, tight spaces. These factors make proper knot construction considerably more challenging. Your hands must still be kept on either side of the knot, parallel with the suture loop, which is horizontally oriented. This requirement necessitates either reversing the hand positions as each throw is run down or crossing the segments before a half-hitch is begun to avoid forming slip knots. When the hands are crossed, your view of the knot is temporarily obscured. Crossing the hands can also interfere with applying equal tension to the two ends of the suture in a plane parallel with the tissue surface.

Extending your index fingers and pressing the tips against the medial sides of the strands during rundown will help lay the knot flat against the tissue and help equalize the tension applied to each segment, thus increasing the likelihood of forming the throw correctly. Always check that your throw lays flat before proceeding to the next because when you are actually suturing in a small, deep space, your view is likely to be at least partially obscured, which can interfere with visually confirming correct placement (Edlich & Long, 2008).

Different methods of tying a square knot: The following pages illustrate three methods of tying a square knot: one-handed, two-handed and the instrument tie. Although the language used is hand-neutral (dominant and nondominant), right-handed ties are illustrated. Offering three methods of tying allows for individual preference and ensures that you have a sufficient repertoire of skills to place square knots in a variety of clinical situations. It is, nevertheless, perfectly acceptable to master only one of these techniques. If you learn only one, I suggest learning the instrument tie as it is most useful for working in small spaces, although many competent practitioners only use hand ties for all their knots.

Surgical square knots can be tied using either a "one-hand" or "two-hand" technique.

In each method, however, both hands are involved; the tying hand makes the knot and the non-tying hand holds the needle (fixed) end and does some manipulation of the free end as well. If you are going to learn a only one hand-tie technique, the two-hand tie is preferred.

Recall that, in both "right-handed" and "left-handed" tying, the hand to which "handedness" refers merely holds, lets go of and regrasps the free end and is usually the same (dominant) hand that manipulates the needle holder. Many right-handed surgeons, however, tie left-handed, grasping the free end with their left hand. The advantage is that most of the manipulations are done with the dominant hand and the surgeon does not have to put down the needle holder to perform a two-handed tie. Just remember that, once the loop is placed in the tissue, the needle will be on your nondominant side and the free end will be on your dominant side. To help remember this very important detail when practicing with string, attach a hemostat or paper clip to the needle (colored) end. This will prevent you from trying to pass the needle end through the knot loop and will help give you more of a feel for what you will be doing during an actual repair.

Lay people tie a square knot by crossing the segments to form a loop and then poking one end of the strand through the loop. Surgeons cross the segments and then poke a finger or fingers through the loop, grasp the free end of the strand and pull or push it through the loop. Keeping hold of the free end during manipulation helps maintain control of the segments.

These illustrations assume you are tying over a longitudinal tear. When you begin with the segments uncrossed for the first throw, your hands must cross to keep the knot flat and square as you tighten it down. You can also begin the first throw by first crossing the segments so that the free end is crossed over the needle end toward your nondominant side. This avoids having to cross your hands when tightening the first throw (DeLancey, 1987). To start, become very practiced at executing the knots as illustrated, then you can move on to experimenting with variations that you may like better.

Make sure each throw is properly placed before starting the next. Once finished, check both sides of the knot to make sure it is tied correctly. Rather than using a long piece of string and tying consecutive knots, practice tying individual knots because that is what you must do during an actual repair. It is easy to tie many knots rapidly until you become quite practiced at doing it wrong. Be scrupulous about your technique to start with, even if it means going very slowly. Your speed will naturally increase as you become more proficient.

One-handed square knot: The one-hand technique is so named because one hand does all the maneuvering to tie the knot, including releasing and regrasping the free end of the strand. The other hand merely holds the needle end of the strand taut. The one-handed method is more difficult to learn than the two-handed method because it is harder to maintain tension on the segments as you form the knot. Thus, the first and second throws often slip, especially when you are just learning. Slippage necessitates retightening the knot, which may cause the strand to break, which, in turn, requires placing a new stitch. Nonetheless, the one-handed technique is useful to know; once mastered, it is the faster method of tying. Step-by-step instructions begin on the next page. Note that each step is illustrated with hand positions as well as a closeup of how the segments should look at that point.

1. One-handed square knot, first throw: Begin with the white segment (free end) on your dominant side. Cross the colored segment over the white.

1. Grasp the crossed segments. Pick up the white segment with your nondominant thumb and index finger, stretching it across your other fingers. Hold the colored segment with your dominant thumb and index finger.	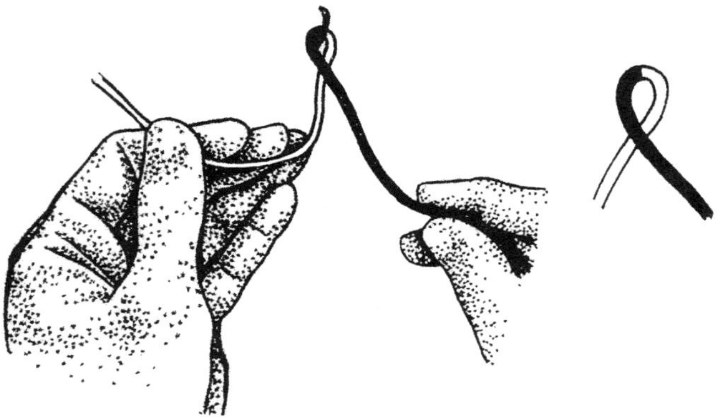
2. Open the crossed segments. Lift the colored segment up and over the middle and ring fingers of your nondominant hand so that the segments form an X.	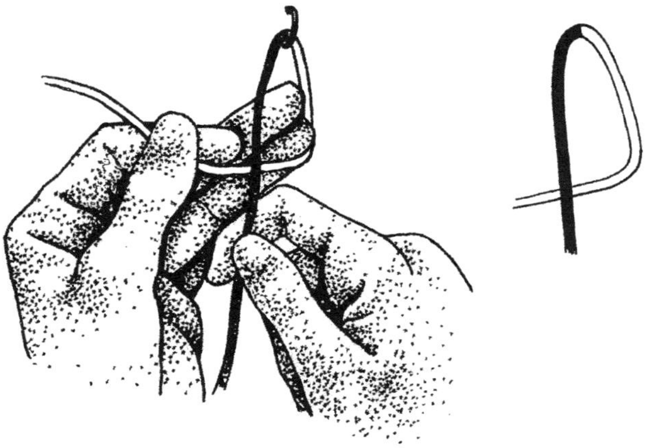
3. Flex your finger. Press your nondominant middle fingerpad against the colored segment as you lift up the white segment with your non-dominant thumb and index finger.	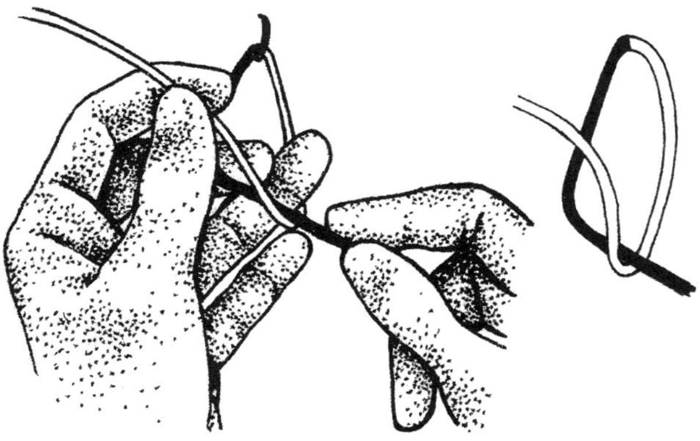

4. Insert your fingertip between the segments. Insert your nondominant fingertip between the white and colored segments so that the white segment winds up behind the nail of your middle finger.	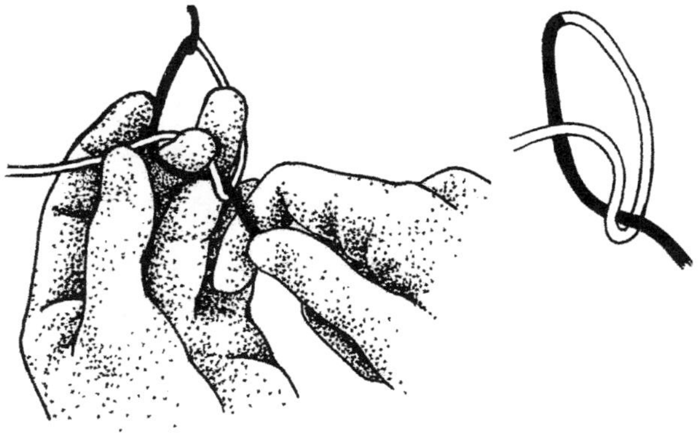
5. Flip the white segment through the loop. Release the end of the white segment as you straighten your finger to push the white segment backward through the loop as you release the end from your dominant hand.	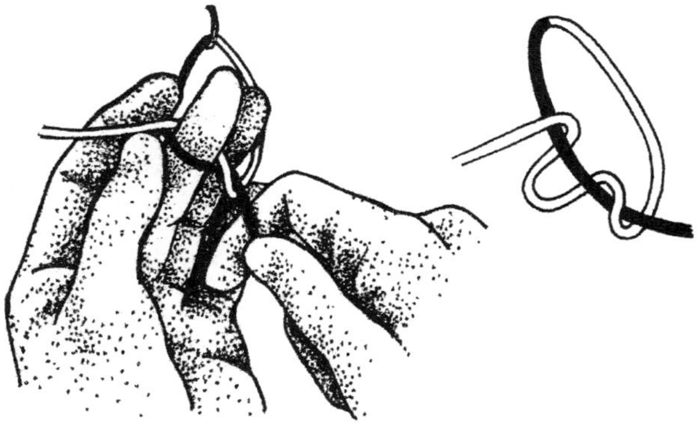
6. Tighten the throw. Press your extended index fingers against the segments to keep the knot as flat and as parallel to the tissue surface as possible as you tighten it down and lay it flat by separating your hands.	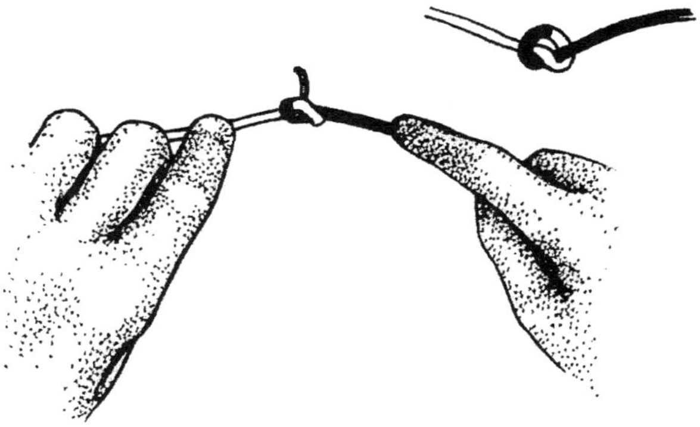

2. One-handed square knot: second throw

1. Grasp the segments. Hold the white segment between your nondominant thumb and index finger and rotate your hand to bring the white segment over your index finger. Pinch the colored segment with your dominant hand.	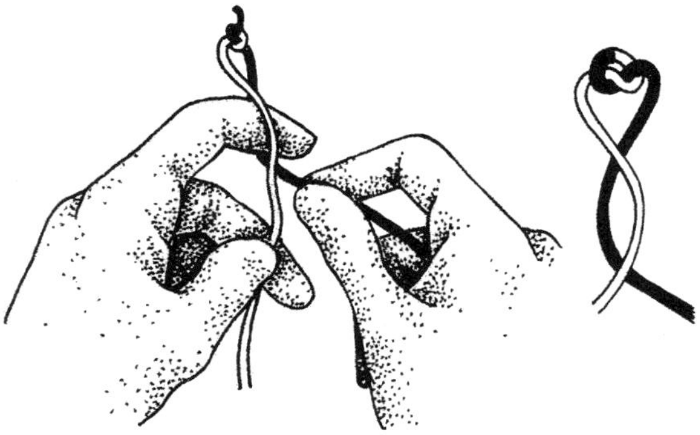
2. Cross the segments. Flex your nondominant index finger as you wrap the colored segment under and around it to form an X.	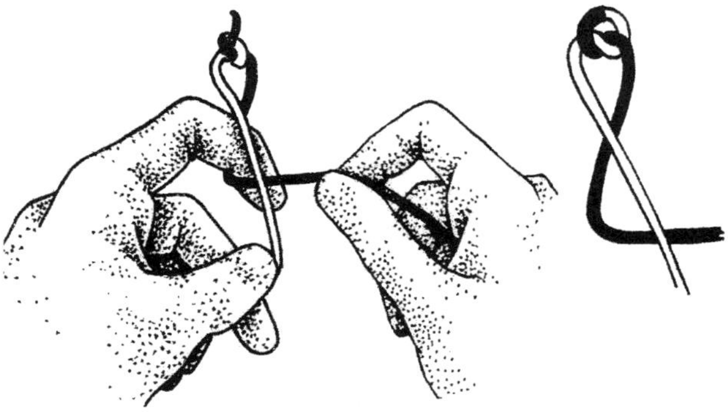
3. Insert your fingernail under the white segment. Use your nondominant thumb and index finger to move the white segment over the nondominant index fingernail. Push your nondominant index fingernail under the white segment.	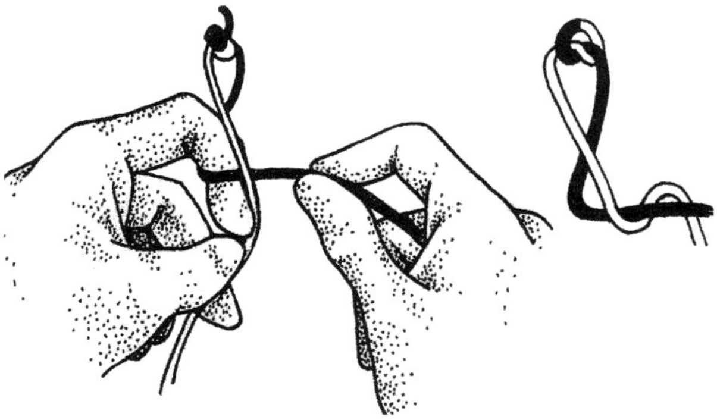

4. Push the white segment through the loop. Let go of the white end and push it up through the loop by straightening your nondominant index finger.	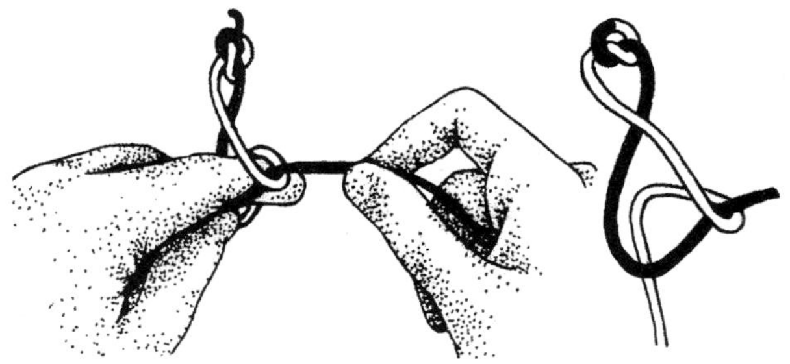
5. Tighten the knot. Cross your dominant hand past your nondominant hand as each hand pulls the segments in opposite directions.	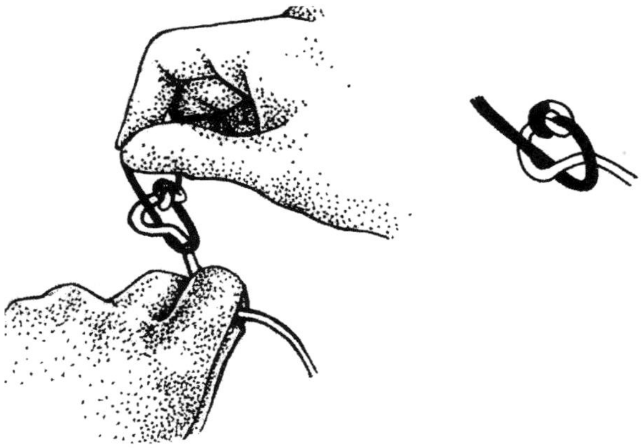
6. Lay the knot flat. Extend your index fingertips against the segments as you tighten the knot down and lay it flat. This completes the second throw of a square knot.	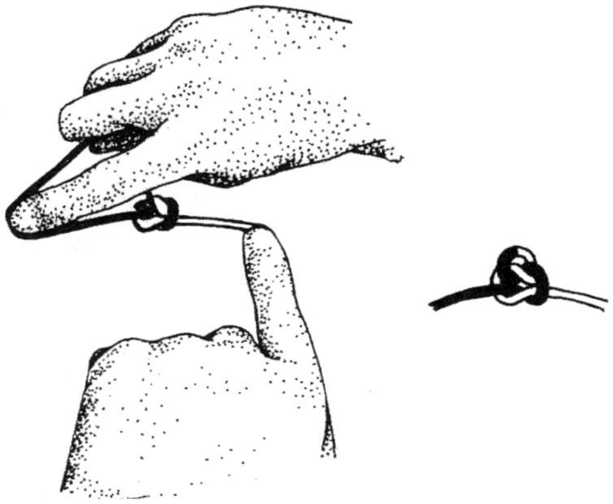

3. One-handed square knot: third throw: To make the third throw, repeat the first throw. This completes three throws (one-and-a-half square knots). Depending upon the suture material, add more throws until an adequately configured knot is formed.

4. Trim the ears: When finished, trim the ends to no less than 3 mm in length.

Two-handed square knot: The two-hand tie is easier to learn than the one-hand method because it relies less on finger action and more on arm and wrist action. It is somewhat slower to perform but gives better control of the knot, allowing you to maintain continuous tension on the segments to form a secure knot.

1. Two-handed tie, first throw: Start with the segments uncrossed (colored end on your nondominant side).

1. Grasp the segments. With palms up and the segments running over the index fingerpads, hold the colored segment in your nondominant hand and the white segment in your dominant hand.	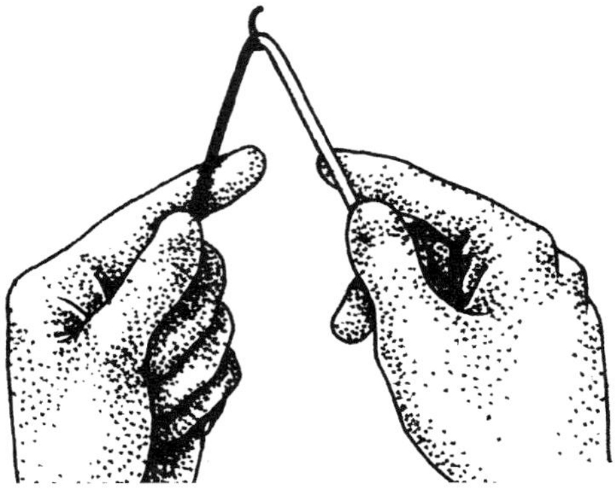
2. Cross the segments. Wrap the white segment over and around the pad of the nondominant index finger so that the segments form an X.	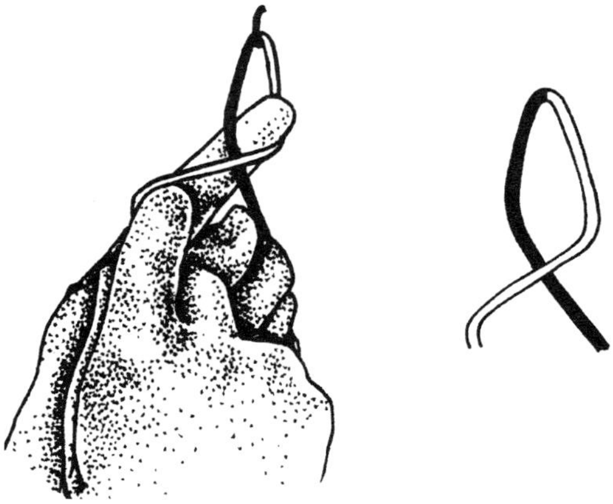

3. Pinch your fingers. Pinch your nondominant thumb and index fingers together inside the loop.	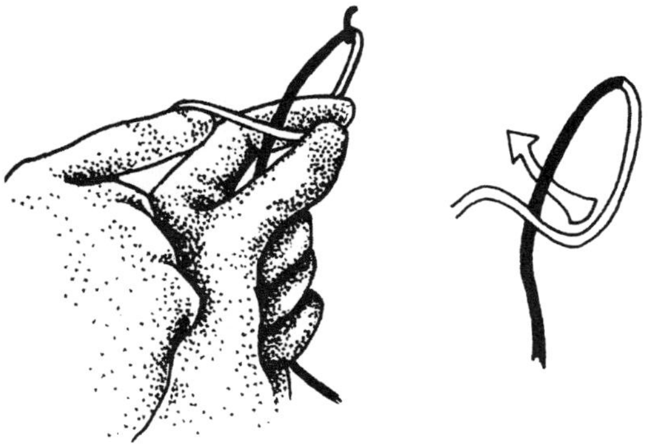
4. Poke your nondominant thumb through the loop. Rotate your nondominant wrist, palm down, so your pinched fingers pass up through the loop. This causes the colored segment to cross over the white.	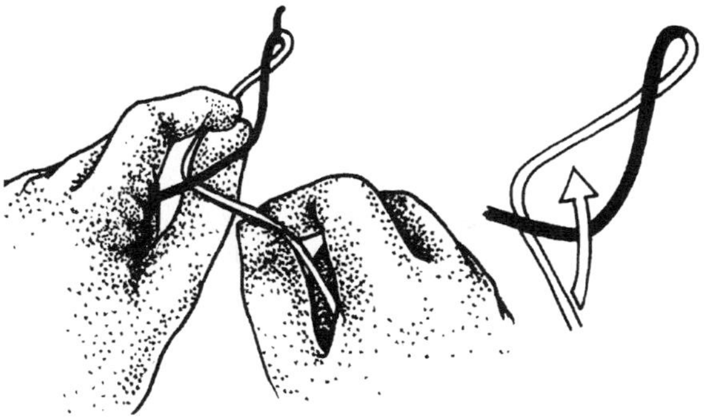
5. Grasp the white segment. Grasp the white segment with your dominant thumb and index finger, bring it around the colored segment and place it between your pinched nondominant fingers.	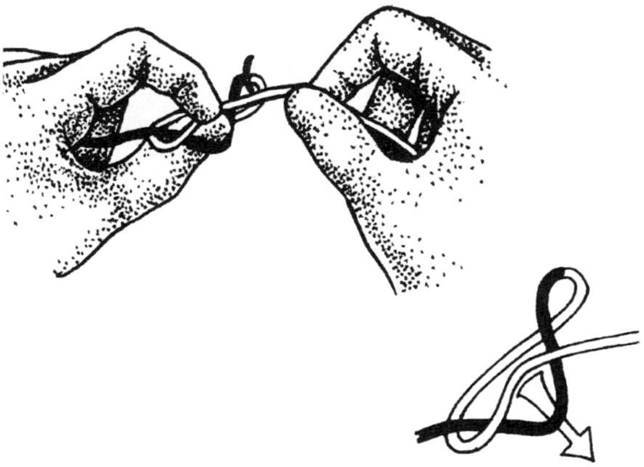

6. Push the white segment through the loop. Rotate your nondominant palm toward you, part your pinched fingers and push the white segment down and through the loop; then grasp the white end with your dominant hand.	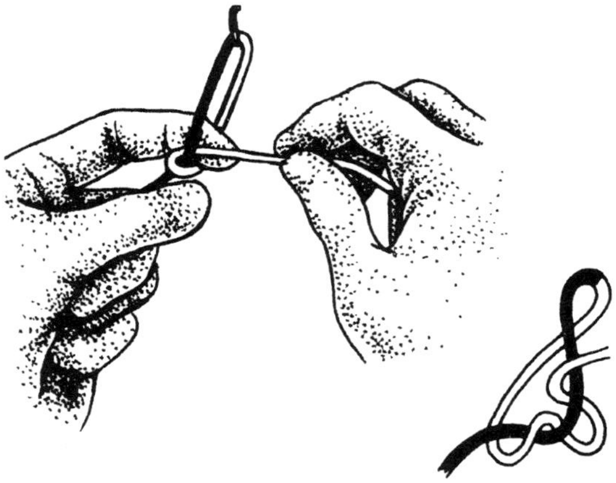
7. Tighten the knot. Tighten the knot by crossing your dominant hand over the other. Extend your index fingers to direct the tension as you snug the knot into place.	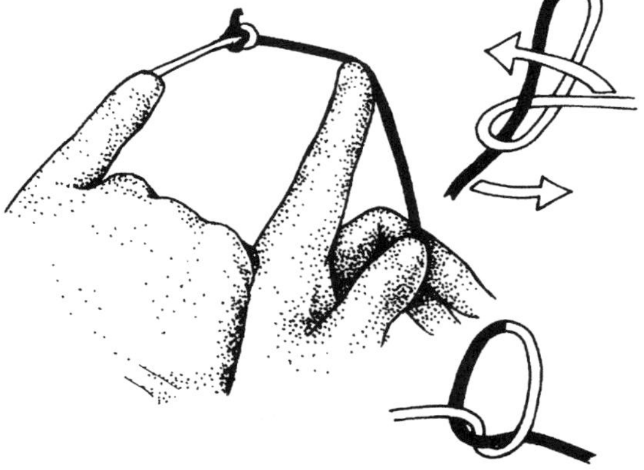

As the first throw is wrapped, the ends wind up on opposite sides from where they started because you cross them in step 4. You then cross yours hands as you lay the throw flat to *uncross* the segments, so that the resulting throw does not become bunched.

2. Two-handed square knot, second throw: Upon running down the first throw, proceed with the second.

1. Grasp the segments. Continue holding the colored segment with your nondominant hand as you move the white end to your dominant side.	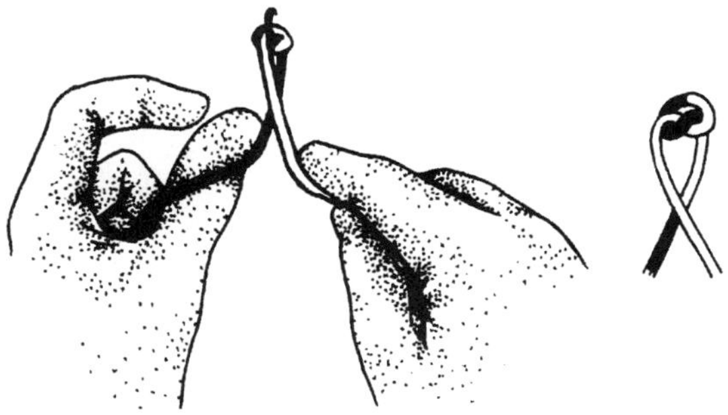
2. Cross the segments. Wrap the white segment up and around the other side of the nondominant thumbnail so that the segments form an X.	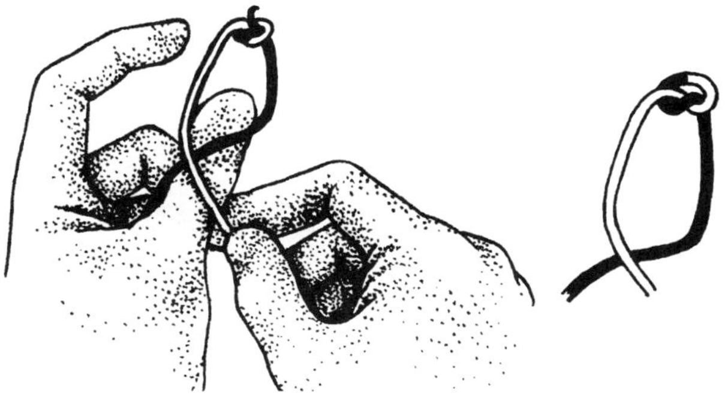
3. Pinch your fingers together. Flex your nondominant index finger over the white segment so that you can pinch your thumb and index fingers together inside the loop.	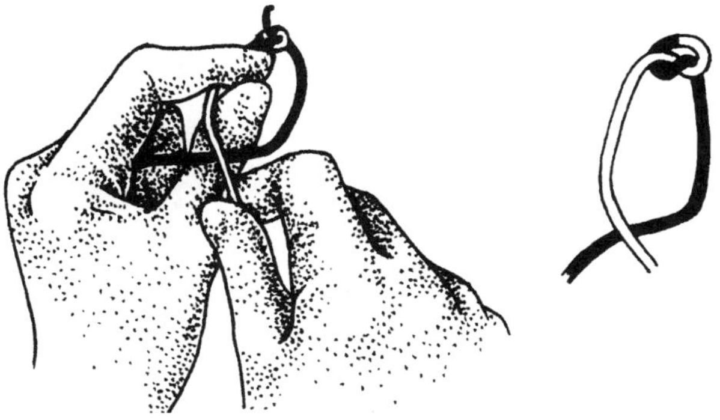

4. Poke your nondominant pinched fingers down through the loop and grasp the white segment. Rotate your palm toward you to push the pinched fingers down through the loop. Release the white segment and use your dominant hand to insert the white segment between your pinched fingers.	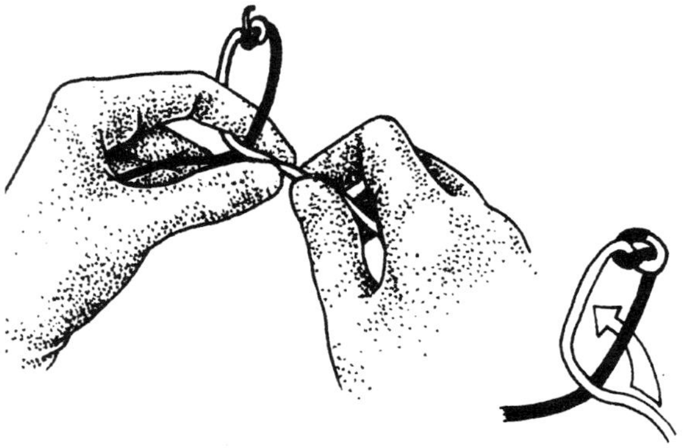
5. Push the white segment up through the loop. Rotate your wrist to bring the white segment up through the loop. Grasp the white end with your dominant hand and pull it completely through the loop.	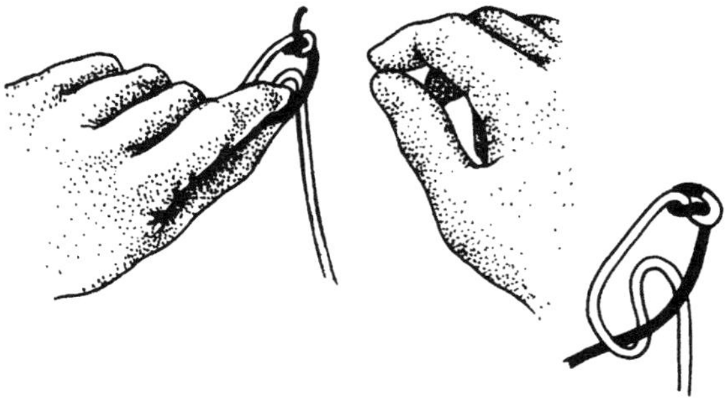
6. Tighten the knot. Extend your index fingers to lay the knot flat and parallel with the tissue surface as you tighten down the knot by separating your hands. (Note that this sequence results in a square knot that is reversed from the rest that are illustrated in this chapter).	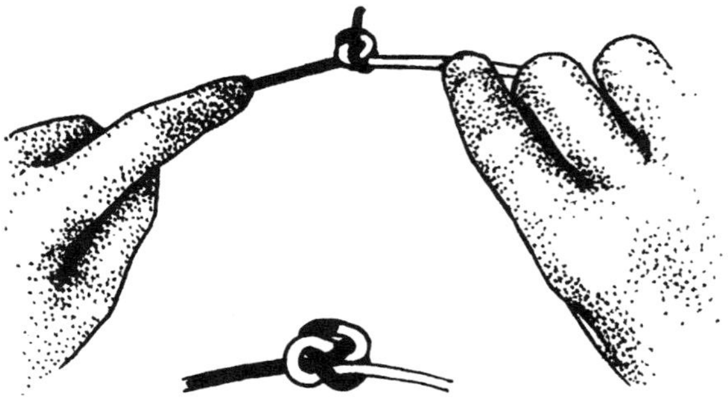

3. Two-handed square knot: third throw: To make the third throw, repeat the first throw. This completes three throws (one-and-a-half square knots). Depending upon the suture material, add more alternating throws until a complete knot is formed.

4. Trim the ears: When finished, trim the ends to no less than 3 mm in length.

***Tying a two-hand square knot in a tight space*:** When forming a two-hand tie in a deep, tight space, you use the same basic technique already described but modified to ensure that you form a well-snugged knot. These considerations are most important when placing a stitch deep within the yoni or the rectum or when tying off a bleeding blood vessel. Before placing the stitch, be sure the ends of the strand will be long enough so that, after you have encircled or sutured the deep structure, both ends will stick up above the cavity. This is important because you will need to hold the segments and form each throw above the wound. Form the first throw outside the cavity using a two-hand tie without applying tension to the segments. Extend a finger or use a closed instrument to push the throw down to the level where the knot is to be placed. Tighten the throw by placing one finger down near the knot location and using it to push down on the strand near the tissue surface, while using the other hand to apply the same amount of force on the other strand from outside of the cavity; this will help the throw lie flat. Alternatively, if there is room in the wound, you can place your extended index fingers against the strands on either side of the narrow space near the knot as you tighten it to ensure that the strands are kept as parallel as possible with the tissue surface.

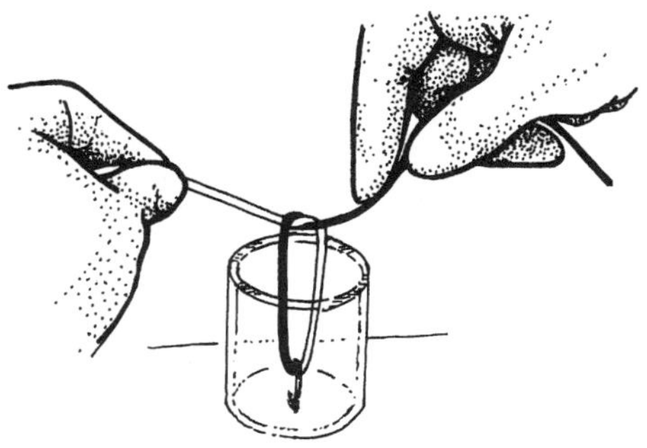

Beginning the throw above the cavity

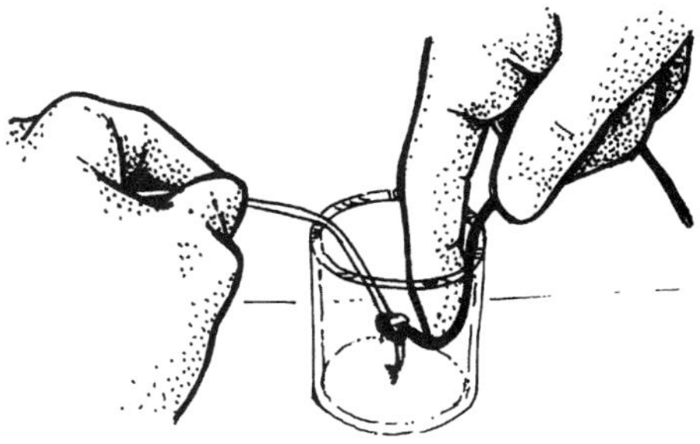

Tightening the throw in the cavity

Instrument-tied square knot: The majority of your knots will be in small places, where using an instrument tie will often be easier than hand tying. To begin an instrument tie, place the colored segment on your nondominant side and get out your needle holder.

Instrument-tied square knot, first throw:

1. Position your hands. Hold the colored segment in your nondominant hand. Hold the needle holder by its shaft in your dominant hand and lay it over the colored segment.	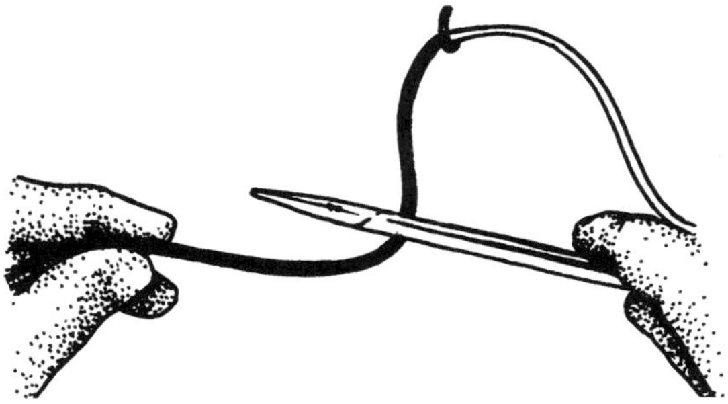
2. Loop the colored segment over the needle holder. Form the first loop by wrapping the colored segment over and around the shaft of the needle holder.	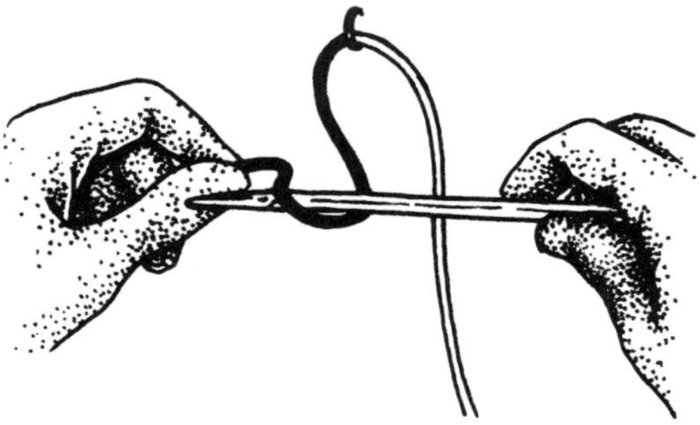
3. Pick up the free end and pull it through the loop. Reposition your dominant hand and place your fingers in the rings. Pick up the white segment with the needle holder and pull it through the loop.	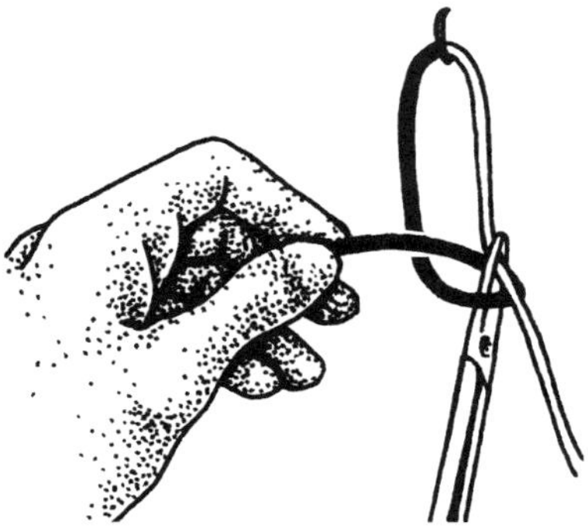

4. Tighten the knot. Tighten the knot and lay it flat by crossing the nondominant hand over the dominant hand.	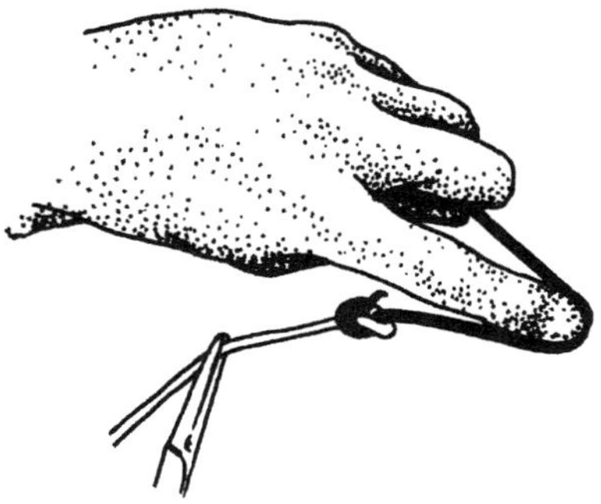

2. Instrument-tied square knot, second throw:

1. Make a loop. Place the needle holder under the colored segment. Wrap the colored segment toward you, around the end of the needle holder.	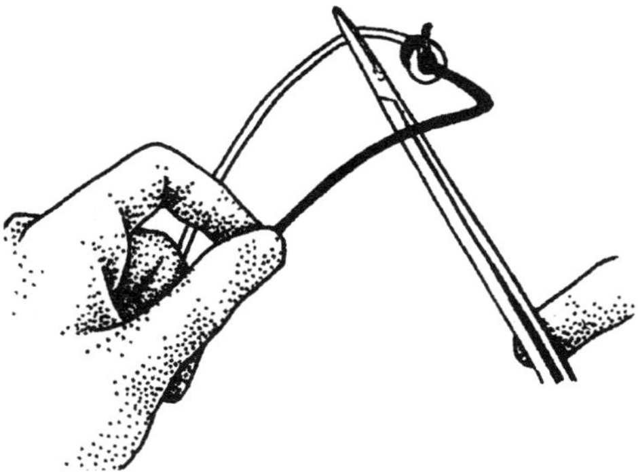
2. Grasp the white segment and pull it through. Insert fingers in the rings; pick up the white segment with the needle holder and pull it through the loop.	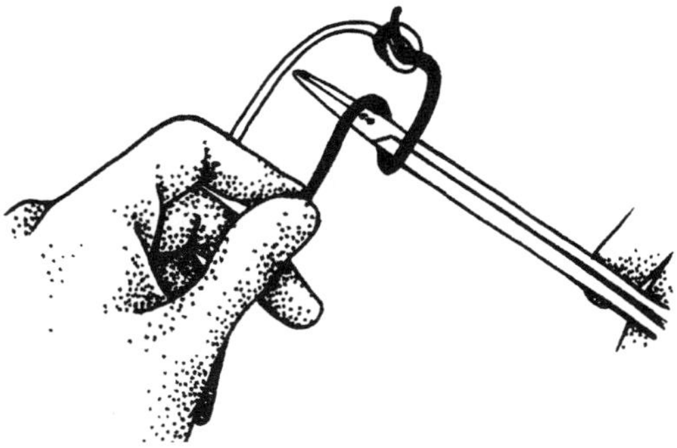

3. Tighten the throw. Keep the segments as parallel to the tissue surface as possible as you tighten the knot by pulling in opposite directions as you separate your hands.	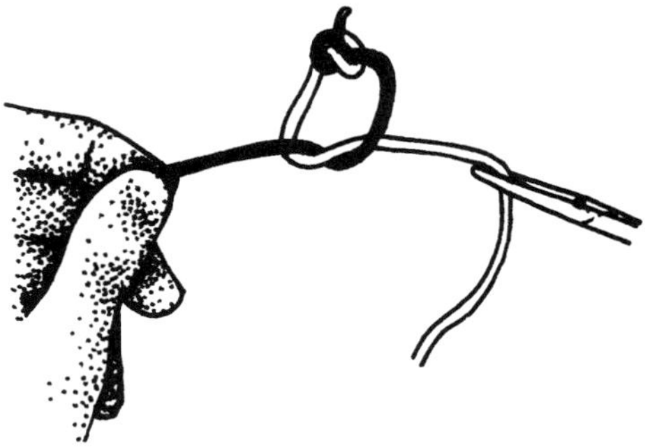

3. Instrument-tied square knot, third throw: To make the third throw, repeat the first throw. This completes three throws (one-and-a-half square knots). Depending upon the suture material, add more throws until a complete knot is formed.

4. Trim the ears: Trim the ends to 3 mm in length. (Anderson & Romfh, 1980; Edlich & Long, 2008; Zikria, 1981)

***Slip knots*:** A slip knot consists of two throws, which can be either mirror image or identical. A square knot can be constructed to slip almost as freely as a granny knot. The slip knot has a mechanical advantage in that only the force vector that pulls the tissue edges together is applied to the knot. A slip knot is created when greater tension is applied to one segment than the other during rundown. This is accomplished by not fully snugging down the first throw during rundown, then applying more tension to the needle end than to the free end when tightening the second throw. The knot's ability to slip depends on having one straight segment along which the loops of the other segment can slide. Applying more tension on one side straightens that segment, causing the other, wrapped segment to curl around it.

At times it may be advantageous to temporarily convert a square knot into a slip knot in order to reposition it more accurately or when a square knot has been tied too loosely. The knot, even though snugged down, can be temporarily converted to a slip knot by letting go of one end and gently tugging several times on the other strand to straighten that end out. Slide the knot into place by applying slightly more tension to the straight strand than to the wrapped one, thus the straight strand forms a cable along which the wraps slide into position. Restore the slip knot to a locked configuration by reversing the strength of tension applied to the strands; pull on the free end more strongly than on the needle end and check to make sure that the knot is now flat and square.

When one end of your suture is very short (a circumstance you will encounter frequently), it is tempting to hold it taut while you tighten the other end. You *must*, however, give the short end slack while taking up the slack in the longer end until the tension is equal or you will wind up with a slipping half-hitch knot. Once the tension is equal, continue to apply equal and opposing tension to both ends to form a true half-hitch.

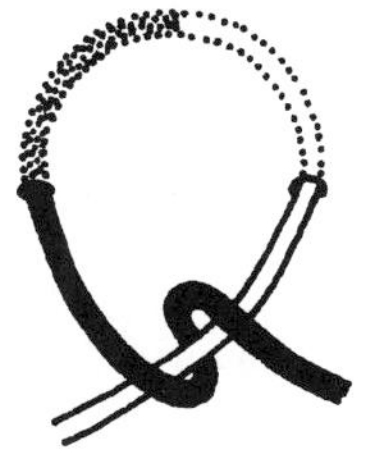

The half-hitch before rundown

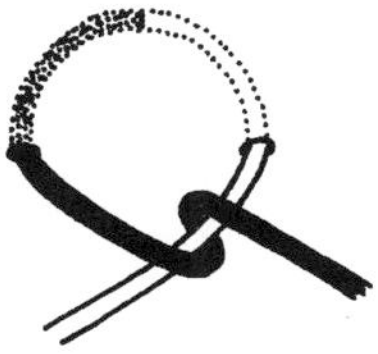

Here, too much tension applied to the white end produces a slip hitch.

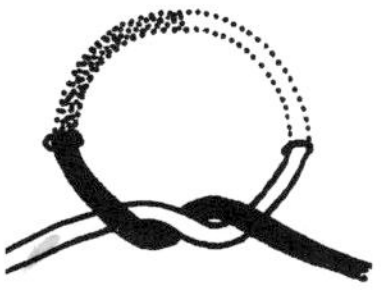

Applying equal tension to each end produces a true half-hitch.

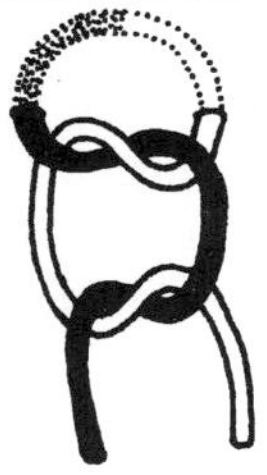

Loose square knot

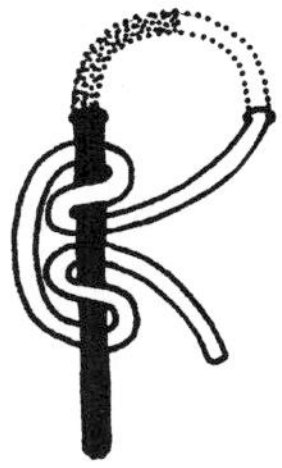

Tension on the black segment . . .

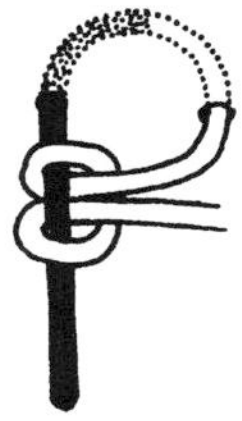

produces a slipping square knot.

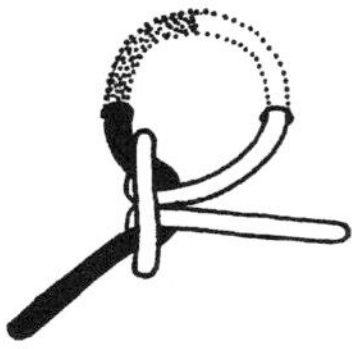

Applying more tension to the white segment. . . .

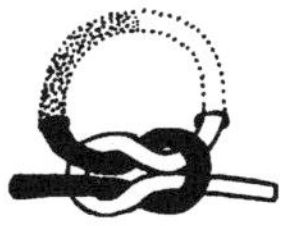

and then equalizing the tension on both segments converts it back to a square knot.

The influence of suture material on the formation of a knot: Once you are skilled in these basic techniques using thick cord, move on to practicing knot tying using different types of material that are similar to sutures. A thick sewing thread or 3-0 silk suture can substitute for braided synthetic. Fishing line can stand in for synthetic monofilament. There is really no substitute for chromic gut, though. Try to obtain some packets of 3-0 chromic gut for practicing (needle size is not important at this juncture because you are not yet practicing stitches).

How many throws are optimal to use with each material is still a matter of debate. You'd think, with knot security being so critical, good studies using standardized testing methods would have settled these questions long ago. In fact, there are only a limited number of studies that have addressed knot security, and these have used different testing methods and thus produced results that are not comparable (von Fraunhofer & Chu, 1996b). It is not uncommon for surgeons to try and improve knot security by simply using a larger gauge suture material or adding extra throws. Both approaches increase the amount of foreign material left in the tissues, with the use of a larger diameter strand leaving much more foreign material in the tissues, greatly increasing the inflammatory zone around the strand, much more so than does an extra throw or two. Therefore, using more throws is the better choice. The following pointers will help form secure knots with different materials.

- **Chromic gut:** Gut exhibits the highest knot security of any suture material and rarely slips regardless of the knot configuration, another good reason to use chromic (von Fraunhofer & Chu, 1996). Each square knot needs at least three alternating throws (i.e., 1½ square knots). Surgical gut is relatively rough and has a moderate amount of memory. It will need to be straightened out frequently during the suturing process to avoid tangles. Even so, experienced midwives report less spontaneous strand knotting when using gut materials.
- **Synthetic materials:** Compared to chromic gut, all coated synthetic materials are smoother and slipperier, and monofilamentgreat thats are the smoothest of all. Therefore, synthetic materials require more throws to hold a square knot securely (at least four throws; i.e., two complete square knots). Vicryl, with its thicker coating, behaves more like surgical gut, and some surgeons only use three throws. Dexon II, on the other hand, does not hold knots as securely as Vicryl, which makes it easier to handle during placement. It requires at least four throws, however, or two full square knots, to hold securely. I am recommending that you use a minimum of four throws (two square knots) with all synthetics, although the Colorado Surgical Assistants program recommends 6 throws (3 square knots) for all braided synthetics and 16 throws (8 square knots) for monofilament materials. While a 2=1=1 surgeon's friction knot will usually hold all these materials securely with only three throws, this type of knot is hard to work with and I do not recommend it. Cut the ears on synthetics no less than 3 mm long straight across the strand, even when against the skin; to avoid unraveling, never trim the ears on synthetics flush with the knot.

Practicing breaking knotted suture: You should apply 80% of the knot-breaking strength to the segments when you run down your throws. To get a feel for the breaking strength of various suture materials, experiment with pieces of real suture to see how hard you must pull to break an unknotted strand and then tie two ends in a 1=1=1square knot and pull on each end to determine the knot-breaking strength.

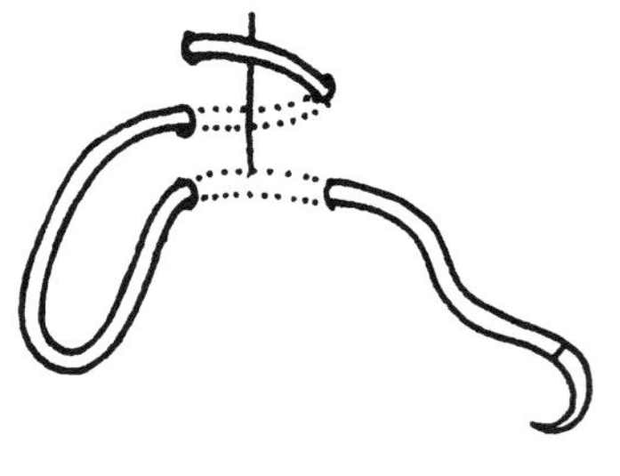

Loop contributes two strands.

Finishing a continuous row of stitches with a final square knot: At the beginning of a row of stitches or when an interrupted stitch is placed, a "double-strand" square knot is created using the segments of the strand from either side of the stitch. At the end of a continuous row of stitches, however, a **"triple-strand" square knot** is used. It is formed by first creating a loop of suture on the needle-end side. This is done by taking a backwardly directed stitch alongside the one you just created by reinserting the needle on the same side you just exited and bringing it out on the other side of the laceration (your dominant side), beside your original insertion point.

The stitch is left loose so that a loop remains open on your nondominant side. Pinch the sides of the loop together, creating a double strand segment, and treat this pinched loop as though it were one thread. Cut the needle off of the dominant-side segment and the pinched loop is then tied to the needle-end.

The triple-strand square knot is markedly different from the double-strand square knot because it has two segments on one side (the pinched loop) that are intertwined with the single segment on the dominant side. Double-strand square knots have two ears that point in opposite directions. A triple strand knot has one ear on one side and two ears (from both ends of the loop) that exit the opposite side of the knot. Triple-strand square knots are thus more likely to slip. Nevertheless, this is a good way to close off a row of stitches and is widely used.

To avoid slippage, additional throws are added to increase knot security. When constructing a double-strand square knot with absorbable synthetic multifilament material, use *at least* four throws. Tying a triple-strand square knot using a synthetic monofiliment material, requires *at least* five or six throws to achieve knot security, leaving a big bunch of suture on the surface of the tissue. Because of this, there is really no advantage in attempting any techniques to bury such a bulky knot. When working with chromic gut, one and a half square knots (three throws) may be used to form either a double- or a triple-strand square knot.

The Aberdeen knot

The **Aberdeen knot** is a variation of a **highwayman's hitch** or **high post hitch knot**. These knots were originally developed to temporarily secure an object to a post and are therefore designed to release easily. The knot has been modified for surgical applications so that it will not come untied and thus lacks a built-in mechanism to unravel it. This knot has gained wide popularity in the United Kingdom, Australia and New Zealand. It was named by James Learmonth (Professor of Surgery, Aberdeen University, Scotland, from 1952 to 1958), who noted that it used less suture than a standard surgeon's knot and therefore must have been invented by a Scot.

This knot can be used as the final knot to tie off continuous stitches and is a good alternative to the triple-strand square knot for this purpose. It is very easy to construct and, if done correctly, offers the best security of all surgeon's knots when used appropriately. After running the strand through the tissue, a knot is formed by creating a loop of thread with the free end and passing another loop created on the needle end through it; each such configuration equals one throw. A wrap is created when the needle end is passed around one side of the final loop one or more times prior to running down the last throw.

Stott and colleagues (2007) found that a maximally strong and slip-free knot could be created using three throws, with two wraps incorporated on the final throw. They used Polydioxanone monofilament (PDS II, Ethicon), size 0, for these tests, which is not recommended for perineal repair. Nevertheless, synthetic monofilament materials are widely regarded as the most difficult materials with which to create a secure knot. PDS-II is considered quite pliable compared to other synthetic materials, but the use of such a thick strand stiffens the material somewhat. Based on this understanding, the three-throw, two-wrap configuration they found to be most secure in this material is likely to be entirely adequate for use in the thinner materials that midwives commonly use. If you are in doubt about this, you could add one more throw before wrapping the last loop.

The Aberdeen knot is self-tightening. As it tightens, the stitch becomes slack. Thus, it is important to snug down the first throw securely before beginning the next.

Practicing the Aberdeen knot: Begin this knot by forming a loop. This can be done by not completing your last stitch or by completing the final stitch and then reentering the tissue on the same side you just exited and coming out on the opposite side, as for a triple-strand square knot, thus creating a loop on your nondominant side and moving the needle end back to your dominant side. Based on my experience, completing your last stitch before creating a separate loop is the best option because I believe it places less tension on the tissues, although it does require leaving more suture in the tissue. A right-handed knot is illustrated here, where the loop will be formed on the nondominant side.

1. Create a loop. Reinsert the needle on the same side you just exited and come up on your dominant side. This leaves a loop on your nondominant side. Whenever needed, reduce the size of the loop by pulling on the needle end with your dominant hand. (You can trim off the needle at this point, here the needle is shown in the closeups to clarify which end you are manipulating.)	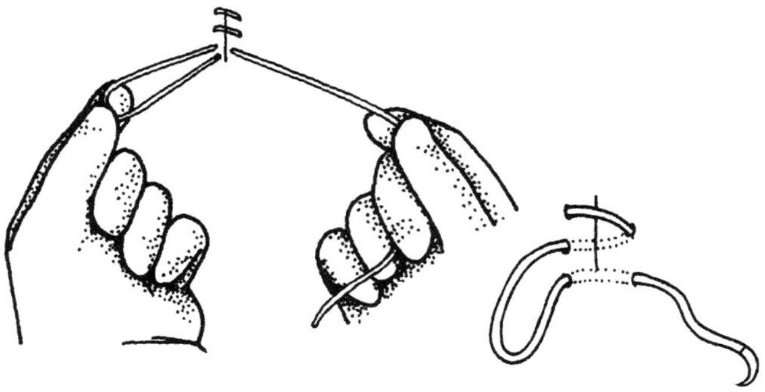

2. Lift the loop toward your dominant side and insert your non-dominant thumb and index finger into it. Spread your fingers slightly to widen the loop.	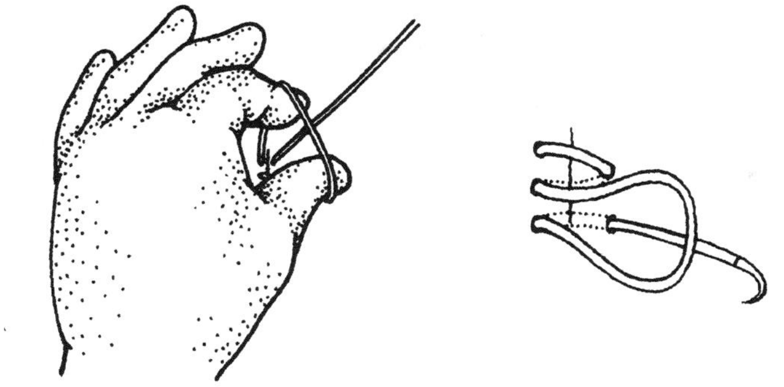
3. Grasp the needle segment between your nondominant thumb and index fingers and pull it through the loop. The process of pulling the straight segment through the first loop creates the first throw. It also forms the second loop.	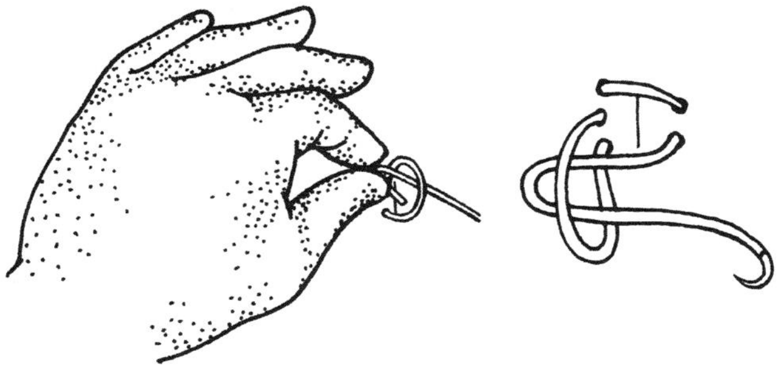
4. Finish the first throw. Continue pulling on the second loop to snug down the first throw. Whenever necessary, adjust the loop's size by pulling on the needle segment with your dominant hand.	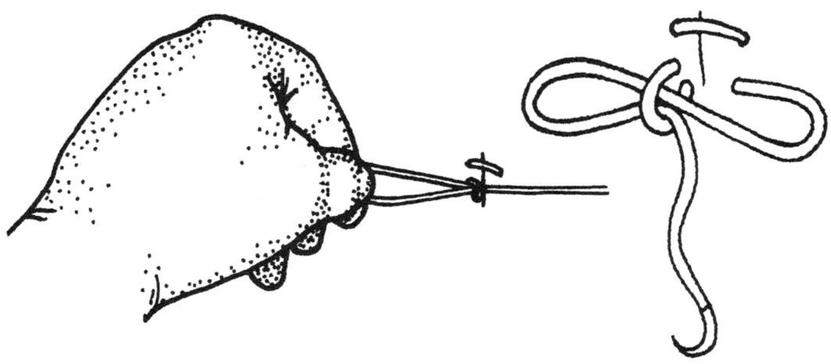

5. Begin a second throw. Lift the second loop toward your dominant side and insert your non-dominant thumb and index fingers into it.	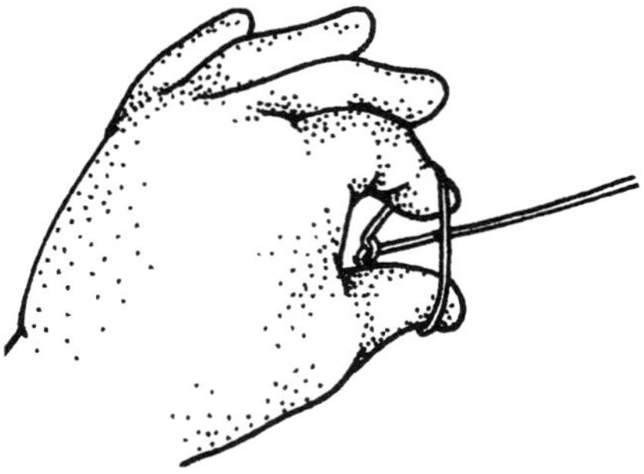
6. Pinch the needle-segment and pull it through the loop. This step creates the second throw. It also forms a third loop.	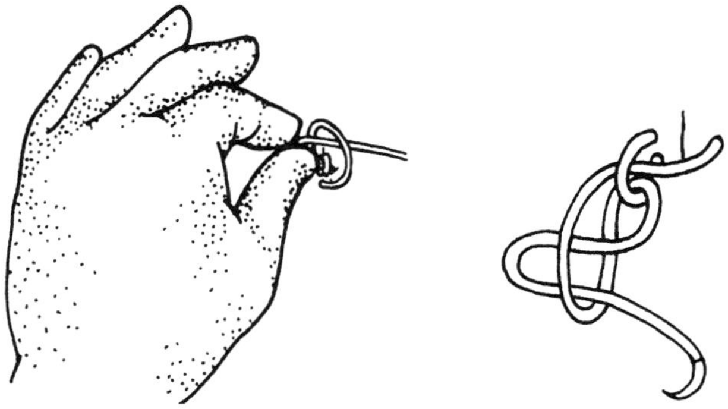
7. Finish the second throw. Continue adjusting the tension on the loop and the needle end to snug down the second throw.	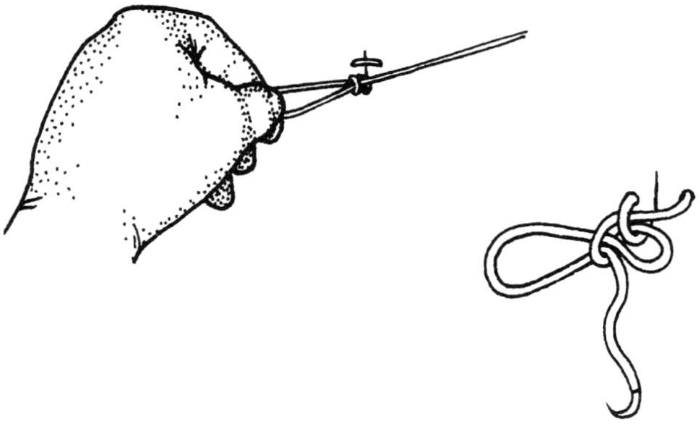

8. Begin a third throw. Lift the loop toward your dominant side and insert your nondominant thumb and index finger through the loop. Reduce the size of the loop by pulling on the needle end with your dominant hand, as necessary.	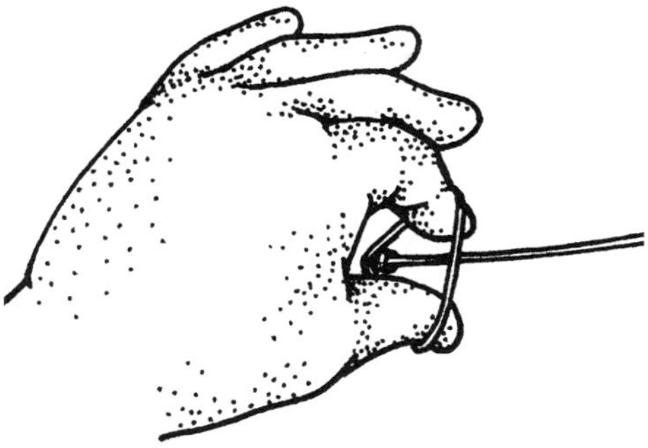
9. Now pinch the needle segment with your nondominant thumb and index fingers and pull it through the loop. This creates the third throw. It also forms a fourth loop.	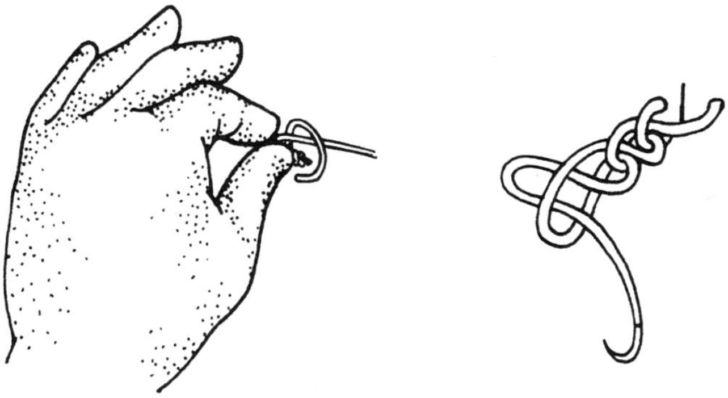
10. Finish the third throw. Continue pulling to snug down the third throw.	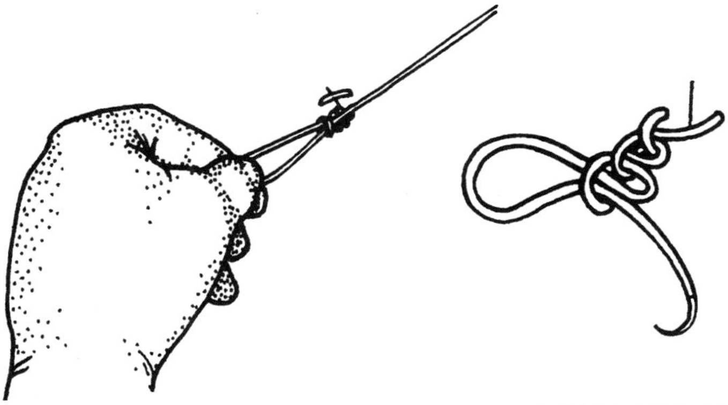

11. Finishing the knot. Start by inserting your nondominant thumb and index fingers into the fourth loop and spread them to open the loop.

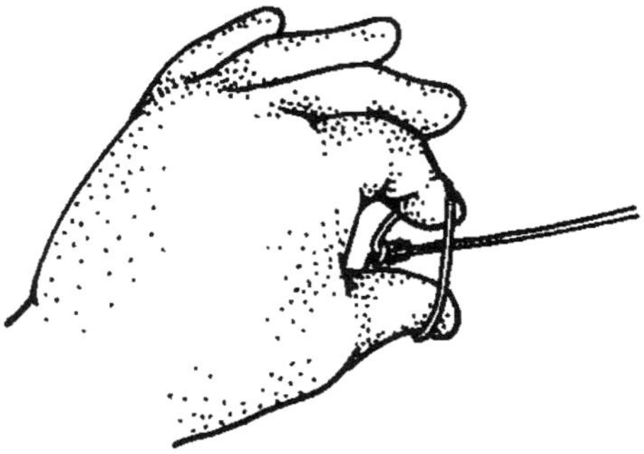

12. Begin to lock the stitch. Pass the needle end of the strand through the loop.

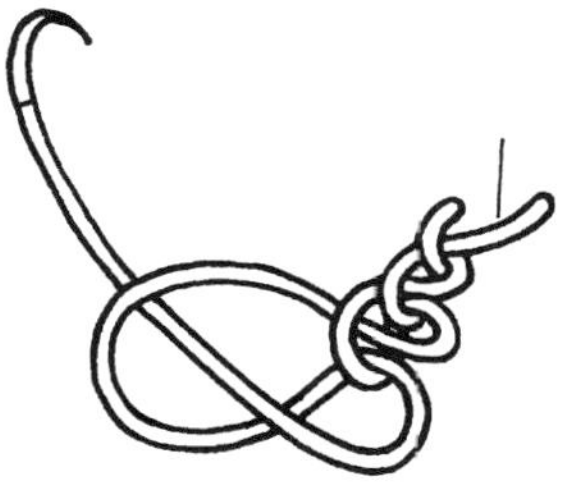

13. Create the first wrap. Wrap (turn) the needle end around one side of the loop.

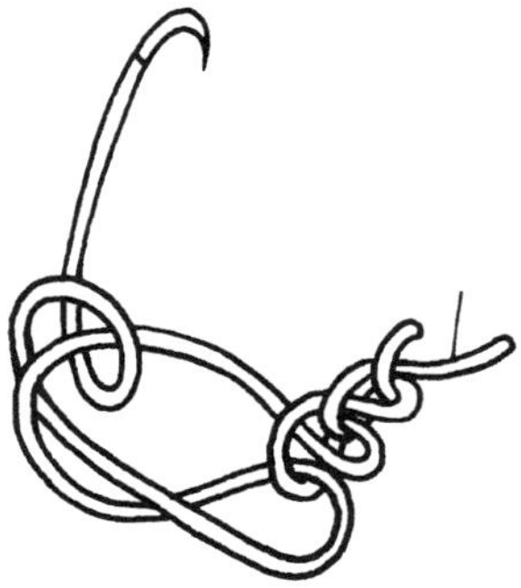

14. Create the second wrap (turn) by passing the needle end around the side of the loop a second time.

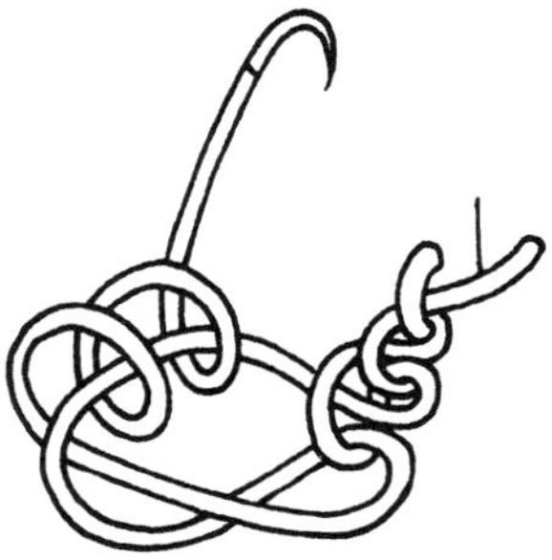

15. Now the knot looks like this.

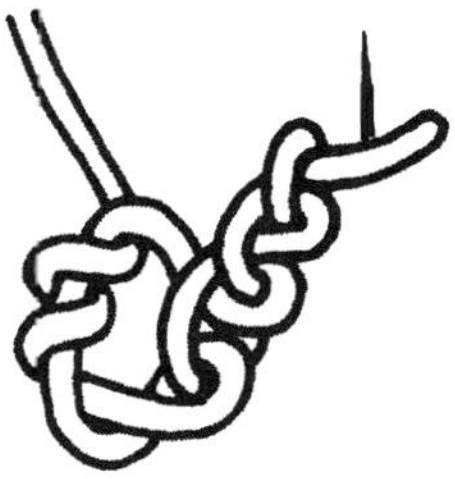

16. As you rundown the knot for the last time, it starts to twist and look like this.

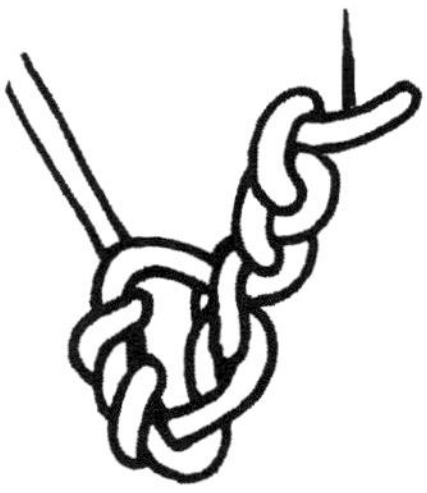

To bury an Aberdeen knot: If desired, you can bury the knot. To do so, you must leave the needle attached. Arm your needle holder and insert the needle tip between the edges of the perineal tear, just below the uppermost perineal stitch. Bring the needle up between the edges of the tear, behind the last stitch in the yoni floor (which will, in most women, also be behind the hymenal ring). Pull up on the needle end, which will drag the knot between the edges of the perineal tear, thus burying it under the tissue surface. The disadvantage to this is that it leaves an additional wad of suture in the tissue. The disadvantage to not doing this is that a longish knot is left on the tissue surface that could become entangled in a sanitary pad and that may be otherwise irritating to the woman.

Trim the ears: Trim the needle-end, leaving a short ear.

General Considerations When Selecting and Using Surgical Instruments

The decision about which instrument to use must sometimes be made on the basis of what is available. When you need to decide based on what you've got rather than what you need, consider the following points:

- Choose the shortest instrument that will comfortably reach the operative site.
- If cutting suture or other nontissue materials, avoid using scissors that are designed to cut tissue. Use larger and blunter scissors or stitch scissors for nontissue materials (the only exception is the umbilical cord, for which a blunt scissors is preferred).
- Choose instruments in good repair. Forceps that cross at the tip, scissors that do not cut easily and needle holders that do not grip the needle securely can be frustrating and dangerous.

The basic principles of all instrument handling include safety, economy of movement, relaxed handling and avoiding awkward movements (RCSE, 2009). When holding instruments:

- Use three-point control: have three points of contact between your hand and the instrument to stabilize the instrument and increase the precision of use.
- When using instruments that open and close, extend your index finger along the instrument to provide extra control and stability.
- Place only the tips of your fingers and thumb through the rings of instruments that open and close. Doing so allows you to use your wrist and forearm to maneuver the instrument, providing a greater arc of control. It also makes it quicker and less cumbersome to pick up and put down the instrument.

Many more tips on specific ways to use the primary instruments needed in midwifery-level surgical care are explained in the chapters that follow.

USING LOCKING SURGICAL CLAMPS

"Locking surgical clamps" refers to a broad category of instruments that have grasping jaws and a mechanism to keep the jaws closed. Such clamps have a wide variety of uses, including occlusion of blood vessels; dissecting, retracting and holding tissue; holding suture or the needle; and driving the needle. Instruments in this category that are used by midwives include hemostats, ring forceps, Allis clamps and needle holders. It will be helpful for you to have some sort of locking surgical clamp on hand as you read through this chapter.

The anatomy of locking surgical clamps

Most hinged clamping instruments share the same basic construction. They consist of two **levers** or **shanks** (a male and a female) that rotate on a common fulcrum. Together these levers form the **shaft** of the instrument. The levers are joined inside a **box lock** that has flat sides, allowing them to pivot freely. The edges of the box lock and the sides of the jaws are **chamfered**, or rounded, to prevent damage to tissue or suture material. The **jaws** are specialized grasping parts located at one end of each lever. At the other end of the levers is the **handle**, consisting of two **finger rings**.

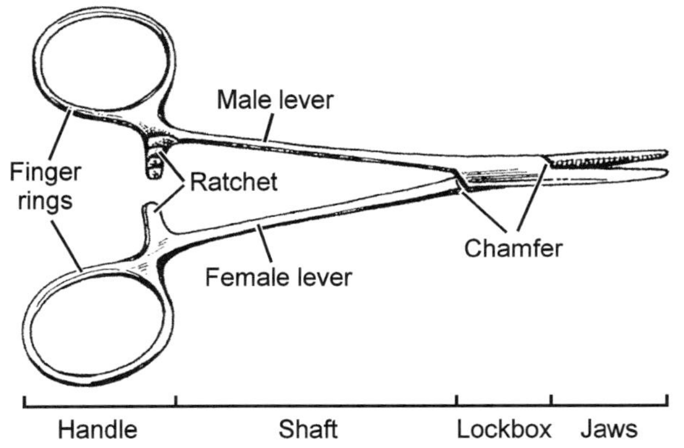

Parts of a locking surgical clamp

The locking mechanism, or **ratchet**, has a series of interlockable teeth that allow the jaws to be fixed at different degrees of tightness. The number of teeth vary depending upon the instrument's design. There are usually at least three sets of teeth. These teeth are arranged in rows that project from the inside of each handle toward the midline at the base of the finger rings. Right-handed instruments are designed so that, when the right palm is facing down, the ratchet operated by the thumb is below the one operated by the fingers, allowing easy closure and release by the thumb. A left-handed ratchet has the thumb-side teeth lowermost when the instrument is used in the left hand. This is easy to understand when you experiment with your instrument. For more information about left- and right-handed closure, see the chapter entitled "Using Surgical Scissors."

Grasping the instrument

The most secure grip involves inserting the thumb and index fingers in the finger rings. Unfortunately, this grip limits mobility, and it can be difficult to remove the clamp from your hand once you are finished with it. The thumb and ring finger grip involves three fingers to control the instrument and is suited to delicate work.

To assist with removal from the finger rings, rest the tip of the clamp on a firm surface, bring the finger rings together and push the clamp off your hand by pressing your index finger down against the closed but unlocked shank. (When several instruments are being used, lock the ratchet on the first set of teeth before discarding to avoid entanglement when it is placed aside with other used equipment.)

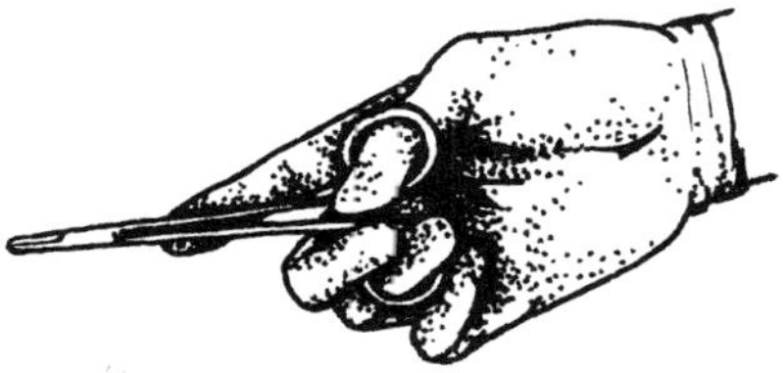 Thumb and ring finger grip	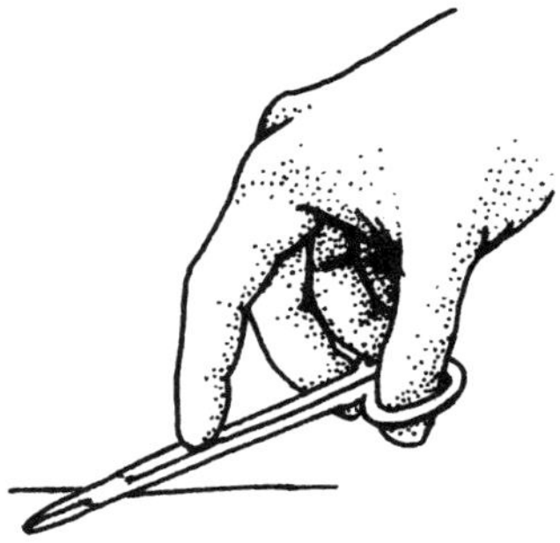 Discarding the clamp
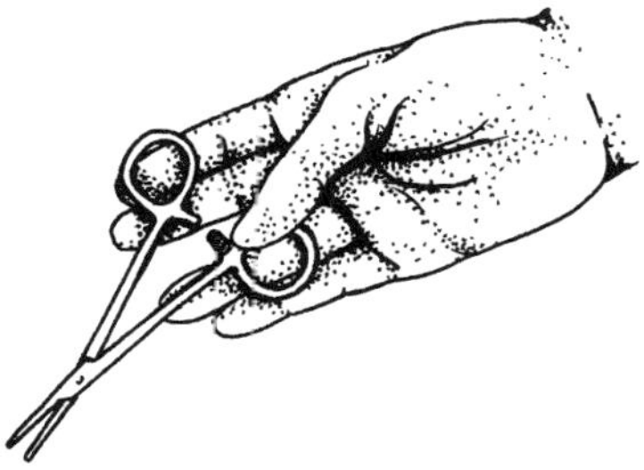 **Right-handed removal:** To release the ratchet without fingers in the finger rings, pinch the bottom ring between your thumb and ring finger and disengage the ratchet using outward pressure from the index finger on the topmost finger ring.	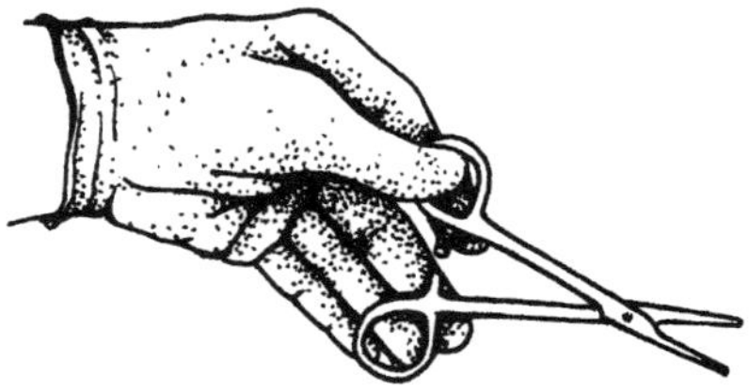 **Left-handed removal:** Grasp the top ring between the thumb and index finger and disengage the ratchet by applying outward pressure on the bottom ring with the middle, ring, and little fingers.

Palming the instrument as the rachet is disengaged allows you to remove it from your hand more easily. This grip also allows a greater range of mobility. The instructions above apply to the use of any instrument equipped with a right-handed ratchet (Anderson & Romfh, 1980). If you are left-handed and have a left-handed instrument, hold it as in the illustration in the left box (right-handed removal).

Manipulating the instrument

Part the finger rings to open the jaws. Position the open jaws on either side of the object to be grasped. Be sure of what you are grasping because, in most cases, any tissue that is grasped in locked jaws can be considered dead, as the gripping action will crush it, especially if the instrument in question is not intended to grasp tissue. Bring the finger rings together to close the jaws and grip the object. Once the jaws are grasping the object, lock the instrument by engaging the ratchet by compressing the finger rings together to bring the ratchet teeth adjacent to each other so that they interlock. This puts tension on each lever, bending them inward slightly. While the ratchet is engaged, the instrument will continue to grasp the desired object without the midwife needing to apply continual force to the handle.

When the clamping action is no longer required, gradually exert closing pressure on the finger rings to release the spring tension of the handles and smoothly disengage the ratchet. Once the teeth are disengaged, prevent them from reengaging by exerting separating pressure on each finger ring to keep the teeth apart. Then relax your hand and the jaws will open, releasing the object.

Hemostats and related instruments

Hemostats are primarily used to grasp blood vessels and other tissue. They have a variety of other uses as well, some of which will be detailed later in this text. Most hemostatic ratchets have three or four sets of teeth. If the goal is stabilization or hemostasis of tissue, engage the ratchet on the first tooth to apply minimally effective pressure. If the goal is to assist in the removal of tissue (such as a skin tag), engage the ratchet on its last set of teeth to apply maximum pressure.

When using a hemostat to hold suture out of the way (as in anal sphincter repair), engage the last teeth to achieve the tightest hold to ensure that the strands do not slip. Be sure the strands are grasped at an angle to the serrations, or the suture will tend to slip out. Take care not to clamp a part of a strand that will eventually remain in a knot or in tissue.

Using the Needle Holder

A needle holder (or driver) is a specialized type of locking clamp that allows you to firmly hold and precisely manipulate a suturing needle in small, slippery spaces while avoiding needlestick injuries. As Anderson and Romfh (1980) point out, there are 11 steps in taking a stitch with a needle holder, all of which are important to a skillful repair. Before studying this chapter, it will be helpful for you to gather a needle holder, a half-circle needle of some kind (preferably a 36 or 37 mm size), a foam or paper coffee cup, a piece of paper and a piece of foam rubber.

1. Matching the needle holder to the needle

Match the size of the needle holder to the size of the needle. If the needle holder is too big for the chosen needle, its grip will be too strong, and the needle may be damaged by the jaws. This should not be a problem if you are using the needle holder with the needles mentioned in this text; the larger needle holders can be used with any size needle midwives typically use, although they are best suited to drive the larger 36 to 37 mm needles. The smaller needle holders are for use with the various smaller needles recommended for periurethral and rectal mucosa repair and should not be used to drive the larger needles.

2. Positioning the needle in the holder

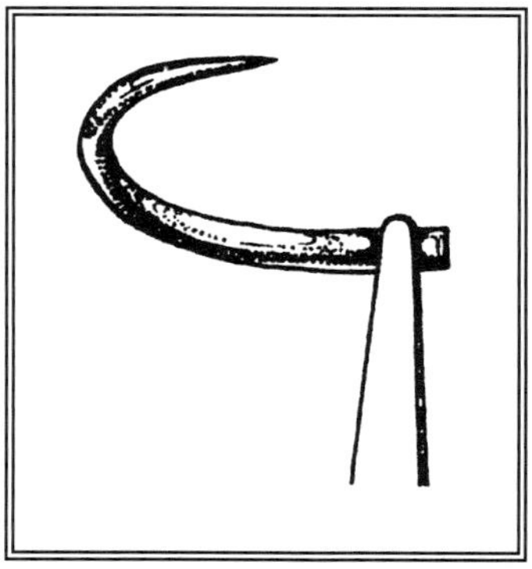

Grasping the needle in the jaws is referred to as arming the holder. There are two things when doing so: at what point to grasp the needle wire along its length and what angle to place the needle in the jaws. To repair soft tissues, grasp the slightly flattened part of the needle near the swaged end. Take care to clamp a little below the swaged end, as the swage is the weakest point in the needle wire and can snap off if stressed. Clamping below the swage also maximizes stabilization and works well for soft tissue repair. It allows more of the needle to pass through the tissue in one movement, poses less chance that the needle will back out of the tissue once it is released and makes the pointed end of the needle easier to retrieve.

The needle may also be grasped at its midpoint or even near the tip. The closer the needle is gripped to its tip, the greater the force available to drive the needle through the tissue. This can be useful when the tissue is very tough, as may be the case with scar tissue in the perineal skin. When gripped this way, the needle must be driven in stages because the holder must be continuously released and the jaws re-positioned to advance the needle through the tissue.

The angle at which the needle is placed in the jaws is the other consideration. For most perineal suturing you will need to position the needle in the jaws so that it is perpendicular (90°) to the line of the handle when holding the needle holder upright in front of you. The sharp end of the needle will be pointing straight at you on one side of the jaws, and the swagged end will be pointing at you on the other side. When the needle is correctly positioned, engage the ratchet to its first or second tooth; this should hold the needle securely. The smaller the needle, the tighter the jaws must be.

Perpendicular placement of a half-circle needle in the holder allows the needle to be driven by simply rotating the holder on its axis, a movement that requires no additional space.

The needle can also be placed at an acute or obtuse angle or even grasped parallel with the shaft. Nevertheless, if the needle is held at an angle of other than 90°, the handles must move through a wider arc to follow the curve of the needle as it is advanced through the tissue. This is hard to accomplish in a small space, and it is usually easier to figure out how to work with the needle held perpendicularly than to move the handle through a wide arc.

3. Grasping the needle holder

Once the holder is armed with the needle, there are four ways to grasp the needle holder. Each grip has advantages and disadvantages and it is a good idea to become familiar with them all. Regardless of the grip you use, it is sometimes helpful to use your nondominant hand to help stabilize your dominant hand as it drives the needle.

Palmed grip: With the needle clamped in the jaws, grasp the needle holder securely by the shaft with the back of your hand facing up; this is called the "palm grip." This is the strongest grip, providing the greatest pressure when driving the needle. The thumb and index finger's position near the needle offer maximal control of needle movement. The disadvantage is that the needle holder cannot be released after a stitch is taken without readjusting your grip.

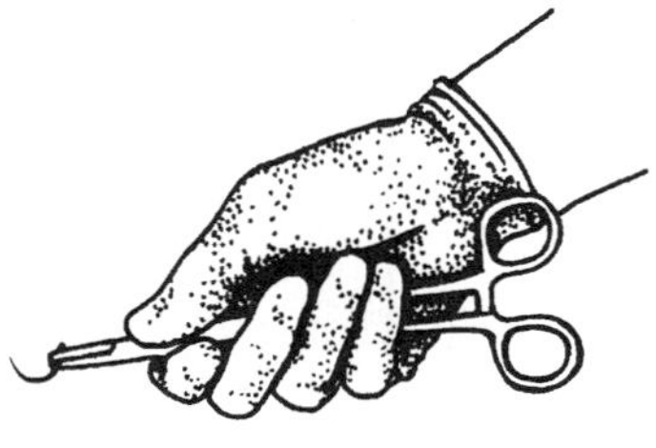

Palmed grip

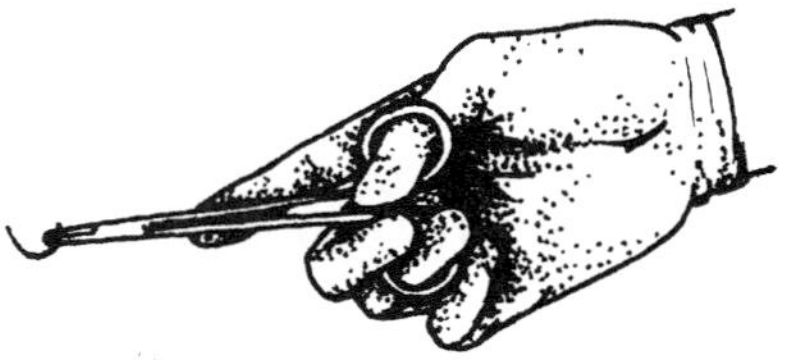

Thumb–ring finger grip

Thumb–ring (third) finger grip: This grip involves simply placing the thumb and third finger in the finger rings, which allows for the precise release of the needle. By exerting closing pressure on the finger rings, the spring action of the handles is relieved before the teeth are disengaged; this avoids popping the teeth apart. Regrasping the needle is also more precise because, with a finger in both finger rings, this grip allows for a greater range of motion, making this the best grip to use for releasing the ratchet in delicate, easy-to-traumatize tissues.

Thenar grip: The needle holder is grasped between the ball of the thumb and the third finger or little finger. This grip saves time when placing continuous stitches because it eliminates some of the repositioning necessary when other grips are used. The needle can be released and regrasped for removal without changing grips, which is necessary with a palmed grip. When preparing to take the next stitch, the needle can be redirected by pivoting the holder clockwise in the palm without needing to readjust the needle in the holder or changing grips, as is required with the thumb–ring grip. The Thenar grip allows as much mobility in supination as the palmed grip, and it offers average strength and direction control compared to other grips. It is less precise, however, for releasing the needle because disengaging the ratchet requires exerting pressure perpendicular to the shafts until the teeth are unlocked, which can cause the handles to pop as the ratchet releases, making it difficult not to move the needle in the process. With practice, this tendency to pop the rachet can nevertheless be overcome by learning to release it smoothly by pressing the ring on the thumb side down and away from the midline, thus disengaging the teeth.

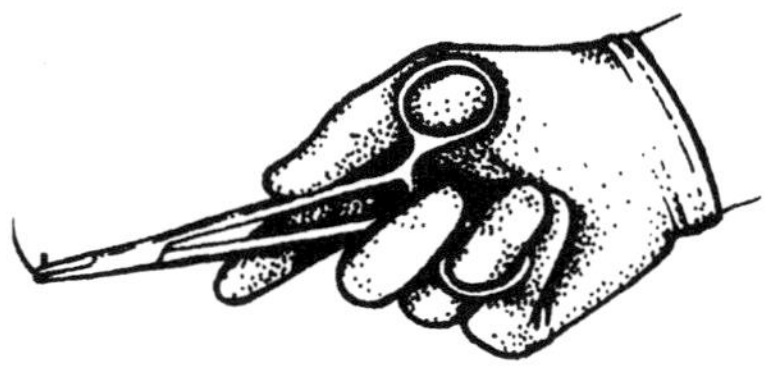

Thenar grip

Pencil grip: The pencil grip is the most delicate and accurate for very fine suturing. Simply grasp the shaft of the needle holder as you would a writing implement. This allows the needle to be driven by rotating the holder on its axis between the index finger and the thumb. Although this grip is most easily used with small needle holders that have either no lock or a pressure–release lock, it could be used to drive the needle during delicate labial repair using one of the needle holders mentioned in this text. This grip, however, requires you to reposition your hand to make the stitch after the needle is locked in the jaws and requires repositioning your hand again to release the needle, so it is an awkward technique to master with a locking needle holder and is rarely needed in midwifery-related repairs. Reserve this technique for the very fine stitching of surface tissue (such as the labia minora) after you are basically competent with using the needle holder.

4. Dealing with the free end of the suture

Be sure that the free end of the suture material is to your dominant side before proceeding with the stitch. This important step is often overlooked. It will help minimize tangling and allow for more efficient knot tying.

5. Placing the needle point where you want to enter the tissue

Carefully place the point of the needle where you want it and position yourself so that your body mechanics will allow you to drive the needle in the desired direction. Try to put the needle tip where you want it the first time. Hand position and direction of approach are important considerations in gaining optimal mechanical advantage. To drive the needle down and around requires a supinating motion of the wrist. Therefore starting with the hand in pronation (i.e., palm down), gives you 180°of maneuvering radius to rotate the needle through the tissue. In most midwifery-related repairs, you will be driving the needle from one side of the midline to the other. This usually involves driving the needle from your dominant side toward your nondominant side. However, if you ever need to drive a needle through a labial laceration that is more parallel than vertical, use a forehand technique, i.e., drive the needle from the far side of the laceration toward the near side, so the needle tip is coming toward you. This approach affords the best maneuverability.

6. Driving a curved needle through tissue

A curved needle is used where deep bites are needed in an area where the point of a straight needle would be difficult to reach after it has passed through the tissue. A half-circle needle works best for perineal repair. Moving a curved needle through tissue involves two force vectors. **Driving force** advances the needle through the tissue. Once the needle enters the tissue, **rotating force** ensures that it is driven along a curved path.

The driving force is in the direction of advancement of a part of the needle that is in the tissue at any given moment. In most perineal repairs, it will be across the tear from your dominant to your nondominant side. When using a curved needle, the driving force does not rotate with the curve of the needle, but has the same direction no matter whether the point, the shaft or the swaged end is in the tissue. Put another way, the driving force is applied to each segment of the needle wire as it moves through the tissue and always moves in the same direction, even though the needle is rotated as it is advanced. Thus, the driving force is not applied in the direction of the point except at the beginning of the stitch.

A half-circle needle must be rotated exactly 180°as it is pushed through the tissue. If the arc of rotation is greater than 180° (called "torquing the needle"), the force will then tend to lacerate the tissue adjacent to the outside (convex) curve of the needle (producing a tear on the lateral aspect of the needle's path). If the arc of rotation is less than 180°, the path of force will deviate from the curve of the needle and the force will tend to lacerate the tissue adjacent to the inside (concave) curve of the needle (producing a tear on the medial aspect of the needle's path). Therefore, to drive the needle through the tissue as atraumatically as possible you must learn to follow the curve of the needle so that the tip, shaft and end traverse the same path that the tip originally created.

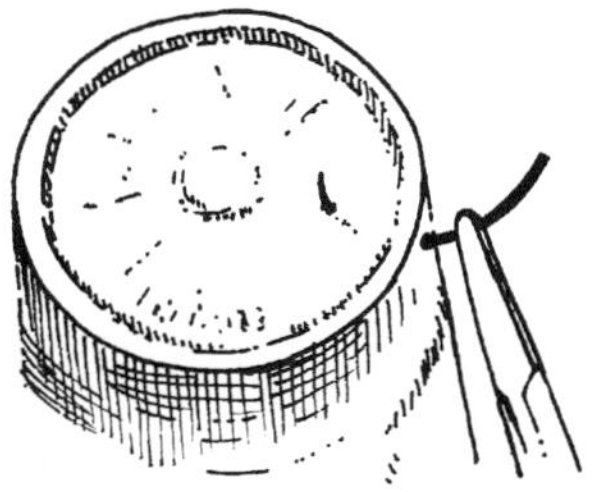	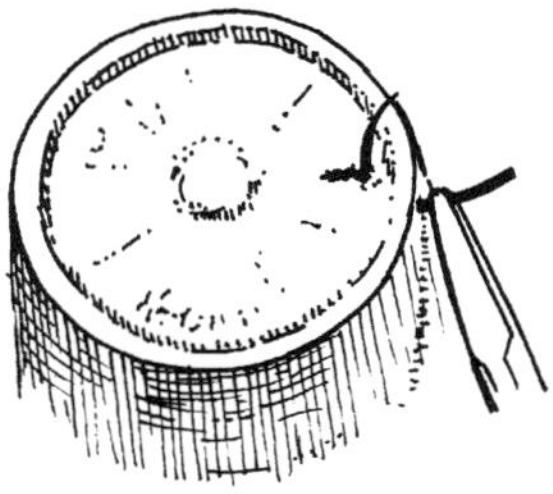	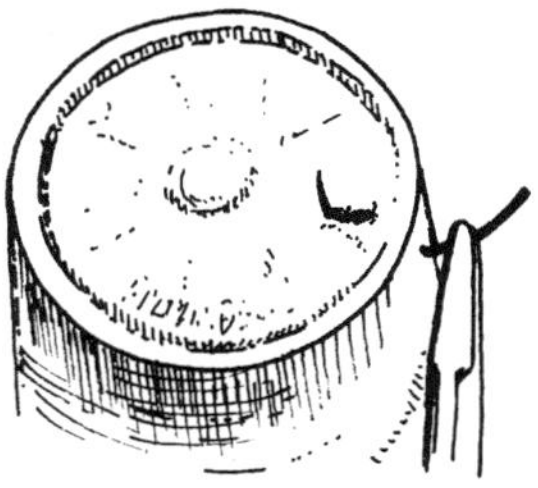
Needle driven correctly along a true half-circle path.	Tear caused by too much rotation (>180°)	Tear caused by too little rotation (<180°)

To begin, learn to form a half-circle stitch. Start with your palm down, place the needle tip at right angles to the surface, and drive the needle by rotating your hand to bring the palm up. In other words, direct the needle through the tissue in a circular motion by rotating your wrist. Practice driving a half-circle needle into the side of and through the bottom of an upside-down Styrofoam (or suitable ecological alternative) or paper coffee cup. By starting from the side of the cup, you can better see where and how you are exiting the surface. When done properly, there will be only two small holes, the entry point on the side of the cup and the exit point on the bottom of the cup; these holes should be the same diameter as the needle. Confirm that the needle has been driven properly by sliding it back and forth through these holes. It will be easy to see if there are tears the cup adjacent to either hole (DeLancey, 1987).

Practice with the cup until you can reliably drive the needle correctly. Then, with the cup still upside down on the table, enter the bottom of the cup and exit the side, the direction you will usually be driving the needle through tissue. Once you have mastered that, practice the same technique with pieces of paper. Driving the needle improperly will tear the paper. Finally, practice with foam rubber. Driving the needle improperly through foam will result in excessive tearing sounds as you rip the foam. Only minimal tearing sounds should be heard as the needle penetrates the foam.

When placing stitches, you will also start by positioning the needle point at a right angle to the surface of the tissue (Figure 1 below). Entering the tissue with the needle perpendicular to the surface ensures that the stitch will neither evert nor invert the wound edges. Now drive the needle (Figures 2 and 3 below) along a curved path by rotating your wrist. Gentle, steady, sustained pressure will provide adequate force, whereas greater force is more likely to break the needle.

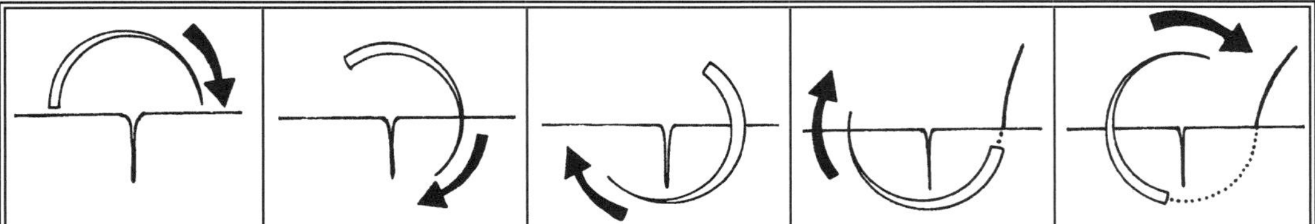

Fig. 1 | Fig. 2 | Fig. 3 | Fig. 4 | Fig. 5

1. Insert the needle tip at a right angle to the tissue surface.
2. Drive the needle in a true half-circle path.
3. Continue to drive the needle along a half-circle path.
4. Release the needle holder while stabilizing the needle tip with another instrument.
5. Complete the stitch by either regripping the needle below the point or by taking it out with another instrument.

Advance the needle though the tissue as far as possible in order to expose as much of the needle's tip as you can; this will facilitate retrieving the needle. When bringing the two sides of a wound together, picking up both sides in the same bite or stitch is permissible and will save time, as long as the needle's tip can be grasped easily once it is exposed on the other side of the wound. Although during continuous stitching, when placing the first stitch or the last stitch through the wound itself (not the anchor stitch) better tissue alignment is accomplished if the stitches at each end are taken with separate bites on each side, in perineal repair this technique is most relevant when the wound is oddly shaped. To accomplish a two-bite stitch, you pass the needle through one side of the tissue to create the first half of the stitch, remove the needle from the tissue completely (just after Figure 2), and repeat steps 6, 7, 8 and 9 as outlined in this chapter to complete the other half of the stitch (Figures 3, 4 and 5 above).

When placing a stitch at the bottom of a deep, narrow space, you will need to grip the needle at an angle in the jaws or use a Heaney needle holder, which has a curved jaw that allows perpendicular placement of the needle. Practice placing the needle in the holder at various angles and passing it through a Styrofoam cup.

If you feel the needle bending and you are using one of the needles recommended on page 318, you may be applying too much pressure or pushing through extremely thick scar tissue. If you are not using a recommended needle, it is possible that you are using one with a wire that is too fine for perineal repair. If the needle's advance is really blocked as you try to drive it through the tissue, forcing it is likely to cause it to bend. This can occur even if the needle size and wire are correct. Bending or even breaking of a needle may also happen because you have taken too large a bite of tissue, because you have continued to try to drive the needle after the needle holder jaws come in contact with the tissue or because you are trying to use the needle to lift the tissue (not recommended). Solutions include exiting the tissue in the midline after placing half the stitch, taking smaller bites or using thumb forceps, rather than the needle, to manipulate the tissue.

7. Releasing the ratchet

After you complete the first two-thirds of a stitch, the needle tip will be protruding through the tissue opposite your entry point. Use tissue forceps, another small needle holder or a hemostat in your nondominant hand to grasp the needle just below the point. Then use your dominant hand to release the needle holder from the swagged end. Using a Thenar grip (described on page 397), release the ratchet smoothly so as not to jerk the needle, which can stress the tissue or dislodge the needle. You may have to use your nondominant hand to stabilize the needle holder as you release the ratchet. If you must do this, keep the needle holder clamped to the swaged end of the needle while you regrasp the tip of the needle with your thumb forceps before releasing the swaged end completely.

It is always safest not to leave the needle free in the tissue, although you can get away with it if you can see the point and you are sure it will stay in place when you release the needle holder. If, however, you must exert any tension *whatsoever* on the needle holder to maintain the needle's position before you release the ratchet, upon release the needle will probably retract into the tissue. In this case, do not release the ratchet until you have grasped just below the needle's point with another instrument. The exception to this is delicate labial tissue, which may be more traumatized from using an instrument to stabilize the needle than by using nothing at all and is so soft and shallow that retraction of the needle is really not an issue. Therefore, you can often leave the needle free momentarily while repositioning the needle holder.

8. Regrasping the needle to complete the stitch

With your palm down, grasp the needle perpendicular to the holder just below the needle point (where the point widens to the full diameter of the wire). Perpendicular placement simplifies the rotational forces required to remove the needle and minimizes the risk of tissue trauma. Be careful: it is possible to snap the point of a needle off if you grip too close to the tip. Also, repeatedly grasping the point itself dulls the tip, leading to more tissue trauma as you complete the repair. Once you have a grip on the wire just beneath the point, engage the rachet only enough to secure the needle (usually just one click).

9. Completing the stitch and removing the needle

The same vector forces come into play when completing the stitch. Begin with your palm down. Grasp the needle holder and rotate your palm up in an arc, curving the needle through the tissue. A circular motion is always required when using a curved needle; pulling the needle straight up will only traumatize the tissue and invite bleeding, as well as prevent its removal. It will also be quite painful to the mother.

Tissue can also be unnecessarily traumatized if you try to remove the needle with your fingers because the needle, which will be slippery with blood, is usually more difficult to grasp with the fingers. Using your hand to remove the needle also increases the likelihood of puncturing your glove or finger, with the consequent danger of contracting blood-borne pathogens. Therefore, make it a rule never to manipulate the needle with your fingers.

10. Pulling the desired length of suture through the tissue

If placing continuous stitches, pull the strand through in one uninterrupted motion by raising your dominant hand, which is still holding the armed needle holder, until the stitch is snugged down. When placing an interrupted stitch, you must leave at least a 2 to 3 inch (4 to 8 cm) tail on the free end to allow you to tie the stitch off.

11. Tying off the stitch and positioning the needle in the holder for the next stitch

If continuous stitches are being placed, rearm the needle holder to prepare for the next stitch. If interrupted stitches are being placed, leave at least two to three inches of suture on the fixed side, cut off the rest (preserve usable suture if there is enough left to take more stitches) and tie off the stitch you have just finished. Then rearm the needle holder.

If you have an assistant, they can help manipulate the free end of the suture strand to minimize tangling and assist in forming certain stitches, such as a locked stitch.

Keep the shaft of the needle holder parallel with the wound's edge as you move down the tear; this helps to prevent a rippled line of stitches.

(Anderson & Romfh, 1980; DeLancey, 1987; Varney et al., 2004)

USING THUMB (TISSUE, DRESSING OR PICK UP) FORCEPS

Thumb (tissue or dressing) forceps are all similar nonlocking grasping tools. (I like the term "thumb" because it is the most generic.) Their basic design resembles a big tweezer, and they come with a variety of tips. They are used to hold tissue during dissection, retract small areas of tissue to aid exposure, stabilize tissue or the needle during suturing, grasp the end of a suture strand or pass it around hemostats deep in a wound, grasp objects for extraction and manipulate gauze or sponges to clear away blood.

Forceps come with or without teeth. Toothed forceps are also referred to as "atraumatic" because their tiny teeth can select and hold a specific piece of tissue with less risk of crushing it. Toothed ends can also be used to manipulate gauze, but they are not very helpful when trying to manipulate the needle or suture because they are not designed to grip these materials. Some styles are more all-purpose, such as Russian forceps. Careful use will minimize trauma to tissues, the suture strand and the needle. As you work through this chapter, have a pair of thumb forceps on hand to practice with.

Thumb forceps versus a surgical clamp

In many cases, thumb forceps or a surgical clamp, such as a hemostat, can be used interchangeably. For example, a bleeding vessel may be grasped with thumb forceps or clamped with a hemostat. The advantage of using forceps is that they can be opened and closed easily and the tension applied to the tissue can be more precisely gauged than with a clamp. Conversely, surgical clamps have a stronger grip and can be locked into place to hold onto an object for an extended period of time without causing hand fatigue, allowing time to position a knot and slide it down over a bleeding vessel or to grasp the end of a torn anal sphincter while placing stitches (Anderson & Romfh, 1980).

Handling thumb forceps

Thumb forceps are usually manipulated by the nondominant hand to assist with maneuvers of the operating hand, eliminating the need to insert fingers in the wound and reducing the incidence of needlestick injuries. Become proficient at manipulating the needle, suture strand and tissue using instruments instead of your fingers.

The forceps are held in a **modified pencil grip** between the thumb and two or three fingers so that the joined end rests in the crook of the thumb and index finger. One blade serves as an extension of your thumb and the other as an extension of your opposing fingers (as shown below). Spring tension at the joined end keeps the grasping tips separated until pressure is applied. This allows one to quickly and easily grasp and release small objects or tissue or to grasp and hold tissue with easily variable pressure. The other useful grip is the **classic pencil grip**. Both allow a wide range of maneuverability.

During surgery thumb forceps are frequently "palmed" to save time consumed in the process of repeatedly picking up and putting down the instrument. Although this consideration is much less of an issue at home, where there is no one waiting to use the operating theater, palming the forceps keeps them at hand, ready for use.

When you are ready to switch to a "hold" position, palm the forceps by pinching them between your thumb and index fingers as you lift your other fingers away from your palm.

Rotate your hand palm up, which allows the shaft to fall into your palm. Transfer your grip on the forceps by bending only the proximal joints of your ring and little fingers. This leaves the index and middle fingers free to move. Since the flexor digitorum profundus muscle attaches to the middle, ring and little fingers, flexing the distal joint of the last two fingers causes the distal joint of the middle finger to flex as well. However, if the distal joints of the ring and little finger remain extended, the flexor digitorum profundus muscle stays relaxed, leaving the middle finger free to move more easily during manipulations. When the nondominant little and ring fingers are needed during a one-handed tie, the forceps can be temporarily shifted to be held in a pinch between the thumb and index fingers.

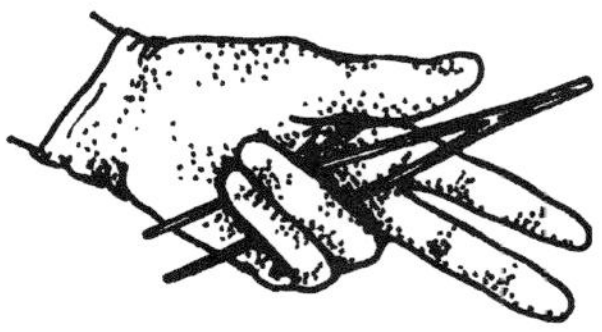 Palming the forceps	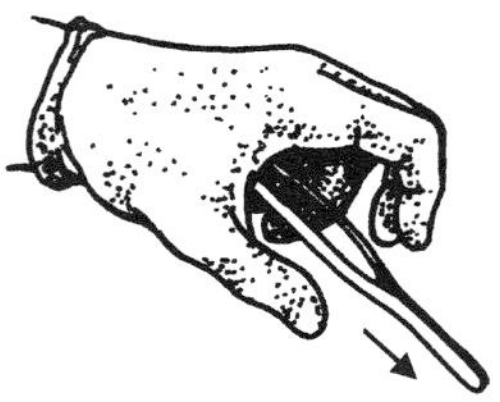 Allowing gravity to assist in moving the forceps to a position for use just before grasping the shaft	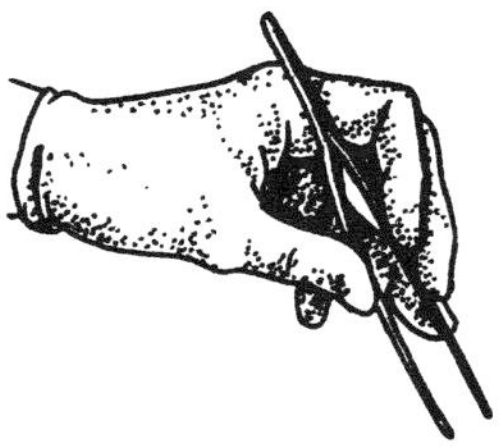 Modified pencil grip for use

To convert the forceps back to a use position, first grasp them in the proper place. Turn your hand palm down, which allows gravity to pull the shaft away from your palm. Then let go of the joined end, flex your thumb and index finger to grasp the forceps low along the shaft (as you would a writing implement) and be ready to pinch the handle with your index finger and thumb at the proper spot without straining.

Using forceps in tissue

You must be very gentle when using forceps to manipulate tissue. Keep tissue manipulation of all kinds to a minimum. It is easy to crush tissue if the grip is not gentle. You might also distort such delicate tissue with forceps and misplace the needle in the process. Tissue forceps come in most handy during the repair of distinct layers of tissue with interrupted sutures. However, such distinct layers are generally absent in the genital area.

Forceps with tiny teeth are useful when a specific piece of tissue needs to be delicately lifted and isolated from the rest. Forceps with ends shaped like tiny serrated paddles, as are those on Russian tissue forceps, are good for grasping the needle point below the tip as it exits the tissue and can be used for holding tissue out of the way, but cannot be used as precisely as forceps with a narrow tip and mouse teeth.

Placing a stitch: Most suturing in the genital area does not lend itself to the use of thumb forceps in the manner described next because the layers of tissue are not very distinct and few interrupted stitches are used. In the perineal area, you will not be lifting or moving the tissue very far, thus these skills are primarily included so that you know how to use forceps to visualize the entry and exit points of the needle when indicated. Thumb forceps are most useful to handle tissue when repairing skin edges, the labia or the rectal mucosa. They are also useful in visualizing what you are doing during cervical repairs and will help prevent accidently suturing an adjacent part of the cervix.

***Approaching the laceration*:** First of all, the hand grasping the forceps should always approach the wound from the side opposite the hand using the needle holder. This leaves you free to move your elbows, increasing the mobility of one arm without cramping the movement of the other.

***Grasping the layer of tissue to be stitched*:** Visualize the point where the needle is to enter the tissue. Then use the thumb forceps to expose and stabilize this point at a comfortable distance away from the site of needle entry by gently grasping the edge of the tissue in line with the intended entry point, but not at the entry point itself. This avoids distorting the tissue.

You can also move the edge of the layer of tissue overlying the one being sutured by gently lifting the upper layer and pulling it up or out to expose the layer underneath. (This motion is like pulling your bottom lip away from your lower teeth.) This maneuver might be useful in some instances when sewing a subcuticular layer in the perineum or when sewing a deep tear involving the rectal mucosa, but it is generally not used in midwifery-related repairs.

Once the needle is in the tissue, lift up the edge of the layer being sutured and turn it back to expose the needle's exit point. (This is the same action as pulling the center edge of your lower lip toward your chin; the midpoint of the curve of your inner lip would be the needle's exit point.) This technique may also come in handy at times when sewing labial tears. But due to the relatively shallow lacerations that you will be sewing and to the running mattress stitch (explained later) that you will probably be using, it will not be needed very often in midwifery practice.

To complete the second half of the stitch, you can reverse these steps on the other side by lifting the deeper layer first to expose the first entry point on that side and then lifting the superficial layer away from the underlying layer to expose the exit point. By moving from the superficial to the deep layer on the dominant side and from the deep to the superficial layer on the nondominant side, the forceps are used as both a stabilization tool and an instrument of exposure.

Grasping tissue for other purposes: Thumb forceps can be very helpful when you need to remove small skin tags. The same principles apply. Use the forceps to stabilize the tissue, straighten it out and expose the area where the scissor blades will do the trimming. Grasp the skin tag near the tip, well away from the where you will trim it off. You might work with the tissue a bit to ensure that your grip is not pulling at the base of the tag and distorting the tissue, which could cause you to cut too deeply.

Manipulating the suture needle

Thumb forceps come in really handy for manipulating the needle. They can be used in two ways during needle extraction. The first is to grasp the needle below the point, perpendicular to the shaft (just as you would with the needle holder) to stabilize it before releasing the ratchet on the needle holder. Doing so requires only a slight shift in the position of the forceps in your hand, not a major repositioning. Keeping the tissue forceps perpendicular to the needle's point results in a more secure grip than when it is grasped at an oblique angle or a parallel position. Forceps with teeth or serrations can both be used to stabilize the needle prior to releasing the needle holder jaws.

Tissue forceps that have serrations rather than sharp, interlocking teeth, however, are best suited to extract the needle, using the same motions you would with a needle holder. If you intend to remove the needle with the forceps, position your palm up before grasping the needle. This allows you to rotate your wrist to extract the needle from the tissue easily. Do not try to use forceps with teeth to extract the needle; they will not grasp it securely. Since thumb forceps cannot be locked, you may need your assistant to hold the forceps (which are grasping the needle) while you release the needle holder from the swaged end.

Using Surgical Scissors

You will primarily use scissors to cut the ends of suture strands as you sew. You may also need to remove skin tags or, very rarely, to perform a clitorotomy. Scissors cut flaccid tissue more accurately than a scalpel because they provide better stabilization. Have a pair of scissors on hand as you study this chapter. If you are left-handed, try to obtain a pair of left-handed scissors.

How scissors work

Scissors consist of two specially designed shanks or levers. At the lower end, the shanks consist of two blades attached at a pivoting joint or fulcrum. Above the fulcrum, the two shanks each terminate in a finger ring. When using scissors of the appropriate handedness, the shanks are designed so that you can see the cutting action of the blades.

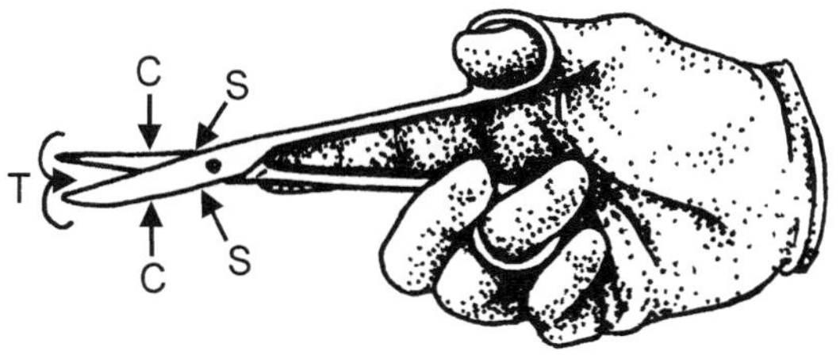

Forces at work in scissors: C=closing force; S=shearing force; T=torque. These scissors are held in a large tripod grip.

Scissors work on a pivot principle that applies three force vectors during cutting: **closing**, **torque** and **shearing**. These forces are transferred from the hand, to the shanks through the fulcrum, and finally to the cutting edges. Closing force (C) is applied as the hand squeezes the finger rings together, causing the blades to move toward each other. Torque (T) is the force that moves the leading edge of each blade into contact. Shearing force (S) pushes one blade flat against the other during closure.

Most scissors are designed to allow the effective combination of these forces to result in precise cuts in right-handed individuals. Right-handed scissors are designed so that, when the palm is facing down, the blade manipulated by the thumb underlies the blade manipulated by the fingers. This arrangement uses the natural pushing force of the thumb and the pulling action of the fingers inserted in the opposite ring to achieve maximal shear and torque forces in the blades. Turn right-handed scissors over and grasp them again. You will see that, regardless of which side is facing up, the thumb blade is always on the bottom.

Control of the direction and accuracy of an incision depends upon a secure grip on the scissors and the stability of the material being cut. The wider the blades are opened and the closer the material to be cut is to the fulcrum of the blades, the more the blades will push the material away, bunching it ahead of the shearing action of the blades. Beginning to cut with the material nearer the tips of the scissors reduces the amount of closing force that can be applied but holds the material more securely and more stably between the blades as they are brought together.

The angle between the plane of the blades and the plane of the material being cut should be 90°; in other words, the flat side of the blades should be perpendicular to the surface of the material being cut. The more obtusely they are held in relation to the material to be cut, the more unstable the material will be and the less accurate the cut.

Manipulating the scissors

For maximum control of the scissors, use a large tripod grip (as illustrated on the preceding page). Place the thumb and ring finger in each of the finger rings, with the tip of the extended index finger resting against the fulcrum. This grip makes the best use of the scissors' force vectors to achieve crisp, clean cuts. While scissors can be grasped in several other ways, most of these grips have disadvantages. The exception is the backhand variation of the thumb and ring finger grip that can be used for cutting to the right, although this grip will rarely be useful in perineal repairs. If you are left-handed and have a left-handed scissor, this grip could be used for cutting to the left.

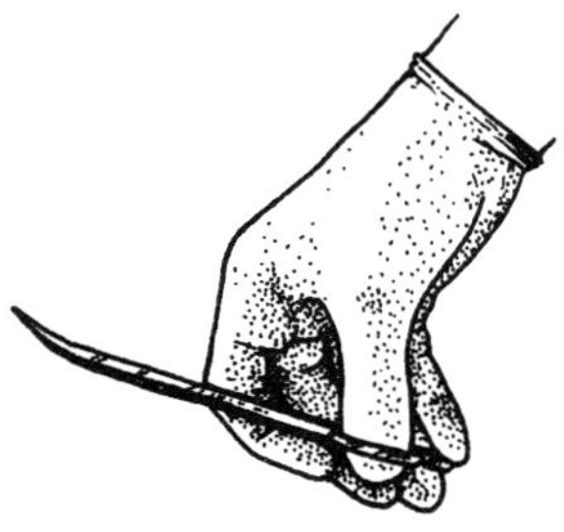

The backhand variation of the thumb and ring finger grip for cutting to the right

If you are left-hand dominant: Most scissors are designed for right-handed persons. If you have a pair of scissors that matches your handedness, transfer them to your nondominant hand as you read through this explanation. When right-handed scissors are used in the left hand (or vice versa), the thumb blade becomes positioned on the far side of the scissors. Closing the finger rings results in a grasping motion that pushes with the thumb. This reverses the pushing and pulling action of the shanks, which significantly reduces control and results in a loss of shear and torque forces.

Right-handed scissors are designed so that the blades come together when used in the right hand. When right-handed scissors are used in the left hand, the motion of cutting actually separates the tips of the blades and widens the space between them, making cutting difficult, if not impossible. In order to cut with right-handed scissors using your left hand, it is necessary to apply pressure to the shanks in a way that brings the blades closer together. Left-handed scissoring with right-handed scissors can be improved using the awkward motion of pulling with the left thumb and pushing with the left middle finger in their respective finger rings; this maneuver results in improved shear and torque on the blades. Pushing with the middle finger, however, does not add useful torque to the blade's leading edge. While it is certainly possible for many people to use right-handed scissors and make reasonably accurate cuts with the left hand, repeatedly having to push the thumb and middle finger together in this unnatural way is an ergonomic disaster that leads to marks on the hand and eventually callouses. Also, you must look over the top blade to see what you are cutting, because the top blade obscures the view, meaning that you usually wind up cutting inside of the desired line of incision.

Therefore, if you are left-handed you must either learn to cut with your right hand or get a pair of left-handed scissors. You can probably get by with using your right hand when trimming easy-to-reach suture ends, but having the wrong kind of scissors will prove a significant problem when you are called upon to cut tissue.

It is not possible to make "ambidextrous scissors," although some manufacturers claim their scissors are "suitable for left or right hand use." This is not generally a claim made for surgical scissors, but in any case only refers to the handles, which have not been moulded to fit the right hand's knuckles, and they offer no real advantage for left-handers whatsoever as the blades are still set right-handed.

There are far fewer choices of left-handed surgical scissors than there are for right-handed ones. Those that I could locate are discussed in the chapters entitled "Selecting Suturing Tools, Related Supplies and Equipment" and "Clitorotomy ('Episiotomy')" (Anderson & Romfh, 1980). Also check the website Anything Left Handed (www.anythingleft-handed.co.uk/acatalog/scissors.html).

Arm, hand and body posture while using scissors

For horizontal cutting, which is required to trim suture strands, the greatest maneuverability as well as visibility of the suture and the knot is afforded when the scissors are held with the palm down. This positions the elbow away from the body and leaves it free to move. The hand can then be rotated toward the midline (supinated) 180° or pronated 90° by abducting the arm without any other changes in torso position.

For vertical cutting, as is needed to perform a clitorotomy, position the forearm midway between pronation and supination, with the palm facing laterally and point the tip of the scissors directly down, which will also cause your thumb to point downward.

Trimming suture ears

The most common occasion for using scissors in perineal repair is trimming the ears on a knot. When cutting suture strands, approach the strand near the knot; do not slide the blades down the strand to the knot, as this will abrade the strand (although the strand's condition is not an issue if the extra length of suture is being discarded). Sliding down the strand could also cause accidental tissue trauma from the scissor tips.

If you have just placed an anchor stitch for a continuous row of stitches, be sure to identify which strand you need to sever (it will be the short, free end, without the needle attached). Hold the scissors blades perpendicular to the strand to be cut to keep the knot in view between the blades. This will ensure that you cut at the right distance from the knot and that you do not cut the knot itself. Do not attempt to visualize the knot by looking underneath the blades.

Avoid "past pointing" by opening the blades only wide enough to get the tip of each blade on either side of the strand to be trimmed and by keeping the tips within view at all times; this also lessens the risk of inadvertently damaging nearby tissues as you cut. Correct positioning is easy to accomplish when you are using small stitch scissors that have a C-shaped cutout on the thumb blade. This cutout is intended to help you isolate a single strand, to gather the strand to the blade as the tips are brought together (rather than pushing it away) and to cut only the intended strand.

Once the strand is identified and the scissors are in place, use your dominant hand to cut the strand while your nondominant hand uses another instrument to hold onto the end of that strand. This will avoid having a small, loose bit of suture that falls into the wound and has to be retrieved. Although such a fragment could dissolve, it will be more foreign material for the mother's body to cope with, and it could poke her and cause discomfort.

For those with impaired vision or poor eye–hand coordination, the scissors blades can be placed right above the knot, and the length of the ear can be gauged by turning the blades slightly, which measures out a short, uniform free end. In most cases, however, cutting strands on a slant is to be avoided to prevent creating a pointed tip on the ear that will cause more tissue irritation.

When trimming the ears on a stitch that is in the bottom of a deep wound, you may want to steady your dominant hand with your other hand or steady your arm against some firm object.

Take your time. Cutting with a hurried jabbing or snapping motion may tear the tissue if the scissors are misplaced and may wind up chewing the strand only partway through.

After cutting the strand, discard the cut piece of suture away from the field so that it does not clutter the area or inadvertently make its way back into the wound.

Using scissors in tissue

Scissors can precisely cut flaccid tissue that cannot be held under tension, and they afford excellent depth control. Flaccid tissue is stabilized between the blades, thereby helping control the direction of the cut. Scissors can make three types of cuts: scissor-cuts, push-cuts and chewed cuts. **Scissor-cutting** involves all three of the force vectors, making full use of the instrument. **Push-cutting**, often used in sewing, uses static shear and torque forces. It involves pushing the slightly open blades through a sheet of tissue and is not appropriate for midwifery applications. **Chew-cutting** involves a crushing action caused by a lack of shear and torque. This results when the cutting edges of the blades are opened and closed one or more times to accomplish the cutting or when widely opened scissors bunch tissue ahead of the closing blades instead of cutting cleanly. Chew-cutting results in ragged incisions of crushed tissue and can be avoided by using sharp scissors with optimal grip. Cutting tissue nearer the tips rather than close to the fulcrum also prevents chewing. Open the blades just wide enough to complete the desired cut. Another technique that deters chewing is taking several bites with the tips rather than one large bite that starts near the fulcrum of the blades.

The primary way you will use scissors in tissue is to remove skin tags. A discussion of how to do so is found in the chapter entitled "Skin Tags." Very rarely, you may find you need to dissect tissue to complete a repair. An example would be the need to cut the perineal skin to reach a severed anal sphincter. Although this sounds like an improbable scenario, such tears do occur. This is discussed in the chapter entitled "Special Tricks and Techniques" under the entry entitled Repairing a "Pocket Tear in the Yoni Floor." Cutting a clitorotomy is discussed in detail in a separate chapter entitled "Clitorotomy ('Episiotomy')."

The Six Stitches Used in Perineal Repair

NOTE: For variations and special stitching techniques see the chapter entitled "Special Tricks and Techniques."

The stitches described in this chapter are the only ones you need to know to successfully repair whatever degree of damage you may encounter. The basic stitches include the simple interrupted stitch as well as the following continuous stitches: the simple running stitch, the locked mattress stitch and the running mattress stitch. In addition, two advanced interrupted stitches are included as well: the horizontal mattress stitch and the figure-eight. To practice, we will start with the easiest stitch and then proceed to the more complex.

Even when "just" practicing, it is important to use the same size needles and suture material that you will use for actual repairs. You cannot learn what the suture and needle will tolerate or how to use them correctly unless you use materials appropriate to the job. More about this can be found in the APPENDICES, where practice materials are discussed.

General considerations when practicing stitches

Observe the following pointers when practicing stitches on foam, fabric or meat.

Spacing stitches: During practice, place all stitches 1 cm apart unless otherwise noted. Use a small ruler to make 1 cm marks on your dominant side (where the needle will be inserted) down your practice material. Measure across the tear and make another mark equidistant from the midline of the incision to show where the needle should exit the foam or chicken.

Depth and width of stitches: For most tissues, create stitches no more than 1.25 to 1.5 cm deep, the maximum depth possible when using a CT-1 or T-12 needle to place a stitch with one motion as you pass the needle from one side of a tear to the other. Frequently, stitches will be a little shallower than this. To create a symmetrical stitch, the distance between the needle entry point and the edge of the wound on one side must be the same as the distance between the needle exit point and the wound edge on the other side. Each stitch loop should consist of at least a half-circle once it is completed.

The edges of the tear should lie flat. If your edges invert (i.e., roll together, turning down toward the wound) or evert (i.e., bunch up and become directed away from the wound, forming a peak in the midline) while practicing on foam, you have either taken too much tissue into that stitch (i.e., the stitch may be too wide) or you are tying the suture too tightly.

Regardless of the location of the stitches, inversion of edges is always undesirable because it can lead to pitting of the scar. This is because, as the wound contracts during healing, the edges flatten out. For the same reason, eversion of the edges is desirable when closing the skin layer with stitches that bridge across the wound, such as interrupted stitches. Wound edges that are not properly everted contract below the skin plane, resulting in a depressed scar. However, eversion is not of particular concern when performing most perineal repairs. This is because the labial tissue is so soft and because the running mattress stitch to close the perineal skin is completely buried, although slight eversion should not interfere with healing.

Accurate placement of the needle: As a general rule, for each stitch, place the needle tip at right angles to the wound at the same distance from the wound edge on either side. This will help equalize tension along the entire length of the wound. Perpendicular placement of the needle as it is inserted tends to evert (rather than invert) the wound edges slightly.

Orientation of the needle holder when placing a stitch: Keep the shaft of the needle holder parallel with the edge of the tear as you place each new stitch. This will help prevent forming a rippled line of stitches.

Appropriate tension in the stitches: Tighten each stitch so that it rests on the surface of the tissue with edges touching. When practicing with foam, a slight puckering at the entry and exit points with the edges of the incision just touching represents appropriate tension (when little anesthetic is used).

Simple interrupted stitches

The simplest of all stitches is the basic interrupted stitch. It employs a single loop that enters the tissue to one side of the wound and exits at a point directly opposite the initial insertion point equidistant from the wound edge, producing what we will call a **horizontal interrupted stitch**. It draws the sides of the wound together and is tied with a square knot with the ears cut short. This basic technique is also used to form an anchor stitch for a series of continuous stitches, leaving the needle end long.

If only one stitch is needed, an interrupted is the obvious choice. In midwifery it is used for muscle, anal sphincter, rectal mucosa and labial repairs as well as to ligate torn blood vessels. When anatomical alignment of tissue is difficult (such as in deep muscle tears; soft, hard-to-align labial tissue; or extremely jagged tears), an interrupted stitch allows the most control over how the edges match. An interrupted can be placed in the center of the tear to help align the tissue so that a continuous row of stitches can be started at the internal apex (or the superior apex if it is a surface wound) to close the length of the wound. When several interrupted stitches are placed, should one stitch come undone, the others usually stay in place, thus normal healing may proceed in spite of the disruption (see below for risks). An interrupted stitch is also useful in situations that increase the likelihood of sewing through the wall of the bowel or the urinary tract, since a misplaced one can be removed without having to undo and replace adjacent stitches.

There are also risks involved when using interrupted stitches; even some of the benefits carry risks themselves. Each interrupted stitch requires a knot, several of which make for a more bulky repair and more irritation during healing. Interrupted stitches are inherently weaker because no matter how perfectly the knots are tied, knotting weakens the strand. Should one knot give way, the remaining stitches are subjected to increased tension and may come loose as well. One missing stitch may create a small pocket where lochia can pool, inviting infection, or a weak point in a stressed wall (such as the bowel or urethral wall) that could allow contaminants to leak into the wound, risking the development of an infection, a fistula or both. This is also the easiest type of stitch to place too tightly, impeding wound healing and ultimately weakening the repair. The flip side of controlled placement is that interrupted stitches can easily wind up distorting the tissue if your placement is not precise, resulting in an anatomically incorrect repair. Tension cannot be readjusted later if a stitch tied too tight: the stitch must be cut out and redone. Interrupted stitches should be used only when necessary, which will not be very often in perineal repair.

Here is step-by-step instruction for how to place a horizontal interrupted stitch:

HORIZONTAL INTERRUPTED STITCH		
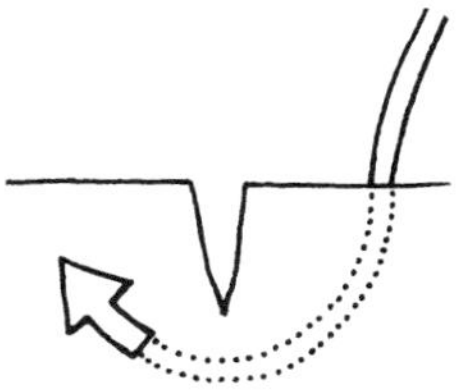	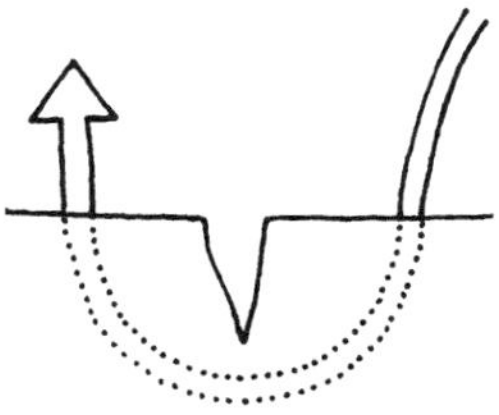	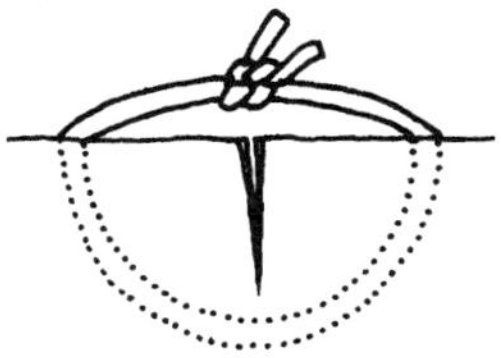
Position the needle tip perpendicular to the tissue surface at a distance that is no more than half the chord length of the needle. Take a deep bite, encompassing the depth of the tear when possible.	Maintain a 180° arc as you pass the needle through the tissue. Be sure your stitch is a true half-circle.	Leave the free end short and tie the stitch so that the knot rests on the surface of the tissue; but does not roll or pucker the edges.

Once the knot is in place, gently slide it over to your nondominant side so that it does not directly overlie the divided tissue. The technique illustrated above is used when a simple, uninterrupted bite is to be taken across the wound from one side to the other. The basic technique described above is also used to begin each stitch described in this chapter except for the running mattress suture.

These stitches can also be oriented "vertically" (that is, longitudinally), for use across a horizontal tear. A vertical interrupted stitch is best accomplished using a forehand technique; in this case by entering the upper part of the tissue and exiting below that point. This approach allows the most maneuverability for your arm. In midwifery a vertical stitch is used only rarely. It is most often called for to reinforce and rejoin horizontal layers of tissue that have split apart from each other (as occurs when the yoni mucosa separates from the yoni muscle layer). They are placed after other stitches have been used to bring the wound edges in the mucosa together.

Adjusting the depth of a stitch: The maximum size and depth of a stitch is primarily a product of the size of the needle. The type of stitch you have been learning so far I will call a "half-circle" stitch, because the bottom half (180°) of the circle constitutes the loop side and the top half (the other 180° of the circle), which is the knot or midwife's side, remains above the tissue surface. A true half-circle (180°) stitch is created (which will be the deepest half-circle stitch the needle can produce) when the needle is inserted half of its chord length from the wound edge, which allows 25% of the needle's circumference (if the needle were a full circle) to be used in creating the first half of the loop.

It is always ideal to choose the needle size based on the stitch size required, but it is not practical to be switching needles as you sew along wounds that vary in depth; such depth variations are often associated with perineal trauma. When you are competent with the basic technique of creating a simple, half-circle interrupted stitch, you can experiment with creating deeper or more shallow half-circle stitches by adjusting the distance at which the needle is inserted into the tissue relative to the edges of the wound. While these techniques can be used to vary the depth of continuous stitches as well, it is easiest to learn this skill using interrupted stitches. The shallower the wound, the shorter should be the distance from the wound edges to the needle entry and exit points. Another way of putting this is that a deeper half-circle stitch is created when the needle is inserted farther from the wound edge and a shallower stitch is created when the needle is inserted closer to the wound edge. To avoid taking shallow stitches that are too wide, be sure that the needle tip is perpendicular to the tissue surface with each bite.

It is also possible to create what I will call a "buried circle" stitch, where most of the circle is below the tissue surface; this will create a considerably deeper stitch. This type of stitch is much trickier to master and requires lots of practice on foam before attempting it in real tissue. When you want such a stitch, you must insert the needle closer to the wound edge (about 25% of the chord length). Position your wrist so that the needle's tip will enter the tissue at a slight, laterally-directed angle. Hold the wound open with your left hand as you *slowly and gently* pass the needle deeply into the tissue so that most of the first half of the loop (circumference of half the circle) will remain beneath the tissue surface. When using a CT-1 or T-12 needle, a stitch up to about 2.5 cm in depth can be created with this technique. Meticulous care must be taken because it is very easy to mismatch the sides when you make the other half of the stitch. As you practice on foam rubber, listen carefully for crackling sounds; any more than the very slight sound the needle produces as it courses along its intended path means the way you are moving the needle is tearing the foam.

Two-Bite Buried Interrupted Stitch		
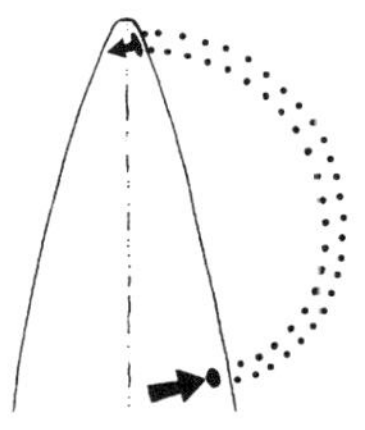	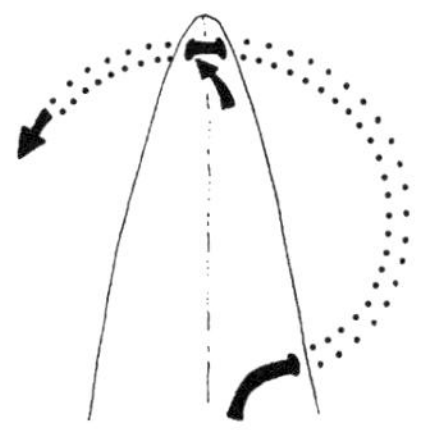	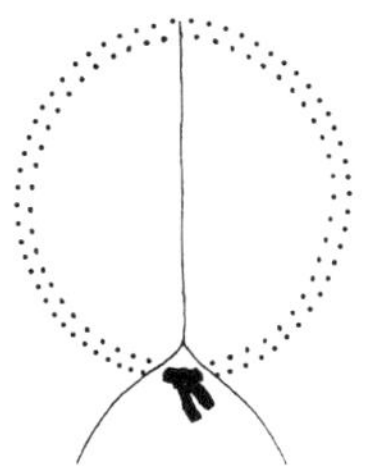
Insert the needle on one side of the wound so that a 3/4 or so-circle bite will reach the trough of the tear.	Completely remove the needle from the tissue when it reaches the trough and begin a second bite on the other side.	Tie off the stitch, notice how most of the circle is now buried.

Whenever you are making a maximally deep stitch with either method, tissue trauma will be minimized when the stitches are made with "two bites." The needle enters on one side of the wound and exits at the trough of the wound (just above bottom of the tear) on that side. The needle holder is released to allow the needle to be completely removed from the tissue. The second half of the stitch is then made; the needle is replaced in the needle holder jaws, and the stitch is continued from the wound's trough (it is reinserted into the tissue immediately opposite your last exit point) and is brought out parallel with the original insertion point on the opposite side of the wound. A two-bite technique allows for a larger stitch and also identifies where the needle tip exits the tissue, reducing the risk of puncturing through the anorectal wall (Fleming, 1990).

Both sides of the stitch must be equal in every respect. The distance between the needle entry point and the edge of the wound on one side must be the same as the distance between the needle exit point and the wound edge on the other side. The same amount of tissue must be included on both sides of the wound, and the angle that the needle enters and exits the tissue must be the same on either side. As long as each individual bite in such a stitch passes easily through the tissue without twisting or tearing, you will not traumatize the tissue (Thomson & Thomson, 2002).

Before you attempt these stitch variations in tissue, gain proficiency with the basic technique by practicing on Styrofoam cup and then on foam to ensure that you technique is as atraumatic as possible (see page 399 for details).

Continuous (running) stitches

Continuous stitches are created using a single strand of suture to form a spiral of suture in the tissue by inserting several stitches of the same type. Compared with interrupted stitches, continuous stitches are quicker to place and pose less risk of being pulled too tight, thereby making strangulation of the tissues less likely. The tension naturally provided by the row of stitches is usually sufficient to provide hemostasis. These stitches are also more watertight than a row of interrupteds and more easily result in a slightly everted wound edge.

Continuous stitches are always begun with an **anchor stitch**, which provides a starting point for several stitches. Pointers to note about placing continuous stitches:

- Make sure the stitches lie correctly. Guide the stitch by holding the loop with a closed thumb forceps and carefully position the strand as you tighten it. If you use your fingers, be sure the needle is held out of the way as you do this. It is *always* safest to use an instrument to manipulate the suture or the needle.

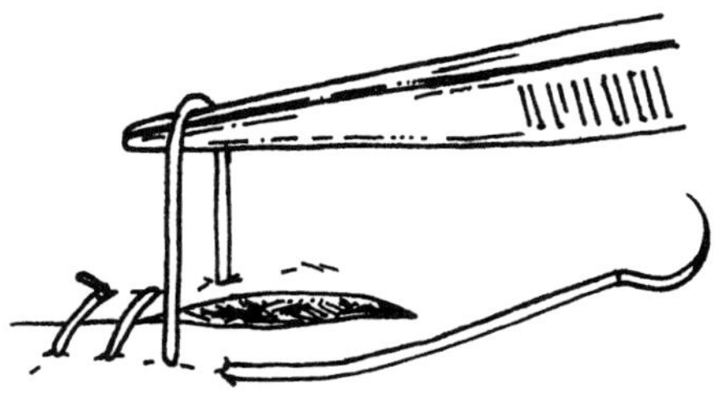

Fine-tuning a stitch with thumb forceps.

- Placing continuous stitches results in twisting the strand. To minimize this, gently straighten and untwist the strand occasionally by leaving the needle in the jaws and manipulating the needle holder.
- The use of a continuous stitch is not advised if there is a significant risk of a hematoma developing directly under the row of stitches. This risk might be increased if trauma is deep, complex or extensive in a woman who has pronounced varicosities, is on blood thinners or has a history of hematomas with previous births. In these cases, placing an interrupted stitch at either end of the

wound and closing the rest of it with a continuous stitch leaves the option of removing an interrupted stitch to drain a hematoma, although not every hematoma can be dealt with in this way (Sherris & Kern, 2004).

Basting (over-and-over/spiral/simple running/baseball) stitches: This is the simplest continuous stitch and the one most commonly used in perineal repair. It can be used to close the yoni mucosa, the skin of the labia minora and periurethral area, the subcutaneous layer in the perineal body and the rectal mucosa. It can also be used when a deep layer of stitches is needed. Its surgical names are given above, but any woman who sews will readily recognize this as one type of basting stitch, so this term is used as the primary reminder about what is meant. This stitch slightly everts the wound edges, so when using it below the skin surface, be *sure* to make it loose!

Begin by placing an anchor stitch at one end of the tear. Start as for an interrupted stitch and pull the suture through the tissue, leaving a 5 cm free end. Tie this first stitch off with a square knot incorporating an appropriate number of throws according to the type of suture material you are using. Cut the free end short, being careful to cut the free end only. This is the starting stitch for a continuous row of stitches, as illustrated below.

Basting (Over-and-Over) Stitches	
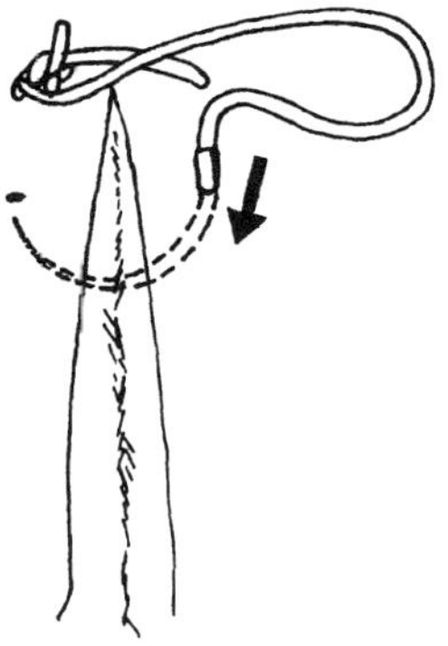	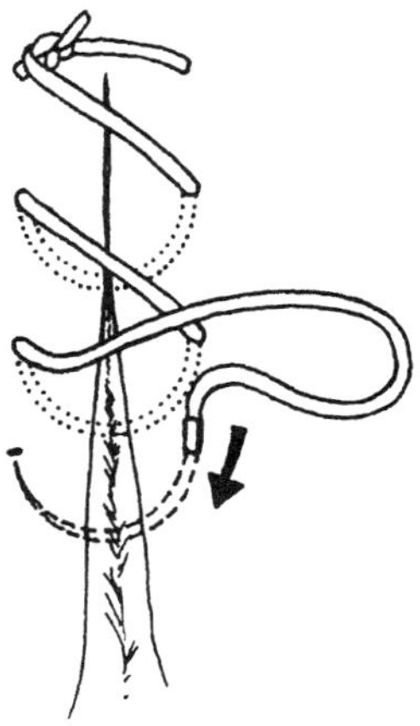
Slide the knot to your non-dominant side. Begin your next stitch about 1 cm below the anchor stitch on the side opposite the knot.	Continue taking basting stitches about 0.75 to 1 cm apart down the tear.

As you place additional stitches, be sure to keep the strand out of the path of the needle as you bring your needle out of the tissue when completing each stitch. This will prevent you from locking the stitch.

Locked blanket (locking/blanket/running-lock) stitch: Because the locked blanket stitch provides more hemostasis than a simple basting stitch, it is primarily used to secure the yoni mucosa when the wound is seeping more blood more than usual. It also results in significantly more tissue eversion than a simple running stitch (Sherris & Kern, 2004). This is, in part, because the lock helps maintain tension on the stitch while the next stitch is being placed. Begin by placing an anchor stitch above the internal apex of the tear. Tie off this stitch and slide the knot to your nondominant side.

Continue by taking stitches as you would for a basting stitch. The only difference is that you bring your needle out inside a loop of the suture strand. To ensure that the stitch locks, hold the strand of suture with your nondominant hand and keep the needle point between the strand and the tear (i.e., inside the strand).

RUNNING LOCKED BLANKET STITCHES		
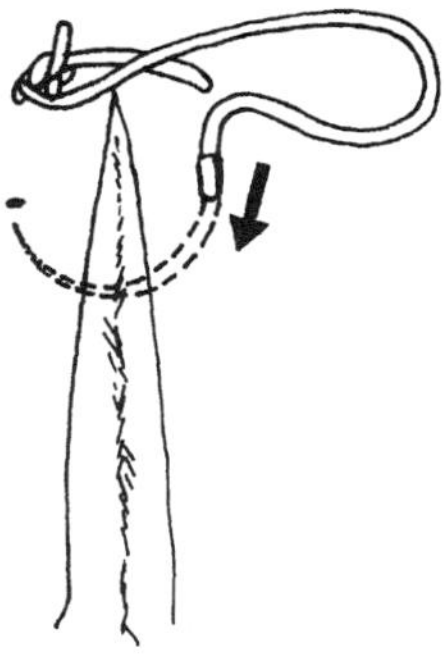	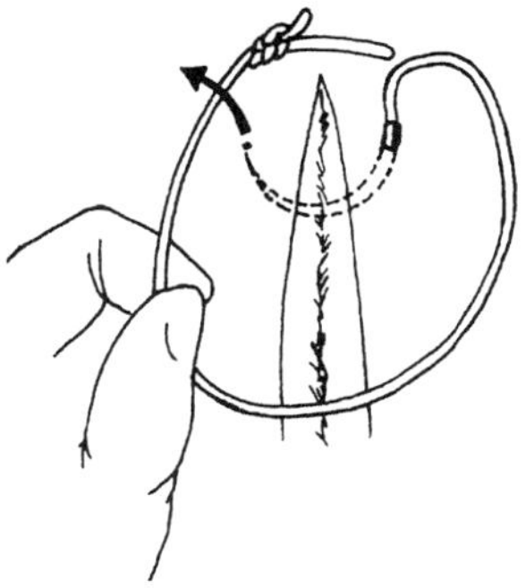	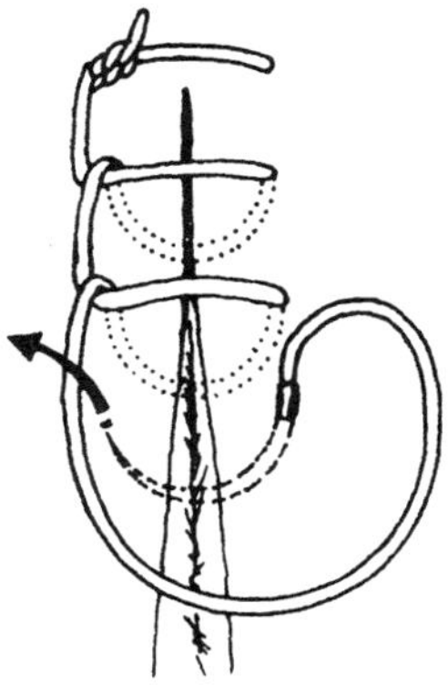
After placing an anchor stitch, go down about 1 cm and enter the tissue on your dominant side.	Hold the loop with the little finger of your nondominant hand so that the tip of the needle comes up inside the loop. Bring the needle out of the tissue . . .	. . . and pull the stitch to secure it. As you do, you lock the stitch. Repeat these steps for each stitch.

Running mattress (intracuticular/intradermal or subcuticular stitches: This lacing stitch gives the appearance of an "invisible zipper." Running mattress stitches are usually continuous with a previously placed row of stitches and are most frequently used to close the skin layer of the perineum. For practice, you may begin by placing an anchor stitch below the surface. This anchoring style is used in certain kinds of repair where this stitch is not continuous with previously placed stitches (for example, when repairing the labia minora). Be careful not to pull the edges together too snugly; they should touch but not pucker.

During practice, place the stitches 2 to 3 mm or so below the surface of the foam. In an actual repair, this avoids directly inserting the needle into the more nerve-rich dermal tissues, where it would create a true subcuticular stitch. In the thin skin of the perineum, this will actually result in a subcutaneous stitch and will result in the skin edges remaining slightly separated (Fleming, 1990) Be sure keep the needle parallel and not to allow it to penetrate the tissue surface at the points where it enters and exits the tissue. To begin practice, grasp the needle in the holder as follows:

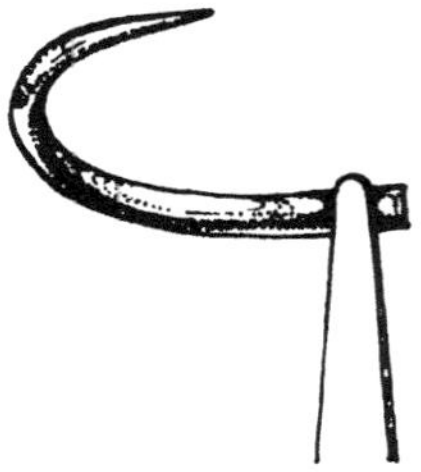	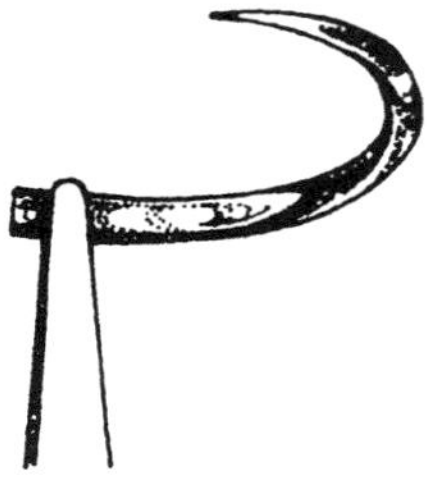
To place stitches on (your) left side of a tear in the perineum, hold the needle like this (tip is pointing toward you).	To place stitches on (your) right side of a tear in the perineum, hold the needle like this (tip is pointing toward you).

Running Mattress Stitches		
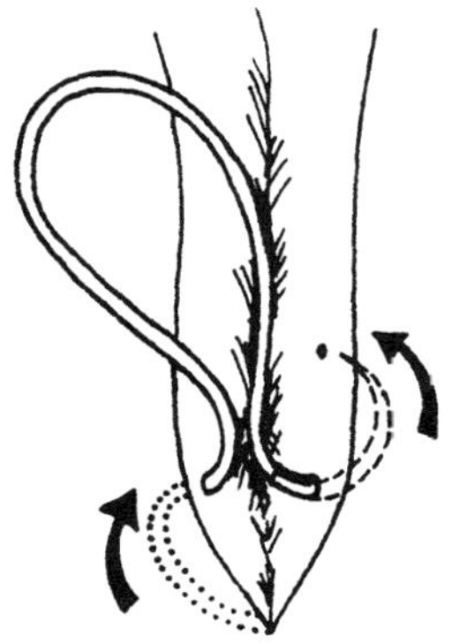	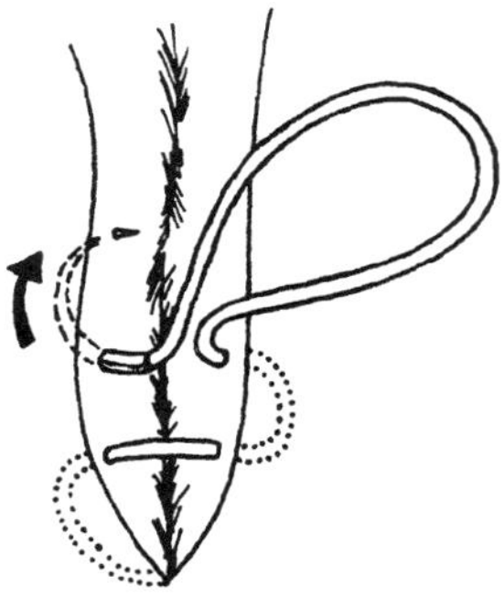	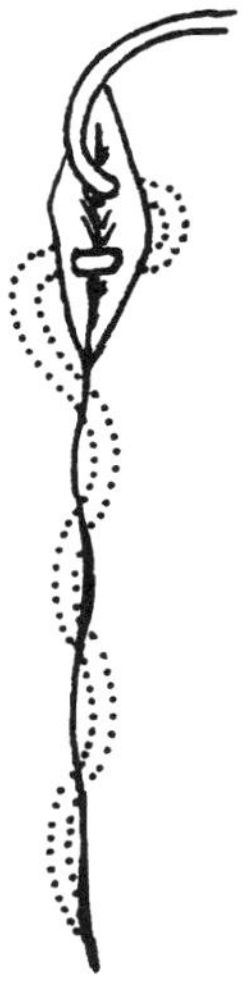
Starting at the apex of the tear, take a C-shaped bite 2-3 mm beneath the skin surface. Exit above that point on the same side you entered.	Reposition the needle so that you can take another bite across from your exit point on the opposite side. For the third stitch go back to the first side, taking a bite parallel to the tear edge as before.	Continue in this manner until you reach the end of the tear.

Special-use interrupted stitches

These stitches are included last because they are more advanced techniques that are optional for midwifery practice. They are useful to know, however, and should be learned once you are skilled with the other types of stitches.

Horizontal mattress stitch: The horizontal mattress stitch is a type of interrupted stitch that uses a two-bite technique wherein each bite is parallel the other, joining the wound from side to side, creating a modified, "double" interrupted stitch. The loop is mostly buried, producing a double loop that is continuous on one side and knotted on the other, leaving no suture crossing the superficial edges of the wound. This type of stitch does a good job of everting the wound edges. In midwifery it can be used to repair the internal or external sphincters. When the entry and exit points are widely spaced, it tends to reduce tension on the wound edges.

To create this stitch, the first bite is taken as for a simple interrupted stitch by driving the needle as for a half-circle stitch from your dominant to your nondominant side, as you usually would. The needle is then removed from the holder and repositioned in the jaws in a mirror image fashion, so it can be driven from your nondominant side. The needle is then reinserted on your nondominant side, parallel to and a short distance away from its exit point. (It will take some practice to learn to drive the needle this way with your dominant hand without traumatizing the tissue; alternatively, you can learn to drive the needle with your nondominant hand, an option that may appeal to those who have some ambidextrous abilities.) Once positioned correctly, another simple "interrupted"– style stitch is taken, this time by driving the needle from your nondominant to your dominant side. The needle exits the tissue parallel with and equidistant from the original insertion point; the stitch is tied and the ears are trimmed (Sherris & Kern, 2004; Trott, 2005).

<table>
<tr><th colspan="3">HORIZONTAL MATTRESS STITCH</th></tr>
<tr>
<td>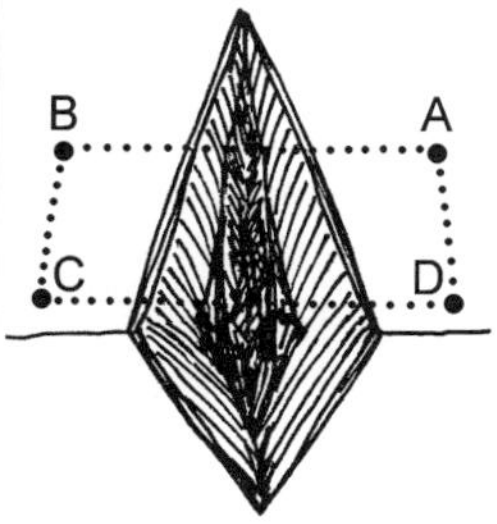
</td>
<td>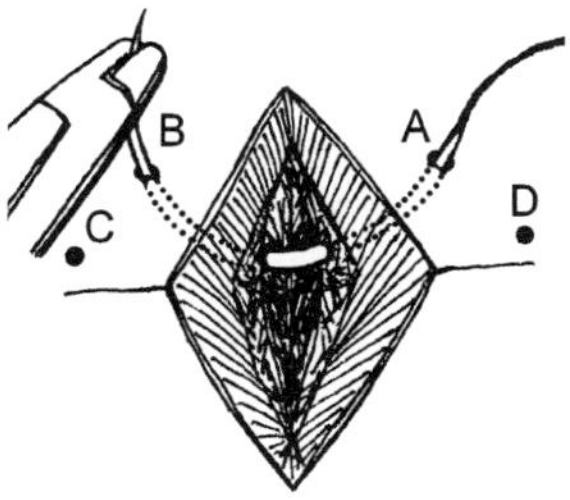
</td>
<td>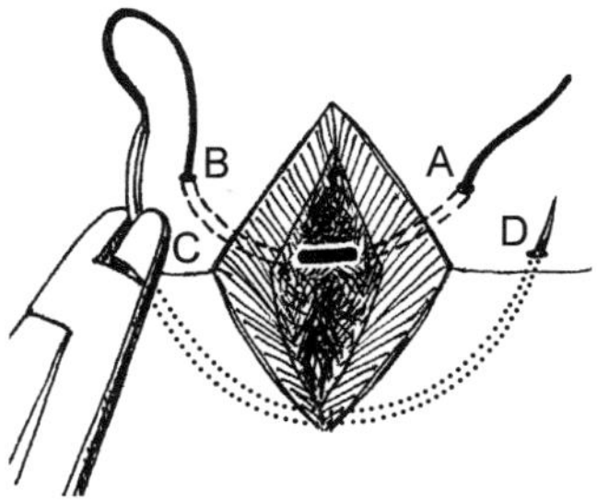
</td>
</tr>
<tr>
<td>Looking straight down at the tear, imagine a rectangle placed across the center with corners marked as shown.</td>
<td>Take a horizontal bite across the tear, entering the tissue at A and exiting at B.</td>
<td>Reposition the needle in the holder and reinsert the needle at C. Take another horizontal bite from C to D. Tie the stitch off.</td>
</tr>
</table>

Figure-eight stitch: This is essentially a horizontal mattress–style stitch that is crossed in the center. It can be used when you need to place for an extra secure stitch or one that provides increased hemostasis. It assists in gathering and ligating bleeding tissue. It may also be used when repairing the external anal sphincter. Be sure the distance from each edge and the depth of both sides of the stitch are equal all around. This stitch can be placed as a vertical eight (8) or a horizontal eight (∞).

Figure-Eight Stitch

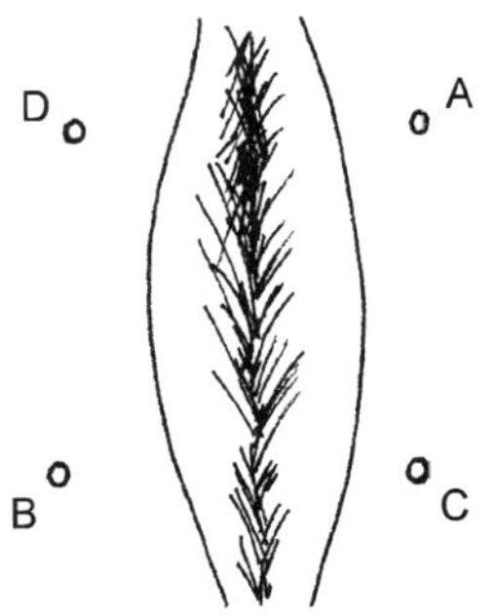

Looking straight down at the tear, imagine a rectangle placed across the wound with corners marked as shown.

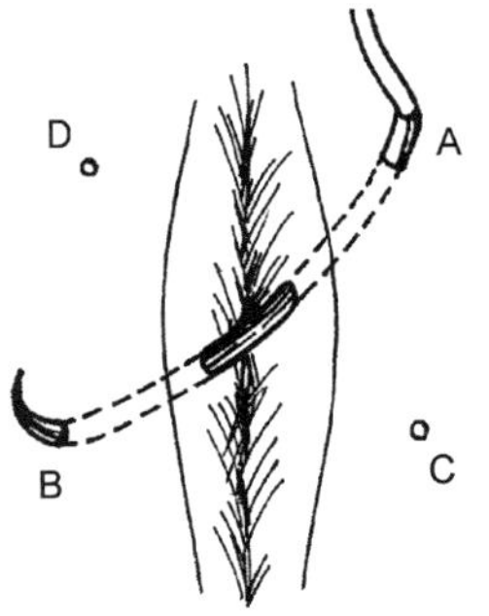

Take a diagonal bite across the tear, entering the tissue at A and exiting at B. Be sure the stitch reaches the depth of the tear.

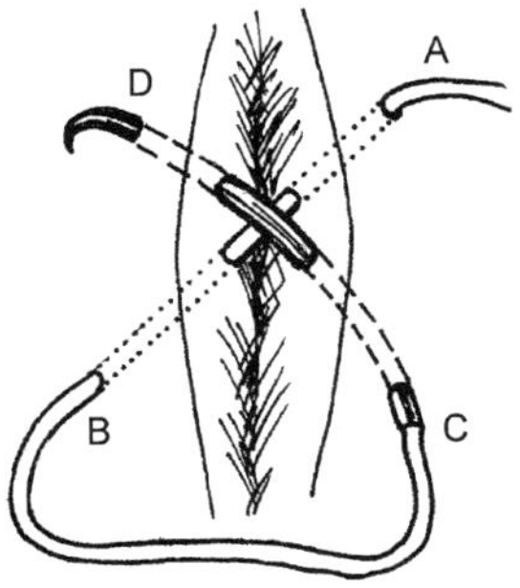

Reinsert the needle at C. Take another diagonal stitch from C to D, passing the needle just above or below the center of the first segment as you do.

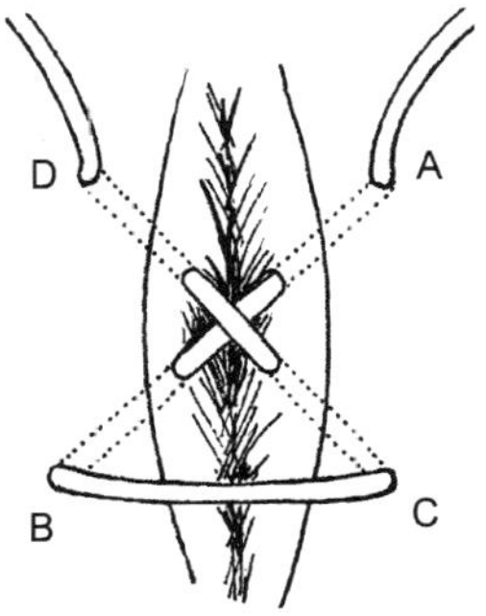

Now pull the wound edges together.

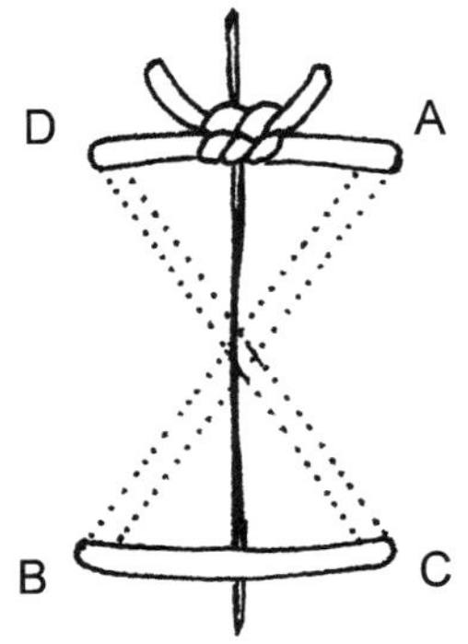

Tie the stitch off using a square knot.

Crown suture

The crown suture was devised to join the severed halves of the bulbocavernosus muscle. In light of the newest understanding of the anatomy of the perineal body, this stitch, at best, joins the severed halves of the superficial transverse muscle and the torn halves of the lower border of the perineal membrane. It is notoriously difficult to place correctly, as its traditional configuration involves a three-dimensional figure-eight stitch placed at a very hard-to-achieve, backwardly directed, oblique angle. If you feel that a separate stitch is required to bring together the superficial transverse perineal muscle, a single horizontal interrupted stitch or a simple horizontal figure-eight stitch can be used instead. I do not routinely recommend this practice, however, as it is too easy to make such a stitch too tight.

(Ethicon, 1977; Oxorn, 1986; Sherris & Kern, 2004; Varney et al., 2004)

Using a Yoni Retractor

The use of a retractor is already somewhat familiar to you, as it is used very much like a speculum.

Using a single speculum blade for unilateral retraction

If using only one blade of a speculum, after detaching it from the assembled speculum, place the lip of the blade in the center of the yoni canal and gently advance it as far as you believe to be necessary for the task at hand. The blade is then depressed against the wall of the yoni that is *opposite* the side you are trying to visualize. When you are done, the pressure on the blade is simply relaxed, and the blade is slowly withdrawn.

Using a double-bladed retractor

If you require better or more complete visualization, use a retractor designed for this purpose rather than a speculum. (If a speculum is all you have, it can serve if you have an apprentice to help hold it where you need it, but it is not ideally suited to this task.) The Guardian vaginal retractor is inserted very much as a speculum would be. First, inspect the edges of the retractor to make sure there are no rough areas that could cause pain or injury.

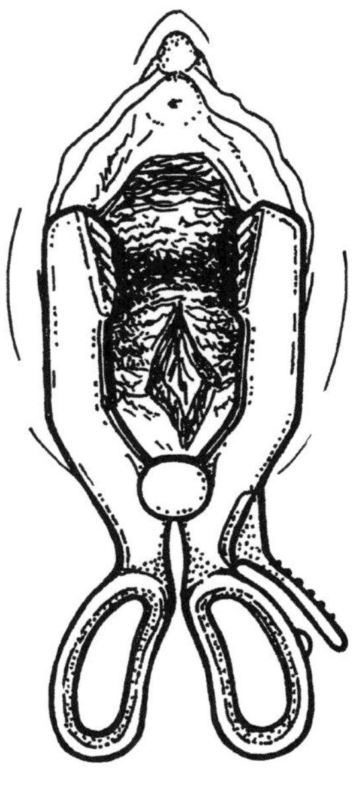

Guardian retractor in place

Inserting the retractor: Close the blades, center them in the yoni opening, and gently and slowly begin to advance them as far as appears necessary to allow you to see what you need to see. Once they are advanced sufficiently, adjust their angle so that when the blades are parted, you will be able to see the desired area. In most cases, vertical alignment of the blades will afford the best view. Once they are in position, slowly squeeze the finger rings to open the blades and lock them into place, all the while making sure you are not pinching tissue and that the mother can tolerate the pressure. Proceed with your repair. If the retractor requires repositioning, insert your fingers in the rings, release the lock, collapse the blades at least part way, and reposition the blades as necessary to complete the repair.

Removing the retractor: Once the deep internal damage is repaired, the retractor can be removed before proceeding to any labial or periurethral repairs. When you are ready to remove it, the pressure on the blades is gently relaxed by disengaging the lock. This is done by inserting your fingers in the rings, unlocking the blades and slowly collapsing them until they meet, being sure you are not pinching tissue in the process. Once collapsed, the retractor is slowly withdrawn.

USING LOCAL ANESTHETIC

The desire to minimize the mother's discomfort during the repair must be balanced with the equally desirable goal of avoiding long-term discomfort as well as optimizing healing. In my experience, the topical use of local anesthetic plays a big role in achieving both of these goals. A local anesthetic is defined as an agent that produces regional numbness in a conscious individual.

The physiology of physical pain and its control

To understand how anesthetics work, it is helpful to review the source of pain sensations. The brain interprets some nerve messages as physical pain. As intra- and extracellular fluids move across the semipermeable membranes of nerve cells, ions in the fluids transmit electrical impulses. Nerve cell membranes normally have a positive charge produced by the sodium ions surrounding it. The interior of the cell is usually negatively charged, a product of potassium ion concentration. Pain causes a temporary change in cellular permeability, allowing sodium to enter and potassium to leave. This shift, called **depolarization**, changes the cell's electrical charge, and causes an electrical impulse to be transmitted to surrounding cells and eventually to the brain. After transmission, **repolarization** occurs when the cell rids itself of sodium ions and returns to its original balance.

Large nerves are coated with myelin (MY-uh-lin), an insulating fatty substance that minimizes leakage of electric current, allowing the transmission of pain messages to the central nervous system faster than the smaller, uncoated nerves in the autonomic (involuntary) nervous system. Both large and small nerves relay messages simultaneously, but each impulse is perceived at slightly different times. The primary sensation of pain is sharp and penetrating, which is then followed by a burning sensation (Baer & Williams, 1988).

Mechanism of pain blockage: Local pharmaceutical agents produce anesthesia by blocking nerve impulses. Prior to suturing, percutaneous infiltration is used to numb the area immediately adjacent to the tear. Upon injection, the drug diffuses across neural membranes where it blocks the conduction of neural impulses along axons by swelling the nerve endings. This blocks sodium from entering the nerve cells and prevents other intracellular fluid exchanges that facilitate the transmission of pain impulses to the brain.

The myelin sheath that covers nerve fibers within most axons varies in diameter and thickness. Fibers carrying pain signals in the skin lack a myelin sheath and have the smallest diameter, so they are rapidly and easily blocked by local anesthetics. Sensations of pressure and touch are carried by larger myelinated fibers. This means that 1% lidocaine may effectively block pain but not sensations of touch and pressure, which some anxious women may interpret as pain. A 2% concentration of lidocaine will often eliminate all sensations.

Onset and duration of anesthetic action: The onset of an anesthetic effect is influenced by the technique of injection, the concentration and total dose of the agent, the diameter of the adjacent nerve fibers, the presence of epinephrine, the pH of the solution as well as that of the infiltrated tissues, and other local physiochemical conditions such as lipid solubility and protein binding. Local infiltration of a wound produces rapid anesthesia, especially when it is injected into the boundary between the dermis and the superficial fascia, where nerve fibers respond immediately to blockage. The use of 2% solutions results in a slightly faster onset of action, but this effect is clinically insignificant.

The duration of action is primarily determined by the protein-binding characteristics of the local anesthetic agent being used. Solutions that have a higher percentage of protein binding, such as Bupivacaine (95% protein bound) have a duration of action ranging from 2 to 4 hours because they remain in the sodium channel longer than those that have a lower percentage. Lidocaine's protein-binding capacity is only 64% and that of mepivacaine is just 78%, with correspondingly shorter durations of action. Duration of effectiveness is also influenced by vasoactivity, blood supply to the region and the presence of epinephrine. The pelvic tissues are highly vascular and well suited to the use of local anesthetics. Of the commonly used local anesthetics, lidocaine produces the most vasodilation, which helps it to disburse from the tissues more quickly but also causes the wound to bleed more.

The pros and cons of using local anesthetic

There are numerous disadvantages to using injected anesthetic, which include the following:

- The administration of anesthetic is somewhat painful to the woman.
- It frequently doesn't entirely eliminate the pain of suturing.
- It swells the tissue considerably, making approximation more difficult (especially if the tissue is already swollen).
- Postpartum pain and swelling are prolonged and healing is impaired because the body must dissipate the extra fluid from the tissues.
- The drug must be metabolized, giving the woman's body one more task after birth.
- Using anesthetic presents the possibility, though remote, of a systemic drug reaction. This creates a potentially life-threatening problem for the woman and a dilemma for you, especially if you are not legally permitted to use the drug in the first place, have no access to epinephrine or are not trained to deal with an adverse reaction.

There are, of course, advantages to using some form of anesthetic. The mother may be less restless and more comfortable during the repair, especially when it involves highly enervated areas such as the labial skin. Highly sensitive women may not be able to tolerate suturing without any anesthetic. A minimal amount of injected anesthetic helps demarcate tissue edges, making it easier to identify swollen and bruised structures. Not using anesthetic and then having the incision or repair be terribly painful may introduce or restimulate trauma in the genital area; this could be especially harmful to women who have a history of sexual abuse or traditional female genital surgery.

Due to the legal status of midwifery where I practiced, local anesthetic was almost impossible for us to obtain and was illegal for us to use. Thus, I sutured without using anesthetic for many years. I never made a big deal of it, and most women did an exceptional job of handling the idea, as well as the procedure, all having been very committed to a homebirth without the use of any drugs. There are relatively few nerve endings in the yoni mucosa, and most women tolerated suturing in this area very well. Although subcutaneous and subcuticular repairs were more painful, postpartum pain and swelling were almost nil.

Then I discovered that topical application of lidocaine or injection of minimal amounts of anesthetic produced adequate numbing in most women and the same almost pain-free postpartum course in the majority of cases. (I never found that women reported less postpartum discomfort during the first day or two when injected anesthetic was used.)

The main purpose of using local anesthesia is to deaden the nerves just below the skin surface. You need not infuse anesthetic into the yoni mucosa or deep inside the yoni. Because of the few nerve endings there, using injected anesthetic causes more swelling than it is worth. The aim is to make the suturing procedure tolerable, not to obliterate every bit of sensation, which can require excessive amounts of anesthetic and is sometimes impossible to completely accomplish in any event. Even when pain is abolished, women will still feel pressure and pulling during the repair.

Anesthetic is very helpful, however, during the repair of superficial skin tears and labial or rectal damage, since these are the most painful areas to suture. These are also the most difficult areas to numb. This is especially true of the outer apex of a tear in or near the perianal skin and in the tissue near the superficial clitoral parts. You might warn the mother that, even with the liberal use of anesthetic, stitches in those areas may still be painful.

Types of anesthetic agents

There are basically two types of chemical compounds used for local anesthesia.

Amide agents: Amide (AM-ide) agents contain radical NH2 and CO molecules and include lidocaine, mepivacaine, bupivacaine and diphenhydramine (Benadryl). Ninety percent of amide solutions are metabolized by the liver, and the other 10% remain unmetabolized and are excreted by the kidneys.

Lidocaine hydrochloride (HCl) (Xylocaine, lignocaine, plain lidocaine) 1% or 2% is an amide anesthetic mixed with sodium chloride (lidocaine HCl 2% consists of 20 mg lidocaine and 4.6 mg sodium chloride per cc [mL]). Sodium chloride is added to maintain isotonicity. The solution also contains water for injection and sodium hydroxide or hydrochloric acid to adjust the pH of the solution to 5.0 to 7.0. Multidose vials often contain 1 gm/mL of methyl-paraben as a preservative (an additive found in many cosmetics that has been implicated as a carcinogen).

Lidocaine is the most commonly used local anesthetic in the United States in general and for perineal repair in particular. Its tissue-spreading properties are good and it readily penetrates nerve sheaths. It begins to act immediately or within 30 seconds after local infiltration and the anesthetic effects typically persist for about 20 to 30 minutes, although a few people seem to metabolize it much quicker and require multiple injections.

A 1% solution contains 10 mg/mL and 2% contains 20 mg/mL. Most of it is metabolized rapidly by the liver; less than 10% of a dose is excreted unchanged in the urine. Although it is considered somewhat toxic, lidocaine is popular because it acts rapidly. It is also the best choice for topical application in the genital area. In normal healthy adults, the maximum recommended dose of lidocaine injection with epinephrine for local anesthesia other than spinal should not exceed 7 mg/Kg, and the maximum total dose should not exceed 500 mg. Lidocaine injection with epinephrine should not be used on fingers and toes. The maximum recommended dose of lidocaine injection without epinephrine should not exceed 4.5 mg/Kg, and the maximum total dose should not exceed 300 mg (you will be using far less than this for repairs). Viscous lidocaine 2% for topical use is typically dosed as 15 ml (300 mg) orally swish and spit/swallow every 3 hours as needed in adults. Patients should not exceed 8 doses in 24 hours. Adverse effects such as dizziness, light-headedness and numbness of the tongue have been reported with 500 mg oral doses of lidocaine. Topical administration of lidocaine in adults and children should not exceed 3 mg/Kg/dose (e.g., 4.2 gm of a 5% ointment for a 70 Kg patient). The maximum dose should not be repeated within 2 hours.

Bupivacaine (Marcaine, Sensorcaine) 0.25 or 0.5% is also an amide that is being more widely used in wound care. It takes effect a bit more slowly than the other amides after local infiltration and takes longer to wear off (2.7 to 3.5 hours) than lidocaine or mepivacaine. There is no significant difference in the pain of injection, onset of action or adequacy of anesthesia between these drugs.

Mepivacaine (Carbocaine) 1 or 2% is another popular wound anesthetic that differs from lidocaine in some respects. It also takes effect immediately after local injection and lasts 30 to 60 minutes. Mepivacaine has less of a vasodilatory effect than lidocaine and usually is not mixed with epinephrine for this reason.

Articaine hydrochloride 4% (Septocaine) is an amide that has been used in Europe and other parts of the world for years that is now approved for use in the United States. Unfortunately, it is only available in combination with epinephrine. It is used in dental procedures but has not been studied for other uses. It takes effect 1 to 6 minutes after injection, lasts about 1 hour and has a similar safety profile as the other amide drugs.

Ester-based agents: Ester-based anesthetics contain an organic acid and an alcohol and include procaine (Novocaine) and tetracaine. They are metabolized by plasma enzymes and the liver and are excreted by the kidneys. Ester agents are not used as much as they once were in developed countries because these anesthetics are more prone to producing allergic reactions. They are included here because those in developing countries may have to use whatever they can get.

Benzocaine is an ester-based agent that can be safely and effectively used on any damaged mucous membrane, although most products are designed for oral use (and may be flavored). It has a very rapid onset (15 to 30 seconds) and short duration (10 to 15 minutes) of effectiveness. It can be reapplied as necessary during the suturing procedure. Hurricane spray is one such product (produced by Beutlich Inc., 800-238-8542). A 2 oz spray can dispenses 200 one-second dispersals. A can with a single application tube that can be resterilized is about $18.95 (US) and kits containing one can and 200 application tubes cost about $32.00 (US).

Procaine hydrochloride (Novocain) is another ester anesthetic and is considered the least toxic of the ester agents. Onset of action is 2 to 5 minutes after administration, and lasts 1 to 1.5 hours. Maximum dosages for peripheral block are 500 mg in up to 200 mL of 0.5%, 100 mL of 1%, or 50 mL of 2%. Novocaine is rapidly broken down by hydrolysis in the plasma.

Cetacaine spray is a combination topical local anesthetic that appears to be the best such anesthetic that is readily available to midwives in many respects. It contains three active ingredients: benzocaine (14%), tetracaine hydrochloride (2%) and butyl aminobenzoate (2%). It also contains benzalkonium chloride (0.5%) and cetyl dimethyl ethyl ammonium bromide (0.005%). Cetacaine effectively numbs mucous membranes and can be applied prior to injection or used instead of injection. It takes effect in 60 seconds and is effective for up to

30 minutes. It is available as a gel, an ointment, a liquid and an aerosol (the gel is available from Cascade HealthCare Products, [www.1cascade.com]). It can be used to lubricate needle tips and suture material. Cetacaine is not absorbed to a significant degree and has no systemic effects. It should not be used, however, in those who have exhibited any type of allergic reaction to any of its ingredients (RxList 2009; Poznar, 2002).

SINGLE LOCAL ANESTHETICS WITHOUT EPINEPHRINE USED FOR INFILTRATION			
AGENT	MAXIMUM DOSE*	ONSET & DURATION OF ACTION	AVERAGE ADULT DOSE (MG)
Lidocaine (Xylocaine)	4.5 mg/kg	Immediate/2 hours	500
Bupivacaine (Marcaine)	3 mg/kg	2 to 5 minutes/4 hours	100
Procaine (Novocaine)	15 mg/kg	2 to 5 minutes/1 hour	1000
Kern's rule: the % concentration of a liquid solution × 10 = mg of drug per cc (mL) of solution.			
*To calculate the maximum dose for each woman, first convert her body weight to kilograms by dividing her weight in pounds by 2.2. Then multiply that figure by the maximum dose value. For example, to find out how much 1 or 2% lidocaine you can give a woman weighing 154 lbs, convert her weight to kg (154 ÷ 2.2 = 70 kg). 70 × 4.5 = 315 mg. Now convert 315 mg to cc. There are 10 mg/cc in 1% and 20 mg/cc in 2%, so you divide 315 by 10 or 20. Rounding down to obtain a maximum dose, 315 mg = 30 cc of 1% lidocaine or 15 cc of 2%.			

Epinephrine (EP-ih-NEFF-rin): Local anesthetics are sold plain or combined with a vasoconstrictor, usually epinephrine (adrenalin). Such additives constrict blood vessels in the area being anesthetized, thus controlling bleeding and reducing the rate of anesthetic absorption. This prolongs the anesthetic effect, as well as providing a less bloody field, enabling you to better see what you are doing.

You could, if necessary, use anesthetic with epinephrine in the yoni mucosa if bleeding were profuse, which is very rare. But epinephrine will also prolong the time it takes for the body to disperse anesthetic from the perineal area, thus prolonging swelling while impairing circulation and oxygenation. A bit of pressure with a gauze pad soaked in an infusion of an astringent herb will usually slow bleeding enough to complete the repair, but even this intervention is rarely necessary. Although some practitioners make limited use of local anesthetics with vasoconstrictors, these drugs are generally contraindicated for use in perineal repair.

Pharmaceutical vasoconstrictor agents are absolutely contraindicated in tissue that only contains small blood vessels such a skin tags and labial or periurethral tears. If the small vessels are constricted, blood flow to the area will be diminished and the tissue may die from inadequate circulation.

The adverse side effects of epinephrine include rapid heart rate (tachycardia), palpitations and chest pain. The use of any vasoconstrictor (vasopressor) drug is therefore contraindicated in those with hypertension or other cardiovascular problems. Neither should it be used if an oxytocic drug has been administered; combining these drugs can lead to severe hypertension and even rupture of cerebral vessels in susceptible individuals. Epinephrine may intensify afterbirth pains as well. Other reactions include anxiety, headache, restlessness, tremors, heart pain (angina) and dizziness. Extreme reactions have caused pulmonary edema and ventricular fibrillation. Use of anesthesia with a vasoconstrictor complicates the drug picture and adds one more variable to the overall situation.

A burning sensation at the injection site is common when vasoconstrictor agents are added. Rarely, a severe allergic reaction may produce localized pain, discoloration of tissue, irritation, swelling, nerve inflammation or destruction, tissue necrosis and sloughing. These symptoms usually appear only after repeated injections.

Adverse reactions and side-effects to local anesthetics

Both amide- and ester-based local anesthetics may cause a variety of adverse reactions. A person who is sensitive to an ester agent will probably not be sensitive to an amide agent (although she usually will be to other ester agents).

ADVERSE REACTIONS TO LOCAL ANESTHETICS	
FREQUENCY	SIGNS & SYMPTOMS
Common (> 1/100 to < 1/10)	**Vascular disorders:** hypotension or hypertension **Gastrointestinal disorders:** nausea, vomiting. **Nervous system disorders:** pins and needles sensation (paresthesia), dizziness **Cardiac disorders:** bradycardia
Uncommon (> 1/1,000 to < 1/100)	**Nervous system disorders:** convulsions, pins and needles sensation around the mouth, numbness of the tongue, sensitivity to sounds (hyperacusis), visual disturbances, tremor, tinnitus, impaired speech, depression
Rare (< 1/1,000)	**Cardiac disorders:** cardiac arrest, cardiac arrhythmias **Immune system disorders:** allergic or anaphylactic reactions **Respiratory disorders:** respiratory depression **Nervous system disorders:** neuropathy, peripheral nerve injury, stinging or burning sensation (arachnoiditis) **Eye disorders:** double vision (diplopia)

Systemic reactions: Systemic reactions may occur as the result of unusually rapid absorption, accidental injection directly into a blood vessel (especially cardiovascular or central nervous system [CNS] reactions) or administration of too much drug at once. Any of these may lead to high plasma levels. Other causes of reactions include hypersensitivity and diminished tolerance for reasons unknown.

With the accidental intravascular injection of lidocaine, the toxic effect will be obvious within 1 to 3 minutes, while with overdosage, peak plasma concentrations may not be reached for 20 to 30 minutes, depending on the site of injection, with signs of toxicity thus being delayed. Toxicity usually presents with excitation of the nervous system or cardiovascular depression or both.

Generally, toxicity manifests initially with subtle signs of CNS excitation including tingling of the tongue and numbness around the mouth. Continued absorption produces progressive symptoms such as tinnitus, lightheadedness, sleepiness and sometimes visual disturbances, clonic hyperreflexes, restlessness and eventually seizures. Unconsciousness, coma, respiratory arrest and cardiac arrest rapidly follow seizures if systemic levels are high enough.

High plasma levels are dose and drug dependent. Local infiltration of the skin and subcutaneous tissues rarely results in toxicity unless intravascular injection accidently occurs.

Cardiovascular collapse occurs at lower doses with bupivacaine than with lidocaine, in part because bupivacaine protein binds with myocardial muscle tissue. Another symptom is ventricular arrhythmia with fatal fibrillation, which is not usually seen with lidocaine toxicity, even when given intravenously. Pregnancy enhances the cardiovascular toxicity of bupivacaine.

Methemoglobinemia (MHb), a state of excess methemoglobin, may result from the systemic absorption of some topical anesthetics, notably prilocaine and benzocaine. Lidocaine overdose is also an associated factor, but only very rarely. Hemoglobin can accept and transport oxygen only when the iron atom is in its ferrous form. When iron becomes oxidized, it is converted to the ferric state (Fe^{3+}) or methemoglobin. Methemoglobin lacks the electron required to form a bond with oxygen, rendering it incapable of oxygen transport. Because red blood cells are continuously exposed to various oxidating stresses, blood normally contains approximately 1% methemoglobin (levels range from 0 to 3%).

Repeated use of 20% benzocaine (Hurricaine spray) on oral mucous membranes can produce methemoglobin concentrations greater than 15%. Symptoms of MHb correlate with the level of methemoglobin in the blood. Oxygenated blood is red, deoxygenated blood is blue, and blood containing methemoglobin is a dark reddish brown color. This dark hue causes clinical cyanosis when methemoglobin levels reach 1.5 g/dL (approximately 10-15% methemoglobin concentration); a level of 5 g/dL of deoxygenated blood due to simple deprivation is required for similar effects. Therefore, when methemoglobin levels are relatively low, it can produce cyanosis without cardiopulmonary symptoms. At concentrations of 3 to 15%, a slight discoloration (i.e., pale, gray, or blue) of the skin may be obvious. Symptoms of difficult breathing and lethargy appear at levels greater than 30%. Standard monitoring parameters do not detect MHb so it is not easily identified. Tests such as pulse oximetry and arterial blood gases can be misleading because circulating methemoglobin interferes with the technology used to determine oxygen saturation. Hypoxia is not relieved by 100% oxygen because the methemoglobin cannot carry oxygen. Some indigenous peoples, such as the Inuit, have a genetic predisposition toward methemoglobinemia. Treatment is with methylene blue, 1 to 2 mg/kg, administered slowly via IV. Methemoglobinemia is an exceedingly rare reaction that is not usually life threatening but is alarming since it causes the person to turn blue all over.

Treatment for other systemic reactions is mostly supportive. Maintain the airway and be sure the woman is breathing. Hypotension and bradycardia usually resolve on their own, a process that can be encouraged by placing her in a Trendelenburg position. If that doesn't help, an IV can be started with lactated Ringer's (Hartman solution). Infuse a bolus of 250 to 500 cc to correct hypotension. Check vital signs frequently. Seizures also typically resolve by themselves but sometimes require control with diazepam (Valium). Any woman who has more than fleeting side-effects such as these should probably be taken to the hospital for observation, just to be on the safe side.

Local complications may arise at the site of injection such as infection, hematoma formation and, uncommonly, permanent nerve damage to peripheral nerves.

Allergic reactions: Allergic reactions to local anesthetics are rare. Even so, you need to be aware of this possibility and what to expect because a severe reaction can quickly turn into anaphylactic shock, which constitutes a medical emergency that is life threatening.

Ask about allergies during prenatal care, and ask again prior to administration. Has she ever had a reaction to numbing medication at the dentist or elsewhere? What was the reaction? Does she know what drug she received? If you have any doubts and cannot confirm what drug caused the problem, play it safe by not giving her any anesthetic.

If the mother has a highly allergic constitution, the safest thing to do is to use no anesthetic. You can also test for sensitivity: rub a cotton swab soaked with anesthetic on the inside of her cheek and wait at least five minutes. Any reaction other than numbness (such as itching) suggests an allergy. (This test is not 100% reliable, and a systemic reaction can still occur after injection even when this test is negative.)

For some, reactions may be more emotional than physiological. If a woman reports any peculiar sensations after you have begun injection, stop and reassess the situation. If you suspect she is experiencing a drug reaction, don't give her any more.

Drug-induced anaphylactic shock is not something you want to be dealing with outside of the hospital if you can avoid it. If a woman begins to have signs of a severe reaction, give oxygen by mask, do CPR if necessary, administer epinephrine and transport. Rescue Remedy (a Bach flower remedy) may be safely given as well to both the mother and the care providers in any crisis situation. Apis. Mel. is a homeopathic remedy used in severe allergic reactions; 30C or 200C may be given every 15 minutes during transport. The pathophysiology and emergency treatment of anaphylactic shock, including the use of epinephrine as an antidote, is covered in detail in HOLISTIC MIDWIFERY, VOL II.

Allergic reactions are less common with amide-based local anesthetics than with ester agents. Multiple-dose vials contain the preservative methylparaben, which is suspected to contribute to allergic reactions. In addition, be aware that parabens, which are widely used in cosmetics, have been implicated as a causative factor in a variety of health-related problems, including cancer, and are best avoided altogether; research into these possible links is ongoing (Darbre & Harvey, 2008). Allergic reactions typically present as either a delayed onset skin rash or the acute onset of localized or generalized hives and itching 24 to 48 hours following administration. More rarely, frank anaphylactic shock can occur with skin symptoms, swelling, asthmatic respirations or respiratory arrest due to tracheal constriction. True allergic reactions occur in fewer than 1% of those receiving local anesthetics.

If you can determine with certainty that a previous drug reaction was due to one type of anesthetic (either amine- or ester-based), you can usually give an agent of the alternate type.

Administering anesthetic

This part of the chapter reviews some aspects of giving injections that are most relevant to perineal anesthesia. Please also review the subchapter entitled "Hypodermic Injections" in HOLISTIC MIDWIFERY, VOL. II, for more complete details regarding the use of syringes and injectable medications in midwifery care.

Timing of administration: Administer anesthetic after you have set up your equipment and just before beginning the repair, taking into account how long the particular agent you have on hand takes to become effective. Even if an agent is said to take effect immediately, depending upon the how and where it is administered, it may take up to a few minutes to take effect, especially when applied topically.

Topical anesthetic: The best way to use local anesthetic is topically in a spray, liquid or gel form. Topical application carries the least risk of a systemic drug reaction (although this can occur) and does not increase edema unless an allergy exists. You don't waste needles, gauze, etc., and it usually takes effect quickly. You must be careful because the dosage is harder to keep track of (for example, a 5% concentration delivers 50 mg/mL; a 10% concentration delivers 100 mg/mL). Topical administration of lidocaine in adults and children should not exceed 3 mg/kg/dose (for example, 4.2 gm of a 5% ointment for a 154 lb [70 kg.] person). Once the maximum dose has been given, do not administer more within two hours. Be sure to clean away blood and expose the raw surfaces, then spray for a second or two. If more is needed during the repair, just spray again, but be careful: the higher the concentration of a spray, the easier it is to administer too much.

If you don't have access to a spray, you can draw up a syringe (see below) and drip anesthetic on, or soak a gauze square or long-handled cotton swab in it and press into the wound, being sure it gets to the raw skin edges. This alone is enough to take the edge off suturing for most women. A nurse-midwife friend, on my advice, started to use anesthetic by opening the vial and dumping it into the tear. She found postpartum pain and swelling remarkably reduced. Try it!

A gel is easiest to apply, since it will stay where you put it. Use your gloved finger to dab it along the edges of the wound or to cover the entire raw area of a labial or periurethral tear.

The next table includes two less desirable topical anaesthetics (Cocaine and Tetracaine) that you may have to use if one of these is all you've got.

LOCAL ANESTHETICS WITHOUT EPINEPHRINE USED TOPICALLY			
AGENT	WHERE USED	CONCENTRATION	MAXIMUM DOSE
Lidocaine (Xylocaine)	Mucosa	4%	200 mg (5 cc)
Cocaine	Mucosa	5%	200 mg (4 cc)
Tetracaine	Mucosa	2%	100 mg (5 cc)

Administering anesthetic by injection

In the hospital, 10 to 15 cc of anesthetic are typically used during repairs. I recommend using much less. Large quantities produce a significant degree of tissue distortion, making it hard to decide how to approximate tissue. Sutures tend to be placed too tightly. This frequently leads to more immediate and long-term pain. If the mother is swelling significantly from tissue trauma alone, it is best to avoid injections altogether, since they will increase the swelling even more. If you use 2% (20 mg/cc) lidocaine for injection, you will get the same anesthetic benefit while using only half the volume you would if you gave 1% (10 mg/cc).

To withdraw anesthetic from a vial: This material reviews that covered in detail in HOLISTIC MIDWIFERY, VOL. II.

- Have your assistant remove the lid and wipe the top of the vial with an alcohol swab. When disinfecting multidose vials, be sure to use either isopropyl alcohol (70%) or ethyl alcohol (70%). Many commercially available brands of rubbing alcohol, as well as solutions of ethyl alcohol, are not of USP grade and contain denaturants that are injurious to rubber. Since there is some discussion of the possible carcinogenicity of these alcohols, a grain alcohol can also be used, either alone or made into an antiseptic tincture (in which case allergies must be ruled out).

- Pull back on the plunger to fill the syringe with air equal to the amount of liquid to be withdrawn from the vial.
- Hold the vial upright. Position the bevel of the needle tip uppermost, hold the needle at a 45° angle against the stopper and apply pressure to slice into the rubber, then reposition the needle so it is perpendicular to the rubber stopper.
- Inject air into the vial. (This makes it easier to draw up the liquid because the air creates pressure, otherwise you are drawing against a vacuum.) Do not remove the needle from the vial.
- Pull back the plunger again to withdraw between 1 to 4 cc of anesthetic, depending upon how much you think you will need. (Use a larger amount if you are using 1% concentration.)
- If you have used the needle in tissue and need more anesthetic, use a new, sterile needle *and syringe* to withdraw more agent from the vial, to avoid contaminating the entire vial. (Using a new syringe avoids contaminating the contents of the vial when the remaining medication is to be saved for use with another woman).

Dribble a little anesthetic along the tear edges to numb the puncture sites or apply some Cetacaine gel. First numb the skin edges, as described in the next paragraph, and then use one of the suggested techniques to infiltrate the deeper tissues.

Infiltrate at the skin edge: Begin by inserting the tip of the needle into the edge of the wound, just under and parallel with the skin surface. Inject a small amount of the agent to create an intradermal wheal. Advance the needle tip into this wheal and slowly continue injecting agent as you expand and enter the subdermal space, spreading the agent around the area to be sutured. Aspirate the syringe periodically to ensure that you are not injecting into a blood vessel. If you get blood in the barrel, reposition the needle slightly and aspirate again before you inject more agent. Allow a few minutes for the agent to reach surrounding nerves and penetrate axonal sheaths to effect a blockage.

Infiltrate deeper tissues: I strongly prefer Method 2.

Method 1. Insert the needle parallel with the inner surface of the torn skin all the way to the outer apex of the tear in the perineum (i.e., keep the needle just beneath the skin edge). Now aspirate by pulling back on the plunger to be sure you aren't in a blood vessel. If you get blood in the barrel, withdraw the needle slightly and aspirate again until you are sure you're not in a vessel. Now slowly draw the needle out as you inject fluid into the tissue (approximately ½ cc of 2% or 1 cc of 1%),

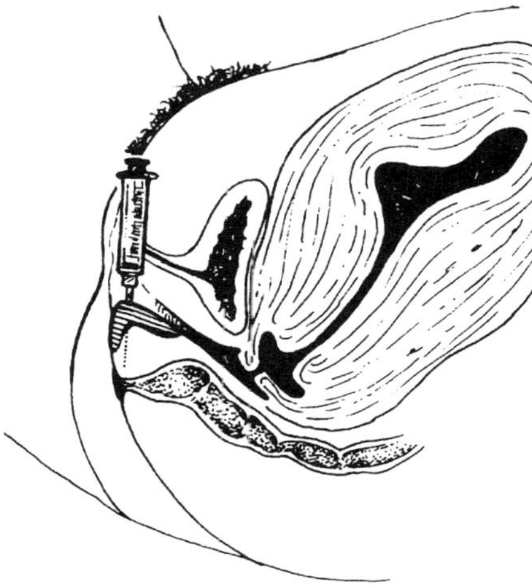

Insert the needle along the dotted line
(Shaded region represents one side of the tear)

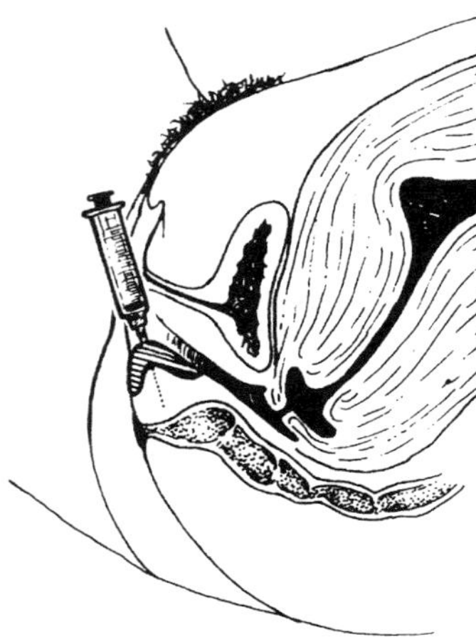

Withdraw the needle almost completely, adjust its angle slightly (along dotted line) and plunge the needle in again to the hub. Inject another 0.5 to 1 cc as you withdraw the needle. Repeat on the other side of the tear.

As the tissue swells slightly, continue to withdraw the needle as you infiltrate tiny bits of anesthetic along the needle's path. Reposition the needle and aspirate again, and repeat the injection. Continue, creating a fan pattern with three or so spokes that radiate from the point of needle entry.

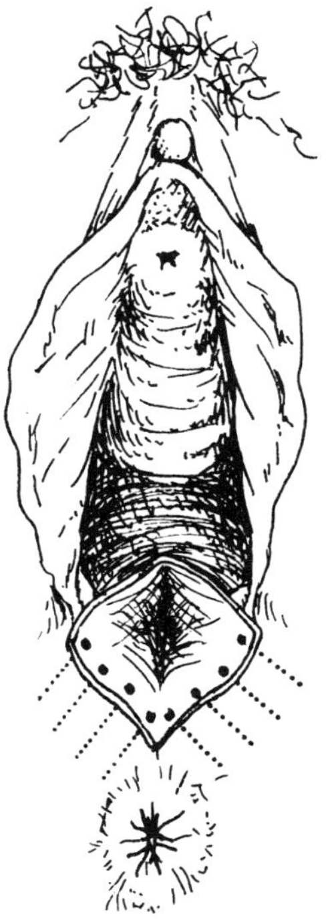

Method 2. Inject anesthetic by infusing very small amounts of drug along the outer wound edge under the skin, using several shallow punctures and the least possible amount. This creates less swelling and you won't use nearly as much of the drug. Even though this method requires more punctures, it is the method I recommend. If the tear involves the skin around the anus, use only method 2 for injecting anesthetic. The same goes for tears near the superficial clitoral structures or the labia minora. The illustration to the right shows the maximum depth of penetration appropriate.

Storage of anesthetics

Store local anesthetics at room temperature between 59 and 86°F (15 to 30°C) away from light and moisture. Do not freeze. Check the expiration date on the container and discard any unused medication after that date. Keep sprays away from heat and open flames. Because contents in canisters are under pressure, do not puncture the container. Before use, inspect all injectable products while holding them over a white surface under bright light. Injectable lidocaine should be clear and slightly yellow. Discard any injectable solution that becomes discolored or contains particulate matter (crystals). Autoclaving a partially used vial will increase the likelihood of crystallization and is not recommended.

HAND HYGIENE, ENVIRONMENTAL HYGIENE AND PREVENTING THE SPREAD OF INFECTIOUS AGENTS

This chapter reviews some general principles of personal and client protection that take into account typical work settings for midwives, with a focus on hand hygiene and maintaining appropriate cleanliness for suturing at home. For more information on workplace safety, see the chapter entitled "Standard Precautions to Avoid Contamination from Infectious Agents" in my UNDERSTANDING DIAGNOSTIC TESTS IN THE CHILDBEARING YEAR, 7th ed. (2007).

Today, it is felt prudent to assume that every person you care for is potentially infected or colonized with an organism that could be transmitted to you and to always apply infection control practices during the delivery of care. Most recommendations are designed for large facilities, such as hospitals, where people with all types of infections are cared for. At home, there will not be the same level of exposure. Nevertheless, I have included protocols for riskier environments so that you can decide what level of precaution makes sense for your practice setting. Knowing what might be needed in a high-risk situation will help you know what to do when faced with such a situation in your normally very low-risk practice.

Whenever you employ other midwives or assistants in the United States, OSHA regulations require you to provide protective equipment and clothing and to conduct your practice in a way that minimizes employee risk. If you work independently, you are not required to adhere to OSHA regulations yourself. You should check with your local government regarding OSHA rules and regulations in your area. The material in this chapter is based on Siegal and colleagues (2007) unless otherwise noted.

Blood-Borne Disease Agents

Blood may communicate hepatitis, HIV, syphilis, and malaria, as well as other organisms. Although hepatitis B is a far less fragile organism than HIV, concern over possible contamination from body fluids did not really mount until knowledge of AIDS became widespread. There is evidence that HIV may not be the root cause of AIDS after all. A growing number of scientists have called for a reappraisal of the HIV=AIDS hypothesis. For more about this controversy, see my UNDERSTANDING DIAGNOSTIC TESTS IN THE CHILDBEARING YEAR, 7th ed. (2007).

Whatever the outcome may be, there are plenty of blood-borne pathogens to be concerned about. Contact with blood infected with syphilis or hepatitis can result in transmission. Syphilis dies when it drys in air but can be preserved in deep cold (such as that used to preserve blood transfusions) and, as is said of HIV, can be communicated via blood contact, including needle-sticks. Regardless of what factors contribute to the development of AIDS, precautions are necessary (Chambers, 1969; Coulter, 1987; Mitchell, 1990).

HIV is said to be a somewhat fragile virus, but it can live outside the body. Experiments with diluted calf's blood and laboratory concentrations of virus (far higher than biological concentrations) showed that HIV can survive 14 days at room temperature and up to 11 days at 100°F (37.8°C). Dried HIV loses about 90% to 99% of its infectivity after a few hours at room temperature, with complete inactivity requiring three days. Biological concentrations (i.e., the virus in human blood) are far lower with HIV than with hepatitis B, and hepatitis B is about half the size. Thus hepatitis is far easier to transmit via blood contamination than HIV.

When sterilizing equipment, keep in mind that heat inactivates HIV, syphilis and hepatitis B in liquid human blood solutions: 10 minutes at 140°F (60°C) destroys HIV (60 minutes to destroy hepatitis B). Disinfectants that destroy HIV (for sure) and hepatitis B (with longer exposure) include:

- •Grain alcohol (ethanol) at 50% solution or higher (usually available at 95%)
- •Isopropyl (rubbing) alcohol at 35% (most is 70%)
- •Household bleach at 1 part per 100 parts water (or 1/4 cup to 1 gallon of water). That's right, 1:100, not 1:10. According to an FDA researcher I spoke with, this is more than strong enough to destroy HIV a few times over.

The alcohols are widely available and the least damaging to rubber and skin. Clean materials with disinfectant soap and water as soon as possible after use and then soak in one of the above solutions for 10 minutes (alcohol is recommended); this should eliminate all HIV virus. Soak for a total of at least 30 minutes to kill hepatitis B. Tissue proteins, such as blood, quickly neutralize the effectiveness of alcohol, so thorough cleaning of used items prior to soaking is important. (In a personal communication with a CDC representative, I was told that soaking like this should kill hepatitis B and syphilis, but, in fact, no real studies have been done on hepatitis in this regard because "people aren't afraid of it." Therefore, there is no research money.)

Freezing has a preservative effect on viruses and on syphilis, causing them to go dormant. Although viral infectivity is lost in the freezing process, freezing cannot be thought of as eliminating risk. All those interesting placentas in your freezer must therefore be considered potentially contaminated and infectious.

Blood and semen are the most likely sources of body fluid contagion with HIV and syphilis. Saliva contains very small amounts of the HIV virus and is not considered infectious, but it may communicate hepatitis. Urine and feces are somewhat problematic with HIV; prolonged exposure is probably required (such as when caring for a sick person or an infant) before it is transmitted. Hepatitis and polio are highly communicable from fecal contact; hepatitis is transmitted via blood and urine as well. Syphilis is usually communicated via direct contact from infected blood or body fluid with mucous membranes, a sore or the bloodstream of a noninfected person. Under normal circumstances, syphilis dies within minutes once outside the body, especially when exposed to air and allowed to dry.

In situations in which body fluids may splatter, goggles are recommended to prevent contamination of your eyes. Alternatively, plain lens glasses can be purchased in many eyewear departments; they provide less obtrusive but somewhat less effective, protection. If body fluid contacts skin surfaces, wash the area with an antibacterial agent as soon as possible. If you should stick yourself with a contaminated needle, make the injury bleed as much as you can, soak the body part in hydrogen peroxide, review the client's records for any concerning history of infections and consult a medical provider accordingly.

Protecting Yourself, the Mother and the Newborn: Sterile Surgical Technique vs. Clean Technique

The basic principle of sterile technique is to touch only sterile things with other sterile things while wearing sterile gloves. When suturing at home, in many situations it is unnecessary to maintain strict sterile technique. Exceptions to this might include working in tropical areas (where infection occurs more easily) or with women in poor health. (Although in the birthing clinic where I trained, women were frequently not very healthy, but sterile technique was not used. There were no perineal infections during the six months I was there.) Sterile technique is much more important in hospitals because of the resistant pathogens present.

"Clean technique" works just fine when suturing at home and does not usually lead to infection. By "clean technique" I mean keeping your washed, gloved hands as clean as possible. Avoid unnecessary touching of surfaces in close proximity to the woman to prevent both contamination of clean hands from environmental surfaces and transmission of pathogens from contaminated hands to surfaces. However, I often do fundal checks or other necessary procedures involving touching the mother's body with the same gloves I use to suture. A new, sterile glove should be used if it is necessary to examine deep inside the yoni. Any glove that has been used to touch the anal area should be immediately removed, discarded and replaced. More about maintaining a clean or a sterile field can be found in the chapter that follows this one, entitled "Maintaining a Sterile or Clean Field."

Hand Hygiene

Aside from being careful about what you touch, washing is the primary means of achieving hand hygiene. Thorough handwashing is usually sufficient to remove transient contaminants from the skin. **Transient contaminants** are microbes that are easily acquired and transferred by direct contact. They lie loosely on the skin surface, are attached by fats and dirt, and are most abundant around the fingertips. Typically, a high percentage of these organisms are pathogenic, and they are an important source of cross-contamination. Examples include *Staphylococcus aureus*, streptococci, gram-negative bacilli such as *Escherichia coli* and *Pseudomonas aeruginosa*, and viruses. Virulence will be determined by a person's environment: as a rule, far more virulent microbes will be picked up in a hospital environment than in the home. Plus, family members are likely to be immune to organisms prevalent in their own home. There are two means of removing transient hand flora: alcohol-based hand rubs and soap and water (May, 2000).

General principles of hand hygiene

Follow handwashing protocols as described in this chapter. Cleanse your hands before touching women or their newborns; after contact with blood, body fluids or excretions, mucous membranes, nonintact skin, or wound dressings; after contact with intact skin (e.g., when taking a pulse or blood pressure or lifting a woman or newborn); when hands will be moving from a contaminated body site to a clean body site during the provision of care; after contact with objects (including medical equipment) in the immediate vicinity of the woman or her newborn and after removing gloves.

Handwashing agents (the short version): Products containing 60 to 95% ethanol or isopropyl alcohol alone or in a 50 to 95% concentration when combined with limited amounts of a quaternary ammonium compound, hexachlorophene, or chlorhexidine gluconate will lower bacterial counts on the skin immediately and more effectively than other agents. Using the proper volume of solution is important to achieve effectiveness. Purchase containers that dispense the recommended portion whenever possible.

Hibiclens with 4% chlorohexidine gluconate (ICI Australia, Operations Pty., Ltd., Sydney) or 7.5% povidone iodine, (Betadine™) are good options for general handwashing or surgical antisepsis. Avagard™D (3-M) is an alcohol-based hand rub that contains 61% ethyl alcohol in a moisturizing base. These products are easily available to the midwifery community through Cascade HealthCare Products and other midwifery practice suppliers. The next most active agents (in order of decreasing activity) are chlorhexidine gluconate, iodophors, triclosan and plain soap. More details on these agents are included in this chapter, beginning on page 446.

Here is a summary of hand hygiene recommendations (CDC, 2009b).

<table>
<tr><th>Hand Cleaning Method</th><th>Agent</th><th>Purpose</th><th>Area</th><th>Minimum Duration</th></tr>
<tr><td>Routine hygienic wash</td><td>Water and non-antimicrobial soap</td><td>Remove soil and transient organisms</td><td rowspan="3">All surfaces of hands, wrists (if soiled) and fingers</td><td rowspan="2">20 seconds</td></tr>
<tr><td>Antiseptic wash</td><td>Water and antimicrobial soap with persistent activity</td><td rowspan="4">Remove or destroy transient micro-organisms and reduce resident flora</td></tr>
<tr><td>Antiseptic rub</td><td>Alcohol-based hand rub</td><td>Rub all surfaces until hands are dry</td></tr>
<tr><td>Surgical antisepsis</td><td>Water and antimicrobial soap with persistent activity</td><td rowspan="2">Hands and forearms</td><td>2 to 6 minutes, follow manufacturer's instructions</td></tr>
<tr><td>Surgical antisepsis rub</td><td>Water and non-antimicrobial soap followed by an alcohol-based surgical hand scrub with persistent activity</td><td>Follow manufacturer's instructions for surgical hand scrub product with persistent activity</td></tr>
</table>

Using an alcohol-based hand rub: If the hands are not visibly soiled and there has been little or no contact with body fluids, an alcohol-based hand rub may be used before care is provided to each woman or newborn and between different care activities for the same mother or newborn. Start with dry hands. Place the volume of solution that the manufacturer recommends or at least 3 mL—a little less than a teaspoon—(A teaspoon is about 5 cc. A cc is the fluid measurement, a mL is by weight) into the palm of one hand. Rub the hands together vigorously, contacting all surfaces, paying particular attention to the tips of the fingers, the thumbs, and the areas between the fingers, until the solution has evaporated and the hands have air-dried. If an adequate amount has been used, drying should take longer than 10 to 15 seconds. Washing with soap and water following the use of an alcohol hand rub is not recommended.

If the hands are visibly soiled and the only antiseptic solution you have is an alcohol hand rub, wash thoroughly with plain soap, then dry your hands thoroughly with a paper towel. Wash your hands again with the alcohol rub as an antiseptic measure, as described above.

Routine hygienic handwashing with soap and water: If contact with body fluids has occurred or the hands are visibly soiled, washing with soap and warm water is recommended. If the hands are soiled with organic material, if you are preparing to perform an invasive procedure or if you are to work with someone who is immune compromised, the use of a liquid antimicrobial soap is recommended whenever available. Whenever plain bar soap is used, drain it well between uses and use small bars to minimize bacterial growth on the bar.

Push your wristwatch and long sleeves above your wrists (or remove the watch). Remove rings. Proceed as follows:

- Stand in front of the sink, keeping your hands and clothing away from the sink surface.
- Turn on the water and adjust it to a warm temperature; avoid splashing water onto your clothing.
- Wet the hands and wrists thoroughly under running water. Keep your hands and wrists below the level of the elbows at all times so that the water flows from the least to the most contaminated areas.
- Apply the specified amount (check label) of liquid soap or antimicrobial preparation to one palm. Rub the hands together vigorously to work up a lather and continue for a minimum of 20 seconds (about the time required to sing the "ABC" song), paying particular attention to the tips of the fingers, the thumbs and the areas between the fingers and under the nails. Rub palms together and use palms to rub the back of each hand. Interlace the fingers and rub palms and back of hands with a circular motion at least 5 times each. Keep fingertips pointed down to help remove transient microorganisms and surface debris.
- Rinse hands and wrists thoroughly in warm, not hot water, keeping the hands down.
- If hands are heavily soiled, wash them again.
- Dry the hands using new, good-quality paper towels. Use a clean, dry towel to turn off the faucet or have an assistant turn it off for you.
- If the hands are dry or chapped, apply a small amount of lotion that does not contain mineral oil or petroleum-based ingredients (CDC, 2009a; Elkin et al., 2000; May, 2009).

Surgical hand antisepsis: There may be times when you will need to perform surgical hand antisepsis, which simply means washing your hands in a prescribed manner to reduce the colony counts of certain organisms on and just beneath the skin surface. This is appropriate when you are going to do anything invasive, such as suturing or before manually removing a placenta (although admittedly there may be no time for it in that circumstance).

Surgical antisepsis is intended to remove resident organisms from the skin surface. **Resident** or **commensal organisms** are present on the skin of healthy individuals (up to 3 million organisms/cm^2). Most tend to live in the deeper layers of the stratum corneum, near the skin scales that they feed on and are not normally shed with desquamation (loss of bits of outer, dead skin cells) (Ross & Chadwick, 2009). Examples include coagulase negative staphylococci such as *Staphylococcus epidermidis*, diphtheroids, anaerobic cocci, and propionibacteria. Most resident organisms are not pathogenic and exist in stable colonies on the skin. Their presence makes it much harder for pathogenic bacteria to survive. Nevertheless, prolonged exposure to resistant organisms, which most commonly occurs when someone is consistently exposed to them (as is the case with hospital staff), can result in a higher percentage of pathogenic microbes becoming resident skin flora.

Thorough handwashing with ordinary soap and running water does not effectively remove resident organisms. Therefore, a surgical scrub using either an antimicrobial soap or an alcohol-based product *with persistent activity designed for surgical antisepsis* is recommended before donning surgical gloves because bacteria multiply rapidly under gloves when hands have only been washed with a nonantimicrobial soap. Bacterial growth is slowed after preoperative scrubbing with an antiseptic agent. Reducing resident skin flora on the hands for the duration of a procedure reduces the risk of bacteria being released into the sterile field if gloves become punctured or torn.

Antiseptic preparations intended for use as surgical hand scrubs are evaluated for their ability to reduce the number of bacteria released from hands at different times, including immediately after scrubbing, after wearing gloves for six hours (persistent activity), and after multiple applications of the product over five days (cumulative activity). Immediate and persistent activity are considered the most important factors when determining the efficacy of a product. US guidelines recommend that agents used in surgical hand scrubs substantially reduce microorganisms on intact skin, contain a nonirritating antimicrobial preparation, have broad-spectrum activity, and be fast acting and persistent.

Although alcohols alone are not considered to have persistent antimicrobial activity, bacteria appear to reproduce slowly on the hands after a surgical scrub with alcohol, and bacterial counts on hands after wearing gloves for 1 to 3 hours seldom exceed baseline (prescrub) values. Alcohol-based preparations containing 0.5% or 1% chlorhexidine gluconate have persistent activity that, in certain studies, has equaled or exceeded that of chlorhexidine gluconate–containing detergents.

Persistent antimicrobial activity of detergent-based surgical scrub formulations is greatest in products containing 2% or 4% chlorhexidine gluconate, followed by hexachlorophene, triclosan and iodophors. Because hexachlorophene is absorbed into the blood after repeated use, it is seldom used as a surgical scrub.

Surgical hand washing: When performing surgical hand antisepsis, scrub the hands and forearms for the length of time with the amount of product recommended by the manufacturer, usually 2 to 6 minutes, using a sponge, rather than a brush, or just friction from rubbing the hands together. Longer scrub times (e.g., 10 minutes) and the use of a brush are not any more effective and damage the skin, which increases bacterial shedding. Scrubbing with a brush or a sponge is not necessary to reduce bacterial counts on the hands of surgical personnel to acceptable levels, especially when alcohol-based products are used (discussed below). Here is a general protocol for water-based surgical antisepsis as recommended by the Centers for Disease Control in the US (Boyce et al., 2002; Sherris & Kern, 2004):

•If your hands are visibly soiled, wash the hands as described on page 438 before you proceed.

- Make yourself comfortable before scrubbing by first attending to any other personal needs. Don your hair covering, if using one. Doing these things now avoids having to rescrub later.
- Assemble supplies near the sink: antiseptic solution, surgical scrub kit, paper towels, a pair of sterile gloves.
- Remove rings, watches and bracelets and put them in a safe place for the duration of the provision of care. Move sleeves up behind the elbows or change to a short-sleeved shirt. Once you are scrubbed, you should not move the sleeves down over your scrubbed arm. You would need to then don a sterile gown, however midwives do not typically don full surgical garb before perineal repair.
- Remove debris from under the fingernails using a nail tool (or new toothpick).
- Turn on the water and adjust it to a warm temperature.
- Rinse hands and arms under warm running water. Keep your *hands higher than your elbows* at all times during a surgical scrub so that the water flows from the least to the most contaminated skin. (This is the opposite of what is recommended for a hygienic hand-wash because here you are removing resident organisms, which are more or less uniformly distributed all over your skin. Once you begin scrubbing, the skin of the hands becomes the least contaminated and you want to prevent soap from the less-clean elbows from running back over the clean hands.)
- Pump the recommended amount of antiseptic solution into one palm.
- Following the product directions, first rub the palms and fingers 10 times and then the backs of each hand. Continue further up the hands and forearms to the level of the elbow. Use a circular motion, either skin-to-skin or with a disposable sponge, stopping 3 cm below the elbows. Interlace your fingers and rub them back and forth for part of this time. This should take a total of 2 to 6 minutes.
- Rinse hands and arms, keeping the hands uppermost.
- Discard the sponge, if used, and rinse off the solution.
- Dry with a sterile paper or cloth towel, starting with one arm from the fingers and hands toward the forearm and elbow. Turn the towel and grasp a clean area; use the same procedure to dry the other arm. Take care not to dry back from the unsterile elbow region toward the clean hands.
- Turn off the water, but do not touch the faucet as you turn it off. Have someone turn it off for you, turn it with your elbow, or turn it off by first covering the faucet with your towel after you have finished thoroughly drying your hands and arms.

Using an alcohol based hand rub for surgical antisepsis: A two-stage surgical scrub using an antiseptic detergent, followed by application of an alcohol-containing preparation, is also effective. For example, a 1- or 2-minute scrub with 4% chlorhexidine gluconate or povidone iodine followed by thorough drying and then the application of an alcohol-based product can be as effective as a five-minute scrub with an antiseptic detergent.

To perform an antiseptic wash using an alcohol-based hand scrub, select a product with persistent activity that is designed for this purpose and follow the manufacturer's instructions. Before applying the alcohol solution, prewash hands and forearms with a nonantimicrobial soap and dry your hands and forearms completely with a new, clean paper towel. Apply the alcohol hand rub as recommended and rub the arms and hands vigorously until dry. Allow your hands and forearms to air dry thoroughly before donning sterile gloves.

Contact with spores: Wash hands with either antimicrobial soap and water or with non-antimicrobial soap and water if contact with spores (such as *Clostridium difficile* or *Bacillus anthracis*) is likely to have occurred. Washing and rinsing hands is recommended because none of the available antiseptic agents are very effective against spores, including alcohol-based agents.

Drying your hands: By far the safest option is to use a new, clean, dry, good-quality, preferably lint-free paper towel each time you must dry your hands. Do not use bath or kitchen towels that are already in use. If you want to use cloth, bring enough freshly laundered hand towels in a resealable plastic bag to supply yourself and your assistants with several clean towels to be used during the birth. (I know of one out of hospital birth where the midwife and her client both got near-fatal infections, and the only thing that anyone could figure out as a cause was that the midwife had repeatedly dried her hands with a kitchen towel that was already in use.)

Skin care after non-surgical handwashing: Apply an emollient hand cream to protect skin from the drying effects of regular hand decontamination. If a particular soap, antimicrobial hand wash or alcohol hand rub is irritating, experiment with others until a suitable one is found. Consult a local medical care supply house regarding lotions that will not interfere with the action of antimicrobial products. Look for products that are free of mineral oil, paraben and other petroleum-based ingredients so that the lotion does not compromise the integrity of glove materials.

Refilling solution containers: Do not "top off" a dispenser of hand cleaning solution, as this can result in contamination. Use it until it is gone and then wash and dry the dispenser thoroughly before refilling (put it through a dishwasher cycle if the container will tolerate it) or use a new dispenser.

Jewelry: The skin underneath rings is more heavily colonized than the skin on fingers without rings. Gram-negative bacilli (e.g., *Escherichia coli, E. cloacae*, *Klebsiella* spp. and *Acinetobacter* spp.) are often found on the skin underlying rings. Whether wearing rings results in greater transmission of pathogens is unknown, however. The mean bacterial colony counts on hands after handwashing is similar among persons wearing rings and those who do not. Further studies are needed to establish if wearing rings results in greater transmission of pathogens in health care settings.

Fingernails and artificial nails: Subungual areas (under the fingernails) can harbor high concentrations of bacteria, most frequently coagulase-negative staphylococci, gram-negative rods (including *Pseudomonas* spp.), corynebacteria and yeasts. While freshly applied nail polish does not increase the colony count, chipped polish may support the growth of larger numbers of organisms on fingernails. Even after careful handwashing or the use of surgical scrubs, the fingers often harbor substantial numbers of potential pathogens in the subungual spaces.

Whether artificial nails contribute to transmission of health care–associated infections is unknown. Those with artificial nails are nevertheless more likely to harbor gram-negative pathogens on their fingertips than those with natural nails, both before and after hand washing. Whether the length of natural or artificial nails is a substantial risk factor is also unknown because the majority of bacterial growth occurs along the proximal 1 mm of the nail adjacent to the subungual skin. Given all these unknowns, it is probably prudent to keep the nails natural and to trim them short, no longer than 0.25".

Personal Protective Equipment (PPE)

Wear personal protective equipment (PPE) (i.e., gloves, eye protection) when the nature of the anticipated care may include contact with blood or body fluids. Prevent contamination of clothing and skin when removing PPE. When you are finished caring for the woman, remove and discard PPE into a plastic bag or contained laundry receptacle.

Examination and surgical gloves

Wear exam gloves when it can be reasonably anticipated that contact with blood or other potentially infectious materials, mucous membranes, nonintact skin or potentially contaminated intact skin (e.g., covered with birth fluids or soiled with stool or urine) could occur. Choose gloves that fit and that are appropriately durable in relation to the task. Wear disposable medical exam gloves or reusable utility gloves for cleaning the environment or medical equipment. Remove gloves after contact with a woman or her newborn or with the surrounding environment (including medical equipment) using proper technique to prevent hand contamination. Don new gloves for the care of each woman or newborn. Do not wash exam gloves for the purpose of reuse since this practice has been associated with transmission of pathogens. Change gloves when providing care if the hands will move from a contaminated body site (e.g., perineal area) to a clean body site (e.g., face).

The protectiveness of gloves: While scrubbing removes organisms for the skin, after a time, the resident organisms in the deeper layers of skin are carried to the surface on perspiration and oil secretion and the bacterial count rises. Thus, gloves form a protective barrier.

It is important to understand, however, that gloves do not provide complete protection against hand contamination. Bacterial flora found on patients has been recovered from the hands of those wearing gloves during patient contact. In such instances, pathogens presumably gain access to the caregiver's hands via small defects in gloves or via contamination as the gloves are removed. Organisms multiply rapidly in the warm, enclosed environment beneath the glove. Therefore, if you puncture a glove during use, it should be removed and discarded, your hands should be rewashed and dried and the glove should be replaced as soon as possible. If it is impossible to wash your hands right away and there is time, dry them thoroughly and then use an alcohol-based product as previously described. If there is no time for that, have an assistant hand you a paper towel to dry your hands quickly, reglove and wash your hands as soon as you can.

Latex weakens when exposed to mineral, petroleum and vegetable oils. In uncontrolled FDA experiments with condoms, air pressure tests show significant weakening with any oil, while stretch tests showed no discernable change. The FDA has noted that mineral oil (a petroleum product) causes rapid deterioration, with splits appearing in glove material shortly after exposure. It is not understood how this weakness occurs. Water-soluble oil-free lotions are thus recommended for use with latex.

Another option is to wear vinyl gloves. Vinyl is generally considered impervious to oil of any kind, but it breaks down rapidly in the presence of alcohol. Therefore, if you are using an alcohol hand rub, it is imperative that your hands be completely dry before donning vinyl gloves. Vinyl is also a good choice when you or the client are allergic to latex.

Donning sterile gloves

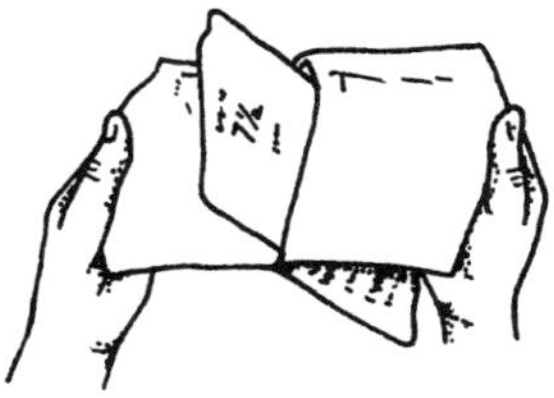 After washing your hands, have an assistant open the gloves by grasping the flaps on either side with thumb and index fingers and rolling her hands apart to expose the inner, sterile wrapper. Now, lift out the inner sterile wrapper.	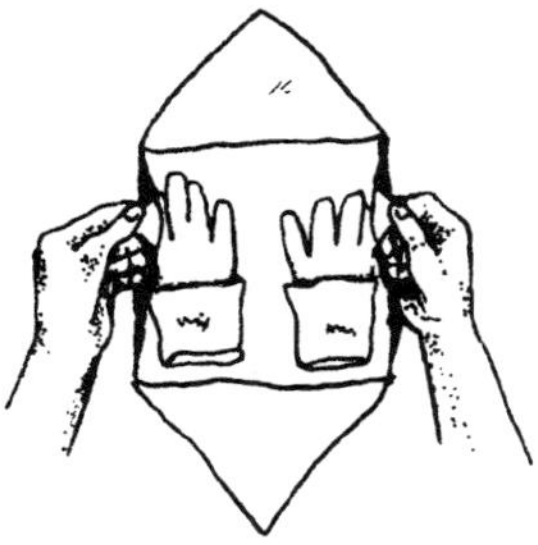 Open the inner wrap and lay it flat, with the cuffs of the gloves pointing toward you. Each glove will have a turned-up cuff.	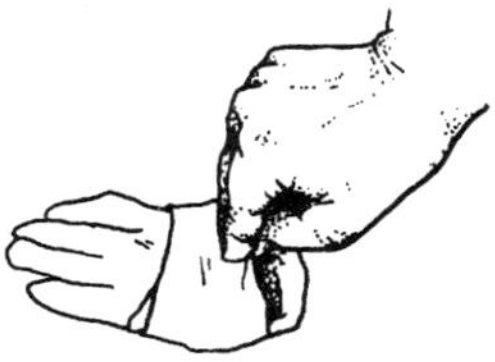 Pick up the first glove by the edge of the cuff with your dominant hand, glove fingers pointing down.
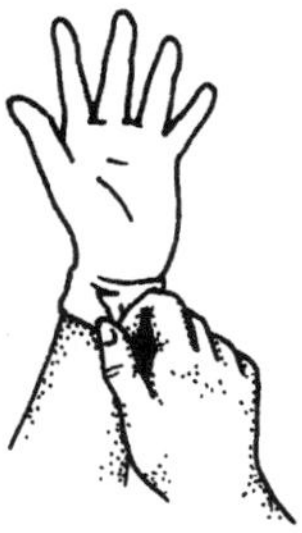 Maneuver the glove onto your nondominant hand without touching the *outer* surface.	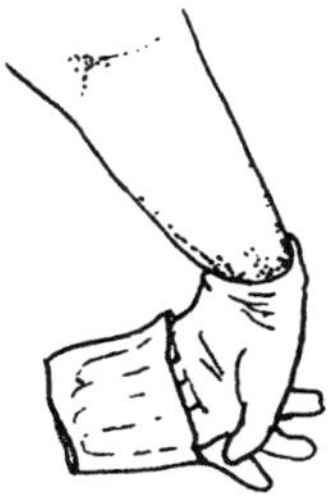 Pick up the other glove by inserting your gloved fingers *inside* the turned-up cuff (so as not to touch the *inner* surface).	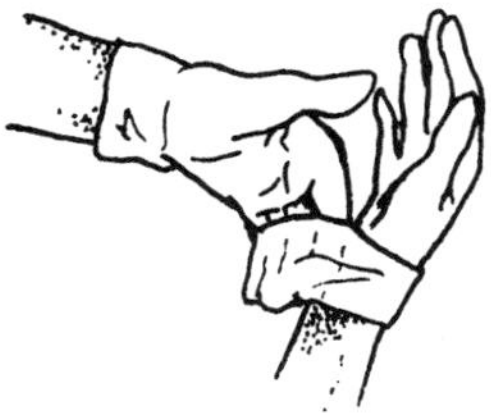 Insert your dominant hand into the second glove without touching the inner surface with your non-dominant gloved hand. Now, turn the cuff right-side out with your nondominant hand.

If no assistant is there, open the outer wrapper, being careful not to touch the inner wrapper, and prop the package in a convenient place. You can then remove the inner wrapper after you have washed your hands.

In short, never touch the outer surface of the sterile gloves with your bare hands and never touch bare skin or the inner glove surface once the sterile gloves are on (Timby, 1989).

Removing used gloves: Gloves should be removed carefully to avoid splattering body fluids. To do so, pinch the outer surface of the cuff and draw the glove over the hand by turning it inside out. Do not touch the outer, soiled portion as you do so. Discard the glove. Remove the remaining glove by slipping your fingers beneath the cuff and removing it as before. If the glove is so soiled that you risk skin contamination during removal, get your assistant to turn the water on for you. Carefully (so as not to splatter fluids) wash and rinse 3your hands with the gloves still on; then remove them as described.

After removing gloves: Hands should be decontaminated with an alcohol hand rub or washed with an antimicrobial soap after removing gloves. Gloves should not be washed or reused if it can possibly be avoided (sometimes in the developing world, it cannot). After using powdered gloves, certain alcohol hand rubs may interact with residual powder on the hands, resulting in a gritty feeling. If powdered gloves are commonly used, various alcohol-based hand rubs should be tested after the gloves are removed to avoid selecting a product that causes this undesirable reaction.

Protective clothing (gowns)

Protective clothing may be in the form of clothes that you don at the birth or a gown; minimally, it may be an apron. It should be washed and ready to use at births. It should protect skin and prevent soiling or contamination of your other clothing during procedures and care activities when contact with blood, body fluids, secretions or excretions is anticipated. Wear protective clothing for direct contact if the woman or newborn has uncontained secretions or excretions. Remove protective clothing and perform hand hygiene before leaving the woman's environment. Clean clothing should be worn for repeated contacts with the same woman or newborn. Routine donning of protective clothing, such as a gown, upon entrance into a high-risk area (e.g., ICU, neonatal intensive care unit [NICU]) is not indicated.

Environmental Considerations

Respiratory hygiene

Take steps to contain respiratory secretions to prevent droplet and fomite transmission of respiratory pathogens, especially during seasonal outbreaks of viral ear-nose-throat respiratory tract infections (e.g., influenza, respiratory syncytial virus [RSV], adenovirus, parainfluenza virus).

If your practice is such that you have a waiting area, provide a separate waiting area for those who have signs and symptoms of a respiratory infection, beginning at the point of initial encounter in your office (i.e., reception and waiting areas). Post signs at entrances and in strategic places with instructions to those with respiratory infections to cover their mouths and noses when coughing or sneezing, use and dispose of tissues, and perform hand hygiene after hands have been in contact with respiratory secretions. Provide tissues and no-touch receptacles (e.g., foot-pedal–operated lid or open, plastic-lined waste basket) for disposal of used tissues.

Provide resources and instructions for performing hand hygiene in or near waiting areas in ambulatory and inpatient settings; provide conveniently located dispensers of alcohol-based hand rubs and, where sinks are available, supplies for handwashing.

During periods of increased prevalence of respiratory infections in the community (e.g., as indicated by increased school absenteeism or increased number of persons seeking care for a respiratory infection), offer masks to those who are coughing and other symptomatic persons (e.g., persons who accompany ill patients) upon entry into your office, birthing center or medical office and encourage them to maintain special separation, ideally a distance of at least 3 feet, from others in common waiting areas. Some facilities may find it easier to institute this recommendation year-round as a standard of practice.

Choosing the right place to care for a woman or her newborn

If you have a birthing center, when deciding upon what exam room or birth room to assign a woman, consider the potential for transmission of infectious agents. Request that women who pose a risk for transmission to others (e.g., uncontained secretions, excretions or wound drainage; infants with suspected viral respiratory or gastrointestinal infections) use the room you have set aside for this purpose, if relevant to your practice. Determine where to place a client based on the following principles:

- Routes of transmission of a known or suspected infectious agent
- Risk factors for transmission in the infected woman or newborn
- Risk factors for adverse outcomes resulting from a healthcare–associated infection (HAI) in other women, newborns or accompanying persons in the area or room being considered for her use.
- Availability of single rooms in your clinic (if relevant)
- If you run a large clinic, assess options for room-sharing (e.g., grouping women or newborns with the same infection).

Keeping the environment clean

If you have a birth center or clinic, establish policies and procedures for the cleaning of environmental surfaces as indicated by the level of client contact and degree of soiling. Clean and disinfect surfaces that are likely to be contaminated with pathogens—including those that are in close proximity to the woman or her newborn (e.g., bed rails, birthing stools, birth tubs, etc.), frequently touched surfaces such as door knobs, and surfaces in and surrounding toilets in prenatal rooms—on a more frequent schedule compared to that for other surfaces (e.g., horizontal surfaces in waiting rooms). Use Environmental Protection Agency (EPA)– registered disinfectants that have microbiocidal (i.e., killing) activity against the pathogens most likely to contaminate the patient care environment. Use in accordance with manufacturer's instructions. Even if you are doing all your visits and births at the mother's home, your equipment can carry pathogens from one home to the next and ideally should to be at least wiped down with an alcohol swab between each use. Clean equipment more thoroughly if the equipment is used in a home where people are sick.

If your waiting area has child play toys, clean the area and the toys at regular intervals. Select play toys that can be easily disinfected by hand and then put into a dishwasher. Do not offer stuffed furry toys if they will be shared. Clean and disinfect large stationary toys (e.g., climbing equipment) at least weekly and whenever visibly soiled. When a toy requires cleaning, store it in a designated labeled container separate from toys that are clean and ready for use.

Clean and disinfect multi-use electronic equipment, especially items that are used by clients, those used during delivery of care and those moved in and out of the woman's space frequently (e.g., daily). There are no official recommendations regarding the use of removable protective covers or washable keyboards.

Textiles and laundry: Handle used textiles and fabrics with minimum agitation to avoid contamination of air, surfaces and persons. Bag soiled linens and transfer them to a washing machine as soon as possible. If you have a clinic with a laundry chute, ensure that it is properly designed, maintained, and used in a manner to minimize dispersion of aerosols from contaminated laundry.

Hand Hygiene Products (the Long Version)

Here follows a detailed review of the most widely available active agents used in hand hygiene products in the United States as of this writing. I include all these details because midwives need to be able to intelligently assess if a product will do what they want it to and many of us do not have a hospital purchasing department to evaluate products for us.

Terminology

First, some definitions: **Antimicrobial** refers to any product or ingredient that destroys or inhibits bacteria, viruses, molds or all three. **Antibacterials** are only effective against bacteria; **antivirals** are only active against viruses. **Disinfectants** are products that destroy infectious agents (usually both bacterial and viral) on objects like counter tops. **Antiseptics** are products for use on the skin, including those intended for cleaning wounds. Another class of products includes objects with embedded antimicrobial agents, usually triclosan. Products labeled "-cidal," as in **bactericidal**, inactivate the microbe specified; while others are labeled "-static," as in **bacteriostatic**, meaning they inhibit, but do not inactivate, the microbe. **MIC** stands for "minimum inhibitory concentration" and reflects the smallest amount of an agent that will inhibit, but not necessarily inactivate, an infectious agent.

Plain (nonantimicrobial) soap

Soaps are detergent-based products that contain esterified fatty acids and sodium or potassium hydroxide. They are available as bars, powders, tissues and liquids. They help remove dirt, soil, and organic substances from the skin. Plain soaps can cause considerable skin irritation and dryness, although adding emollients may reduce this tendency. Regular soaps have minimal, if any, antimicrobial activity but can remove loosely adherent, transient flora. They may not remove resistant pathogens from the hands of hospital personnel and may actually increase bacterial counts on the skin. Plain soaps may become contaminated, which can lead to colonization of hands with gram-negative bacilli.

Alcohols

Most alcohol-based hand antiseptics contain isopropanol (isopropyl), ethanol, n-propanol (approved in Europe) or a combination. They work by denaturing proteins. Solution s containing 60 to 95% alcohol are most effective. Higher concentrations are less potent because proteins are not denatured easily in the absence of water.

Alcohols are active against gram-positive and gram-negative vegetative bacteria, multidrug-resistant pathogens (e.g., MRSA and VRE), mycobacterium tuberculosis, various fungi, certain enveloped (lipophilic) viruses (e.g., herpes simplex, human immunodeficiency virus [HIV], influenza, respiratory syncytial virus, and vaccinia) and hepatitis B and C viruses, these last two are somewhat less susceptible but are likely to be destroyed by 60 to 70% alcohol. Alcohols have poor activity against bacterial spores, protozoan oocysts and certain nonenveloped (nonlipophilic) viruses such as hepatitis A. The inactivation of nonenveloped viruses is influenced by the concentration of alcohol, temperature, disinfectant–virus volume ratio, protein load, and time of exposure to the alcohol. Ethanol has greater activity against viruses than isopropanol.

Alcohols are rapidly germicidal when applied but have no appreciable persistent (residual) activity. Even so, regrowth occurs slowly after use, presumably because of the sublethal effect alcohols have on some skin bacteria. The addition of chlorhexidine, quaternary ammonium compounds, octenidine or triclosan can result in persistent activity.

It is generally advised not to use alcohol when the hands are visibly dirty or contaminated with body fluids. However, when relatively small amounts of body fluid are present, ethanol and isopropanol may reduce viable bacterial counts on hands more than antimicrobial soap.

The efficacy of alcohol-based hand hygiene products is affected by several factors, including the type, volume and concentration of alcohol; contact time; and the presence of water on the hands when the alcohol is applied. Using too little alcohol is no more effective than washing hands with plain soap and water. Using at least 3 mL is recommended, although the ideal volume is not known and may vary among products. Follow manufacturer recommendations, but if hands feel dry after rubbing hands together for 10 to 15 seconds, it is likely that an insufficient volume of product was applied. Alcohol-based hand rinses appear to be more effective than alcohol-based gels. Because alcohol-impregnated towelettes contain only a small amount of alcohol, they are not sufficiently effective.

The drying effect of alcohol can be reduced by adding 1 to 3% glycerol or other skin-conditioning agents, although even hand rubs containing emollients may cause transient stinging in broken skin. Allergic contact dermatitis or urticaria syndrome caused by hypersensitivity to alcohol or to various additives in certain alcohol hand rubs occurs only rarely.

Alcohols are flammable. Flash points of alcohol-based hand rubs are low, ranging from 69.8 to 75.2°F (21 to 24°C), depending on the type and concentration of alcohol. Store hand rubs away from high temperatures or flames. Solutions should be thoroughly rubbed in and hands dry prior to moving on to other activities. Use containers that minimize evaporation.

Contamination of alcohol-based solutions is rare. A cluster of pseudoinfections caused by contamination of ethyl alcohol by *Bacillus cereus* spores has been described.

Chlorhexidine

Chlorhexidine gluconate, a cationic bisbiguanide, is another antimicrobial agent. Chlorhexidine base is only minimally soluble in water, but the digluconate form is water-soluble. Its antimicrobial activity is slower than alcohol's and is likely attributable to attachment to, and subsequent disruption of, cytoplasmic membranes, resulting in the release of cellular contents. It has good activity against gram-positive bacteria, somewhat less against gram-negative bacteria and fungi, and only minimal activity against tubercle bacilli. It is not sporicidal but is active against enveloped viruses. It is substantially less active against nonenveloped viruses (e.g., rotavirus, adenovirus and enteroviruses).

This antimicrobial activity is only minimally affected by organic material, including blood, but can be reduced by natural soaps, various inorganic anions, nonionic surfactants, and hand creams containing anionic emulsifying agents. Aqueous or detergent formulations containing 0.5% or 0.75% chlorhexidine or those containing 1% chlorhexidine gluconate are more effective than plain soap, but they are less effective than antiseptic detergent preparations containing 4% chlorhexidine gluconate. Chlorhexidine has good residual activity and adding low concentrations (0.5 to 1.0%) to alcohol-based preparations results in greater residual activity than alcohol alone.

These formulas have a good safety record, with minimal, if any, absorption through the skin. Avoid contact with the eyes when using preparations with >1% chlorhexidine, because it can cause conjunctivitis and severe corneal damage. The substance is also toxic to internal ear structures. Direct contact with brain tissue and the meninges should be avoided so it should not be used on babies with any kind of exposed organ defect, such as spina bifida. Skin irritation is concentration dependent, with products containing 4% most likely to cause dermatitis when used frequently; allergic reactions are uncommon. Occasional outbreaks of nosocomial infections have been traced to contaminated solutions of chlorhexidine.

Chloroxylenol

Chloroxylenol, also known as parachlorometaxylenol (PCMX), is a halogen-substituted phenolic compound that has been used as a preservative and as an active agent in antimicrobial soaps.

The antimicrobial activity of PCMX is probably attributable to inactivation of bacterial enzymes and alteration of cell walls. It has good activity against gram-positive organisms and fair activity against gram-negative bacteria, mycobacteria, and certain viruses. PCMX is less active against *Pseudomonas aeruginosa*, but adding ethylene-diamine-tetraacetic acid (EDTA) increases its activity against *Pseudomonas* spp. and other pathogens.

PCMX is not as rapidly active as chlorhexidine gluconate or iodophors, and its residual activity is less pronounced than that of chlorhexidine gluconate. In 1994, the FDA stated that there are insufficient data to classify this agent as safe and effective. Further evaluation by the FDA is ongoing.

The antimicrobial activity of PCMX is minimally affected by the presence of organic matter, but it is neutralized by nonionic surfactants. PCMX is absorbed through the skin but appears to be well tolerated, and allergic reactions associated with its use are uncommon. PCMX is available in concentrations of 0.3 to 3.75%. In-use contamination of a PCMX-containing preparation has been reported.

Hexachlorophene

Hexachlorophene is a bisphenol composed of two phenolic groups and three chlorine moieties. Its antimicrobial properties result from its ability to inactivate essential enzyme systems in microorganisms. Hexachlorophene is bacteriostatic, with good activity against *S. aureus* and relatively weak activity against gram-negative bacteria, fungi, and mycobacteria.

As a hygienic handwash, it demonstrates only modest efficacy after a single use. It shows residual activity for several hours and a gradual reduction in bacterial counts on hands after multiple uses. Repeated use results in skin absorption. Regular exposure to 3% hexachlorophene for washing results in blood levels of 0.1 to 0.6 ppm hexachlorophene.

In the early 1970s, infants bathed with hexachlorophene developed neurotoxicity (vacuolar degeneration [a small cavity in the cytoplasm that becomes swollen]). After its routine use in nurseries was discontinued in 1972, however, the incidence of health care–associated *S. aureus* infections in hospital nurseries rose substantially (in fact, vernix has been found to contain polypeptide antibiotics that help prevent skin problems in neonates [Tollin, 2005]). In several instances, the rate of infections decreased when hexachlorophene bathing was reinstituted. Despite these occurrences, current guidelines still recommend against the routine bathing of neonates with hexachlorophene because of its neurotoxic effects.

This agent is FDA classified as not generally recognized as safe and effective for use as an antiseptic handwash. Do not use it to bathe open wounds or extensive areas of susceptible, sensitive skin. Soaps containing 3% hexachlorophene are available by prescription only.

Iodine and Iodophor

Iodine is an effective antiseptic. Iodine molecules rapidly penetrate the cell wall of microorganisms and inactivate cells by forming complexes with amino acids and unsaturated fatty acids, resulting in impaired protein synthesis and alteration of cell membranes. Because it often causes irritation and discoloring of skin, iodine has been largely replaced by iodophors as the active ingredient in antiseptics.

Iodophors are composed of elemental iodine, iodide or triiodide and a polymer carrier of high molecular weight. The amount of molecular iodine present (so-called free iodine) determines the level of antimicrobial activity. "Available" iodine refers to the total amount of iodine that can be titrated with sodium thiosulfate.

Typical 10% povidone-iodine formulations contain 1% available iodine and yield free iodine concentrations of 1 ppm. Combining iodine with various polymers such as polyvinyl pyrrolidone (i.e., povidone) and ethoxylated nonionic detergents (i.e., poloxamers) increases its solubility, promotes its sustained release and reduces skin irritation.

Iodine and iodophors have bactericidal activity against gram-positive, gram-negative, and certain spore-forming bacteria (e.g., clostridia and *Bacillus* spp.) and are active against mycobacteria, viruses and fungi. In concentrations used in antiseptics, however, iodophors are not usually sporicidal.

Iodophors reduce the number of viable organisms on washed hands. Their antimicrobial activity can be affected by pH, temperature, exposure time, concentration of total available iodine, and the amount and type of organic and inorganic compounds present (e.g., alcohols and detergents). Povidone-iodine in 5 to 10% concentrations has been tentatively FDA classified as an effective agent for use as an antiseptic handwash for health care personnel.

The extent to which iodophors exhibit persistent antimicrobial activity after they have been washed off the skin is unclear. Persistent activity has been noted for periods ranging from 30 to 60 minutes to six hours. Bacterial counts obtained after gloves were worn for 1 to 4 hours after washing, show poor persistent iodophor activity. The in vivo antimicrobial activity of iodophors is substantially reduced in the presence of body fluids.

The majority of iodophor preparations used for hand hygiene contain 7.5 to 10% povidone-iodine. Formulations with lower concentrations also have good antimicrobial activity because dilution can increase free iodine concentrations. As the amount of free iodine increases, though, the degree of skin irritation also rises. Iodophors cause less skin irritation and fewer allergic reactions than iodine but still cause more irritant contact dermatitis than other antiseptics commonly used for hand hygiene. Occasionally, iodophor antiseptics have become contaminated with gram-negative bacilli as a result of poor manufacturing processes and have caused outbreaks or pseudo-outbreaks of infection.

Quaternary ammonium compounds

Among the quaternary ammonium compounds, alkyl benzalkonium chlorides are the most widely used as antiseptics. Others include benzethonium chloride, cetrimide, and cetylpyridium chloride. The antimicrobial activity of these compounds is probably attributable to absorption into the cytoplasmic membrane, with subsequent leakage of low molecular weight cytoplasmic constituents.

These compounds are primarily bacteriostatic and fungistatic, although they are microbicidal against certain organisms at high concentrations. They are more active against gram-positive than gram-negative bacilli, have relatively weak activity against mycobacteria and fungi, and have greater activity against lipophilic viruses. Their effectiveness is adversely affected by organic material, and they are not compatible with anionic detergents.

Quaternary ammonium compounds are usually well tolerated. Because of weak activity against gram-negative bacteria, however, benzalkonium chloride is prone to contamination by these organisms. Several outbreaks of infection or pseudoinfection have been traced to quaternary ammonium compounds contaminated with gram-negative bacilli. For this reason, these compounds have been seldom used for hand antisepsis during the last 15 to 20 years in the US, although newer handwashing products containing benzalkonium chloride or benzethonium chloride have recently been introduced. Cleaning hands with antimicrobial wipes containing a quaternary ammonium compound has been found to be about as effective as using plain soap and water for handwashing; both were less effective than decontaminating hands with an alcohol-based hand rub. One laboratory-based study reported that an alcohol-free hand rub containing a quaternary ammonium compound was efficacious in reducing microbial counts on the hands. Further studies of such products are needed to determine if newer formulations are effective in health care settings.

Triclosan

Triclosan (2,4,4'-trichloro-2'-hydroxy-diphenyl ether) is a nonionic, colorless substance that can be incorporated into antiseptic soaps and has been widely used in other consumer products, such as toys. Concentrations of 0.2 to 2% have antimicrobial activity. Triclosan enters bacterial cells, where it affects the cytoplasmic membrane and synthesis of RNA, fatty acids and proteins. Its antibacterial activity is attributable to binding to the active site of enoyl-acyl carrier protein reductase.

Although triclosan has a broad range of antimicrobial activity, it is often merely bacteriostatic. MICs range from 0.1 to 10 μg/mL, whereas minimum bactericidal concentrations are much higher, ranging from 25 to 500 μg/mL. Triclosan's activity against gram-positive organisms (including MRSA) is greater than against gram-negative bacilli, particularly *P. aeruginosa*. It possesses reasonable activity against mycobacterial and *Candida* spp., but has limited activity against filamentous fungi. In a 0.1% solution, triclosan reduces bacterial counts on hands by 2.8 $\log_{10}$ after a one-minute hygienic handwash. In several studies, log reductions have been lower after triclosan is used than when chlorhexidine, iodophors or alcohol-based products were applied.

Triclosan has persistent activity on the skin. Its activity in hand care products is affected by pH, by the presence of emollients or humectants, and by the ionic nature of the formulation. Triclosan's activity is not substantially affected by organic matter, but it can be inhibited by surfactants present in certain formulations. The majority of products containing < 2% triclosan are well tolerated and seldom cause allergic reactions. The use of triclosan- containing products for hand antisepsis may be related to decreased MRSA infections. Triclosan's lack of potent activity against gram-negative bacilli has resulted in occasional reports of contamination.

In 1994, the FDA classified triclosan <1.0% as an agent for which insufficient data exist to classify as safe and effective for use as an antiseptic handwash. Triclosan appears to be low in toxicity, but it is structurally similar to the herbicide 2,4-D (2,4-dichlorohenoxyacetic acid) and 2,3,7,8-TCDD, the most toxic form of dioxin. Some are concerned that this similarity could give rise to contamination of triclosan with dioxins, since dioxin contamination of 2,4-D and other chlorinated phenolic compounds has occurred. When triclosan in water is exposed to ultraviolet light, a type of dioxin is formed, although not the most toxic form. Triclosan has been detected in breast milk and in the aquatic environment, and it may be an endocrine disruptor (Dickey, 2008). Triclosan is probably best avoided altogether.

Hypochlorite

Aqueous hypochlorite solution (4% w/w [weight to weight]), which was first recommended by Semmelweis in 1861, and has been found to be 30 times more effective than a 1-minute rub using 60% isopropanol. Nevertheless, because hypochlorite solutions are often irritating and have a strong odor, they are seldom used for hand hygiene today.

Alternative antimicrobials

As midwives, we want to use the most effective agents with the least risk of harmful effects. Therefore, we are very interested in alternative products for cleaning. We must be careful, however, about taking the word of a manufacturer about the efficacy of any product.

Common household substances like vinegar and borax are often suggested as "alternative" disinfectants. The basis of the claim for vinegar is its low pH, which is hostile to some gastrointestinal bugs when ingested. While safe and effective as household cleaners, none of these substances is registered as a disinfectant with the EPA and should not be depended upon to disinfect.

Similarly, several plant oils (i.e., tea tree oil, grapefruit seed extract) have disinfectant properties, and there are some commercial products based on these ingredients. Look for an EPA registration number on the bottle; if there is none, do not assume that these products can truly disinfect. One such registered product is based on thymol (from thyme oil) as an active ingredient: Sol-U-Guard™ by Melaleuca.

Hydrogen peroxide is also a recognized disinfectant and is found in some products, though most are not available to consumers. One that can be obtained easily is H2Orange2, a combination of hydrogen peroxide and orange oil. This is a low-toxicity product, although citrus oils may not be tolerated by some people with chemical sensitivities. Hydrogen peroxide is one of the safest disinfectants available, provided the concentration is not above about 3%, which is the concentration available in over-the-counter antiseptics (concentrated hydrogen peroxide is a potent oxidizer and may be dangerous). You had probably better not depend upon ordinary, medicine-cabinet hydrogen peroxide alone to disinfect, however, unless it is all you have access to, since there are no label instructions for that use. It is better to stick with a registered product; if you have questions, call the manufacturer. You can usually find a phone number on the label.

The activity of antiseptic agents against spore-forming bacteria

The widespread prevalence of diarrhea caused by *Clostridium difficile* (*C. diff*) and the exposure of postal workers to human *Bacillus anthracis* (anthrax) has raised concern regarding the activity of antiseptic agents against spore-forming bacteria. None of the agents (including alcohols, chlorhexidine, hexachlorophene, iodophors, PCMX and triclosan) used in antiseptic handwash or antiseptic hand-rub preparations are reliably sporicidal against *Clostridium* spp. or *Bacillus* spp. Washing hands with nonantimicrobial or antimicrobial soap and water may help to physically remove spores from the surface of contaminated hands. Providers should wear gloves when caring for patients with *C. difficile*–associated diarrhea or during a general outbreak. After removing gloves, hands should be washed with plain soap or an antimicrobial soap and water or disinfected with an alcohol-based hand rub. Providers with suspected or documented exposure to *B. anthracis*—contaminated items should be encouraged to wash their hands with a plain soap or an antimicrobial soap and water.

Antiseptic-resistant bacteria

Resistance of bacteria to antiseptic agents can either be an intrinsic characteristic of a species or an acquired trait. Several reports have described strains of bacteria that appear to have acquired resistance (when defined by MICs established in vitro) to certain antiseptics (e.g., chlorhexidine, quaternary ammonium compounds and triclosan). Nonetheless, because the antiseptic concentrations that are actually used are often substantially higher than the MICs of resistant strains, the clinical relevance of these in vitro findings is questionable. More studies are needed to see if resistance to antiseptic agents is of epidemiologic significance and if it influences the prevalence of antibiotic-resistant strains.

When Prions Diseases are a Concern

The measures in this section hit the high points of dealing with prions and are included to give you some idea of what dealing with potential prion contamination looks like. Prion protocols may have changed since this printing: please Google "CDC prion" to find out what the complete and current recommendations may be.

In the US as of this printing, it is not recommended to sterilize for prions unless prion contamination is likely due to a known or suspected infection. In the UK however, it is postulated that there is a reservoir of undiagnosed prion disease in the population due to the outbreak of bovine spongiform encephalopathy (BSE) or "mad cow disease," that started to surface in the 1980s. The National Health Service has therefore recommended that midwives use disposable suture kits to eliminate the concern of cross-infectivity. These instruments are used once and incinerated. Even though such instruments are of poor quality, they can usually withstand a single use without a problem. Since prions are so hard to deactivate, this is considered the very best protection when actual infection has been identified or is suspected.

When non-disposable instruments are used, sterilization requires denaturation of the misfolded prion proteins to a state where the molecule is no longer able to trigger normal proteins to misfold. The challenge is that prions are generally quite resistant to proteases, heat, radiation, and formalin treatments, although their infectivity can be reduced by some of these treatments. In fact, infectivity is strongly stabilized by drying or fixation with alcohol, formalin or glutaraldehyde. As a consequence, contaminated materials should not be exposed to fixation reagents, and should be kept wet with water between the time of use and disinfection by immersion in chemical disinfectants (WHO, 1999).

Effective prion decontamination relies upon protein hydrolysis or reduction or destruction of the protein's tertiary structure. Autoclaving at a temperature of 273.2°F (134°C) maintained for 18 minutes in a pressurized steam autoclave may not be enough to deactivate prions. Thus, chemical disinfection and heat are used. The list of effective chemicals is short; it includes bleach and soda lye, as recommended by WHO (1999).

Protecting yourself: There is no risk during routine care. In the presence of an open wound or at the time of birth, disposable barrier protection should be worn at all times and discarded immediately after use. All disposable items from the birth, including fluid-soaked underpads and the placenta should be double bagged in biohazard bags for later incineration. Sharps should be separately packaged and marked as prion contaminated. These should be given to your biohazard waste management company and they should be informed that they are potentially contaminated with prions.

Cleaning of surfaces: Strive to keep everything contained by covering working areas with large disposable sheets and pads that can be discarded. For soiled surfaces that can tolerate it, first mob up as much material as possible using disposable towels and toss these into the double biohazard bag. Then flood with sodium hydroxide (2N NaOH concentration) or undiluted bleach. Let stand for 1 hour; then mop up and rinse with water. For surfaces that cannot tolerate either of these solutions, thorough cleaning will remove most infectivity by dilution and some additional benefit may be derived from the use of one or another partially effective method such as chlorine dioxide or glutaraldehyde.

Presterilization of instruments: The World Health Organization (1999) recommends either of the following procedures for the pre-sterilization of all heat-resistant non-disposable surgical instruments to remove most, if not all infectivity under the widest range of conditions. These options have been selected because they are the easiest for midwives to use. This is the one exception to the rule of never soaking your instruments in these types of strong solutions, although doing so will be hard on them and shorten their life.

1. Wipe the instruments to reduce gross contamination and discard the wipes. Immerse the instruments in 1N NaOH (sodium hydroxide) or bleach (sodium hypochlorite in a 2% concentration [20,000 parts per million available chlorine]) for 1 hour; rinse throughly; transfer instruments to a water bath; heat in a gravity-displacement autoclave at 249.8°F (121°C) for 1 hour; clean; and then perform routine sterilization procedures.
2. Prepare instruments as above. Then immerse them in either 1N NaOH or bleach (sodium hypochlorite–20,000 parts per million available chlorine) for 1 hour; remove and rinse in water, then transfer to an open pan and heat in a gravity-displacement autoclave at 249.8°F (121°C) or in a porous-load autoclave at 273.2°F (134°C) for 1 hour; clean; and then perform routine sterilization procedures.

After you go through your routine sterilization procedures, autoclave them again at a temperature of at least 249.8°F (121°C) for 18 to 30 minutes. Higher temperatures may actually fix the proteins and make them more stable, so more heat is not necessarily better (Mason & Day, 1999).

All of the recommended chemical disinfectants are toxic. Wear disposable protective clothing, eye protection and gloves. Use them in a well ventilated area.

Sodium hydroxide readily reacts with carbon dioxide which neutralizes it, diminishes its disinfective properties. The working solutions of sodium hydroxide should be prepared fresh for each use either from solid NaOH pellets, or by dilution of 10 N NaOH stock solutions. To make 1N (N=normal) solution of sodium hydroxide dissolve 40 grams of NaHO in distilled water and then fill container with more distilled water to create 1 litre of solution.

Sodium hypochlorite bleach (NaOCl) can be prepared in a well ventilated area from industrial grade or commercially available bleach. Dilute the bleach to provide a final concentration of 2% (20,000 ppm) available chlorine. Most commercially available bleaches in the US have a 5.25% concentration, which contains 25,000 ppm available chlorine; it can be used straight.

Prion contamination of the skin: Intact skin exposure to potentially prion-contaminated materials should be followed promptly by washing with 1N NaOH or 5.25% bleach for two to three minutes, followed by extensive washing with water. For needle sticks or lacerations, gently encourage bleeding, wash with warm soapy water, rinse, dry and cover with a waterproof dressing. In the event of a splash to the eye, rinse the affected eye with copious amounts of water or saline only. In the instance of a splash or puncture, the exposed individual should then report the event to their supervising midwife.

Maintaining a Sterile or Clean Field

At home, away from pathogenic, resistant hospital organisms, midwives can often use what is called "clean" technique when dealing with perineal wounds. The concept of clean versus sterile technique is somewhat hard to quantify and, over the years, a variety of definitions associated with wound care have filtered into the literature. Many terms employed have been used interchangeably and are all subject to individual interpretation. The Wound, Ostomy and Continence Nurses Society (WOCN) (Wooten & Hawkins, 2009) have proposed the following definitions in an attempt to establish some continuity in terminology:

- **Sterile technique** involves strategies that reduce exposure to microorganisms and that maintain objects and areas as free from microorganisms as possible. It involves meticulous handwashing, the use of a sterile field and sterile gloves for application of a sterile dressing, and the use of sterile instruments. "Sterile to sterile" involves the use of only sterile instruments and materials in dressing change procedures. Contact between sterile instruments or materials and any nonsterile surface or product must be avoided. Adhering to sterile technique is intended to reduce the risk of infection for the person being cared for during surgery or other invasive procedures such as blood drawing or urinary catheterization.
- **Clean technique** involves strategies to reduce the overall number of microorganisms or to prevent or reduce the risk of transmitting microorganisms from person to person or from place to place. Clean technique involves meticulous handwashing, maintaining a clean environment by preparing a clean field, using clean gloves and sterile instruments, and preventing direct contamination of materials and supplies. No "sterile to sterile" rules apply. This technique may also be called "nonsterile."

For most perineal repairs, you will achieve a very clean field if you strive to maintain a sterile field, with the knowledge that, even if the sterile field is breached (for example, you reach across the field to get an instrument or you touch the mother's thigh and then touch the field), you will maintain a field that is clean enough to prevent an infection in most healthy women. Recall that the genital area is normally populated with a variety of organisms and cannot be rendered sterile itself.

A **sterile field** is an area that is draped with sterile surfaces for the placement of sterile equipment. Creating and maintaining a sterile field involves the following principles:

- A sterile field is established immediately before the procedure because the longer the field lies exposed, the more likely it will become compromised by airborne contaminants.
- The sterile field must always be visible to avoid unobserved contamination.
- The sterile field should not be covered because it is too difficult to uncover it without introducing contaminants.
- Only sterile items are to be placed on a sterile field. If there is doubt about the sterility of an item, assume that it is not sterile.
- Moisture contaminates a sterile field and renders it unsterile because it provides a breeding ground for microbes.
- Once a sterile packet is opened, the edges of the cloth or paper drape that covered it

are considered unsterile.

- Sterile gowns are considered to remain sterile in front and from chest to waist or table level as long as precautions are taken to avoid touching anything that is not sterile with those parts of the gown; sleeves are considered sterile from 5 cm (2 inches) above the elbows to the fingertips of gloved hands.
- Persons wearing sterile barriers, such as sterile gloves, should only touch sterile items.

Maintaining the sterility of supplies

Sterile cloth instrument packs: A nonsterile practitioner first places a clean underpad or towel down on the work surface. Place the closed instrument pack down on the surface. Remove any indicator tape from the pack. Open the first flap of the outer (dust cover) wrapper by lifting and opening it away from yourself. Then open the flaps to either side and finally open the last flap toward yourself. When ready to begin, the inner sterile pack is opened in the same manner by the sterile practitioner, while she keeps her arms to the side and avoids reaching over the sterile packet.

Sterile paper or plastic instrument packs: The end can be opened and the instruments poured out onto a sterile field without reaching across the field. If the instruments are double wrapped, the outer wrapper is opened and the inner sterile packet is dumped out onto the sterile field.

Prepackaged materials: Disposable surgical supplies generally come in packages designed to be opened by someone who is "not sterile" with items to be removed by someone who "is sterile" while maintaining the sterility of the contents within as well as the operator's gloves.

Delivering prepackaged sterile items (such as gauze or suture) to the sterile field: Pull back the edges of the outer wrapper and gently toss the contents of the packet onto the sterile field without reaching across the field to do so.

Pouring sterile solutions: Verify the contents and expiration date of the bottle. Remove the seal and cap, taking care not to touch the inside of the cap or the top of the bottle. Hold the bottle with the label against the palm (to avoid smearing it) a safe distance above the sterile field and pour the solution slowly into a sterile container without splashing (Elkin et al., 2000).

References and Further Reading on Essential Surgical Skills for Midwives

References Used in Multiple Chapters

Adusumilli P, et al. "Left-handed surgeons: are they left out?" CURRENT SURG, 61(6):587-591, Nov-Dec 2004.

Anderson M. "Principles of wound healing in the repair of the episiotomy" (unpublished paper), Hawthorne NY, 1975.

Anderson R, Romfh R. TECHNIQUE IN THE USE OF SURGICAL TOOLS. Appleton-Century-Crofts, New York NY, 1980.

Colorado Surgical Assisting (CSA), Inc. Workshop handout: "A special hands-on workshop on wound closure: suturing and tying techniques," Colorado Surgical Assisting, Inc., Denver CO, Jun 2, 2002.

DeLancey J. BASIC EXERCISES: SURGICAL TECHNIQUE. Davis-Geck, Wayne NJ, 1987.

Dunn D. WOUND CLOSURE MANUAL. Ethicon, Inc., Johnson & Johnson, Somerville, NJ, 2008.

Edlich R, Long W. SURGICAL KNOT TYING MANUAL, 3rd ed. Covidien, Norwalk CT, 2008.

Edlich R, Long W. SYNETURE SURGICAL KNOT TYING MANUAL. US Surgical/Tyco Healthcare, Norwalk CT, 2005.

Elkin M, et al. NURSING INTERVENTIONS AND CLINICAL SKILLS, 2nd ed. Mosby. St Louis MO, 2000.

Ethicon, Inc. ADVANCED WOUND CLOSURE (product brochure). Johnson & Johnson, Somerville NJ, 2005.

Ethicon, Inc. WOUND CLOSURE MANUAL. Johnson & Johnson, Somerville NJ, 1999.

Ethicon, Inc. VICRYL RAPIDE (product brochure). Johnson & Johnson, Somerville, NJ, 1995.

Ethicon, Inc. WOUND CLOSURE MANUAL. Johnson & Johnson, Somerville, NJ, 1994.

Ethicon, Inc. WOUND CLOSURE MANUAL. Johnson & Johnson, Somerville, NJ, 1985.

Ethicon, Inc. SUTURE USE MANUAL: USE AND HANDLING OF SUTURES AND NEEDLES. Ethicon, Inc., Somerville NJ, 1977.

Kirk R. BASIC SURGICAL TECHNIQUES, 5th ed. Churchill Livingstone, London UK, 2002.

Lin K, Long W. SCIENTIFIC BASIS FOR THE SELECTION OF SURGICAL NEEDLES AND SUTURES. US Surgical/Tyco Healthcare. Norwalk CT, 2005.

Lin K, Long W. SCIENTIFIC BASIS FOR THE SELECTION OF SURGICAL NEEDLES AND SUTURES, US Surgical/Tyco Healthcare, Norwalk CT, 1999.

Royal College of Surgeons of Edinburgh (RCSE). Intercollegiate Basic Surgical Skills Course, Basic surgical skills: Module one: "Open surgery," www.medkaau.com/bssc, accessed Mar 18, 2009.

Sherris D, Kern E. ESSENTIAL SURGICAL SKILLS, 2nd ed. Saunders, Philadelphia PA, 2004.

Thomson T, Thomson C. ASSISTING AT PODIATRIC SURGERY: A GUIDE FOR PODIATRIC SURGICAL STUDENTS AND PODIATRIC THEATRE ASSISTANTS. Churchill Livingstone, Edinburgh Scotland, 2002.

Trott A. WOUNDS AND LACERATIONS: EMERGENCY CARE AND CLOSURE, 3rd ed. Elsevier Mosby, Philadelphia PA, 2005.

Varney H, et al. Chapter 79: "Cutting an episiotomy and repairing episiotomies and lacerations," in their VARNEY'S MIDWIFERY, 4th ed. Jones & Bartlett, Sudbury MA, 2004.

Zederfeldt B, Hunt T. WOUND CLOSURE: MATERIALS AND TECHNIQUES. Davis & Geck, Wayne NJ, 1990.

Tying Surgical Knots

Alzacko S, Majid O. "'Security loop' tie: a new technique to overcome loosening of surgical knots," ORAL SURG ORAL MED ORAL PATHOL ORAL RADIOL ENDOD, 104(5):e1-4, Nov, 2007.

Annunziata C, et al. "Technical considerations in knot construction. Part I. Continuous percutaneous and dermal suture closure," J EMERG MED, 15(3):351-360, May-Jun, 1997.

Behm T, et al. "Flat square knots: are 3 throws enough?" AM J OBSTET GYNECOL, 197(2):172.el-172.e3, Aug, 2007.

Chu C. Chapter 4: "Classification and General Characteristics of Suture Materials," in Chu C, et al., eds. WOUND CLOSURE BIOMATERIALS AND DEVICES. CRC Press, Boca Raton FL, 1996.

Ethicon, Inc. KNOT TYING MANUAL. Johnson & Johnson, Somerville NJ, 2005.

Fong E, et al. "Tensile strength of surgical knots in abdominal wound closure," ANZ J SURG, 78(3):164-166, Mar, 2008.

Giddings F. SURGICAL KNOTS AND SUTURING TECHNIQUES, 2nd ed. Giddings Studio Pub., Fort Collins CO, 2002.

Hogston P. "Suture choice in general gynaecological surgery," OBSTETRICIAN & GYNAECOLOGIST, 3(3):127-131, Jul, 2001.

Rosin E, Robinson G. "Knot security of suture materials," VET SURG, 18(4):269-273, Jul-Aug, 1989.

Sanz L. "Wound management: Matching materials and methods for best results," CONTEMP OB/GYN, 30(5):86-114, Nov, 1987.

Schubert D, et al. "Mechnical performance of knots using braided and monofilament absorbable sutures," AM J OBSTET GYNECOL, 187(6):1438-1442, Dec, 2002.

Shaw A, Duthie B. "A simple assessment of surgical sutures and knots," J R COLL SURG EDINB, 40(6):388-391, Dec, 1995.

Stott P, et al. "The ultimate Aberdeen knot," J R COLL SURG ENGL, 89(7):713-717, Oct, 2007.

Swindle M. BASIC SURGICAL EXERCISES USING SWINE. Praeger Scientific Pub., New York NY, 1983.

Trimbos J. "Security of various knots commonly used in surgical practice," OBSTET GYNECOL, 64(2):274-280, Aug, 1984.

von Fraunhofer J, Chu C. Chapter 6: "Mechanical Properties," in Chu C, et al., eds. WOUND CLOSURE BIOMATERIALS AND DEVICES. CRC Press, Boca Raton FL, 1996a.

von Fraunhofer J, Chu C. Chapter 3: "Surgical Needles," in Chu C, et al., eds. WOUND CLOSURE BIOMATERIALS AND DEVICES. CRC Press, Boca Raton FL, 1996b.

Walker J. Comment on "A simple assessment of surgical sutures and knots," J R COLL SURG EDINB, 41(6):425-426, Dec, 1996.

Zikria B. MANUAL OF SURGICAL KNOTS. Ethicon Inc., Sommerville NJ, 1981.

THE SIX STITCHES USED IN PERINEAL REPAIR

Dietz U, et al. Chapter 16: "Suture Materials and Techniques," in Téot L, et al. SURGERY IN WOUNDS. Springer-Verlag, New York NY, 2004.

Fleming N. "Can the suturing method make a difference in postpartum perineal pain?" J NURSE MIDWIFERY, 35(1):19-25, Jan-Feb 1990.

Galli S, et al. "Wound closure technique," www.emedicine.com/ent/topic35.htm, accessed Aug 13, 2008.

Kettle C, Johanson RB. "Continuous versus interrupted sutures for perineal repair," COCHRANE DATABASE SYST REV 2000;(2):CD000947, 2000.

Kettle D, O'Brien PMS. "Methods and materials used in perineal repair," ROYAL COLLEGE OF OBSTET GYNAECOL, Guideline No. 23, revised June 2004, www.rcog.org.uk/resources/Public/pdf/perineal_repair.pdf, accessed Aug 31, 2007.

Materson B. "Taking steps to promote wound healing," CONTEMP OB/GYN, 31(3):119-130, 1988.

Morano S, et al. "A randomized comparison of suturing techniques for episiotomy and laceration repair after spontaneous vaginal birth," J MINIMALLY INVASIVE GYNECOL, 13(5):457-462, Sep-Oct, 2006.

Munsick R. "Introital operation for dyspareunia," CLIN OBSTET GYNECOL, 23(1):243-271, Mar, 1980.
Oxorn, H. Chapter 34: Episiotomy, lacerations, uterine rupture, inversion," in his HUMAN LABOR & BIRTH, 5th ed. Appleton-Century-Crofts, Norwalk CT, 1986.
RCOG (Royal College of Obstetrics and Gynecology). "Methods and materials used in perineal repair,"ROYAL COLLEGE OBSTET GYNAECOL, Guideline No. 23, www.rcog.org.uk/resources/Public/pdf/perinealth _repair. pdf, accessed Aug 31, 2007.
Stone K, et al. "The biomechanical effects of tight suture closure on fascia," SURG GYNECOL OBSTET, 163(5):448-452, 1986.

USING A YONI RETRACTOR

Cooper Surgical, Inc. GUARDIAN VAGINAL RETRACTOR (product brochure). Cooper Surgical, Inc., Trumbull CT, revised Apr 2005.

USING LOCAL ANESTHETIC

Baer C, Williams B. CLINICAL PHARMACOLOGY AND NURSING. Springhouse Pub., Springhouse PA, 1988.
Cunningham F, Burk M. "A guidance on the use of topical anesthetics for naso/oropharyngeal and laryngotracheal procedures," Feb 2006. www.pbm.va.gov, accessed Nov, 2007.
Darbre P, Harvey P. "Paraben esters: review of recent studies of endocrine toxicity, absorption, esterase and human exposure, and discussion of potential human health risks," J APPL TOXICOL, 28(5):561-578, Jul 2008.
Kastrup E, et al., eds. "Injectable local anesthetics," in their DRUG FACTS AND COMPARISONS 2005, 59th ed. Wolters Kluwer Health, St. Louis MO, 2005.
Murhammer J, et al. "Rx Update: December 2004: Licocaine–maximum dosing recommendations," www.healthcare.uiowa.edu/pharmacy/RxUpdate/2004/12rxu.html, accessed Feb 20, 2009.
Murray J. Chapter 1: "Anesthesia," in Lynge C, et al., eds. 20 COMMON PROBLEMS: SURGICAL PROBLEMS AND PROCEDURES IN PRIMARY CARE. McGraw-Hill Pro., New York NY, 2001.
Peyton V. Chapter 20: "Episiotomy and obstetrics tears," in Lynge C, et al., eds. 20 COMMON PROBLEMS: SURGICAL PROBLEMS AND PROCEDURES IN PRIMARY CARE. McGraw-Hill Pro., New York NY, 2001.
Poznar J. PHARMACOLOGY FOR MIDWIVES, 2nd ed. Bellpine Pub., Monroe OR, 2002.
RxList. Cetacaine. http://www.rxlist.com/cetacaine-drug.htm, accessed Mar 28, 2009.

HAND HYGIENE AND PREVENTING THE SPREAD OF INFECTIOUS AGENTS

American College of Surgeons. MANUAL ON CONTROL OF INFECTION IN SURGICAL PATIENTS. JB Lippincott, Philadelphia PA, 1976.
Association of Operating Room Nurses (AORN). "Recommended practices for maintaining a sterile field. Association of Operating Room Nurses," AORN J, 64(5):817-821, Nov, 1996.
Bond, W. Microbiologist, Centers for Disease Control. Telephone conversation regarding HIV and HBV contamination, Mar 26, 1990.
Boyce J, et al., "Guideline for hand hygiene in health-care settings: recommendations of the healthcare infection control practices advisory committee and the HICPAC/SHEA/APIC/IDSA hand hygiene task force," MMWR, 51(RR16):1-44, Oct 25, 2002.
Centers for Disease Control. "Salmonella: handwashing instructions," www.cdc.gov/salmonella/typhimurium/handwashing.html, accessed Feb 4, 2009a.
Centers for Disease Control. "Infection control in dental settings: hand hygiene," www.cdc.gov/OralHealth/infectioncontrol/faq/hand.htm, accessed Jan 13, 2009b.

Centers for Disease Control. "Guidelines for the prevention of infection in surgical wounds, 1981." CDC, Atlanta GA, 1981.

Chambers RW, et. al. "Transmission of syphilis by fresh blood components," TRANSFUSION, 9(1):32-34, Jan-Feb, 1969.

Coulter H. AIDS AND SYPHILIS: THE HIDDEN LINK. North Atlantic Books, Washington DC, 1987.

Davis D. "Choosing and using the right surgical glove" Workhorse Pub., 2001. www.cardinal.com/mps/brands/gloves/selection/surgglove.asp, accessed Oct 14, 2008.

Dickey P. "Antimicrobial products: who needs them?" www.watoxics.org/homes-and-gardens/factsheets/antimicrobials, accessed Jul 16, 2008.

Faller N. "Clean versus sterile: a review of the literature," OSTOMY WOUND MANAGE, 45(5):56-60, 62, 64 passim., May, 1999.

Garner J, Favero M. "CDC guidelines for the prevention and control of nosocomial infections: guidelines for handwashing & hospital environmental control, 1985," AM J INFECT CONTROL, 14(3):110-129, Jun, 1986.

Gruendermann B. "Brush-free surgical hand asepsis," CEU handout, eChapter continuing education, Dallas TX, 2006, www.echapter.org/BFScrub-online.pdf, accessed Jan 13, 2009.

Lin K, Long W. "Postexposure prophylaxis for deadly bloodborne viral infections," US Surgical/Tyco Healthcare, Norwalk CT, Sep, 2005.

Mason I, Day M. "Sterilizing surgical instruments," NEW SCIENTIST, Feb 13, 1999, http://www.mad-cow.org/99feb_late_news.html, Accessed Jun 22, 2010.

May D. "Handwashing Guidelines," Daniele Healthcare, 2000. http://209.85.173.132/search?q=cache:wpZev-mf1rYJ:www.daniels.co.uk/image-bank-download.php%3Fid%3D7+surgical+handwashing+keep+hands+than−elbows&hl=en&ct=clnk&cd=5&gl =us, accessed Feb 4, 2009.

Michigan State U. "Recommended biosafety practices for handling prions and prion-infected tissues" Updated May 2007, www.biosafety.msu.edu, Accessed Jun 22, 2010.

Mitchell RB. SYPHILIS AS AIDS. Banned Books, Austin TX, 1990.

National Collaborating Centre for Nursing and Supportive Care. Infection control. "Prevention of healthcare-associated infections in primary and community care,": National Institute for Clinical Excellence (NICE) (London, UK);1-257. www.guideline.gov/summary/summary.aspx?doc_id=5069&nbr=003553&string=soap, Jun, 2003, accessed Jul 16, 2008.

Pereira L, et. al. "The effect of surgical handwashing routines on the microbial counts of operating room nurses," AM J INFEC CONTROL, 18(6):354-364, Dec, 1990.

Ross J, Chadwick S. "The human body's innate nonspecific defense," http://www.jdaross.cwc.net/nonspec.htm, accessed Mar 4, 2009.

Semmelweis I. THE ETIOLOGY, THE CONCEPT AND THE PROPHYLAXIS OF CHILDBED FEVER. Translated from the German by Murphy F. Edited with commentary and translation of the Semmelweis "Open Letters" by Nuland S, Gyorgyey F. Facsimile reprint. Gryphon Editions, Classics in Obstetrics and Gynecology Library, New York NY [1861] 1990.

Siegel JD, et al. and the Healthcare Infection Control Practices Advisory Committee. "2007 Guideline for isolation precautions: Preventing transmission of infectious agents in healthcare settings," Centers for Disease Control and Prevention (CDC);1-17, Jun, 2007.

Sutton JM, et al. "Methods to minimize the risks of Creutzfeldt-Jakob disease transmission by surgical procedures: where to set the standard?" CLIN INFECT DIS Vol 43(6):757–764, Sept 2006.

Tollin M, et al. "Vernix caseosa as a multi-component defense system based on polypeptides, lipids and their interactions," CELLULAR MOLECUL LIFE SCI, 62(19-20):2390-2399, Oct. 2005.

Wikipedia contributors. "Prion." Wikipedia, the Free Encyclopedia, http://en.wikipedia.org/wiki/prion, Jun 5, 2010, accessed Jun 7, 2010.

Williams V. "Sterile (?) techniques and home birth," unpublished paper (n.d., ca. 1985).

World Health Organization "WHO infection control guidelines for transmissible spongiform encephalopathies. Report of a WHO consultation, Geneva, Switzerland, Mar 23-26, 1999.

Maintaining a Sterile or Clean Field

Wooten M, Hawkins K. "WOCN position statement clean versus sterile: management of chronic wound," Rev. 2005. Guidelines of the Wound, Ostomy and Continence Nurses Society, Glenview IL, www.wocn.org/pdfs/WOCN_Library/Position_ Statements/clvst.pdf, accessed Feb 4, 2009.

NOTES:

CHECKING FOR PERINEAL DAMAGE AFTER BIRTH

EXAMINING THE PERINEUM AFTER BIRTH

Reassess the condition of the genital tissues and perineum during pushing and remind yourself where any lesions such as painful scars, inclusion cysts or varicose veins may be located. If there is scar tissue, notice if it is stretching nicely or being strained and correct these problems if possible (see the chapter entitled "Preparing the Perineal Tissues for Birth").

After the Birth and Before You Check for Tears

A tear is usually not a life-threatening problem. Therefore, if the mother is stable and not continuously bleeding, it is important to allow uninterrupted time after the birth for the mother and baby to connect and to allow the mother to deliver the placenta. Ideally, at least one hour is allowed for this quiet time. The first several hours following birth have been recognized as a sensitive period when certain genetic "keys" that are related to attachment are being turned on in the baby's DNA. Once these precious, irretrievable, first minutes have past, be sure all of the following questions are satisfied before you inspect the perineum for damage. Many of these tasks can be performed relatively unobtrusively while the mother remains focused on her baby.

- Are baby and mother stable?
- Is the placenta out?
- Is bleeding normal and under control?
- Is the uterus low and firm?
- Has the mother been hydrated, cleaned up (with a quick bed bath of her pelvic area) and made comfortable?
- Has the baby nursed?
- Has the bed been tidied up?
- Does the mother feel ready to be checked?
- Are you ready to suture if need be?

Changing the bed and the herbal bath can usually wait until after any necessary repairs have been completed. But you should be able to say yes to these preliminaries before checking for tears. The exception is the woman who is bleeding with a low and firm uterus. In this case, bleeding is likely to be from a yoni or cervical tear and needs to be assessed more quickly. After such bleeding is under control, wait to perform additional perineal care until the mother and baby are ready.

Timing of Inspection and Repair

The timing of inspection and repair is dictated by the needs of the individual situation. The need to leave mother, baby and partner alone to bond should always take precedence over your desire to get everything done and cleaned up. However, if the mother is to remain at home and you believe a repair will be needed, you must also take into account your fatigue level and how much the mother is swelling from the trauma of birth when deciding how to proceed.

While you are waiting to examine the mother, give her at least one dose of oral homeopathic Arnica to minimize bruising and edema. Since every woman has some tissue trauma from the stretching of birth, this is a reasonable and safe routine precaution for the immediate postpartum period. When a woman has a history of swelling or is at high risk (blondes, redheads and fair-skinned women are more prone to the rapid development of edema, as are those who have experienced a prolonged pushing phase), you can administer one pellet of 30C Arnica (available at most health food stores) every 10 to 15 minutes after the birth. While this may seem a bit intrusive, it is far less so than interrupting the bonding period much more intrusively to move quickly to perineal inspection. Arnica will help minimize swelling so it is less of an issue by the time you are ready to suture. (See the chapter entitled "Postpartum Care and Comfort Measures" for more information.)

If the initial postpartum hour has passed and a repair is needed, give the mother a choice regarding timing, but remind her there will be less numbness from the pressure of birth the longer you wait to suture. Therefore, it may hurt more. If the mother wants to wait awhile, inspect her perineum first to assess how realistic this is, considering the damage and swelling you find. If you inspect sooner (rather than later) and the happy news is that there are no tears (or at least none that need repair), the new family can relax, and you can go about cleaning up and relaxing yourself. As you move into the second hour, arrange the mother so that you can inspect her perineum while she focuses on the baby; the baby should not be physically separated from the mother unless it is absolutely unavoidable for as many of the first 6 hours after birth as possible.

If you are practicing illegally, you may wish to wait until the placenta has been out for at least two hours before proceeding with repair. Waiting longer lessens the chance that a complication such as hemorrhage will arise during the early postpartum period (when they are most likely to occur). This will considerably reduce the chances you will need to transport after the repair has been completed.

When you examine the perineum, should you find yourself unable to identify landmarks or are sure the damage is beyond your skills, in ideal circumstances you should wait no longer than six to eight hours (the "golden period") from time of injury to make other arrangements and have the repair completed. This time period is especially important if the anal sphincter is damaged, because the potential for wound contamination rises the longer the tissues are left unrepaired. These time constraints on when a wound that is to heal by primary intention can be repaired are an additional reason not to postpone your inspection for too long after the birth.

While this timing is ideal, if you feel incompetent to perform the repair and it takes more time to arrange for another practitioner to do it, it is comforting to know that Nordenstam and colleagues (2008) studied two groups of women, 78 of whom had their torn sphincter repaired immediately and 87 of whom had a delay of 8 to 12 hours before having their sphincters repaired using an end-to-end technique (see the chapter entitled "Repairing the External Anal Sphincter" for an explanation of this technique). They found no significant differences in rectal incontinence between the two groups; in fact, the delayed-repair group had a slightly lower rate of problems. (They also found that increasing maternal age correlated significantly with increased symptoms of fecal urgency and the inability to distinguish between flatus and feces.)

While a six-hour time frame is best when muscles are damaged, the repair of simpler tears may be postponed for as long as 24 hours. Any injury that has no visible contamination or debris and no devitalized tissue and that can be converted to a fresh-appearing, slightly bleeding wound after aggressive cleansing, irrigation or débridement is a candidate for primary closure (Trott, 2005).

Timing inspection and repair for a multiple birth

A special situation presents itself when you are attending a multiple birth. Although the vast majority of multiple births will be completed within six hours after the birth of the first baby, should this not be the case, it seems pointless to proceed with repair until all the babies are out and the placentas are delivered.

The one exception to this is when the first baby is born preterm. If the first placenta delivers, the second baby's chorioamnionic membranes remain intact, contractions stop and do not resume after many hours, and all is well, you could choose to let the other baby remain in utero until he reaches term. (Of course, it is possible that the first baby could be term and the second early, but it is hard to know if this is true.) Although this situation is very rare, it does happen (Hellman & Pritchard, 1971). If you find yourself faced with this unlikely scenario, a full discussion of all the variables (including back-up options) should take place with the parents. If the decision is to wait for labor to resume, I recommend leaving the yoni unrepaired unless serious damage has resulted. If rectovaginal, anal sphincter, upper yoni wall, or extreme labial or cervical damage has occurred, the pros and cons regarding early delivery of the second baby must be weighed against the possible risks to the mother, which are primarily poor healing and infection, the risks of which must be weighed with the risk of repairing the tear only to have it restressed when the next baby is born. If the mother has sustained a serious tear with the first baby (an unlikely scenario if the first baby is small and early), I'd recommend delivery of any other babies within the six- to eight-hour time frame, although, if the other baby is estimated to be fewer than 36 weeks gestation, the decision may not be so clear cut. If the option to wait for the other baby is chosen, meaning birth may be a month or more away, repair of severe damage within the first six to eight hours after birth is probably the best alternative. The risks and benefits of waiting versus repairing the tear must be thoroughly discussed. If there is a friendly back-up doctor involved, discuss it with that person as well.

Postpartum Perineal Examination: Step by Step

The importance of a thorough examination

Historically, incomplete perineal exams have been common in the independent midwifery community. Early on, part of the reason for this was the lack of concrete information about how to perform an exam. Incomplete exams lead many midwives to believe that they have very few tears. Others only count tears that they deem require sutures, while leaving many tears unsutured; this kind of reporting skews their data. I encourage all birth attendants to perform complete exams and to meticulously record and tabulate the actual damage that is found and if and how it is repaired. (See the chapter entitled "Assessing the Degree of

Damage and the Need for Repair" and the one in the APPENDICES entitled "Record Keeping.") In this way, you will begin to get a better idea of when tears actually occur, the extent of the damage women are sustaining and how well various tear prevention techniques really work.

Checking for tears should be done systematically to ensure that nothing is left out. Even if a superficial inspection does not reveal tears, check thoroughly. Sometimes tears are hiding. Keep in mind that the easiest birth can produce a bad tear, while a very manipulated birth might leave everything intact. Therefore, it is important to check carefully inside and out, despite how well the birth went or how intact the external tissue may first appear upon cursory inspection. I learned this lesson well when a very easy birth resulted in a totally intact perineum and a pocket tear behind the perineal skin at the bottom of which was a completely severed external anal sphincter (thanks to a nuchal hand, causing an elbow to slice down on the way out). At the very least, the labia, the periurethral area and the lower third of the interior of the yoni and anal area should be examined if the birth was easy and apparently tear free.

Positioning the mother and yourself for the exam

If the bed is firm enough, you can simply expose the mother's perineum, spread her feet to either side and sit between her legs, although this posture is hard on your back and although many beds are too soft for this to be practical. Therefore it is ideal to have the mother reposition herself so that her bottom is at the edge of the bed with her legs spread. Place two chairs with bed-level seats to either side on which she can rest her feet. Sit in a chair placed squarely between the mother's legs. If you still cannot see well, place a fracture pan or a large book (even a phone book wrapped in plastic and a towel will do) under her bottom to lift her up so you can adequately visualize her perineum.

Setting up for the exam

Position the brightest light you have so that it shines directly on the perineum and into the yoni. After you and your assistant have both washed your hands and donned fresh sterile gloves, proceed with the exam. Have your assistant stand beside you, ready to retract tissue if necessary. Explain the procedure as you go for the benefit of the mother and any students present. Warn the mother that the exam may hurt and to breathe through it. If the exam is too uncomfortable, you can spray the perineum with aerosol anesthetic beforehand.

Pointers on handling and visualizing the tissue

It is best to handle the tissue as little as possible, but comprehensively enough to enable you to do a thorough job. Gentleness is especially important when examining women in poor health because you can easily cause more damage to very friable tissue.

Bleeding: Use gauze to gently blot up minor blood seepage in the area you are trying to examine. Rubbing hurts the mother and disturbs clotting. If there is significant bleeding, you must first locate the source and get it under control before you continue.

Possible sources of bleeding include either an atonic uterus (hemorrhage) or just normal lochia as well as a cervical, periurethral or perineal tear. If there is too much blood to see what you are doing, first be sure it isn't coming from the uterus. If you have ruled out abnormal uterine bleeding, check to see if a torn blood vessel within the laceration requires attention. The vulva has an extensive vascular network that becomes considerably engorged during pregnancy. During pushing, pressure from the presenting part compresses these vessels so that any damage to them is often not readily apparent until after the baby is born and the pressure is relieved. Thus, you must always check carefully to see if any larger blood vessels have been severed, especially if the perineum has been cut. If the bleeding is coming from a vessel and pressure does not staunch the bleeding, you will need to ligate any bleeding vessels prior to repair to avoid burying the vessel and inviting the formation of a hematoma. More information on how to identify and deal with a torn vessel can be found in the chapter entitled "Dealing with Bleeding Vessels". If no torn vessel is found and the uterus is contracted and firm, the blood could be coming from a cervical tear. See the section in this chapter on inspecting the cervix for more details.

Sometimes a visible area in a laceration is oozing blood, even though you cannot find a specific vessel that is torn. To stop the oozing, apply pressure with herbal compresses (you can dip a gauze pad in the steeping infusion for the herbal bath, which is described on page 584), finish your inspection and repair the laceration as quickly as possible. If that doesn't work, wrap a gauze pad soaked in a water-based herbal solution around a piece of ice and hold it firmly against the area, applying pressure until the oozing subsides enough to continue. It is best to use a water-based infusion for this purpose. However, if a grain alcohol–based tincture is all you've got, place a few dropperfuls in a small amount of boiling water. Allow it to sit at least five minutes to burn off the alcohol, then soak a gauze pad and apply. In the meantime, apply pressure with a plain gauze pad. Properly prescribed homeopathic remedies given orally can also arrest this kind of bleeding.

Distinguishing tissue layers: Recognizing what tissues are damaged in a tear is, by far, the most difficult part of learning to suture. There is just no substitute for actually examining a large number of tears slowly and thoroughly so the tissue layers begin to make sense.

When you are beginning to learn, watch every examination and repair that you can. Ask questions. When appropriate, ask that the person doing the repair pause from time to time to allow you to orient yourself and really understand what you are seeing. Pay attention so that you can visually examine the tissues during natural pauses as the repair is being done. A thorough understanding of perineal anatomy will help tremendously, even though most of the muscle tissues in the perineal body cannot be distinguished with the naked eye.

Be sure to have the person doing the suturing point out the mucosal surface of the yoni and the edges of the tear, any bruises, the hymenal tags, any labial tears, and any anal sphincter or rectal mucosa damage and to explain how she plans to do the repair.

It is often very difficult to distinguish tears from bruised tissue and at first glance you are likely to think "Yikes, this all looks the same!" Take a deep breath and look closely. Begin by examining the sidewalls of the yoni, which are likely to be intact. Just after birth, intact mucous membrane will form soft mounds, will look and feel smooth and will be a mostly uniform deep bluish- or even reddish-purple color, whereas torn mucous membrane will appear bumpy and mottled, with a dark purple-burgundy color interlaced with lighter strands of connective tissue. Move toward the midline of the lower yoni wall, looking carefully to see if and where the visual texture of the tissue changes; the closer you get to the midline, the more likely you will encounter torn edges. The edges of tears in the yoni mucosa will often curl inward slightly. Torn skin will be easier to see since it runs along the external margin of the tear; the raw edges will appear lighter pink and may also curl inward slightly.

Torn muscle looks deep red and feels tougher and more resistant to the touch (Anderson, 1975). It will be beneath the skin and mucosa layers.

When the tear is extensive, look for specific damage that makes a deep wound high risk if not properly repaired, such as anterior damage that communicates with the urethra or bladder, damage that has opened a passage into the posterior cul-de-sac or damage that involves the anal sphincter or rectal mucosa.

The anal sphincter muscle will be immediately behind the perineal skin around the anal opening and, if exposed but untorn, may appear as a rounded intact, band that runs side to side. If torn, the external anal sphincter may appear stringy, meaty, rough or chunky, with any exposed but intact fibers running from side to side. The ends and surface of the sphincter look meaty; if intact it may be a dark rose pink. The internal sphincter will underlie the external sphincter and appear much lighter in color, white-pink, more like fish meat. These color differences can be very subtle. Remember, tears may not divide perineal muscles, but clitorotomies almost invariably do.

When, as a student, you finally have an opportunity to perform an inspection yourself, look carefully. Take your time. Carefully inspect the laceration until the various tissues become obvious. Do not hesitate to discuss what you are finding and how best to proceed with the repair with your midwifery partner. The woman wants you to do a good job and will not mind if you confer on these important points.

Landmarks are altered in a short perineum. The sphincter damage I have seen has almost all been due to spontaneous lacerations in short perineums, with perineal skin tears otherwise so shallow I hardly had enough room to put in the two layers of perineal suture I usually use. In most cases there was minimal yoni mucosa damage as well.

The order of examination

To inspect for damage, begin from the top down and from the outside in because the majority of the damage you see will be shallow. I begin with an explanation of how to examine the external structures first: the anterior structures near the clitoral hood and the perineum. I follow this discussion with the posterior yoni wall, the anterior yoni wall, the cervix, the hymen, the anal sphincters and the rectal mucosa.

Locating the apexes of a tear

You are evaluating the depth of damage and are looking for both ends, or the **apexes**, of each tear you find. Typically a simple perineal tear has two apexes, one at the internal extremity of the tear, usually in the posterior yoni wall, and the other at the external extremity of the tear, usually in the skin of the perineum. Sometimes a tear is forked, resulting in one end having two or more internal or external apexes. For any tear, its apexes must be accurately identified and followed until you are sure you have found the end before the repair is begun. Tears that are completely external will also have two apexes and sometimes more: an anterior apex (nearer the pubic bone) and a posterior apex (nearer the sacrum) or a lateral apex (furthest from the body) and a medial apex (nearest the body).

Examining the periurethral/superficial clitoral/labial area

Periurethral and labial tears are often not obvious until the labia are parted. Labia majora damage due to birth-related trauma is exceedingly rare unless a varicose vein ruptures, in which case a hematoma will be the likely result. The labia minora, however, often sustain damage during birth, although thankfully most of this trauma is minor and does not require repair. To examine the labia minora, use your fingers to gently open the lips. Check for tears by starting at the top, at the clitoral hood. **Skid marks** and **skin splits** or **rents** may be found in the periurethral area or, more commonly, in the labia minora, the clitoral hood or the clitoral frenulum. "Skid mark" is a midwifery term that refers to the most superficial kind of skin separation or abrasion. "Skin split" is a similar term for a slightly deeper tear. Both types of tears may occur anywhere, are too shallow to stitch and usually heal well. Skid marks and skin splits are typically only painful for the first 24 hours or so after birth.

Longitudinal labial tears appear as dark pink to red, meaty lines; many such tears can be left to heal on their own. Labial tears that usually heal better if repaired include tears where the tissue peels back to form a flap of skin on one side; tears that run across the width of the labia that leave a chunk of tissue that sags away from the rest; or tears that have a chunk of tissue that is nearly torn away and hanging down. Labial repair is discussed in the chapter entitled "Periurethral and Labial Repairs."

Typical configuration of yoni tearing

Usually tears in the yoni floor constitute the horizontal plane of a tear. They form a wedge shape that is deepest in the region of the introitus and becomes increasingly shallow as it nears the internal apex. Tears in the perineum constitute the vertical plane of a tear. They also form a wedge, which is usually deepest at the introitus and increasingly shallow as they approach the anus. Many tears go along the yoni floor and then extend down the perineum (a sideways "L" shape when thought of in cross-section). When a tear is L-shaped, the angle of the L typically overlies the "corner" of the introitus, where the perineal skin meets the yoni mucosa. This is also usually the deepest point of the tear. In the sagittal section of a tear illustrated here, the area above the dotted line indicates a typical L-shaped tear that is shallow enough to require a single layer of stitches in the yoni floor. Remember, however, that just because a tear is shallow does not necessarily mean the sphincter isn't damaged. (See the entries entitled "Distinguishing tissue layers" and "Examining the anal sphincters and the anorectal wall" in this chapter.)

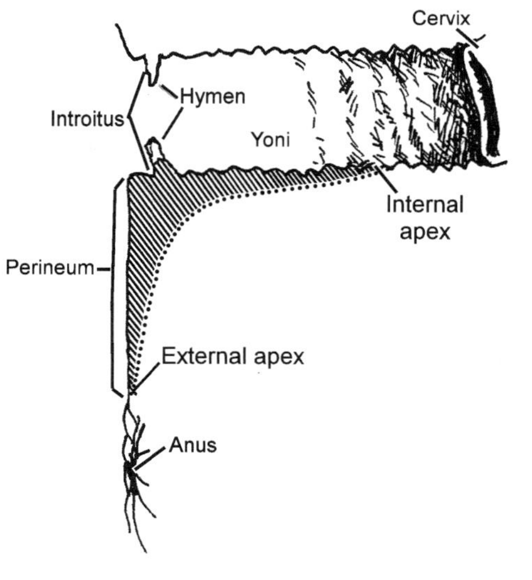

Sagittal schematic of a typical perineal tear
Tear=shaded area

Anything can happen however and, much more rarely (at least among attended women whose genitals are intact), other types of tears may occur. One type occurs when a central rupture of the perineum begins in the midline yoni wall, above the perineal body, before significant stretching takes place. The advancing presenting part enters the yoni tear, widens it, and descends through the perineal body where it begins to bulge the center of the perineum. An external tear begins that extends up toward the introitus and down toward the anus. If the tear starts in the lateral yoni wall, it can extend to one side of the introitus. While a baby can be born through such ruptures, most of the time the tear extends toward the yoni canal and thus the baby is born through a large yoni tear. When such a tear is oriented toward the rectum, the rectal wall may be torn through, creating a spontaneous fistula through which the baby may be born or through which a small part may prolapse (Herman, 1910).

It is also possible for a tear in the perineum to occur adjacent to the yoni introitus, leaving the introitus intact. A tear in the rectal mucosa may also occur, leaving the perineum intact. The baby is born through the unusual laceration. With proper attention to the perineum during birth, this should not occur. However, if the introitus is quite rigid, the mother in poor health or the birth goes unattended of a woman with significant genital scarring, such an accident could happen, particularly in developing countries. Such tears require dissection of the introitus and the perineal body to facilitate proper repair.

Examining the perineum: Perineal skin tears are usually obvious. Check to see how deep a tear is from the skin surface toward the central point of the perineum. Frequently, a shallow longitudinal split down the perineal skin is all you will discover. Look at the edges of the tear. In the unlikely event that they are very ragged, you may have to remove tiny tags of tissue along the edges before you sew. Check the mouth of the yoni to see if the edges of the tear at that level lie together or are mismatched or lying at an odd angle.

Also check the introitus for iatrogenic skin tags. These usually occur when a previous repair has been sewn too tightly and the stretching of birth results in a tear that opens the introitus to its original larger size. This typically creates a short skin tag below a raw place that is larger than the skin tag from which it has separated, as illustrated on the next page. (More on this type of tear can be found in the chapter entitled "Skin Tags.")

Be sure to positively identify the most posterior end of the external apex of any perineal skin tears, which means you must separate the tissue and follow the tear to its visible end. It is possible to have a tear go over, around, and beneath an intact or partially torn external sphincter into the anal mucosa, damage that is likely to be missed if you do not check. When a perineal tear exposes or severs the sphincter, follow it down into and

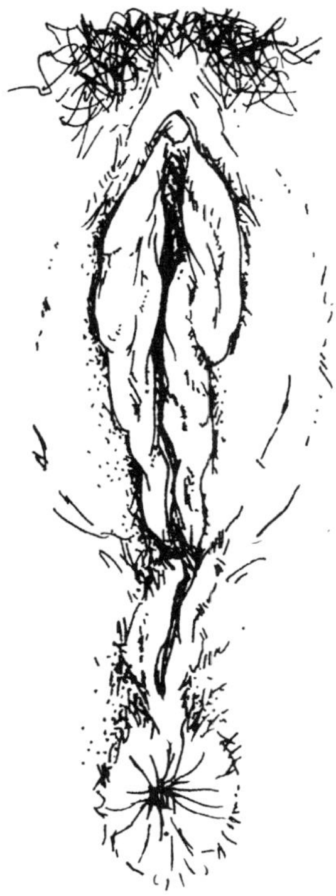

Typical appearance of a torn perineum just after birth, although swelling is usually present even without a tear.

through the folds of the corrugator cutis ani to confirm whether it extends around and under the sphincter and, if so, how far.

Remember how the layers are "stacked": In the posterior midline, you have the yoni canal, the wall of the yoni consisting of a mucosal layer and a muscle layer (which often remain fused in spontaneous tears but can separate into two layers in some cases). At the approximate depth of the hymen most superficially there is the tiny bridge that joins the two sides of the banded portion of the perineal membrane, below that band lies the superficial transverse perineal muscle. Also underlying the yoni wall behind the hymen lies the urethrovaginal sphincter, inferior to that is the puboperinealis muscle, then the rest of the perineal body, the external anal sphincter (shallow, posterior region of perineal body), then the internal anal sphincter and the anorectal wall, below which is the anal canal. Keep these layers in your head as you perform your exam.

Examining the yoni floor: An internal examination will be hindered by the tendency of the just-distended yoni walls to collapse unless firmly held back and out of the way. Your view will also be obscured by lochia. First, you must identify if the tissue is damaged. To do so, get an overview of the region by opening the yoni with either one or two hands.

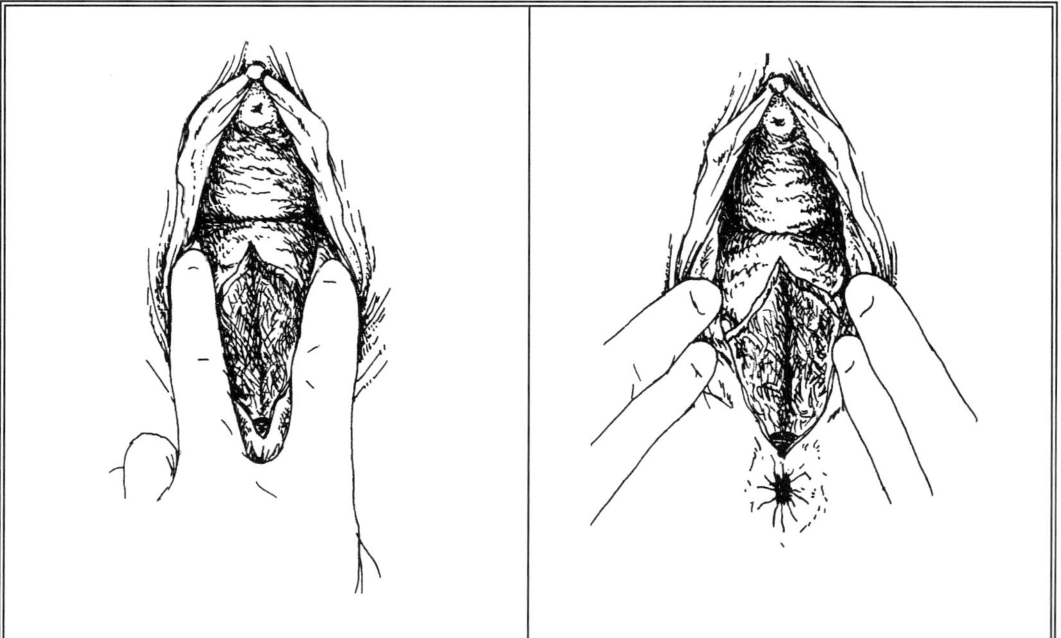

Using one hand for examination	Using two hands for an exam

It can be hard to identify where damage begins. Try placing the length of your index finger against the upper side-wall of the yoni and gently pressing against the tissue. Since high sidewall tears are relatively rare, the sidewalls are very likely to be intact so closely examine the color and texture of these walls. Apply your finger firmly but gently, then slowly sweep it down to the posterior midline of the yoni wall, noting if and when the color and texture of the tissue changes. Feel for a cleft in the posterior yoni wall where the appearance of the tissue changes: this is a tear. After you have identified one side of a tear, finding other landmarks should not be so hard. Once you are oriented and a tear is discovered, begin to examine the tear at the introitus and work your way back toward the cervix, to assess how deeply into the tissue as well as how far back into the yoni any tearing extends. Blot the posterior wall and open the yoni with your extended fingers to visualize any damage.

Shallow skid marks may also occur inside the yoni, and lacerations of the anterior yoni wall that lie close to the urethra are relatively common. Typically these types of tears do not bleed much and can often be left unrepaired (Cunningham et al., 2005).

It is essential to find the internal apex (inside end) of the tear. Do not rely on touch alone to distinguish the soft, intact tissue from lacerated tissue. Look carefully for where tissue shape and color changes. The tear is usually widest at the introitus and narrows to a point at either apex. Beginning at the introitus, follow the damage, looking and feeling for where the edges of the tear come together at the internal apex. If you cannot see the internal apex, insert two fingers of your nondominant hand into the yoni, open your fingers, and press down gently. The internal apex of any tears as well as the cervix should come into view. Also examine the posterior sulcus groves for tears at this point in your exam.

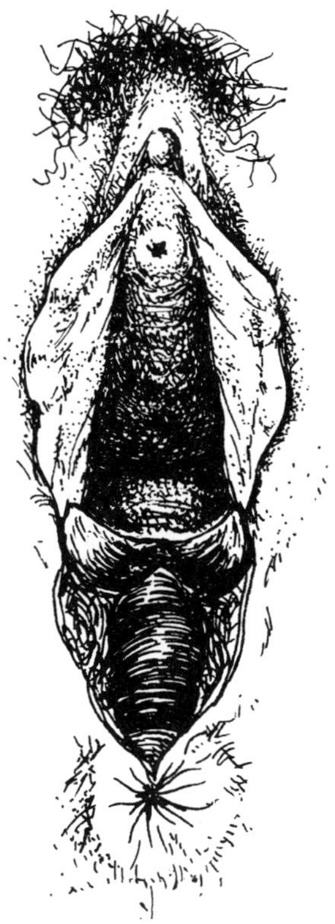

Deep tear with separated yoni floor lifted up. The rectal wall and external sphincter are intact.

The floor of the yoni may split into a separate layer, causing the two layers to appear as bilateral shelves above the anorectal wall, which may or may not also be torn. This occurs when the floor of the yoni wall tears away from the adventitia between it and the anterior anorectal wall, although such damage is more likely to happen when the yoni mucosa is cut rather than torn. This fibromuscular layer is still erroneously referred to as the "rectovaginal septum" in many sources.

Isolated lacerations involving the middle or upper third of the yoni floor occur less often. These are usually longitudinal and may not be associated with either perineal or cervical lacerations. This type of tear usually occurs during an instrumental delivery but may develop with a spontaneous birth as well. Such tears are often deep and may cause significant bleeding, which can usually be controlled by repairing the damage. Unless the upper yoni wall is inspected, this kind of damage may be overlooked. Recall that bleeding in the presence of a firmly contracted uterus is evidence of genital tract laceration of some sort, retention of placental fragments or both (Cunningham et al., 2005).

If you know an inclusion or sebaceous cyst exists, check it now to see if it has been exposed by any tearing or ruptured by the pressure from the birth. Traces of milky fluid or thick, pasty material may be apparent if a large cyst has ruptured.

A pocket tear may have formed, presenting as a variably sized cavity that is deeper than the surrounding tear or that is an isolated area of damage surrounded by intact tissue. Check immediately behind the perineum for pockets in the mucosa. Pockets may be caused by elbows or a difficult shoulder rotation, but they sometimes occur without any obvious precipitating event. If the pocket is in the floor of the yoni right behind the perineum, be sure it does not involve the sphincter capsule, with a torn sphincter retracted inside. It is very rare for a pocket tear to occur in the anterior yoni wall, but if one is found you must rule out urethral or bladder involvement by catheterizing the mother. How to do this is described in the chapter entitled "Repairing the Anterior Yoni Wall."

Identify the hymenal ring: With a few rare exceptions, the hymenal ring in a first-time mother will be torn during birth. (You will often note a trickle of blood during crowning as this occurs.) In multiparas, the hymen will usually appear as healed tags 0.5 to 2 cm inside the introitus. The hymenal ring is an important landmark when you are doing the repair, but the hymen itself is never reconstructed.

If you have incised the hymen during the birth, check to see if the incision has extended below the level of the yoni floor and, if so, how far. If damage is minor and the tissue is not bleeding, no sutures are necessary.

Checking for perineal muscle damage: With the exception of the anal sphincters, the muscle fibers that intermingle in the perineum are usually only distinguishable microscopically. Division of the midline connection in the perineal membrane will cause the structures that are attached to it to separate without necessarily having caused much muscle damage per se. Thus, the muscle fibers most likely to be severed by a tear are fibers of the ureterovaginal sphincter muscle that underlie the distal, posterior yoni wall, the superficial transverse perineal muscle; the smooth muscle fibers within the banded portion of the perineal membrane, the few fibers of the bulbocavernosus and the winged part of the anal sphincter that may cross in the midline in a few women, and the puboperinealis muscle.

For perineal muscle damage to impact the way you will do the repair, the only thing you need to know from a practical point of view is whether the tear can be closed with a single layer of stitches made with a 36.4 or 37 mm half-circle needle. A second layer of deep stitches is required only if the tear is too deep to allow closure with a single layer of stitches.

There is a technique in the literature for identifying a severed bulbocavernosus muscle. However, it is predicated on the erroneous assumption that the muscle fibers pass across the perineal body. You can use the same basic technique to assess for damage to the superficial transverse perineal muscle, although if the tear is more than about a quarter of an inch deep to the perineal surface it probably does involve some transverse fibers.

First, identify the muscle by palpating on one side of the perineal body. Place two fingers inside the yoni at either 3 or 9 o'clock and use your thumb to gently palpate to one side, just below the level of the labia majora and minora on that side. Now, use your inside fingers to follow along the yoni wall and floor to one side of the tear. Press down into the perineum slightly with your fingers and ask the mother to constrict her muscles. Note if it feels like an intact band of muscle runs across the midline of the perineum; most of the time this will be very subtle. If you are unsure, open the tear to its depth and ask her to contract the muscle again while you look at the sides of the tear. If you can see muscle retracting slightly on either side as she does so, this is probably one side of a torn superficial transverse perineal muscle. Sometimes these techniques may reveal damage, but this is also a very subtle exam and this muscle is often composed of only a few sparse fibers that may not be obvious during this exam.

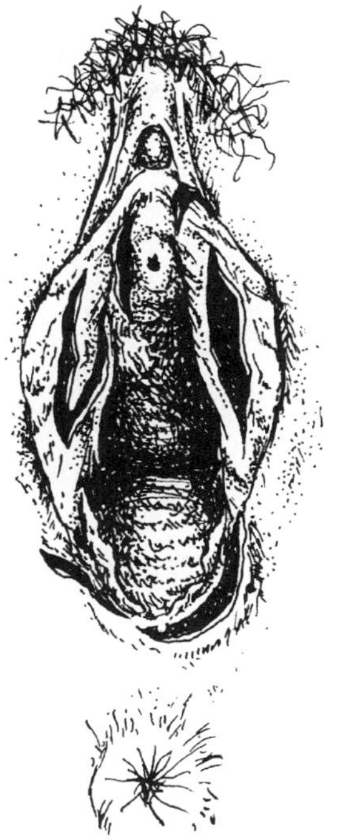

Labial and perineal splits

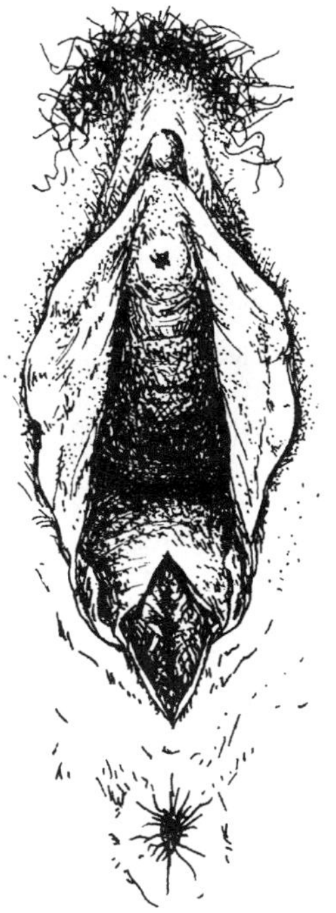

Shallow midline tear with the edges parted

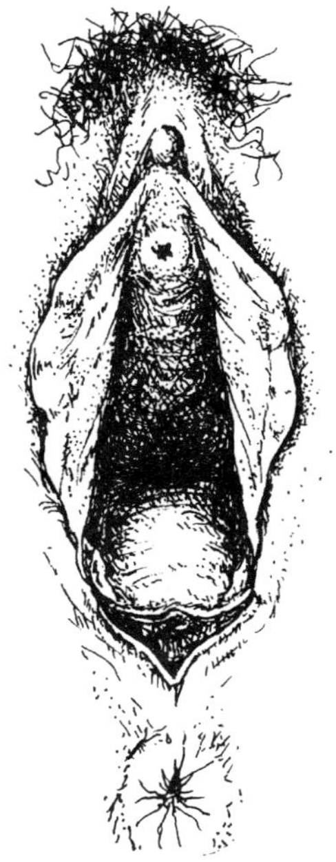

Shallow introital tear

You can also evaluate the depth of interior damage by placing your thumb on the perineum and two fingers in the yoni at 6 o'clock, well behind the central point of the perineum (about 5 cm in). Now pull down and forward with your fingers as you press your thumb into the perineum just above the anus. See if you run into muscle in the perineal body, indicating that it is mostly intact. This exam is more uncomfortable for the woman, so do not do it unless you have an apparently deep tear, requiring a more probing exam (many exam techniques are commonplace in the hospital, where women have frequently received local anesthetic or an epidural, reducing the discomfort of such probing exams). For these very rare tears that leave the perineum intact but produce long, deep tears inside the yoni, this technique may come in handy when determining how deep and extensive the tear really is. For this exam to be informative, you must first practice it a lot on women whose perineal bodies are intact so you know what you are feeling for.

Injury to the muscles due to over-stretching may also occur, but such damage will not be detectable at the time of your exam (Cunningham et al., 2005).

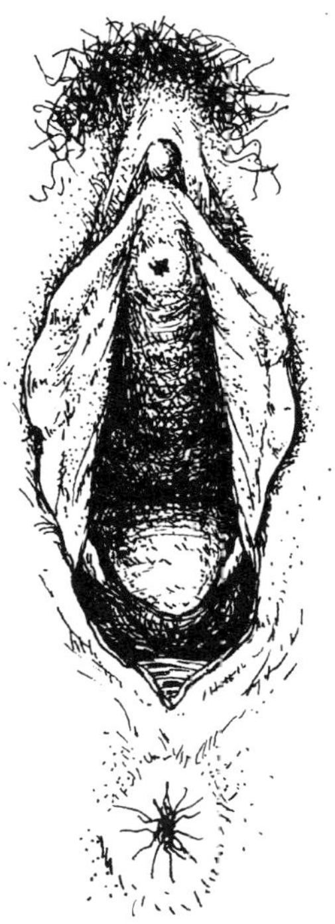	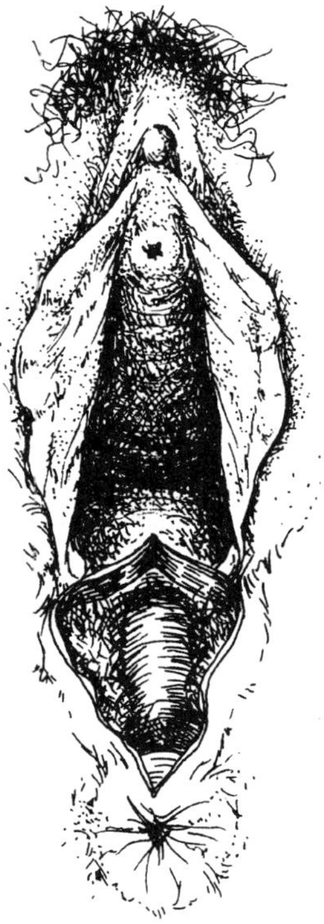	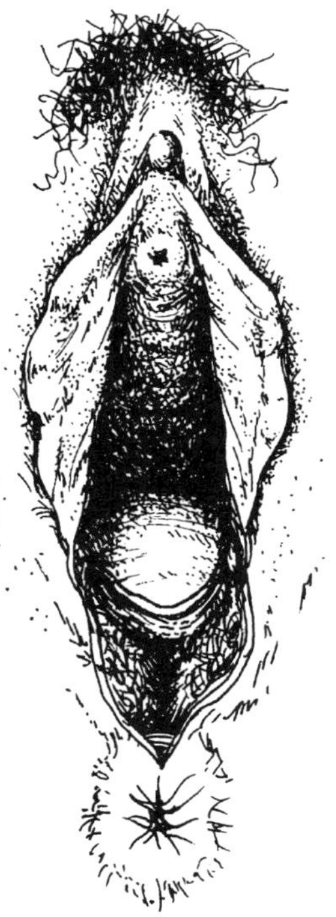
Midline tear extending to sulcus grooves that uncovers transverse perineal muscle fibers (will not be visible)	Deep tear revealing an intact rectal wall and anal sphincter	Sulcus groove and perineal tears extending to reveal an intact external sphincter

Checking for damage to the anterior yoni wall (ceiling) and bladder: The upper wall of the yoni is rarely damaged during a spontaneous birth; lacerations in this area most often occur with forceps births. Upper wall tears should be ruled out, however, as you examine the side walls of the yoni. Check both the anterior sulcus grooves and wall of the yoni for tears. Tears in the upper yoni wall are frequently difficult to see and often bleed profusely. Usually this exam can be accomplished during a visual inspection alone, as long as you can see the anterior wall. If you cannot or what you can see suggests damage, place two fingers deep in the yoni. Press the floor of the yoni down, out of your way, and hold it there while you look and feel for anterior wall damage with your other hand. This inspection may require a focused light source. If you suspect damage, you must examine more thoroughly, in which case the use of a retractor will help a lot.

Bleeding during an anterior wall exam: If there is upper wall damage, you may need to use a ring forceps with a gauze in the jaws to blot up blood, as these tears can bleed profusely. Fold a gauze into a manageable size and clamp it in a long ring forceps. Insert two to four fingers, palm down, as far back into the yoni as you can, and press them down firmly into the yoni floor. Slide the ring forceps holding the gauze into the yoni along the surface of your fingers, while avoiding scraping the gauze against the yoni wall. Identify the end of the forceps with the fingertips of the hand in the yoni. Use the forceps to displace the cervix, which could get in your way. If the gauze becomes saturated with blood, replace it before you proceed. Maneuver your forceps and fingers so that portions of the upper yoni wall become visible. Be sure to check the upper sulcus grooves as well, especially if a deep tear in the labia minora curves around and enters the yoni (Varney et al., 2004).

Check for bladder damage: If upper yoni wall lacerations are discovered, you will need to catheterize the mother to make sure no blood is in her urine. If blood is found, this indicates a tear into the bladder or urethra and the possibility of a fistula (a permanent hole from poor healing) forming. Transport or call for physician consultation. Since upper wall damage is usually not limited to skid marks, it is necessary to rule out damage that penetrates through the yoni wall. Catheterization technique is described in the chapter entitled "Repairing the Anterior Yoni Wall."

Examining the cervix

Identifying and dealing with a swollen cervix: A large, purple-red, smooth mass that protrudes into the middle of the yoni canal is probably the cervix (although not invariably it could also be a hematoma, a cervical polyp, a fibroid or a prolapse of some other kind). You may encounter the cervix if there has been cervical swelling or a stubborn anterior lip during labor. Localized swelling may be due to a small hematoma or a localized cyst-like swelling that can sometimes develop in the anterior lip during labor.

Use a ring forceps as described above to hold the cervix out of your field of view, if necessary. Then, with two fingers placed in the lateral fornices on either side, gently push the cervix toward the uterus. If it is extremely swollen it may not retract very much. If it doesn't, gently move it aside as you complete your inspection of the yoni walls. Give homeopathic Arnica pellets orally to relieve the trauma.

Inspecting for cervical damage: It has been estimated that cervical lacerations occur in as many as half of all births (Fahmy et al., 1991). Tears of up to 2 cm in length can be regarded as a common occurrence.

When indicated, carefully examine the cervix for tears. Examining the cervix is somewhat invasive and can be painful. It should be reserved for situations when you know the cervix was stretched down to the introitus during the birth and thus may have been torn or when the woman has significant bleeding from an as-yet-unidentified source (cervical bleeding is often brighter red and more fluid than uterine bleeding). If the cervix is positioned normally and bleeding is normal, you needn't routinely perform an elaborate inspection after spontaneous homebirths. In most cases, I recommend visualizing it as best you can in the process of doing the rest of the exam. Tears are typically small, not exceeding 0.5 cm in length. Cervical lacerations less than 0.5 cm long that are not bleeding will usually heal well on their own and do not require repair. One exception would be a woman who has a history of loose cervix (called "cervical incompetence" by the medical model). She may benefit from having cervical tears repaired as the ability of her cervix to remain closed is already compromised.

When called for, an examination of the cervix includes looking for obvious tears as well as feeling for areas of mucosa near the edges that are empty of muscle because the muscle has torn and retracted beneath the cervical mucosa, leaving an intact sheath of mucosa. Follow any tears to their upper end, as large tears may involve the fornices, the upper third of the yoni or the lower uterine segment; the uterine artery and its major branches; or even the peritoneum. These types of tears may present no symptoms, but more often there is significant bleeding or hematoma formation. Such deep tears are much more common after instrumental delivery, when inspection should be done routinely.

To visually inspect the cervix begin by inserting three or four fingers of your nondominant hand, palm down, along the posterior wall of the yoni to the point just anterior to the lower edge of the cervix. Apply firm downward pressure to the posterior yoni wall. Maintain your nondominant hand in this position to help orient yourself in the tissues and to avoid accidently poking your fingers into the cervical os. Very gently clamp the edge of the cervix with ring forceps to the first ratchet teeth, taking care to grasp only the anterior cervical lip at about 12 o'clock; do not include a fold of the bladder or the upper yoni wall by mistake.

Now, slide your nondominant fingers into the posterior fornix and apply strong downward pressure again. Insert another ring forceps to grasp the posterior lip of the cervix at about 6 o'clock. Leaving each forceps in place, apply slight traction to them and use the handles to move the cervix to one side of the introitus. This will pull the cervix over so you can inspect one side. Reverse this maneuver so you can examine the other side (Varney et al., 2004). Avoid pulling forcefully on the cervix; if you need to see better, it is preferable to open the yoni wider instead. If necessary, confirm your visual impressions by palpating the cervix in suspicious areas using the index finger of your internal hand. If there is no cervical damage, remove the forceps and your internal hand. If there is a cervical laceration, remove the ring forceps and reposition them on either side of the tear so you can steady the tissue for repair.

If this method of examining the cervix proves too difficult or too painful, you can try using one of the following techniques:

- If the cervix is large and floppy, as would be the case in a grand multipara, use two ring forceps as you move around the cervix, "leap frogging" them as you go to ensure that the entire cervix is examined (Varney et al., 2004).
- Alternatively, you can inch your way around the cervix using two ring forceps. First identify the cervical lip. Then grasp an accessible area of the edge with a ring forceps. Position the other ring forceps beside the first one; now open the jaws and slide the instrument on your dominant side over about a half inch. Then open and slide the forceps on your nondominant side over next to the first instrument and continue in this manner until you have inspected the entire circumference of the cervix. As you reposition the instruments, open the jaws wide enough so that rings completely clear the cervix. This avoids catching the rings on any tears or otherwise further traumatizing the tissue.

As you move around the cervix, look for areas that appear thin or irregular compared to the adjacent tissue. Such an area may be where the underlying muscle has been torn away and retracted from the overlying cervical mucosa. If you find such an area, position the forceps on either side of it. Now palpate the cervix for a lack of muscle tissue in that area. To confirm an occult tear, you must compare the feel of the suspicious area with an adjacent area that appears normal. If you still have questions after your instrumental exam is completed, don a fresh sterile glove and carefully palpate the entire circumference of the cervix for an area of retracted muscle beneath an intact sheath of cervical mucosa. This type of damage is fortunately rare.

If a large tear is found that extends into the fornices or uterus, peritoneal perforation may have also occurred, with either retroperitoneal or intraperitoneal bleeding. In such deep tears, it would be best to transport the woman for laparotomy to determine the true extent of the damage and for a hospital-based repair. Intrauterine exploration to rule out uterine rupture is also warranted. For these serious tears, surgical repair under anesthesia is required and blood replacement may be necessary as well.

Rarely, annular or circular detachment of the cervix occurs, where a portion of the cervix or even the entire circumference tears away. Look for ragged, irregular edges and missing portions as you perform your exam. If only a piece comes loose it is usually part of an anterior lip that got caught between the presenting part and the pubic bone. You may have noted an odd scrap of tissue that was expelled at the time of birth (look for it now). If this has occurred, the woman should be transported for repair (Cunningham et al., 2005).

When you have finished your exam, reposition the cervix back inside the yoni by splinting it with two fingers, one placed in each of the lateral fornices and pushing the cervix up on either side. If you find cervical tears or bleeding, see the chapter entitled "Cervical Lacerations."

Examining the anal sphincters and the anterior rectal wall

Damage to the anal sphincters is uncommon in the absence of a clitorotomy that extends, and it may seem like an unnecessary invasion to check it in every woman. However, you should always, at the very least, visually inspect the sphincter. If you check every time, you will have a much better reference for the normal parameters of the condition of the tissues right after birth. You will thus be more likely to recognize a damaged or severed sphincter should you encounter one. Also perform a digital exam unless you have absolutely no doubt whatsoever about the sphincter's integrity. Nevertheless, if there is a deep tear in the posterior yoni wall or a pocket tear immediately behind the perineal skin, you must rule out sphincter and rectal mucosa damage with a digital exam, even if you think there is none.

The woman with a short perineum is most likely to have a tear that initially appears shallow but is into or through the sphincter.

Anatomy review: The anal region presents multiple layers of tissue that begin below the superficial transverse perineal muscle and immediately behind the perianal skin. Starting with the most superficial anal structures as they are stacked within the perineal body and moving to the deepest, the first anal structure you will encounter is the "capsule of the sphincter," consisting of the connective tissues that enclose the main and subcuticular parts of the external sphincter. Under that, you will find the main part of the external sphincter; beneath and slightly distal to it as well (because the tip pokes out a little from under the main part of the external sphincter), you will find the subcuticular part of the external sphincter. If the main and subcuticular parts of the external sphincter are fully divided at least 6 mm or more from the anal orifice, the internal sphincter will be revealed and may be torn. The layer below the anterior internal sphincter will be the rectal mucosa, which extends from the level of the perianal skin into the anal canal. Because the internal sphincter can be set back slightly from the anal verge (especially in parous women [Frudinger et al., 1999]), you could have a very shallow external sphincter tear that even reveals the rectal mucosa, intact or not, with no involvement of the internal sphincter.

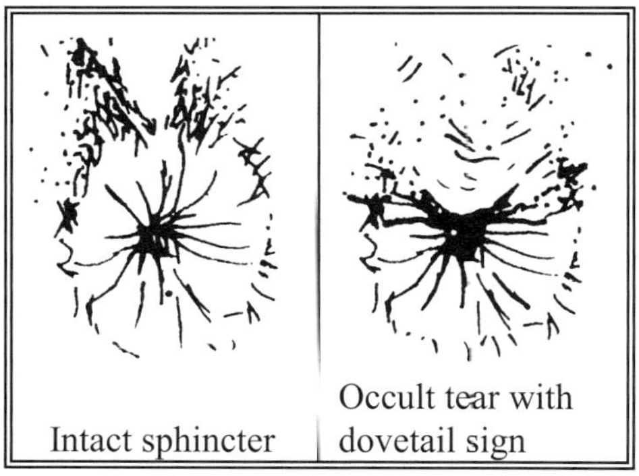

Visual inspection: Start by asking an assistant to check the mother's prenatal records to determine if you noted anything unusual about her anal region during your initial pelvic exam. Then, begin this exam by looking carefully at the anus. Assess the distance between the introitus and the anterior anal margin. There should be a normal amount of skin between them (although it may be damaged in this instance).

Study the corrugator cutis ani; it should be evenly puckered all around the anal circumference (or at least look the same as it did before the birth). Pay particular attention to the anterior quadrant of the anus; disruption of the puckering in this area (the Dovetail sign) usually indicates an underlying torn external sphincter or, more rarely, a fistula. This sign can also appear when a torn sphincter has healed with the ends apart. Frequent anal intercourse may also change the anal opening to mimic a dovetail sign. Ask the mother to contract her sphincter, and observe how the corrugator cutis ani behaves; you should see a circumferential response. If puckering is uneven or absent, you must check further to discover if the sphincter is damaged: in most cases it will be. It is possible, however, to have some degree of sphincter damage that may not produce obvious defects in the corrugator cutis ani because it is not extensive enough to alter the puckering. For this reason, if there is any other indication that there might be sphincter damage, you must proceed with a digital exam as well.

Digital exams: If a visual inspection of the external anus is not conclusive or there is a deep hole or other damage behind an intact perineum, next place your gloved index finger at the introitus of the yoni, press the pad of your finger down firmly and ask the woman to tighten her sphincter. Rock your finger slightly to palpate for the intact muscle. If the muscle is intact, you should feel a band of tissue, but this may be subtle just after birth and a bimanual exam (described below) may be necessary.

Checking the rectovaginal wall: Note that it is possible to have intact internal and external anal sphincters with a tear that somehow involves the anterior anorectal wall. This occurs when a tear goes right down the perineal skin, over, around and under the intact sphincters and extends into the rectal mucosa. If a clitorotomy has been cut, if there is a deep tear at the introitus, if the perineum is quite short or if, for any other reason, you suspect there may be either sphincter or rectal mucosal damage, check the integrity of the rectovaginal wall. This exam will also clarify what is going on when the posterior yoni wall appears to have split into layers.

Explain to the mother what you plan to do and why. Put a larger, clean glove over the glove on the hand you will use for a rectal exam. Lubricate either the index or little finger of the double-gloved hand. (Use the finger you feel will be most sensitive for the examination.) Inform the mother first and then insert this finger into her anal canal. Insert a finger of the other hand into her yoni. Use both fingers to perform a bimanual exam of the rectovaginal wall by simultaneously drawing your fingers forward, beginning just above the internal apex of the tear in the yoni mucosa. Press your fingers together as if to cause them to meet through the tissue. Check any pockets to see if they are really button holes; if fingers touch, there is a tear through the yoni floor into the rectal mucosa. Be sure you have done a thorough exam. Rarely, there are discrete rectovaginal holes in several places. (This is more likely if you have done a clitorotomy, the tissue is extremely friable or getting the baby out involved unusually aggressive manipulations.) Of course, depending on the location of the hole, intervening layers of tissue will also be divided and this may include the internal sphincter, the external sphincter or both.

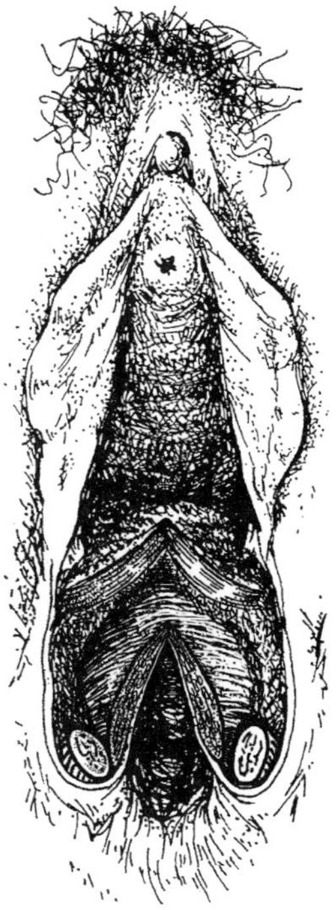

Extensive (4th degree) tear with a torn external and internal sphincter and a torn anorectal mucosa

Discovering an intestinal prolapse: Very rarely, you may discover loops of small intestines that have slipped through a rectal mucosa tear or a deep yoni tear. This indicates that the mother has an enterocele with a tear that goes through the posterior cul-de-sac. In order to prevent strangulation of the loops of bowel and avoid accidently pricking the bowel wall with a needle (a major complication), repairs that involve small bowel prolapse should take place in a hospital and should be done prior to the repair of any other birth-related damage (Lawrence, 1992).

Bimanual rectovaginal examination of the perineal muscles: If you still have questions concerning the depth of the tear in the yoni mucosa or the integrity of the perineal muscles, this is a good time to reexamine from another angle since you are already performing a rectal exam. Have the mother tighten her perineal muscles and see what the perineal body feels like from below. Use your yoni finger to assist your rectal finger in identifying any damage.

Bimanual and visual inspection of the anal sphincters: Most of the time, anal sphincter damage follows a predicable course of severity, first occurring in the most superficial fibers that pass beneath the distal introitus. More extensive damage frays or divides the muscle to a greater anteroposterior depth. Tearing usually occurs this way because during a normal birth, the muscle is stretched side to side and the most shallow, most anterior fibers are stretched the most and therefore are most prone to tearing. When the perineum has been cut, however, the sphincter may be nipped by the scissors; when this occurs, it is much more likely to tear in half.

With this in mind and your two hands still in place, ask the mother to tighten her sphincters around your finger. Can you feel the muscle? If you are unsure, you can use both your yoni and rectal fingers to feel from either side for the firm band of tissue that is the intact main part of the external sphincter. After the birth, most women do not have very much sphincter sensation, and the tissue is soft. It is often hard for either of you to feel the sphincter tighten; at the same time, if the muscle is severed, a gap may be detected as she tightens it.

Alternatively, you can do a one-handed exam by inserting your index finger into the anal canal and your thumb in the yoni. Roll these fingers back and forth over the sphincter.

Now, remove your yoni finger and look down into the yoni. Position your rectal finger at a slightly upward angle and press toward you. Have the mother tighten her sphincter again. Look and feel for the muscle. A fully severed external sphincter will often retract and pucker the tissue on either side of your finger, just behind the skin layer. Sometimes the external sphincter and its enclosing capsule has been exposed but not torn. In this case, when the mother tightens the muscle contracts all the way around your finger, it will appear as a distinct, fat band of firm, smooth, light rose-pink tissue. If the sphincter itself is exposed or partially severed, it will look round and meaty-red and the ends may be stringy.

If the external sphincter is more than 50% severed, you may sometimes find just a cavity on one side because half of the muscle has retracted down inside its capsule and may therefore be difficult to find, while the other half is visible across from the hole as a large, round, rough, meaty or stringy chunk. The retracted half will need to be retrieved before you proceed with repair. Rarely, one torn half will not retract, but will be found partially attached to the inner wall of the capsule resulting in an empty and palpable pocket with no retrievable sphincter down inside. In other cases, both ends will retract, or both may be visible. Regardless of where each end may be, you must find them both before you can do the repair. (See the chapters covering anal sphincter repair in the part entitled "Third- and Fourth-Degree Repair" for more details.)

The internal sphincter lies between the external sphincter and the rectal mucosa and begins about 6 mm above the lower border of the external anal sphincter (DeLancey et al., 1997). It is taller and flatter than the external sphincter. It may tear along with the external sphincter, it may stay intact under the external sphincter, or it may tear separately from the external sphincter and retract in a separate layer. It is made of circular smooth muscle that appears paler than the external sphincter (similar to raw fish). If the internal anal sphincter is torn, you should assume that the external sphincter is torn as well. Likewise, if the external sphincter and rectal muscosa are torn, the internal sphincter may have torn as well, especially when the damage to the rectal muscosa extends more than 6 mm above the anal orifice.

Before removing your rectal finger, palpate the anterior rectal wall one more time while looking down at the floor of the yoni to see if any buttonhole tears in the rectovaginal wall become evident.

When you finish, carefully remove the cover glove used for the rectal inspection so as not to contaminate your other gloves and discard it.

Identifying a hematoma (HE-ma-TOE-ma)

A hematoma is a blood blister caused by a broken, bleeding vessel beneath the tissue. Hematomas usually develop over the course of hours or by the next day after the birth but can develop quite quickly, particularly when a large vessel is involved. Women with very fragile tissue, a very rapid fetal descent, an instrumental or manipulated birth, or genital varicosities are prone to develop hematomas.

As you do your exam, note any distinct, smooth, dark purplish swellings in or near the damaged tissue or on the anterior lip of the cervix. Deep hematomas may not present a visible purple mass. They may develop a tender swelling that is too far under the skin to appear purple. They may produce an internal swelling that is painful when disturbed during your exam. Palpate gently and to help locate the region of pain or tenderness. A hematoma may be out of reach and sight behind the yoni or between the yoni and rectum. The mother senses increasing pain and pressure as it enlarges. Signs of shock out of proportion to visible blood loss are also a tip-off that you have some sort of concealed bleeding. (See the chapter entitled "Hematomas" for more information.)

Assessing the Degree of Damage and the Need for Repair

Measuring the tear

If you have a Peri-Rule or have scratched measuring marks on an instrument, now is a good time to measure the tear. In a typical tear you will take three measurements, recalling the L shape of most tears. The first (1) is the depth of the tear through the center of the perineal body from the midline "corner" of the fourchette (the angle of the sideways L where the perineal skin meets the yoni mucosa), to the depth of the tear in the perineal body. The second (2) is the internal length of the tear, defined as the depth from the fourchette to the internal apex of the tear in the yoni mucosa (the horizontal arm of the L). The third measurement (3) is the external length of the tear, which is assessed by measuring from the fourchette to the external apex of the tear in the perineal skin (the vertical arm of the L). The recommended sequence of measurement is intended to minimize contamination of the wound, with the part of the tear nearest the anus being measured last.

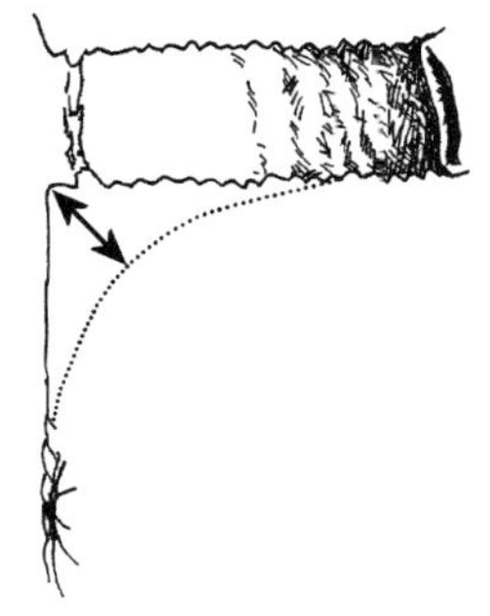
1. Depth of tear

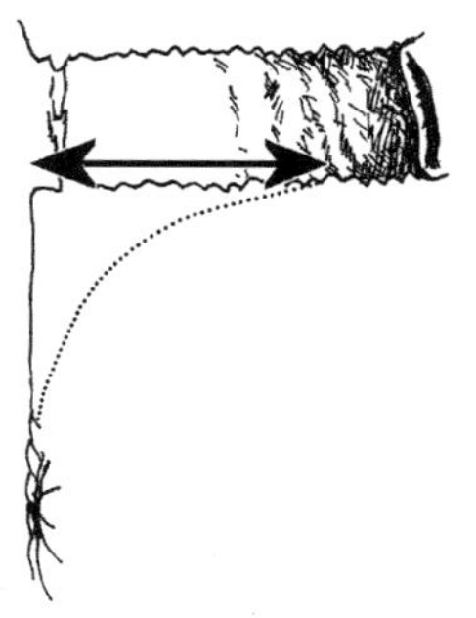
2. Internal length of tear

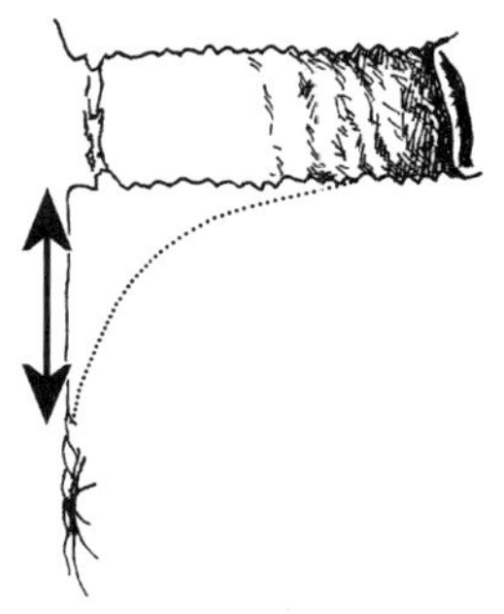
3. External length of tear

If the tear is more complex, you will want to measure each torn area, beginning near the clitoral glans, moving to labial tears, then 1, 2 and 3 above and finally any tears in the rectum last of all. Do not reuse a Peri-rule that has been used near the anus to measure in other areas. Always describe and diagram the tear in your records.

Assigning a degree of damage

Next, assign a degree to the damage. This designation helps you accurately record your findings and discuss the tear with others. Several different classification schemes have been used over the years, leading to much confusion. Three degrees are recognized in most textbooks; some classify a fourth as well. In 1999, Sultan proposed standardizing the classification of perineal trauma, and this chapter presents his recommendations. His scheme has been adopted by the Royal Collage of Obstetricans and Gynecologists and by practitioners internationally, although it is not mentioned in current US sources as of this writing.

First degree: First-degree damage involves the yoni epithelium or perineal skin only and should be identified by location. The tear is shallow at each apex and does not involve perineal muscles. This is the type of tear you will see most frequently. First-degree tears include very minor damage (such as abrasions, skid marks and skin splits) and other shallow tears, many of which do not require repair.

Second degree: A second-degree tear involves the muscles of the perineum. A complete second-degree tear extends through the muscle fibers of the perineal body but does not involve the anal sphincter.

Third degree: Third-degree damage involves injury to one or both of the anal sphincters. If there is any doubt about the grade of tearing, the next highest classification should be assigned when describing any type of anal sphincter injury. Third-degree damage is subcategorized as follows:
3a: A tear that involves less than 50% of the thickness of the external sphincter
3b: A tear that involves more than 50% of the thickness of the external sphincter
3c: A tear that involves both the external and internal anal sphincters

Fourth degree: Officially, fourth-degree damage includes third-degree damage as well as disruption of the anal mucosa. Tears that involve only the anal mucosa with an intact anal sphincter complex (buttonhole tear) should be classified as fourth-degree with the actual injured parts described in detail.

You will note that these definitions focus on the posterior yoni wall, perineal body and anus. They do not refer to tears in the anterior or lateral yoni walls or to tears in the labial or periurethral tissues. These sorts of tears could be classified as either first- or second-degree based on your best guess as to whether they involve muscle tissue.

Moreover, there is no provision for classifying odd tears in the perineal area, for example one that includes yoni mucosa, sphincter and anal mucosa, but are so very shallow that no there is no other perineal muscle involvement. What about a buttonhole tear into the rectal mucosa with completely intact sphincters? Special situations such as these need to be described specifically in your records. The categories described above were obviously designed with incisions that produce much more predictable varieties of damage and extensions in mind.

Deciding if sutures are necessary

Labial tears can usually be left to heal in their own unless they are deep and form a flap or a dangling chunk, are very unsightly or are bleeding uncontrollably. More about deciding whether labial tears require suturing can be found in the chapter entitled "Periurethral and Labial Repairs." Shallow skid marks and skin splits cannot be sutured because they just aren't deep enough. While management in these cases is relatively straightforward, most perineal injuries require a judgement call regarding suturing. The woman has the right to refuse suturing, but she will be depending upon your assessment of the damage to make an informed decision.

For centuries midwives and other birth attendants have debated when and whether perineal lacerations require repair at all. Not suturing first- or second-degree lacerations is widespread among North American direct-entry midwives and among some midwives in the UK, even though there is not really any good, evidenced-based research to support this practice. US-based certified nurse-midwives have, by in large, not jumped on this band-wagon (or at least have not done so as vocally).

Midwives that advocate this practice report some short-term benefits—these include no stitches right after the birth, less postpartum pain, less infection and faster healing—when women are not stitched. Some homebirth midwives in the US have reported remarkable short-term results following large tears that are left to heal naturally with the assistance of herbal compresses. I have even heard of reports of third-degree tears that healed well. Nonetheless, the possible long-term consequences may be less appealing, such as poorer cosmetic results; problems with sexual function; weakening of the pelvic floor; pelvic, perineal or yoni pain and eventual incontinence and organ prolapse.

The few studies that have looked at the short-term results of not suturing the torn perineum (Clement & Reed, 1999; Head, 1993; Leeman et al., 2007; Wood, 1999) were generally favorable to the practice. In addition, two randomized controlled trials have attempted to weigh the benefits and risks of not suturing by studying two groups in which one group of women was sutured and another was not. A Swedish study (Lundquist et al., 2000) found that women have more short-term discomfort when they are not stitched, which has been my observation as well. A Scottish study (Fleming et al., 2003) looked at pain levels at 10 days and again at six weeks and found no significant differences between two similar groups of women. Fleming and colleagues did find that women who were sutured had better wound approximation at six weeks. Note, however, that no study to date has looked at the long-term consequences of leaving perineal lacerations to heal entirely on their own.

With as many women as we now have suffering from pelvic prolapse from the routine practice of clitorotomy, the obvious first solution is to do everything we can to bring the tear rate down to an irreducible minimum. I am not equally convinced that the obvious answer to tearing is to leave it unsutured. While very shallow tears will usually heal very well if left alone, if there is significant muscle involvement or if the perineal membrane has been divided, the wound is unlikely to heal well unless it is reapproximated. I must point out that no one is advocating not suturing third- or fourth-degree tears. Leaving deep or extensive tears to heal without sutures is a very big gamble. Once healed, they are very hard to reconstruct, and the risk of anal incontinence or the formation of a fistula is not something I would want to leave to this level of chance.

Checklist for decision making

Some considerations that might make you lean more toward suturing:

•The woman wants sutures.

•The woman is concerned about a good cosmetic result.

•There is second-, third- or fourth-degree damage.

•The wound is ragged or oddly shaped.

•The edges of the wound do not meet when the legs are together.

•The wound is deep or extensive internally or externally.

•A piece of tissue is hanging away from the vulva in a chunk.

•The wound is bleeding excessively.

•There is a pocket tear that may collect lochia, increasing the likelihood of infection.
•Tissue from a prolapse behind the torn area bulges forward, separating the edges of the laceration (as might occur with a rectocele).
•The woman is (or has been) poorly nourished or is otherwise in poor health.
•The woman has little postpartum help and will be on her feet a lot shortly after birth.

Some circumstances that might sway you in the other direction:
•The woman refuses sutures
•The woman has adequate, ongoing support at home, can realistically manage to stay mostly in bed for the coming 2 to 3 weeks and is able to avoid using stairs on a daily basis for up to 4 weeks (Baldwin, 2010).
•The tear is very short and shallow throughout.
•The edges of the tear are straight and lie together without assistance.
•The tear is along an old scar that was painful, even after healing had occurred.
•No more than two stitches are needed to close the tear (i.e., the tear is no more than 2 cm long and no more than 1 cm deep).
•Periurethral or labial damage has not left chunks hanging and is not bleeding.
•You are quite certain that the rectal mucosa and anal sphincters are intact.

Ultimately, the decision rests with the mother. There are tears that I definitely encourage women to let me repair and others I am more flexible about. (I feel sure I have repaired many tears that other midwives would leave to heal on their own because I do feel comfortable with suturing.) The woman needs to know that suturing will largely eliminate the pain and burning of raw, exposed edges, especially during the first 24 hours.

When women want to decline suturing but their damage is extensive, a compromise may be to offer to suture the deepest or most critical damage, such as a deep perineal tear or an injury to the anal sphincters, rectal mucosa or anterior yoni wall. You could restore the tissues so that deep damage is converted to a shallow tear. This is much more likely to heal well and provides some insurance that the tissues she cannot afford to have heal apart do not. There is also the theoretical risk of lochia seeping down into the sutured part of the laceration and encouraging infection. This is not as much of a risk with a truly shallow tear because the tissue underneath it is really intact; with a deep tear that is partially repaired, the crevices that will inevitably result from having stitches placed may provide an avenue for lochia to seep down into the depths of the tear. I have never done this myself and there are no studies on this issue because most of the time women are either completely repaired or not. However, we do know that Nancy Fleming's 1990 study showed that leaving the skin layer unrepaired resulted in no increased risk for infection.

Circumstances that call for transport to the hospital for repair or consulting with a back-up practitioner with more suturing experience:
•The landmarks are not obvious or you are not sure exactly what structures are damaged.
•The tear is quite a bit more extensive than any you have repaired before, and you are uncertain of your skill.
•You do not have the appropriate suture materials or equipment to do the job properly.
•There is extensive tearing deep in the yoni that requires retractors to repair properly.

- There are extensive cervical tears.
- You cannot locate one of the apexes of a tear.
- Bleeding from the tear is uncontrollable, or the source cannot be identified.
- Repair requires dissection of intact tissue.
- There is a deep upper yoni wall tear.
- There is anal sphincter or rectal mucosa damage.
- There is blood in the urine upon catheterization.
- There is (or you suspect) an extensive or expanding hematoma.
- There is deep and extensive periurethral damage, especially near the clitoris or urethra.

Experience will eliminate some of these considerations, but one of the most important characteristics of a good midwife is humility. If in doubt, transport or call for backup.

References and Further Reading on Checking for Perineal Damage after Birth

Examining the Perineum after Birth

Anderson M. "Principles of wound healing in the repair of the episiotomy" (unpublished paper), Hawthorne NY, 1975.

Cunningham F, et al. Chapter 35: "Obstetrical hemorrhage," in Cunningham F, et al. WILLIAMS OBSTETRICS, 22nd ed. McGraw-Hill, New York NY, 2005.

DeLancey J, et al. "Internal and external anal sphincter anatomy as it relates to midline obstetric lacerations," OBSTET GYNECOL, 90(6):924-927, Dec, 1997.

Fahmy K, et al. "Postpartum colposcopy of the cervix: injury and healing," INT J GYNECOL OBSTET, 34(2):133-137, Feb, 1991.

Frudinger A, et al. "Changes in anal anatomy following vaginal delivery revealed by anal endosonography," BR J OBSTET GYNECOL,106(3):233-237, Mar, 1999.

Groom KM, Paterson-Brown S. "Can we improve on the diagnosis of third-degree tears?," EUR J OBSTET GYNECOL REPROD BIOL, 101(1):19-21, Feb 10, 2002.

Hellman L, Pritchard J. WILLIAM'S OBSTETRICS, 14th ed. Appleton Crofts, New York NY, 1971.

Herman GE. Chapter 21: "Injuries to the genital canal in childbirth," in his DIFFICULT LABOR: A GUIDE TO ITS MANAGEMENT FOR STUDENTS AND PRACTITIONERS, 5th ed. Cassell & Co., Ltd., London UK, 1910.

Lawrence L. Personal correspondence, Win, 1992.

Nordenstam J. "Immediate or delayed repair of obstetric anal sphincter tears—a randomized controlled trial," BJOG, 115(7):857-865, Jun, 2008. (Comment in BJOG, 115(13):1718-1719, Dec, 2008).

Trott A. WOUNDS AND LACERATIONS: EMERGENCY CARE AND CLOSURE, 3rd ed. Elsevier Mosby, Philadelphia PA, 2005.

Varney H, et al. Chapter 75: "Postbirth inspection of the cervix and upper vaginal vault," in their VARNEY'S MIDWIFERY, 4th ed. Jones & Bartlett, Sudbury MA, 2004.

Assessing the Degree of Damage and the Need for Repair

Baldwin, Eiris, editing notes, 2010.

Cioffi J, et al. "Clinical decision-making for repair of spontaneous childbirth trauma: validation of cues and related factors," JMWH, 54(1):65-72, Jan-Feb, 2009.

Clement S, Reed B. "To stitch or not to stitch? A long-term follow-up study of women with unsutured perineal tears," PRACT MIDWIFE, 2(4):20-28, Apr, 1999.

Fleming E, et al. "Does perineal suturing make a difference? The SUNS trial," BR J OBSTET GYNAECOL, 110:684-689, Jul, 2003.

Fleming N. "Can the suturing method make a difference in postpartum perineal pain?" J NURSE MIDWIFERY, 35(1):19-25, Jan-Feb 1990.

Head L. "Midwife's Journal. Dropping stitches," NURS TIMES, 89(33):64-65, Aug 18-24,1993.

Leeman L, et al. "Do unsutured second-degree perineal lacerations affect postpartum functional outcomes?" JABFM, 20(5):451-457, Sep-Oct, 2007.

Lewis P. "Poor science makes poor practice," MODERN MIDWIFE, 7(6):4-5, Jun, 1997.

Lundquist M, et al. "Is it necessary to suture all lacerations after a vaginal delivery?" BIRTH, 27(2):79-85, Jun, 2000.

Metcalfe A, et al. "A pragmatic tool for the measurement of perineal tears," BR J MIDWIFERY, 10(7):412-417, Jul, 2002.

Peri-Rule. www.peri-rule.bham.ac.uk, accessed Dec, 2008.

Peri-Rule. "Instructions for use" and "Assessment of perineal tears record form." (product inserts). Birmingham Health Science Devices, Edgbaston UK, Sep 17, 2004.

Sultan A. "Obstetric perineal injury and anal incontinence," CLINICAL RISK, 5:193-196, 1999.

Tohill S, Metcalfe A. Chapter 6: "Perineal tear assessment and the development of the Peri-Rule," in Henderson C, Bick D, eds. PERINEAL CARE: AN INTERNATIONAL ISSUE. Quay Books, London UK, 2005.

Wood T. "Not suturing is safe," PRACT MIDWIFE, 2(7):15, Jul, 1999.

PREPARING TO SUTURE

SETTING UP FOR SUTURING

Arranging the mother and yourself for suturing

Take a few minutes to figure out a suitable arrangement for the mother and yourself that will ensure that she is comfortable, that you are able to see what you are doing and that you are reasonably comfortable as well. Always strive to make it comfortable for the mother to continue to hold and focus on her baby; leaving the baby skin-to-skin optimizes genetically directed, hormonally mediated attachment in the first hours of life. There are several options.

By far, the easiest for both examination and repair is for the mother to move to the edge of the bed, spread her legs, and position her feet on chairs that have seats that are level with the bed. You would then sit in a chair placed between her legs and not have to work scrunched over on the bed. This is the best arrangement for most repairs, particularly if the tear is deep or complex, requiring light deep inside the yoni. If there are lacerations of the cervix or upper yoni wall and you are not going to transport to the hospital to have them repaired, suturing is best done with the mother on a study table such as an exam or massage table.

Another option is to leave the woman in the middle of the bed and place something firm (like an inverted fracture pan or a firm pillow such as a sofa cushion) underneath her bottom to provide elevation. A drawback to this position is that it promotes pooling of blood in the yoni; this not only obscures your ability to see what you are doing, but it also makes assessment of uterine bleeding difficult.

If there are no suitable chairs available, the bed is too soft and there is no sturdy table for the mother to lie on, sweep the floor, spread some sheets and blankets, and move her to the floor for repair.

If you must suture while sitting on a bed or the floor in front of the supine mother, find the least taxing position that still allows enough arm mobility for you to work.

Arranging your equipment

1. Assess your equipment needs. You may need some or all of the following items:
    - Suture instruments
        - Needle holder(s)
        - Stitch scissors
        - 4 hemostats
        - 2 Allis clamps
        - Thumb forceps
        - 2 ring forceps
    - Tray or other container on which to place equipment
    - Receptacle for used instruments
    - Local anesthetic
    - Goggles and other protective clothing
    - Suture packets containing suitable sizes and lengths of suture swaged to appropriate needles
    - Several packets of sterile 4"×4" gauze
    - Syringes & extra needles
    - Sterile and nonsterile gloves in the appropriate size

•Sterile barrier towel (if desired)
•Water-based lubricant for lubricating gut suture (if desired)
•Urinary catheter or catheterization kit
•Urine collection pan (your placenta pan will do just fine)
•Povidone iodine or similar product
•Alcohol swabs or grain alcohol and cotton or gauze swabs
•A pint of sterile saline and a sterile basin.
•Good, portable, light source
•Mirror for the mother's use if she wants to see what you are doing

2. You and your assistant can wash your hands now.
3. Have a chair beside the bed or a space cleared either between the mother's legs or to her side, where you can put your equipment. A cookie sheet covered with an underpad or clean towel makes a great portable instrument tray. Clear off any other equipment before arranging your suturing instruments. If you are not using a cookie sheet, spread out a clean underpad to use as a field.
4. Place clean underpads beneath the mother's bottom. Put one on her lower belly over the pubic bone if you expect to need an upper area to put instruments or sutures during the repair. (You'll understand this provision more as you read about complicated repairs.)
5. Arrange your light source or have your assistant do so.
6. Have an assistant place your instrument pack on the underpad that is on the chair and have her open it. Do not touch the instruments.
7. Have an assistant open a few 4" × 4" gauze squares and toss them onto the sterile field (you'll use them for blotting up blood). If you do not have an assistant, open the tops of the packages by peeling the flaps apart or rip into them from the side. Do not touch the gauze itself. You may either prop the packages or dump the gauze onto your sterile field.
8. Some midwives like to rinse the preservative from chromic gut. To do so, have your assistant dump a bottle of warmed sterile saline into a sterile container.
9. Some midwives like to lubricate gut suture with water-based lubricant (such as a freshly opened packet of K-Y gel or Astroglide; *do not* use oil) before inserting the needle into the skin. If you prefer to do so, get out a new, unopened container of whichever you plan to use. Do not lubricate synthetic suture materials.
10. Packets of suture are designed with two flaps on either side of one end. Open the outer packet by grasping a flap between the thumb and index finger of each hand, press the heels of your hands together. Now pull the flaps open by rolling your hands away from each other to expose the inner, sterile, foil packet. You can then empty the foil packets onto a sterile field prior to donning your sterile gloves. You can also wait until you don sterile gloves and then have your assistant open the outer pack so you can remove the inner packet. Be prudent and do not open more suture than you know you will use: one packet of 27" (70 cm) suture is sufficient to repair most perineal lacerations.
11. If you plan to inject anesthetic, open the syringe wrapper in the same manner and dump the syringe onto the sterile field.
12. Have your assistant don gloves. (See instructions for donning sterile gloves on page 443).
13. Perform a surgical hand wash at this point. Don sterile gloves. Use the inner sterile glove wrapper (or a sterile disposable barrier towel) as an additional sterile field. Place it on the tray beside your instruments.

14. If you have placed a field above the pubic bone (for complicated repairs), place the inner wrapper from your assistant's gloves on the underpad already in place above the pubic bone. Arrange it so you have a second field for your equipment.
15. Have your assistant peel open your sterile instrument pack. Remove each instrument as you need it. When you need to put an instrument down, place it on the glove wrapper already on the tray; do not put it back into the sterile pack.

Before You Begin Your Repair

Assess whether to remove skin tags

If there are skin tags around the mouth of the yoni that need removal, do this now, unless you are unsure about whether the tag can be repaired. If so, waiting until you have some of the surrounding tissue sewn together should help clarify the decision. (For a complete discussion of when and how to remove tags, see the chapter entitled "Skin Tags.")

Insert a gauze tampon

Normal uterine bleeding can be a nuisance during inspection or repair. A homemade tampon is usually not necessary during the repair of small tears, but can come in handy if the tear is extensive, the internal apex is deep, or the tear is otherwise hard to visualize. Tampons are particularly useful if the cervix is low and in the way. I do *not* recommend using a regular commercial menstrual tampon for this purpose. They are so small and relatively thin that they may more easily enter the cervix by accident and will probably not be sufficient to plug the just-stretched yoni to minimize bleeding into the torn area.

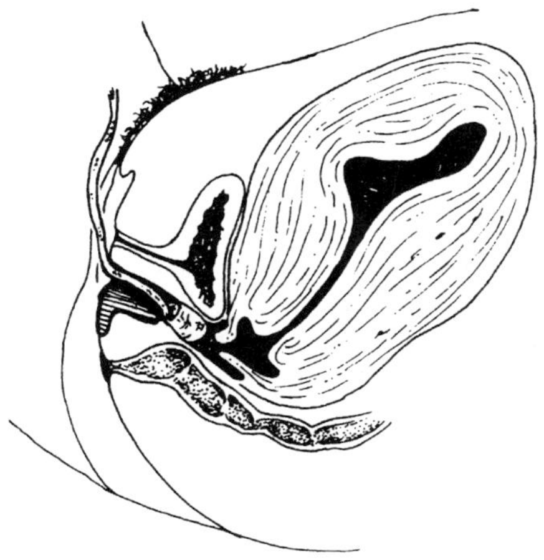

Gauze tampon in place with a locating tail (tear is shaded)

If you are concerned about excessive uterine bleeding, don't insert a tampon unless you can get the repair done quickly. It is easy to get so wrapped up in the repair that you lose track of the bleeding concealed behind the tampon.

Rarely, the source of bleeding is so high up that it appears to be uterine but is really seepage from a tear in the upper yoni or in the cervix. If the uterus is small and firm and low, examine the cervix and upper vault of the yoni to rule out a bleeding tear. If the uterus is softer and high or is big and firm, it is probably full of clots, or it may be displaced and clamping down ineffectively due to a full bladder and thus bleeding more. See the part entitled "Maternal Problems That Can Occur during Placental Delivery and the Hours following Birth" in HOLISTIC MIDWIFERY, VOL. II, for more details as to how to deal with such problems. Also rule out a torn blood vessel as the source of bleeding. Inserting a homemade tampon may clarify the source of bleeding as well. If nothing else is found, do the repair and see if that stops the bleeding.

To insert a tampon before or after administering anesthetic:

- Examine the posterior yoni and cervix first, to avoid missing any damage behind the tampon. Damage in these areas must be repaired before a tampon is inserted.
- Clean out any clots in the yoni and make sure the uterus is low and firm.
- Fold a 4" × 4" gauze square in quarters to stuff into the yoni. Alternately, roll a 4"

× 4" that is folded in half. It is a good idea to attach a drawstring to the tampon, which will help you remove it as well as remember that it is in place. The string can be made of a strip of gauze or unflavored dental floss (from a spool you carry exclusively for this purpose) tied securely around the middle of the tampon. A drawstring can get in the way and become contaminated, however, so be sure it doesn't touch the anus. To avoid this and to prevent sewing it into the repair, make it long enough to attach to the drape above the mother's pubic bone.

•Moisten the gauze with a little lochia or sterile water-based lubricant (such as Astroglide or K-Y jelly).

•Hold the tampon with the drawstring cupped in your palm in one hand and insert two fingers of the other hand along the posterior yoni wall. Press into the yoni floor with the length of your fingers at a slightly upward angle.

•Slide the tampon against your fingers toward the posterior fornix, beyond the internal apex of the tear. Avoid pressing it against the anterior yoni wall. If the cervix is normally placed, be sure it is above and behind the tampon and not trapped between the tampon and the yoni wall. However, if the cervix is low and gaping, be sure the posterior (lower) lip *is* between the tampon and the yoni wall to avoid pushing the tampon up inside the uterus! (This is when a short, securely attached drawstring is required.)

•Check the fundus from time to time to be sure it isn't filling up behind the tampon.

Administer local anesthetic

Apply or inject anesthetic just a few minutes before you plan to start the repair. This will give it plenty of time to take effect.

Final checks before beginning your repair

Recheck the mother's condition next. It is best if she remains occupied with the baby while you work. Someone can sit beside her and help her cope with the suturing. The assistant should record when suturing begins and anything else that occurs during that time.

Clear the area of any clots of blood. Checks for uterine firmness must not be forgotten during suturing, especially if a tampon is inserted. Your assistant is the best person to do this. (Be sure she knows how and that she pays attention to what she touches with which gloves if you are trying to maintain a strictly sterile procedure.)

Rarely, long pubic hair may be in the way. Trim it; grasp several hairs and cut them shorter. Carefully remove them from the field so that hair is not sewn into the repair. Do not shave the hair. Rinse the perineum with warmed sterile saline, if necessary, to remove any bits of hair that remain.

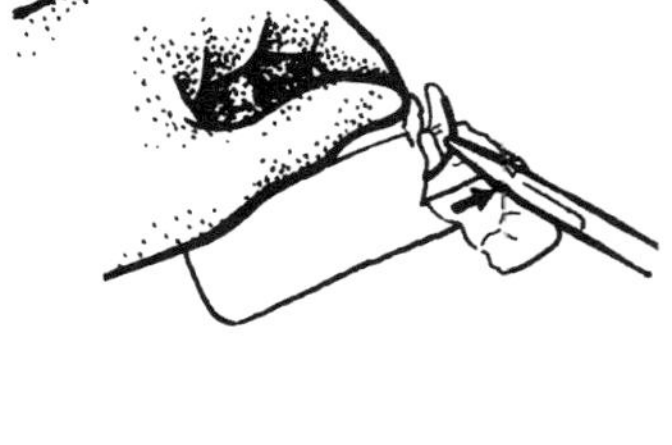

Removing the needle from the foil packet

Preparation of the suture and needle

Before you begin, proceed as follows:

1. Have an assistant open the outer suture wrapper. Withdraw the inner pack with your gloved hand.
2. Tear open the foil wrapper and remove the card

holding the suture and needle. Rinse a card loaded with chromic suture in sterile water. (Chromic is packed in isopropyl alcohol. If it has dried out, the suture will be inflexible. Although it can be softened by immersion in sterile saline solution [¼ tsp salt to 1 cup water], it is far better to discard it, as its tensile strength is likely to be compromised.) Synthetic materials are packed dry and should not be rinsed.

3. Remove the suture from the card around which it is wrapped by grasping the needle with your needle holder and pulling it out from the side of the card. Grasp the free end of the strand with one hand and below the swaged end with the other and straighten the strand with a gentle pull (do not tug or jerk) on each end. If you are using double-swaged suture (with a needle on each end), divide the length as necessary for use in and outside the yoni (keeping in mind where you will use each needle). To do so, hold both needles in one hand, and use your other hand to straighten the suture and snip it in half.
4. If you intend to use Cetacaine for suture lubrication, have your assistant make a puddle on your sterile glove wrapper so you can moisten the strand during suturing.
5. Use your fingers to lubricate the suture, applying only a tiny bit of gel to the needle. Trying to drag it through a puddle is messy, and it gets contaminated easily.
6. Next, place your needle in the needle holder.

Holding the tissue so you can see

If you have no assistant, you can expose the internal apex of the tear in the yoni in either of the following ways:

- Depress the posterior yoni wall by placing your nondominant middle and index fingers on either side of the tear. Your dominant hand will hold the needle holder. The extra suture lies across and to your nondominant side, tucked into the nondominant palm with the ring and little fingers. Spread the labia from above with the thumb and index finger of the nondominant hand. Hold the strand of suture up over the tear with the middle finger of your nondominant hand.
- If manual retraction provides inadequate exposure, insert a yoni retractor, although I don't recommend the routine use of a yoni retractor at home. For one thing, they hurt. For another, if a repair requires retractors, the tear is probably extensive enough to warrant transporting for repair. If you are going to use a retractor, see the chapter entitled "Using a Yoni Retractor."

If you have an assistant, she can hold the tissue open in whatever way you like. Both of your hands are then free to work.

Overview of the repair

Stitches placed in the floor of the yoni are directed down and deep to the surface. Directing the mucosal layer down and deep helps to encompass the depth of the tear and assess whether a layer of deep interrupted stitches are necessary. If the tear can be closed to its depth with a single layer of stitches in the mucosa and the basting layer placed in the deep perineum alone, there is no need for deep interrupted stitches. If a space is left beneath the sutures in the yoni floor that cannot be closed with the basting layer down the perineum, a deep interrupted stitch or, if more than one stitch is required, a deeper layer of running stitches are necessary to close this open space. These stitches are placed back and deep to the perineal surface (rather than deep to the surface of the yoni mucosa) to avoid penetrating the lumen of the bowel. More details about when and how all of these layers are created will be found as you read this section.

Basting stitches placed down the perineum are directed back and deep from the vertical plane of the perineal surface to close any dead space in this area not closed by the stitches already placed in the floor of the yoni mucosa.

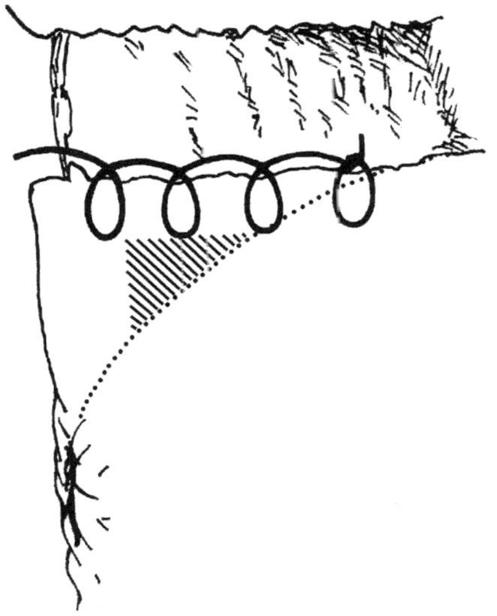

Shaded area represents an unrepaired dead space left beneath continuous basting stitches in yoni mucosa

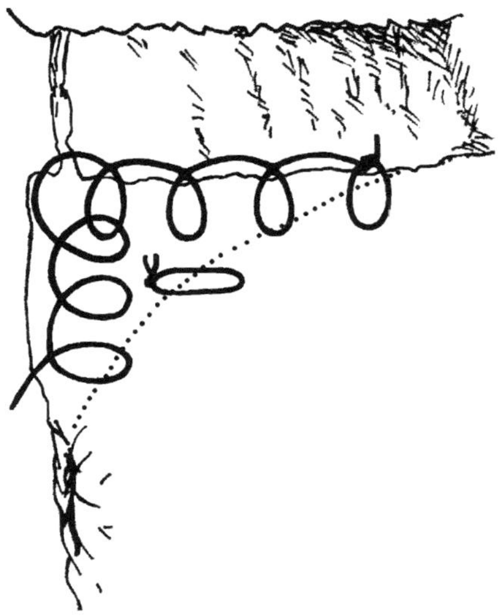

Deep space closed with a single interrupted stitch

<u>If it has been more than six hours since the birth</u>: Make every effort to have repairs completed as soon after the initial postpartum hour as possible, preferably within six hours of the birth. However, if it has been more than six hours between the tear and the repair, apply topical anesthetic and abrade the sides of the tear by rubbing them with a gauze pad soaked with normal saline solution, povidone iodine solution or an infusion of rosemary or echinacea, until they begin to bleed; rinse the tissue thoroughly with warmed sterile saline. Rubbing will débride the tissue, allowing fresh edges to be sewn together. Use Vicryl for the repair for its longer staying power.

Débriding as described will usually work if the raw edges have not been healing for more than 36 hours (i.e., when it is still in the fresh wound to mottled light pink stage of healing). Once the tissue takes on a beefy red appearance, granulation is established and débridement may not be very effective. The sooner a repair is done, the better. Make every effort to get extensive muscle, rectal mucosa or sphincter damage repaired within the six-hour limit.

Whenever a tear has been débrided, antibiotic agents of some kind should be given to help prevent infection. Use either a broad spectrum biotechnical agent, such as ampicillin, or use herbs. Also have the woman follow the precautions to prevent infections that are described in the chapter entitled "Postpartum Care and Comfort Measures."

Planning Your Repair

When performing the actual repair, the deepest, most internal and hardest to reach damage should always be repaired first, except as otherwise noted. The chapters covering first- through fourth-degree repair are laid out with this in mind. This ensures that you will be able to find the deepest apexes of each layer of the wound, will have full access to the tissues and will avoid stressing more superficial stitches already placed. If the tear does not involve one or more of these structures or layers, simply skip to the next relevant layer.

Cervical or anterior yoni wall damage

On the rare occasion that there is damage to the cervix or anterior yoni wall that you can see well enough and you feel skilled enough to repair, repair the cervix and then the anterior yoni wall first, before anything else. For one thing, these areas may be bleeding profusely, obstructing your field. You want maximum room to work, and you don't want to stress a repair in the floor of the yoni as you manipulate these deeper and harder to reach tissues. Be sure to pass a catheter to rule out a buttonhole into the urethra or bladder before you begin. For details, see the chapters entitled "Cervical Lacerations" and "Repairing the Anterior Yoni Wall." For further details regarding how to proceed, see the master list in the chapter entitled "How to Use This Manual."

Tears involving anorectal structures

When repairing deep posterior tears that involve one or both of the anal sphincters, the rectal mucosa or all three, you also start with the deepest layer of the tear. When the perineum is short, sphincter exposure or involvement is more common even in an apparently minor tear; be certain that you have landmarks correctly identified before you proceed. The sequence of repair, from deepest to most superficial layers, will be as follows:

- Rectal mucosa
- Internal anal sphincter
- External anal sphincter and its capsule

Once these repairs are completed, proceed as for a first- or second-degree tear.

First- or second-degree damage

In the vast majority of cases, you will only need to repair the posterior yoni wall, subcutaneous tissues and, if you or the mother prefers, the subcuticular tissues of the perineum. Assuming the cervix and anterior yoni wall are intact or have been repaired, you will repair a first- or second-degree tear, proceeding as follows:

- Begin at the internal apex of the tear in the posterior yoni wall.
- Insert the first two or three stitches.
- Assess whether deep stitches (below the level of the ones just placed) are needed.
- Insert deep stitches, if necessary.
- Resume repair of the posterior yoni wall to the level of the hymen
- Place subcuticular basting stitches down the perineum
- If desired, stitch back up the perineum to close the skin layer using running mattress stitches.

•Tie the repair off behind the hymenal ring.

Superficial damage

Repairs involving skin tags at the introitus, as well as repairs to the labia and in the periurethral area can be performed once all deeper lacerations have been closed *unless* they are bleeding. Most of the time they can wait. Saving them until last means that you will not be stressing the superficial tissues while trying to reach what you are doing deeper inside.

General considerations when placing stitches

Selecting the right needle: Use of a needle of the appropriate size and strength will shorten the length of time it takes to perform the repair and will minimize tissue trauma.

Handling the suture material: Suture material must always be handled with care to preserve its tensile strength. A review of these guidelines follows.

- Store suture packets at room temperature and avoid prolonged exposure to high heat (which might occur if suture sits in a hot car, for example) or moisture.
- Never soak absorbable sutures after they are removed from their packaging; rinse chromic gut only briefly with plain sterile water or sterile saline.
- Absorbable synthetic must be kept dry because it breaks down by a process of hydrolysis (i.e., it is water soluble).
- Avoid excessive handling of the suture strand as this will lead to fraying, especially when using chromic gut.
- Depending upon the type of material being used, the strand may retain some package memory. To straighten it, grasp the needle end of the strand about 1 inch below the swage and grasp the free end of the strand with the other hand and stretch it with a gentle, steady, even pull. Never jerk or tug the strand, which can weaken it. Never hold the needle in one hand and the free end in the other when straightening the strand because this can weaken the swaged attachment point.
- Do not "test" strand strength by pulling or tugging it forcefully, as this can weaken a perfectly good piece of suture. If you are in doubt about the condition of a piece of suture material, discard it.

Assessing where to start: Recheck the tear or incision and make sure you see how it should go together before you proceed. Reidentify all relevant landmarks such as the internal apex(es) of the tear, the hymenal tags, the junction where the yoni mucosa meets the skin, the wound edges, and the external (perineal) apex of the tear. These are your landmarks for correct reconstruction. Gently align the wound edges so you have a good idea of how to go about the repair. Carefully reposition any skin tags until you are certain where they were originally located.

Don't be embarrassed to discuss the tear and the repair with your assistant or partner. For as long as I remained in clinical practice (over 17 years as of this writing), I discussed how to do a repair correctly. As you see more tears, discerning tissue layers from bruised areas will become more clear. Be sure to look for dark purple lines or swellings. These are blood vessels or hematomas and should be avoided.

Assessing the number and spacing of stitches: Before you begin to suture each part of the tear, you need to estimate how many stitches you will need in that part of the wound so that you can assess how to space them. Do this by eyeballing the length of the tear and then dividing it as nearly as possible into 1 cm increments. You could use a Peri-Rule or marked instrument to assist with this. Place only enough stitches to secure the tissue, spacing them no more than 1 cm apart. This maximum 1 cm distance applies whether you are repairing muscle or mucosa. Often, you will find that you need to place stitches slightly closer together to avoid spacing the stitches too far apart. Spacing will also vary depending upon the area being repaired. Due to the highly mobile nature of the tissue of the labia minora, for example, stitches should be placed much more closely together. This is also true for small stitches in the rectal mucosa and in the anterior yoni wall that close tears in the urethra because in both cases you are trying to prevent leakage.

Depth and width of stitches: For most tissues, create stitches no more than 1.25 to 1.5 cm deep, the maximum depth possible when using a CT-1 or T-12 needle and creating a stitch with one motion as you pass the needle through the midline of the tear. Frequently, stitches will be a little shallower than this. Each stitch should be at least as deep as it is wide. Wound edges that lie flat or that are slightly everted are both acceptable in perineal repair.

Accurate placement of the needle: When creating half-circle stitches, place the needle tip at right angles to the tissue surface, at an equal distance from the wound edges on either side and an equal distance apart in order for tension to be evenly distributed along the entire length of the wound.

Orientation of the needle holder when placing a stitch: Keep the shaft of the needle holder parallel with the edge of the tear as you place each new stitch. This will help prevent creating a rippled line of stitches.

Appropriate tension in the stitches: Placing stitches that are too small, too tight and too close together are mistakes frequently made when learning to suture. Excessively tight stitches produce tissue overlap that results in hypoxia, poor healing and probably increased pain as well. In combination, this actually makes for a weaker healed repair (Stone et al., 1986). You are not sewing fabric, but living tissue that requires circulating oxygen and nutrients in order to heal.

At the time of birth, the tissues are engorged due to the extra blood volume of pregnancy and localized swelling from tissue trauma. The traumatized tissue will swell somewhat more after the repair is completed because suture material itself will prompt some additional inflammation. The tissues will then reduce in size as the blood volume returns to nonpregnant levels and the edema resolves postpartum. All this fluctuating tissue fluid strains the stitches. When there is minimal natural or artificial swelling, you may simply tighten the stitches so that they rest on the surface of the tissue with edges touching, and you need not worry about compensating for excessive swelling. When practicing with foam, a slight puckering at the entry and exit points with the edges of the incision just touching represents appropriate tension (when little anesthetic is used). This is not true of tissue, however, and there should be no blanching or puckering where the strand exits the tissue.

In perineal repair, strive to create stitches that result in the edges of the wound lying flat as they meet in the midline. However, if the edges are not flat, they should be slightly everted, rather than inverted. Inversion of the wound edges will interfere with healing.

Pay attention to scraps of suture: Whenever you trim suture, be sure to keep hold of the ends during trimming, remove them from the wound and dispose of them promptly to avoid leaving suture pieces that will irritate the tissues.

PUTTING IT ALL TOGETHER: FIRST- AND SECOND-DEGREE REPAIR

Note: A thorough understanding and mastery of the part entitled "Pertinent Anatomy" and of the part entitled "Essential Surgical Skills for Midwives" are required before proceeding with this section. For better understanding, read this entire section through to the end before beginning to practice.

REPAIRING THE POSTERIOR YONI WALL

NOTE: If the tear angles severely to one side of the perineum, refer to the section in the chapter entitled "Special Tricks and Techniques" that covers the repair of mediolateral tears. If there is cervical, anterior yoni wall, anal sphincter or rectal mucosa damage, see the master list in the chapter entitled "How to Use This Manual" for how to proceed.

We begin our discussion here because first-degree tears are the most common, typically involving damage to the mucosa of the posterior yoni wall and to the perineal skin. Many tears don't even require repair, as they are shallow and will usually heal well on their own with a minimum of commonsense precautions.

When a mucosal laceration is more than superficial, however, bringing the sides of the wound together will greatly facilitate healing (even though mucosal tissues heal by regenerating the same type of tissue that was destroyed). Repair of the posterior yoni wall may involve closing yoni mucosa, connective tissue and muscle tissue.

Suturing materials for repair of the posterior yoni wall

You can use 3-0 chromic gut or 2-0 braided synthetic on a CT-1 or T-12 taper point needle for most of these repairs. If the tear is shallow, a small taper point needle (SH or T-5) will work nicely. If the mouth of the yoni requires reconstruction due to a ragged skin tag, use 2-0 multifilament synthetic for the entire repair.

When it is obvious that shallow stitches will be needed, it is best to use a smaller half-circle needle than to attempt to create significantly smaller stitches with a large needle. Making small stitches with a big needle is tricky and should not be attempted until you are experienced in placing stitches using a properly sized needle. If a larger needle is used to make small stitches, it is easy to produce a shallow but too-wide stitch or an unequally proportioned stitch that does not encompass the depth of the wound.

If very large, deep stitches are called for, use heavier suture. Unlike the yoni mucosa, muscles tend to pull away from the midline. This requires stronger suture material to ensure that the edges will stay together under stress. You can use 2-0 chromic gut or 1-0 absorbable synthetic swagged to a standard (CT-1, T-12) taper point needle for these repairs. Ask your assistant to get out the appropriate suture (to maintain your clean or sterile field).

Special considerations when repairing the posterior yoni wall

Begin by repairing the posterior yoni wall first. Doing so begins closure in the deepest part of the yoni tear, allowing full access to the internal apex; helps minimize seepage of lochia to the bottom of the wound; aligns the edges of the tear and enables you to better visualize what goes where.

Traditionally, it has been considered best surgical practice to close each tissue layer individually, especially the fatty layers. The perineal body is composed of many intermingled tissues and lacks a fatty layer. For these reasons, stitching loosely without regard to reapproximating specific tissue layers and focusing instead on creating large, loose stitches that close all dead space works well in this area. It *is* imperative to eliminate dead space because it encourages the wound to separate, which invites seroma or hematoma formation (i.e., the collection of serous fluid or blood in the space), which, in turn, provides a medium for bacterial growth.

Assessing whether a deep layer of stitches will be needed

If a tear is no more than 1.5 cm deep, you can encompass it to its depth or nearly so in one pass of the needle using a half-circle stitch by inserting the needle on one side of the tear, removing the needle from the tissue, and taking a mirror-image bite on the opposite side, equidistant from your entry point, while making sure the needle enters the opposite side just above the trough of the wound.

Tears of an intermediate depth (between 1.5 and 2.5 cm deep) can be closed using a buried circle stitch (this technique is explained on page 413). If you cannot encompass the depth of a tear using a CT-1 or T-12 needle and a buried circle stitch, the tear is more than about 2.5 cm deep in that area. Such deep tears that do not involve the rectal mucosa can occur when the perineal body is quite long. If the tear is only a little more than 2.5 cm deep, you can usually get away with closing it using only one layer of buried circle stitches. But if it cannot be closed or nearly so with a buried circle stitch, the tear is too deep and you will need to place a second, deeper layer to close the dead space. Evenly spaced stitches promote circulation and healing, so in such a case, placing half circle stitches and then a single centered deep stitch may be the best choice.

Even if you suspect you will need a deep stitch or two, it is a good idea to begin your repair at the internal apex of the tear in the posterior yoni wall. First, doing so will line up the tissue layers, thus minimizing the chances that you will mismatch the sides when you place the deep stitches. Second, you want to take as deep a bite as possible when you place your first few stitches to assess how many deep stitches you actually need. Because the tear in the yoni wall and perineal body is usually wedge shaped, the internal apex is likely to be more shallow than the external apex, meaning that the first few stitches at the end nearest the internal apex will usually close the tear to its depth without any problem. It is always best to close the deepest and hardest to reach part of a tear first, even if the tear itself is shallow. In nearly every case, you will be able to close even deep tears with a single layer of buried circle stitches in the posterior yoni wall. If the anorectal muscosa is damaged, you should start by repairing it first, to ensure you can reach the depth of the tear, and then repair the anal sphincters next before beginning closure of the yoni mucosa.

If the edges of the tear are not flush with each other, refer to the entry entitled "When one longitudinal edge of a tear protrudes more than the other" in the chapter entitled "Special Tricks and Techniques" for a method to fix them.

Repair procedures

The anchor stitch: Traditionally an anchor stitch is placed about 1 cm above the internal apex of the tear to ligate any retracted blood vessels. This helps prevent hematomas. If the tear is not bleeding and the upper end is hard to reach, it is acceptable to place this stitch less than 1 cm above the apex. Both Leo Sorger (1991) and I agree that starting repairs at the level of the internal apex is also acceptable if the wound is not bleeding. It is never acceptable, however, to guess the location of the internal apex of a tear; it must be accurately identified before you proceed with the repair.

Tie the anchor stitch using a square knot, constructed with three throws if using chromic and at least four if using a braided synthetic, as described in the chapter entitled "Tying Surgical Knots." Cut only the short, free end, since you will continue to use the suture still attached to the needle. Check with your fingers to see that the first knot is secure against the tissue and slightly moveable at the same time. There should be no puckering of tissue on either side. Slide the knot to your nondominant side so that it is opposite your needle holder hand (i.e., to the left if right-handed, to the right if left-handed).

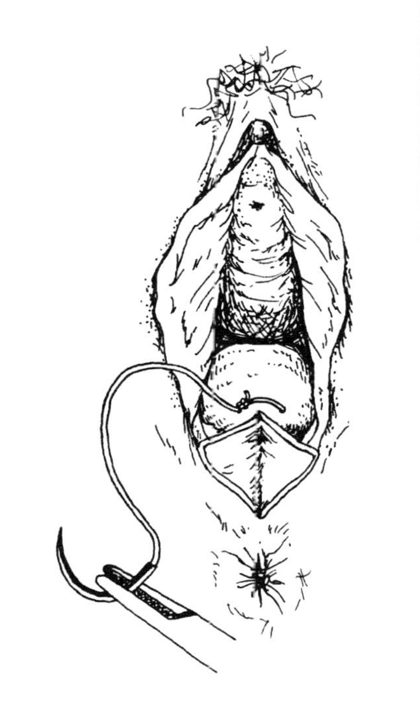

All repairs using continuous stitches begin with an anchor stitch.

Needle work for each stitch: When the depth of the tear allows, insert the needle in one side and bring it up on the other side, thus completing the needlework for that stitch in one motion. Stitches should never exceed the chord length of the needle from entry point to exit point, should include the same amount of tissue from both sides and should be at least as deep as they are wide.

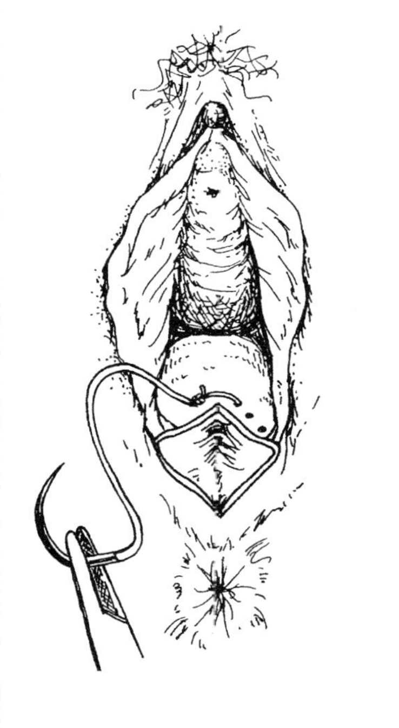

The dots to your right represent the proposed spacing of the stitches.

Spacing stitches in the yoni wall: Now see how much space there is between your anchor stitch and the hymenal ring. Stitches should be approximately, but no greater than, 1 cm apart. (For example, if three stitches are obviously too few and four will be somewhat more closely spaced than 1 cm, use four.) The 1 cm rule avoids creating dead spaces. If the hymen is deeply placed, plan your last stitch to be in front of it. If the hymen is relatively shallow (as most are), plan your last stitch to be behind it. Count how many basting or locked blanket sutures you will place to the level of the hymenal ring. Never sew through the hymenal tags themselves and don't attempt to reconstruct the hymenal ring. This will cause extreme pain and is totally unnecessary. Be sure not to strangle hymenal tags as you secure each stitch.

The tendency is to place too many stitches, especially when you are first learning. If you are in doubt about the appropriate number to use in the mucosal repair, it is probably best to err on the side of too few, as long as you make sure they are equally spaced. Remember, each stitch has to be absorbed, and each puncture creates a new injury.

What kind of stitch to use: A simple, half-circle basting (over-and-over) stitch is ideally suited for most yoni mucosa repairs. This stitch is fast and easy to place and reduces the risk that sutures will be too tight (Fleming, 1990).

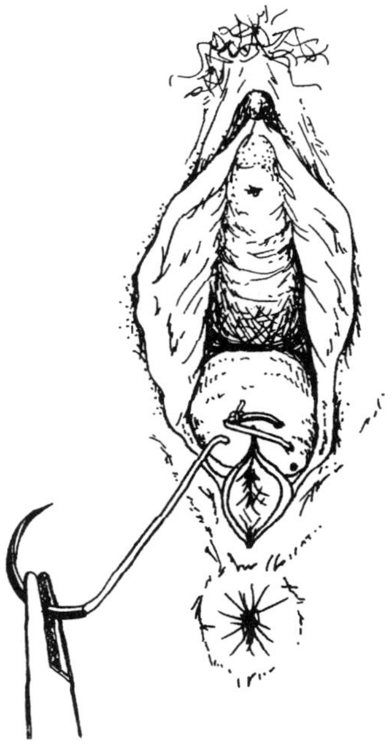

Here a basting stitch is being used to close the yoni floor.

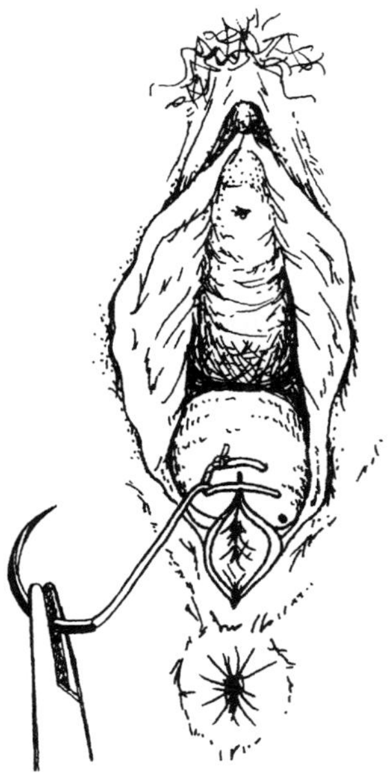

Here a locked blanket stitch is chosen due to seepage of blood from the wound.

The use of locked blanket stitches should be reserved for repairing the posterior yoni wall when the wound is seeping more blood than is usually the case. If the tear is unusually complex or jagged, a locked stitch may also help to better align the tissues. Note, however, that it is *not* appropriate to try and stop active bleeding from a torn blood vessel with a row of overlying stitches whether locked or not (in such a case, before proceeding with the repair, place a ligating stitch around the vessel, described in the chapter entitled "Dealing with Bleeding Vessels"). Limit your use of locked stitches because they tend to shorten as healing takes place and as maternal blood volume reduces over the postpartum period (Anderson, 1975). Thus, locking stitches runs the risk of creating a too-tight line of stitches that could impair healing. So, if you decide to use locked stitches, tighten them only enough to accomplish your goal of eliminating blood seepage or aligning the tissue.

Dealing with separation of layers of the yoni wall: In some tears, you may find that the muscular layer of the posterior yoni wall has separated from the yoni mucosa and from the underlying perineal body, with the layers of torn yoni wall suspended on either side above the perineal tissues or, if the tear is deep enough, above the intact anorectal canal. If this has happened, sew the layers back together by holding the needle holder shaft parallel with the surface of the posterior yoni wall and catching all layers in your stitch. If it is easy, also gather some of the perineal body (or connective tissue overlying the rectal canal) into each stitch. This will help tack the two layers back together, but you must be very careful not to penetrate the anorectal wall and not to tear the delicate adventitial tissue.

If, after using the above technique, any kind of gap is left between the most distal tissue layers, Rogers and colleagues (2001) recommend further restoration of the tissue by tacking the two layers together after you place the last stitch in the posterior yoni wall (or after placing the last deep stitch, if such is required) by taking one or two vertical interrupted stitches through all the yoni wall layer that underlies the yoni mucosa to tack it to the perineal body. This technique is further discussed at the end of this chapter.

Reassessing the need for a deep layer of stitches: If the tear is deep, use the two bite technique to place the first stitch. After taking the first half of the first bite and with the needle still in place, do a digital exam to be certain you have encompassed the depth of the tear. Do so by feeling for an open space below the tip of the needle in the midline of the tear. Since most tears are shallow at each apex, chances are you will have closed it to its depth with the first stitch. If a space is found that is large enough to easily admit the tip of your finger, a two-bite or buried circle stitch should easily close this small gap. Remove the needle and use a buried circle stitch. If the first stitch was too shallow, use buried circle stitches to complete the repair of the yoni floor. If a buried circle stitch still leaves a significant gap below your first layer of stitches, meaning you have a really deep tear, you may need to place one or deep stitches. You will have to judge whether spacing is best accomplished with half circle stitches in the floor of the yoni or buried circle stitches, taking into account how much room is left that needs closing with a deep stitch. In that case, place two or three stitches in the yoni floor, discontinue yoni mucosa repair before you reach the hymenal ring and refer to the next chapter, entitled "When a Deep Layer of Stitches Is Needed Below the Posterior Yoni Wall." If a deep layer is not needed complete your stitching of the yoni floor, then skip to the chapter entitled "Repairing the Perineum."

Placing sutures in a lax pelvic floor: Stitches should be just tight enough to bring the tissues together. If the tissue behind the sutures is bulging against the repair, you can place the stitches slightly closer together to compensate. It is very tempting to think that tighter stitches will shore up a sagging pelvic floor, and indeed traditional approaches to repair have encouraged this notion. Stone and colleagues (1986), however, found that loose stitches foster stronger bonds in fascia. Tight stitches do not provide additional support, except when the stitches are first placed, of course, and raise the risk of repair breakdown because too much tension strangles the tissue and tends to overlap wound edges rather than matching them, increasing the risk of hypoxia and poor healing. At the very least, too-tight stitching increases the risk of infection and can result in less-than-optimal healing. Tight stitches can result in dysfunctionally tense (but not stronger) tissues leading to a mighty uncomfortable yoni during healing and, afterward, during sexual penetration.

Crown suture (to reapproximate the bulbocavernosus muscle): The Crown suture is a complicated, three-dimensional figure-eight-style stitch intended to reunite the severed halves of the bulbocavernosus muscle, thus maintaining its integrity as the "sphincter of the yoni." The newest research finds that bulbocavernous anatomy differs significantly from what has been classically taught. It does not serve a primary sphincteric function for the introitus since the vast majority of its fibers pass straight down through the perineal body rather than crossing in the midline. Therefore, the Crown suture is not a valid technique. (See the chapter entitled "The Urogenital Triangle and Related Structures" for more detailed anatomical information.)

Many practitioners have never used the Crown suture. It is difficult to place correctly and easy to make too tight. You run the risk of puncturing blood vessels and nerves as you go around the muscle with your needle. The swing around each muscle half is difficult, and no doubt, the sides are often reapproximated poorly. This may leave tissue somewhat twisted, increasing the likelihood of postpartum problems.

In addition, it is a hard suture to tie because the knot is supposed to be placed deeply behind the front of the stitch. This placement, when done correctly, is intended to reinforce the anterior edge of the muscle. However, it leads to inevitable difficulty in assessing how tight the knot should be, frequently resulting in an overly tight stitch. While some may contest that the Crown suture still has a place for reuniting the sides of the superficial transverse perineal muscle, it is an unnecessarily complicated stitch for this purpose. For all these reasons, the Crown suture can be relegated to the growing pile of medical techniques that are now of historical interest only.

Finishing repair of the posterior yoni wall: It is usually not necessary to sew right up to the mouth of the yoni (where the mucosa and skin surface meet). It is better to leave a little leeway (at least 0.5 cm or so) between the last stitch and where the yoni mucosa meets the perineal skin, than to risk sewing the mouth of the yoni too tightly. If you make the hymenal ring your landmark for stopping yoni mucosa repair, for beginning perineal repair and for finishing the repair, you can easily avoid sewing the introitus too tightly. (How to repair the perineum and finish the repair are described in the chapter entitled "Repairing the Perineum.") The exceptions to this general rule are skin tags needing reconstruction at the introitus (see the chapter entitled "Skin Tags") or an irregular tear leaving the edges of the introitus mismatched when they rest together even though they are supported by the rest of the repair.

When tissue layers have separated: If you need to reattach separated layers of the yoni wall to the perineal body, proceed as follows. Once you have finished repairing the yoni wall, Rogers and colleagues (2001) recommend placing two vertical stitches, one on either side of the tear at about the level of the hymen, to reattach the separated layers of the yoni wall to the perineal body (but never through the skin). Place a vertical interrupted stitch by passing the needle in a top-to-bottom direction through the muscularis layer of the yoni mucosa and then through the perineal body. Tie the stitch off. Repeat on the opposite side. Tie these stitches loosely to avoid distortion of the tissue. These stitches are placed prior to suturing the perineum. They should only be used, however, when the separation is significant and a gap is left despite your repair thus far. While such a gap may be more common when the perineum has been cut, in the vast majority of tears, the stitches you have placed in the posterior yoni wall and the layer of basting stitches you normally will place down the perineal body will hold any separated layers together just fine.

When a Deep Layer of Stitches Is Needed Below the Posterior Yoni Wall

NOTE: If your first row of stitches closed the yoni tear throughout its depth, skip to the chapter entitled "Repairing the Perineum."

Fleming (1990) pointed out that nearly all second-degree repairs can be completed with a single layer of stitches in the posterior yoni wall. Tears in very long perineums, nonetheless, may require two layers. Therefore, this advice on placing a deep layer is a "just in case" offering.

I am no longer referring to a deep layer of stitches as being placed in the "muscle layer" because it is quite possible for the first layer of stitches in the posterior yoni wall to include some muscle fibers. The perineal body is interlaced with several different types of tissue, and since there are relatively shallow muscle fibers below the yoni floor (urethrovaginal sphincter and puboperinealis muscle), some tears in the yoni floor are likely to involve some muscle fibers.

Suturing materials for a deep layer of stitches

Use 3-0 or 2-0 chromic gut or 2-0 or 1-0 absorbable synthetic swaged to a standard (CT-1, T-12) taper point needle for deep repair. Ask your assistant to get out the appropriate suture (to maintain your clean or sterile field).

The purpose of a deep layer of stitches

A deep layer, when needed, is added to close any dead space that would otherwise remain beneath the layer in the yoni wall and behind the layer you ordinarily place in the perineum. You cannot simply close the yoni mucosa and the perineum, leaving a big hole underneath. Such a hole may involve some muscle fibers. Recall that the perineal muscles are toned when at rest; once severed, the fibers act like elastic, with a tendency to retract into the surrounding tissue. Retracted muscle ends could heal apart, without rejoining their opposite half. This can leave perineal floor support weakened or absent and may eventually result in a rectocele. Moreover, whether muscle fibers are involved or not, the dead space created by a hole leaves a gap that must fill in with scar tissue in order to heal (thus first intention healing does not occur) and a space for lochia to pool deep within the tear, inviting pain, infection and impaired healing.

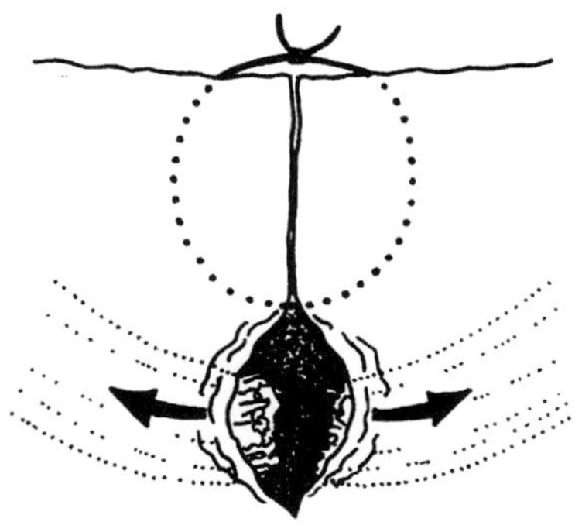

Schematic showing how this buried circle stitch still leaves unsutured dead space below it, where any torn muscle fibers will tend to retract to the sides.

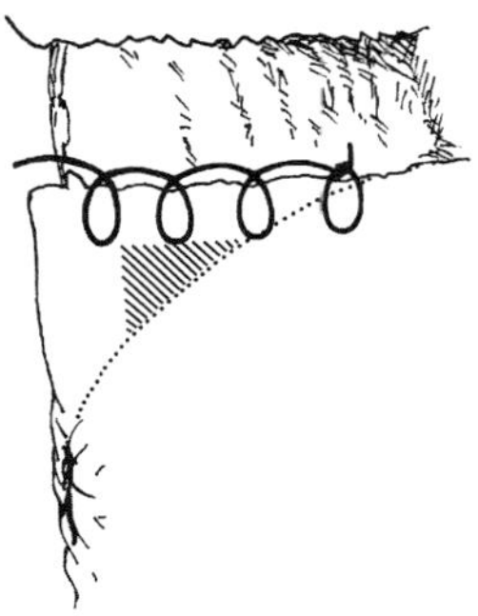	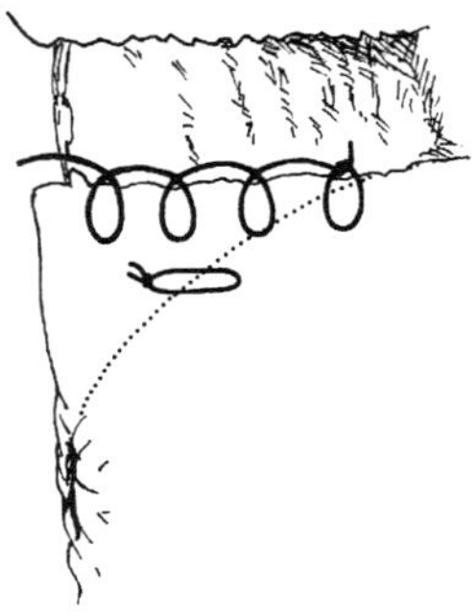	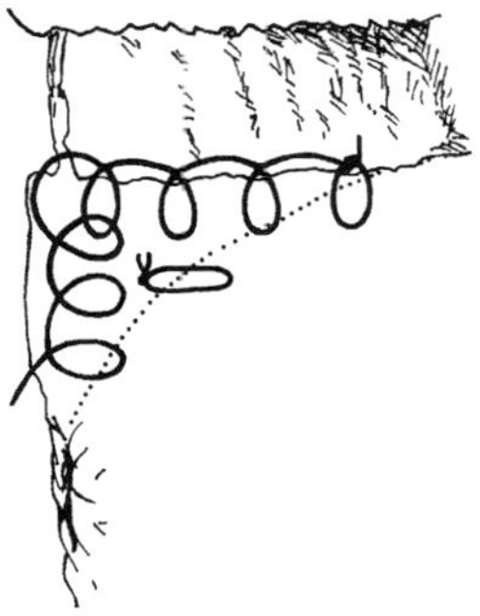
Dead space left under stitches in the yoni mucosa	In most cases, a single deep stitch closes this space (note that the stitch is placed horizontal to the yoni floor).	The basting stitches placed down the perineum complete the closure, eliminating all dead space.

What type of stitch to use

Traditionally, interrupted sutures have been used when deep stitches are needed. The huge advantage, especially for midwives who very rarely need to place a deep layer, is that an individual stitch can be removed without disrupting the rest, should you accidently pass the loop through the anterior wall of the anorectal canal. But a deep layer of basting stitches can give equally good, if not superior, results when there is no bleeding, when you make sure that you do not penetrate the anorectal wall as each stitch is placed and when all the dead space is obliterated (Fleming, 1990).

Following the theory that closing individual layers of perineal muscles is possible and desirable, some care providers still place several layers of interrupted sutures. This is not only unnecessary, but actually rejoining specific muscle fibers is, for the most part, pretty impossible given the indiscrete confluence of tissues within the perineal body. A loosely woven, well-aligned, adequately approximated tear with the fewest possible layers of suture material will heal best.

What to do with the suture left in the yoni mucosa

If you decide a deep layer of sutures is needed, put aside the needle and suture that is still attached to the stitches in the yoni mucosa. The easiest thing to do is pin it to an underpad placed across the mother's pubic bone. You can hold the needle in place with a hemostat, if you wish; if you do, clamp the needle through the pad to protect the wire from damage.

How to hold the needle for deep tissue repair

Be sure the plane of the needle in the needle holder is held at an angle that will allow you to complete the stitch. This will depend on your angle of entry. If the needle is not held properly, you may puncture into the anorectum.

Whenever possible, position the mother so her bottom is hanging slightly off the edge of the bed or table upon which she is lying, with her feet supported on chairs or on a table. This position allows you to grip the needle in the jaws at a 90° angle to the handle, as you

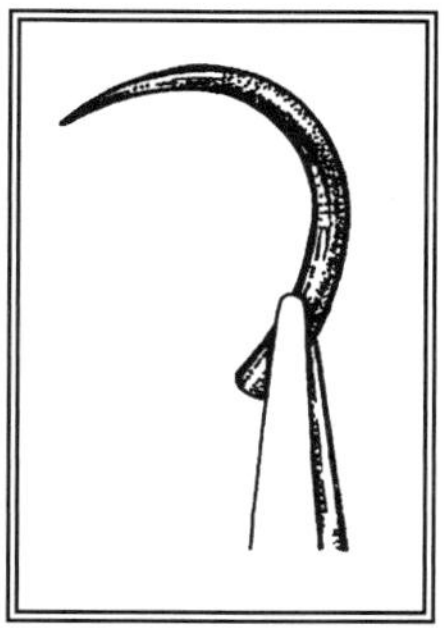

normally would. With the needle so positioned, the shaft of the needle holder is held parallel with the perineal surface (not parallel with the surface of the yoni floor) as you stitch.

If you must sit on the bed or floor with the supine mother in front of you, you may find it easier to hold the needle at a much different angle, as illustrated here. Positioning the needle like this makes it much more awkward to place a stitch without traumatizing the tissue adjacent to the needle's path and is therefore best avoided whenever possible.

Either way, each stitch is made by directing the needle toward the sacrum and parallel with the yoni floor, not down and deep as with yoni floor repair.

Spacing deep stitches

Most of the time you will need only one, or very rarely two, deep stitches. The 1 cm spacing rule still applies, even when spacing deep stitches. In this case, spacing is gauged from the level of the lowermost part of the last loop in yoni floor suture to the lowermost part of the tear that will not be closed by the basting stitches you normally place down the perineum. For example, if there is 0.75 cm of space below your last loop and the part of the tear that will be otherwise closed by basting stitches, you probably only need 1 interrupted stitch in the center of that space. Interrupted stitches, when properly tied, allow good circulation and, if one should come out or must be removed, it will not affect the others; they are the obvious choice when a single deep stitch is all that is required. A figure-eight stitch can be used as well, especially if there is much diffuse bleeding. Continuous basting stitches can also be used and are the better choice if two or more deep stitches are required.

Place deep stitches *parallel* with the yoni floor to avoid penetration into the rectal wall. In other words, your mucosal sutures are placed deep to the surface of the yoni floor (down and deep) while your deep sutures are placed back and deep to the surface of the perineum, and are thus parallel with the surface of the posterior yoni wall.

When only one stitch is needed, place it in the center of the damaged area below the lower part of the last suture loop in the posterior yoni wall. A buried circle stitch may be sufficient, eliminating the need for a deep stitch. If a buried circle stitch would still leave a significant space below it that is not quite large enough to warrant a stitch but too large to leave as is, it may be better to place half-circle stitches in the yoni floor and then center an interrupted stitch in the deep open space that remains below it. When more than one deep stitch is needed, place a deep anchor stitch close to the top of the damaged deep tissues and continue the stitches with a simple basting (over-and-over) style.

In most tears you will find that the closer you get to the external apex (on the perineum), the more shallow the tear will be. Once you reach a point that the tear is shallow enough to be closed with the basting stitch to be placed down the perineum alone, stop placing deep stitches. (See next chapter for details.) If you have used a continuous technique, tie off the last stitch using either an Aberdeen knot or a three-strand technique. (See the chapter entitled "Tying Surgical Knots" for details.)

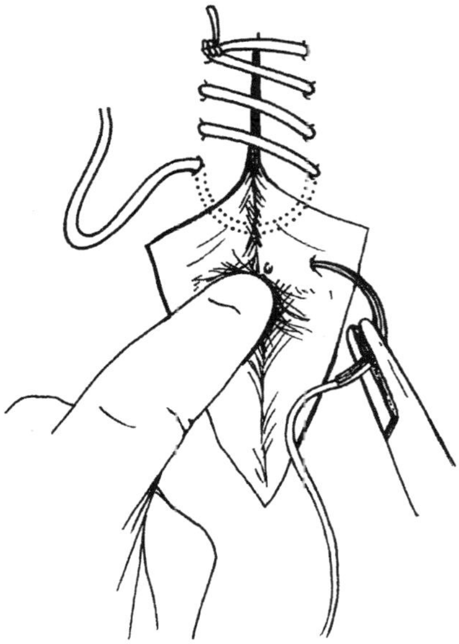

Palpate to locate the bottom of the last suture loop placed in the yoni mucosa and palpate for the trough of the tear. This will help you position the deep stitch. Insert the needle into one side of the tear and bring the tip out just in front of the trough of the tear.

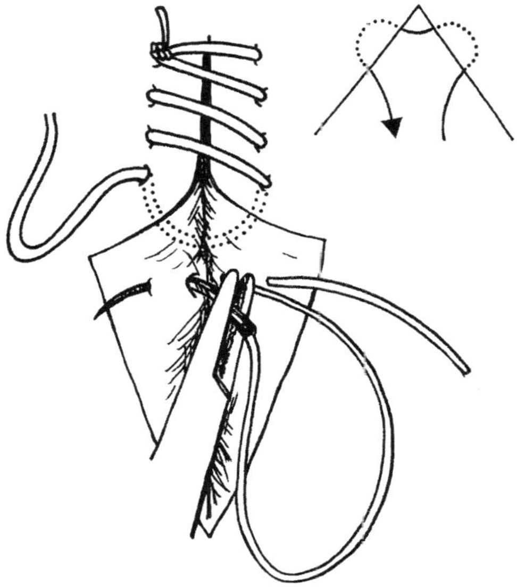

Remove the needle completely and reinsert it opposite its exit point. (The insert shows a schematic view from above.) Keeping the point of the needle visible in the center helps to prevent the needle from penetrating the bowel wall.

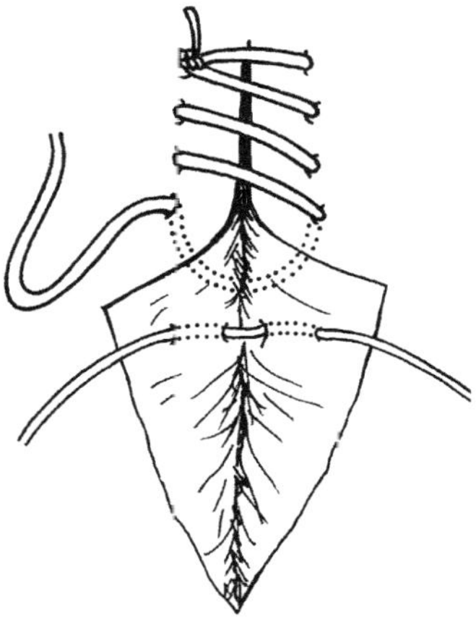

Now the suture is threaded through the tissue like this.

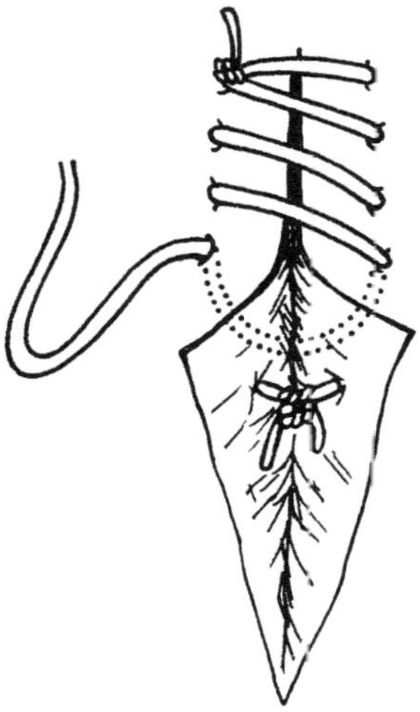

If only one stitch is needed, cut both ears and tie it off. If more are needed, use this stitch as your anchor and place additional continuous stitches, as needed.

Examine the anorectum for misplaced stitches

Whenever a deep layer of stitches is required, examine the anterior anorectal wall to determine if any of the stitches have penetrated it. If any have, they must be removed and replaced. See the chapter entitled "Examining the Anorectum for Misplaced Stitches" for full details.

Securing the muscle wall of the yoni to the perineal body

If the wall of the yoni was split into two layers at the time of the tear, Rogers and colleagues (2001) recommend reattaching the posterior muscle wall of the yoni to the perineal body at this point with a single vertical interrupted stitch on either side of the tear (two stitches in all). For more details on the separation of the yoni wall into layers, see pages 507 and 509.

Repairing the Perineum

The perineum can be closed using the following techniques. Keep in mind that in spite of a tear's being short and shallow, the sphincter can still be involved.

Do you need another pack of suture?

If you used at least a 27" (70 cm) strand of suture to close the yoni mucosa, there is usually enough left to allow you to close the perineum as well. You could also use a new packet of 3-0 chromic or 2-0 synthetic, perhaps on a smaller needle. Your choice will depend upon how extensive the internal repair has been and how much more suture you anticipate needing to complete the job. It is better to open a new pack now than to be almost done and run out of suture at the end. The disadvantage is that opening another pack of suture at any point necessitates tying an extra knot, creating an additional weak link in the stitches.

Another reason to open another packet at this point would be when a skin tag at the mouth of the yoni needs repair. If the edges of the introitus are very uneven, use 3-0 or 4-0 synthetic, which can also be used for shallow perineal repair. Synthetic's longer staying power means it will not break down under the stress that the introitus is subjected to during daily activity. Note that some synthetic is packaged in shorter lengths than chromic. If perineal damage is extensive, be sure to use a new strand that is long enough to finish the repair.

To bring continuous suture to the perineum to continue repair

In most repairs, you will continue to suture down the perineum with the same strand you used to repair the mucosa of the yoni floor. To do so when you have used continuous unlocked stitches in the yoni floor, place your last stitch at the level of the hymenal ring. Direct the needle segment of the suture down to the perineal portion (vertical plane) of the tear by dropping the strand down toward your dominant side between the edges of the tear; keep the strand loose. Now the needle is where it needs to be to begin basting down the perineum. (In the drawing, the first basting stitch is holding the suture strand in place, and the second basting stitch has been started.)

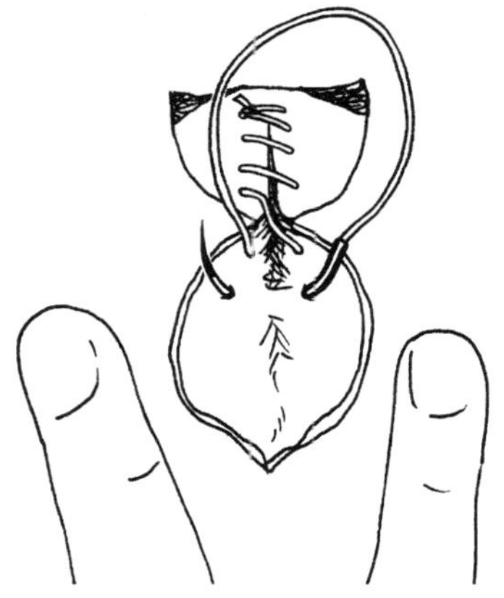

Moving to the vertical plane of the tear and continuing a basting stitch when a basting stitch has been used to close the yoni floor

If you have used locked blanket stitches to close the yoni floor, use the Hobbs maneuver (named for Valerie Hobbs, who introduced this technique to me) as illustrated on the following page, to bring the suture you've been using from inside the yoni to the vertical plane of the tear. This technique preserves your last locked stitch. It is not always possible to do this maneuver perfectly; it depends upon the shape of the tear.

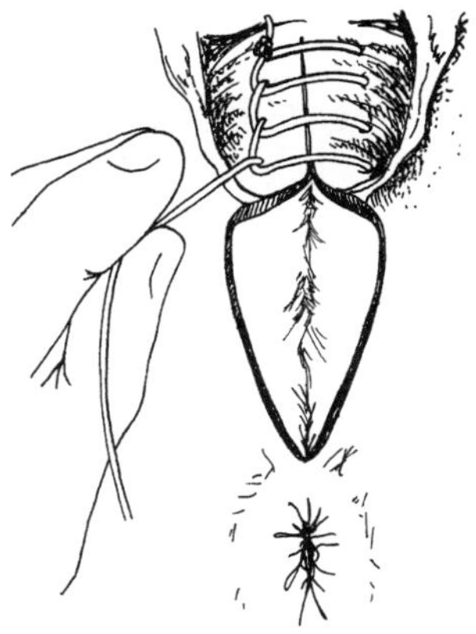	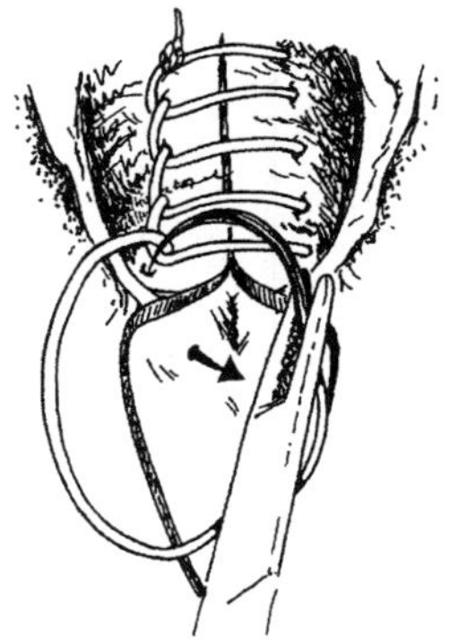	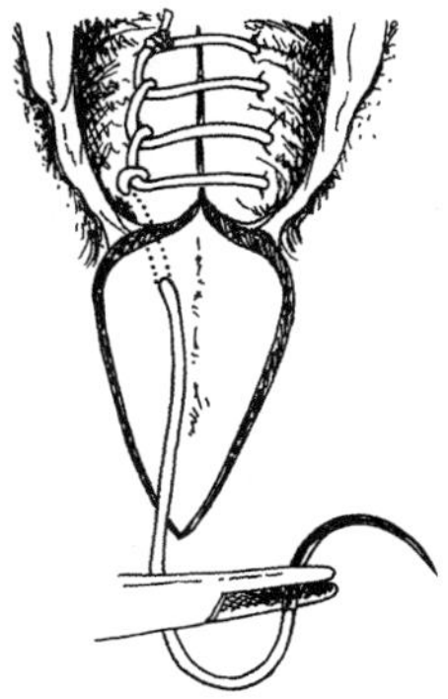
Complete your last locked stitch.	Insert your needle just outside the lock of the last stitch in the yoni floor.	Bring your needle out where you want to begin closure of the perineum.

Continuing the repair when a new pack of suture is needed

If you need to open a new pack of suture to repair the perineum, deal with the strand used for the mucosal layer in one of the following ways:

1. Use a three-strand knot to tie off your last stitch. Insert the mucosal needle beside the last exit point (outside the corner of the last lock if you have locked the stitches) and come up on the opposite side, parallel with your insertion point (i.e., in front or behind the hymenal ring). Leave a long loop on the nondominant side and, using that as one thread, tie and trim your suture. Then, start a new pack of suture by placing an anchor stitch at the top of the perineal body. This is your first basting stitch in the subcutaneous layer. Tie it and cut the tail short (just as you did to begin the repair).
2. If you will be using suture of the same material, you can pin the mucosal suture to the field above the mother's pubic bone and wait until you are done to use the alternative method of tying off the repair described at the end of this chapter.
3. If you are using the same type of suture material, you can also tie the end of the mucosal suture to the end of the new suture. To do so, take the first stitch with the new suture by inserting the needle beside the last exit point (or, if using locked stitches, outside the corner of the last locked stitch). Then tie that end to the end of the mucosal suture. If you choose to use synthetic suture down the perineum, do not tie it to chromic material, because they dissolve at different rates.

Subcutaneous closure

A layer of continuous subcutaneous basting stitches is now placed. This layer helps to control capillary bleeding and prevents the more shallow parts of the wound from becoming disrupted during the healing process.

Have your assistant hold the edges of the tear apart. If you have no assistant, hold the edges of the tear apart with the thumb and middle finger of your nondominant hand from below or above, as it suits you. Now begin closure by starting a row of basting stitches in the perineal body, beginning about 0.5 cm below the introitus. The entry and exit points for these stitches should be at least 8 to 10 mm from the skin edge. The depth of the stitches can vary so that each closes the depth of the tear at that level. Remember to manipulate the tissue with your hand but to remove the needle from the tissue with your thumb forceps.

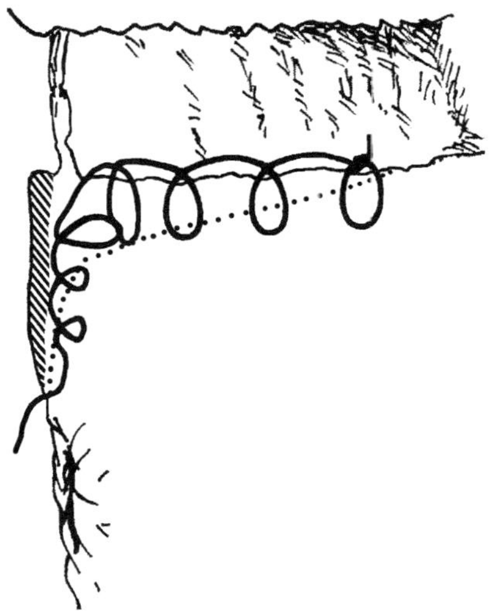

Sagittal schematic showing size, depth and extent of basting stitches

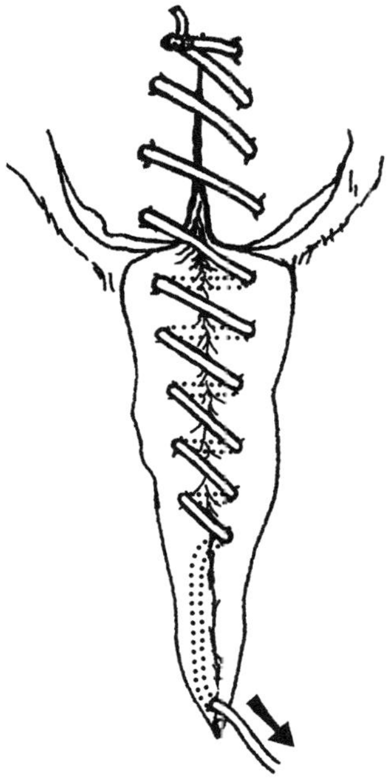

A row of basting stitches down the perineum

As with deeply placed sutures, this layer is placed parallel with the surface of the yoni floor (or deep to the surface of the perineum). Be sure to encompass the depth of the tear. Remember, these stitches are not locked. It is important to keep the distance from the skin edge equal on both sides. A subcuticular layer of stitches will go between this layer and the skin surface (unstitched shaded region in front of basting stitches in the schematic above). If the underlying tissue is bulging outward (as with a rectocele), you can place loose stitches slightly closer together to compensate but do not strangulate the tissue.

Continue these stitches down to the external apex of the tear. Most tears are deepest at the introitus, forming an increasingly shallow wedge as you approach the external apex. Thus, stitches will be increasingly superficial as you near the external apex of the tear (the end above the anus). Once you have gotten to the point that your basting stitches will be less than a quarter of an inch from the skin edge, run your needle under the tissue and bring it out inside the posterior external apex of the tear (also shown in schematic) so that you can begin outer closure. Do not to bring the needle through the skin surface; keep the suture inside the external apex.

If the tear is very shallow and does not necessitate a subcutaneous layer of sutures, you may simply move your needle to begin outer closure by inserting the needle behind the hymenal ring, running it through the tissue all the way down to the bottom of the perineal tear and bringing it out just inside the external apex of the tear.

Closing the skin layer

Interrupted stitches and skin closure: For centuries, interrupted stitches were used to close every type of perineal tear, including those in skin. Current practice recognizes that interrupted stitches are quite a bit more painful than buried stitches. In my experience, it appears that enzymes in the lochia dissolve externally placed chromic sutures more quickly and that internal closure minimizes wound breakdown. In addition, there are several important reasons to avoid placing any type of stitches that penetrate keratinized skin, such as that of the perineum. Like muscle, skin heals by forming scar tissue. When skin is torn, epithelial cells in the basal layer at the margins of the wound flatten and move along the surface of the wound until they find raw, undamaged tissue. They then traverse the raw tissue until they contact cells migrating from the opposite side of the wound. When suture material passes through the skin surface, skin cells can migrate along the path left by the needle. Once the suture is removed or has dissolved, a healed epithelialized channel may remain. Eventually, it may disappear, but some may persist and leave a punctate scar. A punctate scar is usually seen on the skin surface, leaving a "railroad track" or "crosshatch" scar pattern, although this is relatively rare if the skin sutures are not excessively tight when placed and are removed after seven days. Punctate scars are especially likely to develop when chromic gut is used, as it can promote the formation of more scar tissue due to the increased inflammatory response it stimulates. Skin cell migration along the suture tract may also result in cysts, patent sinus tracts (fistulas) or pinholes (blind sinuses) that develop along the line of the repair (Anderson, 1975).

Modified "subcuticular" closure: Once the basting stitch is completed, a deep "subcuticular" (anatomically, a subcutaneous) running mattress stitch is placed beneath the skin to hold the edges closer together. Running mattress stitches are ideal for closing the outer skin layer because they eliminate the irritation caused by interrupted stitches since none of the strand is exposed. There is also much less chance of rolling the edges of the skin inward toward the midline as you sew, a distinct deterrent to proper healing.

Traditionally running mattress stitches are placed as close to the skin surface as possible, resulting in a true subcuticular closure. For midwifery-related repairs, place them parallel with, but 2 to 3 mm below, the skin surface, in the subcutaneous fascia (Fleming, 1990). This avoids placing passing the needle through and leaving stitches in the more nerve-rich tissue of the dermis and still provides entirely adequate closure of the skin overlying the perineal body, resulting in less postpartum pain for the mother. This closes the skin, but not as tightly as a true subcuticular stitch would do, leaving a 2 mm or so gap during healing that may look like a problem until you get used to it.

While some midwives leave the skin unsutured, in my experience, women reported that leaving the skin unrepaired resulted in burning on urination for at least the first 24 hours. Whether to place subcuticular stitches or not can be decided on an individual basis according to the appearance of the wound and the preferences of the mother. (If a subcuticular stitch is not to be used, you can simply tie the stitches off at the external apex of the tear using a triple strand square knot.)

The suture material you will use is the same strand used to close the yoni floor and subcutaneous layer. After the last subcutaneous stitch is completed, the suture will be in the space just inside the external apex of the tear.

Here are some points to keep in mind with this style of stitch:

- •Arm the needle holder so that the needle is at a 90° angle to the shaft of the holder, then hold the *needle* parallel with the skin edge to make the stitch. To make the next stitch, reverse the direction of the needle in the holder (the mirror image). You may want to experiment with other ways of holding the needle.
- •When taking a stitch, it may help to stretch the skin slightly taut from above and below to assist needle insertion. The skin layer can be tough! You may have to apply a fair amount of pressure as you push the needle's tip into the tissue, especially when you are using a taper point needle.
- •If the perineal tissue is bulging from behind the skin layer (as it might with a rectocele), place the stitches slightly closer together to compensate for the pressure, thus providing more integrity during healing. Smaller stitches are usually used near the external apex because that end of the tear is typically the most shallow.
- •Check every stitch to be sure you are closing the tissue adequately. Do so by pulling the suture in the opposite direction from the side you just exited to see how the edges come together; they should not overlap or be staggered.
- •The needle enters the tissue as close as possible to the lower border of the skin layer while staying underneath it; leave 2 to 3 mm between the line of stitches and the skin surface (Fleming, 1990).
- •The needle will enter and exit the subcuticular tissue, but as you curve it through the tissue be sure to take a deep enough bite so the stitches won't pull out.
- •Do not pull the stitches too tightly; allow for swelling. The skin edges should just touch.
- •Ordinarily, you do not place your last stitch at the mouth of the yoni (at the junction of the perineal skin and the yoni mucosa) to avoid sewing the introitus too tightly. Place your last subcuticular stitch about 0.5 cm below the introitus, unless the introitus is very unevenly matched (i.e., the edges do not line up evenly without assistance). If this is the case, sew up to the very top but do not pull this stitch tightly. This type of mismatching can usually be avoided by aligning the tissues carefully at each step of the repair before you begin and making sure that each stitch is parallel in relation to the others or that entry and exit points for each stitch are parallel in the case of subcuticular stitches.
- •If you have had to start with a new piece of suture to complete the skin layer, you may begin a subcuticular layer by creating an anchor stitch with the new strand inside the external apex of the tear and then continuing up the perineum as already described.

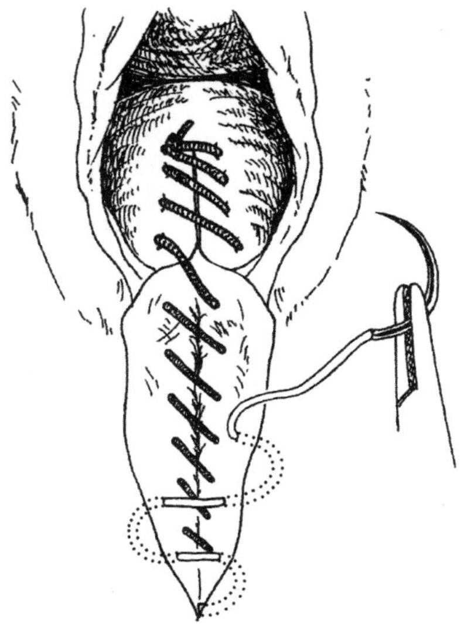

Subcuticular closure

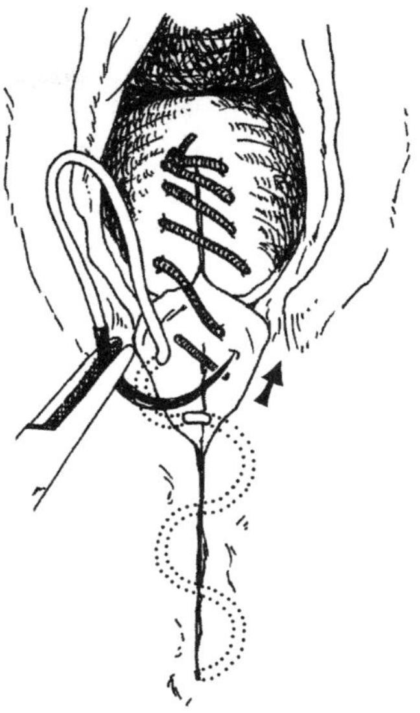

Finishing up subcuticular closure

To finish the repair

When you finish the subcuticular layer, you will again be near the mouth of the yoni. You will use the same technique to tie off the repair, whether you have used unlocked or locked stitches in the yoni mucosa,

- •Begin by inserting the needle between the edges of the skin tear and passing it back inside the yoni for one last stitch. Bring the needle out of the tissue near the hymenal ring. Which side you bring the needle up on will depend upon where you stop inserting running mattress sutures, the location of your final running mattress stitch, perhaps the shape of the tear and other factors. The technique is the same, whether the loop is created to your left or to your right.
- •The last stitch may be placed either in front of or behind the hymenal tags. Use your judgment regarding which seems best.

When skin tags are present: If you have skin tags near the yoni opening, you will have to put some stitches around the introitus. (In some cases you may have to repair tags with another packet of synthetic suture on a small needle before going back inside to tie off the main part of the repair as described below.)

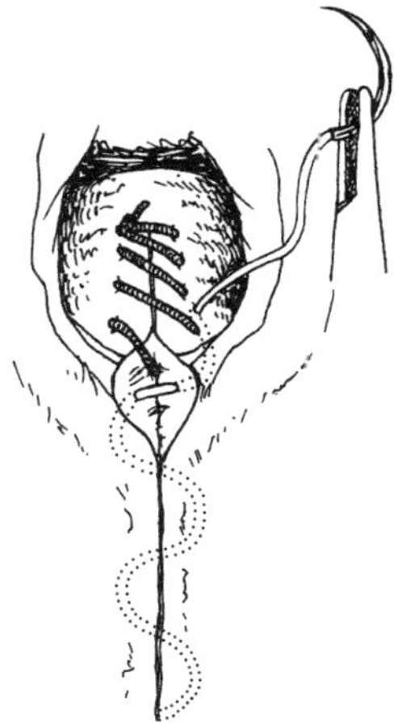	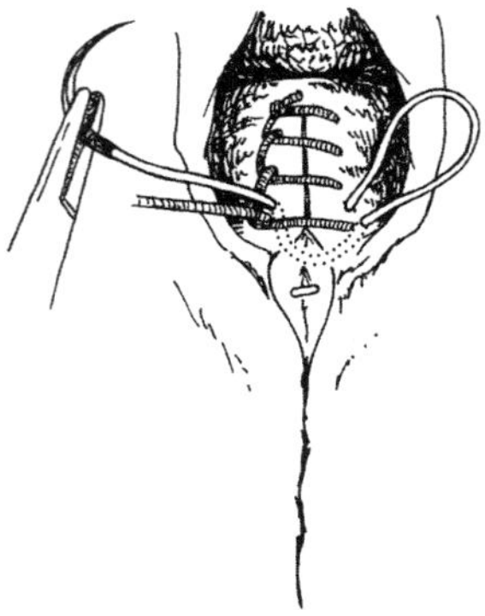	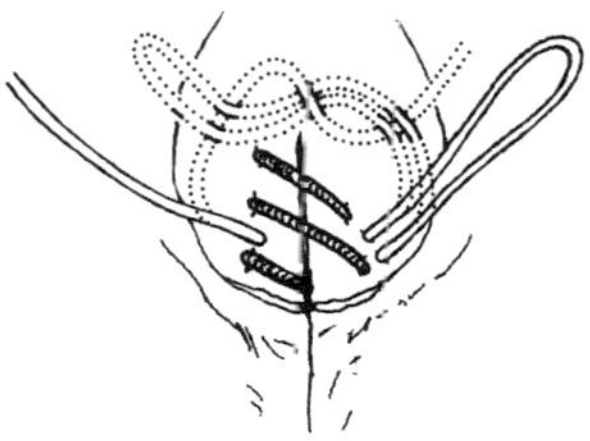
Bring the needle up inside the yoni near the last yoni stitch.	Create a loop on the same side.	Tie a square knot using the loop as one segment.

Finishing when you have used two packs of similar suture

> **NOTE:** Do not use this technique to tie synthetic and chromic together because they break down at different rates.

In you chose to open a new pack of suture for perineal repair, carry your perineal suture up behind the hymenal ring, then bring the second strand out opposite the strand that was left in the last stitch in the yoni floor. Insert the perineal needle on the same side you just exited, parallel with the suture from the yoni floor and exit beside the yoni floor strand (exit outside the last locked stitch if locked stitches were used in the yoni floor). Now you should have a loop on your dominant side and two strands on your nondominant side. Tie the stitch off–this will create a quadruple strand square knot.

Trim the ears

Be sure to trim the ends of suture to a length of no more than 0.5 cm.

Remove the gauze tampon

If you have used a tampon in the upper yoni, remove it now with your fingers or an instrument, being careful not to pinch tissue as you do. Check to be sure no clots have collected behind it during the suturing process.

Remove debris from the area

Be sure that every needle, piece of gauze and all suture fragments are accounted for and discarded; sharps should go into a sharps container.

Developing Your Own Style of Repair

As you learn techniques and gain experience with suturing, you may find yourself experimenting with various approaches to repairs, different suture equipment or materials, and so forth. Like any other creative endeavor, suturing lends itself to innovation. Every woman's perineal area is unique, and each laceration will present slightly different challenges. When repairing tears, a willingness to experiment is a necessity. Once you have the basic techniques down, you should be competent to apply them in individual situations.

I have shared everything I know and have done a great deal of research. No doubt, this will make learning easier for students and clear up many questions from experienced midwives who have limited opportunities to discuss technique with others. These are my major goals in writing this book. If, however, a practitioner you trust makes a reasonable suggestion which you want to try, go ahead. This is a manual, not a bible.

It is likely that you will need to experiment. A certain technique may be difficult for you, or you may find that you get better results with one type of stitch or technique over another. Be sure that you understand the basic anatomy involved, as well as the principles of repair and how tissues heal. Use this knowledge to evaluate different approaches. Do not merely copy a technique because someone more experienced than yourself suggests it, lest you mimic the weak points of your teacher.

I learned much of the suturing information contained in this text on my own, after having read all the books I could find and having had the most rudimentary basics explained to me. Later on, a wonderful CNM gave me a few more pointers. Everyone who has reviewed this book has had different suggestions about types of suture materials to use and styles of repair. In some places I have mentioned these differences, especially when the suggestions deviated significantly from my personal experience.

As you watch other practitioners suture, you will discover that styles are very individual. One person does a meticulous repair while another does what looks to you like a slap-dash job. You may have never heard of a technique, or perhaps you were told by someone else that a particular technique doesn't work. All may report that their repairs heal fine. You should ask detailed questions such as "How many times have you have used the technique? Any problems? How did they resolve?" When another practitioner tells you that she has few tears or that a nonsuturing technique works just as well to close the wound as do stitches, ask questions and observe whenever possible to find out how thoroughly she examines the perineum after births and what kind of follow-up care she provides. If she is not, it will be hard to know if her approach is really effective. You should consider the risks and benefits of any new procedure or technique. The proof, of course, is how the women experience their healing and the types of problems they encounter.

REFERENCES AND FURTHER READING ON PUTTING IT ALL TOGETHER: FIRST- AND SECOND-DEGREE REPAIR

REFERENCES USED IN MULTIPLE CHAPTERS

Anderson M. "Principles of wound healing in the repair of the episiotomy" (unpublished paper), Hawthorne NY, 1975.

Canavan T, Wilke A. ALSO: SYLLABUS UPDATE N: PERINEAL LACERATIONS, Jan 20, 2006.

Ethicon, Inc. WOUND CLOSURE MANUAL. Johnson & Johnson, Somerville, NJ, 1994.

Fernando R, et al. Green-top Guideline No. 29: "The management of third- and fourth-degree perineal tears," Royal College of Obstetricans and Gynaecologists (RCOG), Mar, 2007.

Fleming N. "Can the suturing method make a difference in postpartum perineal pain?" J NURSE-MIDWIFERY, 35(1):19-25, Jan-Feb, 1990.

Galli S, et al. "Wound closure technique," www.emedicine.com/ent/topic35.htm, updated Aug 1, 2006, accessed Aug 13, 2008.

Good Hope Hospital. Guideline No. 30: "Guideline for perineal trauma," Version 2.1.1, Aug, 2005, http://www.benpct.nhs.uk/_aboutus/boardpapers/Eastern/2002/08/30%20Guideline%20for%20Perineal%20trauma.pdf, accessed Aug 31, 2007.

Gordon B, et al. "The Ipswich childbirth study: 1. A randomized evaluation of two stage postpartum perineal repair leaving the skin unsutured," BR J OBSTET GYNAECOL, 105(4):435-440, Apr, 1998.

Hale R, Ling F. EPISIOTOMY: PROCEDURE AND REPAIR TECHNIQUES. American College of Obstetricians and Gynecologists, Washington DC, 2007.

Henderson C, Bick D, eds. PERINEAL CARE: AN INTERNATIONAL ISSUE. Quay Books, London UK, 2005.

Kettle, C. "The management of perineal trauma," in Henderson C, Bick D, eds. PERINEAL CARE: AN INTERNATIONAL ISSUE. Quay Books, London UK, 2005.

Kettle C, Fenner D. Chapter 3: "Repair of episiotomy, first- and second-degree tears," in Sultan A, et al., eds. PERINEAL AND ANAL SPHINCTER TRAUMA. Springer-Verlag, London UK, 2007.

Leeman L, et al. "Repair of obstetric perineal lacerations," AM FAM PHYSICIAN, 68(8):1585-1590, Oct 15, 2003.

Morano S, et al. "A randomized comparison of suturing techniques for episiotomy and laceration repair after spontaneous vaginal birth," J MINIMALLY INVASIVE GYNECOL, 13(5): 457-462, Sep-Oct, 2006.

Nisbet M, Brown R. PERINEAL REPAIR. Davis and Geck. Cyanamid Australia, 1992.

Olsson A. "Perineal repair," DVD. Braun Fotogruppen, Södersjukhuset, Stockholm Sweden, 2005.

Oxorn, H. Chapter 34: "Episiotomy, lacerations, uterine rupture, inversion," in his OXORN-FOOTE HUMAN LABOR & BIRTH. 5th ed. Appleton-Century-Crofts, Norwalk CT, 1986.

Parker L, Brunner J. Chapter 32 "Gynecologic surgery for obstetric patients," in Rock J, Jones H, eds. TE LINDE'S OPERATIVE GYNECOLOGY, 9th ed. Lippincott, Williams & Wilkins, Philadelphia PA, 2003b.

Rogers R, et al. "Repair of second-degree obstetrical lacerations," DVD. American College of Surgeons, Ciné-Med, Chicago IL, 2001.

Royal College of Obstetricians and Gynecologists (RCOGG). Green-Top Guideline No. 23: "Materials and methods used in perineal repair," Jun, 2004.

Sherris D, Kern E. ESSENTIAL SURGICAL SKILLS, 2nd ed. Saunders, Philadelphia PA, 2004.

Stone K, et al. "The biomechanical effects of tight suture closure on fascia," SURG GYNECOL OBSTET, 163(5):448-452, 1986.

Trott A. WOUNDS AND LACERATIONS: EMERGENCY CARE AND CLOSURE, 3rd ed. Elsevier Mosby, Philadelphia PA, 2005.

Varney H, et al. Chapter 79: "Cutting an episiotomy and repairing episiotomies and lacerations," in their VARNEY'S MIDWIFERY, 4th ed. Jones & Bartlett, Sudbury MA, 2004.

REPAIRING THE POSTERIOR YONI WALL

Sorger L, MD. Editing comments, Feb, 1991.

NOTES:

THIRD- AND FOURTH-DEGREE REPAIR

NOTE: Be sure you have studied the chapter entitled "The Anal Triangle and Related Structures" before studying this part. Regardless of the apparent extent of the damage, familiarize yourself with each chapter in this part so that when you are contemplating whether to repair such a serious tear, no important consideration is overlooked.

REPAIRING THE RECTAL MUCOSA

Unfortunately, the literature devotes very little attention to the repair of the rectal mucosa. Today, all specific references I could find only mentioned a single row of stitches, so that is what is described here.

Even though fourth-degree tears are rare without a clitorotomy, I begin this part of the text with a discussion of rectal mucosal repair because it will be the deepest layer you may have to reconstruct. Rectal mucosa damage presents a serious risk of infection. If repaired incorrectly, or if the repair is complicated by suture breakdown, there is a very real possibility that a fistula will form. Do not attempt repair of the rectal mucosa unless you are sure of how to go about it. It is important to be *absolutely certain* that you have located the internal apex of any rectal mucosal tear. Make no assumptions; you must be able to see the apex to be sure. If you neglect this and you start stitching below it, you will leave an open space that invites fecal contamination, infection and the formation of a fistula. IF IN DOUBT, TRANSPORT TO THE HOSPITAL FOR REPAIR!

If a severe rectocele is present, a tear extending into the rectal mucosa may allow loops of bowel to prolapse through it. If this should occur, hospital transport is called for to correctly repair the enterocele and prevent puncture or strangulation of the prolapsed intestines (Lawrence, 1992).

Suture materials to repair the rectal mucosa

Use 4-0 absorbable synthetic on a very fine (RB-1, T-31) taper point needle. Some care providers use 3-0 or 4-0 chromic gut. I recommend using synthetic suture in this area because it will stay longer and produces less inflammation (Sultan & Thakar, 2002). Do not attempt to repair this delicate tissue with a cutting needle.

Preventing contamination in the wound

Most of the contents of the lower rectum will have been emptied by the pressure of fetal descent during pushing. However, there may be tiny traces of fecal matter in the lower bowel or anal canal, which can encourage infection if sewn into the repair; if there are visible traces of feces, remove them first. To do so, carefully cleanse any obvious fecal matter from the lumen of the bowel using a gloved finger and a gauze pad. If there is no visible fecal matter, do not attempt to wipe out the area. Next, rinse the area thoroughly. Place an absorbant towel and then a large bowl or bed pan beneath the woman's bottom. Irrigate the area with warm normal saline (1 tsp salt to 1 quart of water). Forcefully squirt solution into the area, holding the edges of the tear open (with a retractor if you have one) so that the fluid flows down from the yoni side. Direct the stream above the internal apex of the rectal tear, using the entire bottle of solution. Gently blot this tissue dry with sterile gauze pads, or dry the area lightly with a hair dryer.

An overview of rectal mucosa repair

The rectal mucosa is repaired using a single layer of small stitches to ensure that the repair seals off the lumen to prevent fecal contamination in the wound and maintains its integrity under the stress of normal bowel function. You are placing stitches in the ceiling of the anorectal canal.

Choice of stitch: Some practitioners use tiny, closely spaced interrupted stitches to do the first part of the repair while others use continuous running mattress or basting (over-and-over) stitches. The advantage of interrupteds is that, should one accidently penetrate the anorectal lumen, it is easier to remove and replace. In addition, the chance of an infection developing is higher in this area than anywhere else you will be suturing. A continuous stitch increases the risk that, should an infection occur, bacteria will be transmitted along the entire length of the strand (Ethicon, 1994). In most situations, midwives will rarely be called upon to repair the rectal muscosa. This is an important consideration when deciding what stitch is best since it means that you will have few opportunities to become experienced with this type of repair. Interrupted stitches may thus be the most practical type for most midwives to use and is therefore what I discuss in this chapter. However, if you are in a circumstance that calls upon you to become more experienced with rectal repair, continuous stitches can certainly be placed more quickly, require far fewer knots and will give excellent results when placed correctly and the terminal knots are secure (Sorger, 1991; Sultan & Thakar, 2002).

Insert a retractor: Insert a yoni retractor to allow full visualization and to minimize using your hands to do this. The Guardian retractor can be carefully inserted with the handle up so that it is not in your way as you work (take care not to pinch the labia).

Placing the stitches: There are two ways to ensure that you close the tear above the internal apex. The first option is to attach an Allis clamp (just clamp it to the first click) where the tear begins (in the crotch of the tear) and leave it there until you have placed your anchor stitch (Sorger, 1991). Then quickly remove the clamp. (Although this suggestion came from an experienced OB, I am a little worried that it might increase the risk of tissue necrosis in this delicate area.)

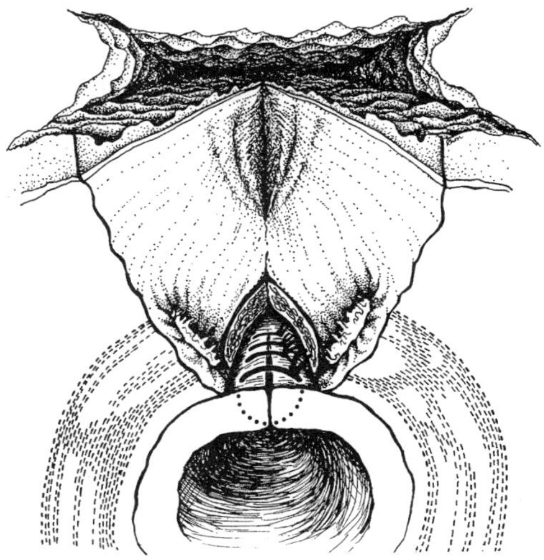

A row of interrupted stitches in the rectal mucosa

Alternatively, you can place a small interrupted stitch as close to the apex as possible, leave the ends long and have an assistant apply just enough traction to the stitch to allow you to get your anchor stitch in place. Then cut the ends of the locating stitch short (this technique, too, could be problematic, as the tissue here is delicate and this stitch might rip out). Regardless of which method you use, you must be gentle.

Once the apex is in view, place a tiny interrupted stitch starting 0.5 cm or so above it. It must be deep enough to hold the tissue, but shallow enough not to go through the rectal wall into the lumen (center space) of the bowel (as illustrated here in cross-section).

Tie off the anchor stitch, remembering to use two full square knots (4 throws) for synthetic suture. Cut the ends, leaving them about 4 inches long. Use a hemostat to grasp the ends and have your assistant hold it up out of the way, or attach the hemostat that is holding the ends to the sterile field on the mother's belly. Take care not to put traction on these threads, or the stitch may be pulled out. These threads will serve as a marker when you begin to repair the internal sphincter.

I suggest placing each stitch so it is tied on the superior side of the tear. Successful repairs have been described using interrupted stitches tied in the lumen of the rectal mucosa, a technique which leaves less foreign material in the tissue, where it may raise the risk of infection. However, placing and tying a stitch like this in the ceiling of the bowel involves both gymnastics on the part of the midwife to see what you are doing as well as more stress on the tissues. Moreover, numerous exposed knots left in the lumen of the anal canal can trap fecal matter, which could creep up the suture strand and become imbedded in the healing wound: a setup for infection and abscess.

Place additional stitches close together to prevent bowel contents from penetrating the line of sutures. The second interrupted stitch is made right in front of the first, leaving only a few mm space between them. Tie this one off (using 4 throws) and cut the thread close to the knot, but be sure the ends are long enough so it won't come undone.

Continue with a row of tiny, closely spaced stitches (3 to 4 per cm) down to the anal opening. Place stitches around the curve of the tissue of the perianal skin to the point where you will later begin placing running mattress stitches beneath the perineal skin.

If you decide to place continuous stitches, be sure to visualize the tip of your needle in the center of the repair before you complete the other half of your stitch. This will help to prevent accidently leaving exposed suture material in the lumen of the anal canal. Tie off the last stitch using the three-strand technique described for closure of a first-degree tear, being careful not to tie it too tightly (this technique is described in the chapter entitled "Tying Surgical Knots.") I would not use an Aberdeen knot here, as it will leave a quantity of suture material in this very delicate tissue.

Examination/removal and replacement of misplaced stitches: If you believe you may have just misplaced a stitch, check immediately before placing any more. Once you are done with a layer, confirm that the first layer is placed correctly before proceeding with the next layer. See the next chapter, entitled "Examining the Anorectum for Misplaced Stitches" for details.

Is a second layer necessary? In previous editions of this text, a second layer of sutures was recommended at this point. This layer of continuous basting stitches was to overlie the first and be spaced slightly wider than the first. It was intended to reinforce the first layer.

This technique was taught to me by an experienced physician who repaired one of my own clients many years ago and it made sense at that time. However, now the standard of care is to place stitches in the internal sphincter, which effectively provides an additional layer of support right above the stitches in the rectal muscosa. For this reason, and because too many layers of stitches can do more harm than good and because I cannot find any reference in the current literature to a two layer repair in this tissue, I am no longer recommending the placement of a second layer.

<u>Check for misplaced stitches</u>: See the next chapter for how to go about this.

<u>Tidy up</u>: Be sure all suture scraps, needles, gauze, etc. are removed from the area and discarded. Double check for any traces of fecal matter and clean it up if found. Replace used underpads before you proceed. Change your gloves. These precautions will help prevent an infection.

Now proceed with the rest of your repair: repair the internal and external anal sphincters, and then proceed as for a first- or second-degree tear.

EXAMINING THE ANORECTUM FOR MISPLACED STITCHES

NOTE: This step is necessary after each layer of deep yoni mucosal, anal sphincter or rectal mucosa repairs.

If you are doing deep yoni repair or have placed stitches in either the sphincter or the rectal mucosa, you must examine the anterior anorectal wall frequently to make sure that no stitches have penetrated into the lumen of the rectum. Misplaced sutures may encourage infection or heal to form a larger passage between the yoni and rectal walls (rectoyoni fistula) or a pinhole passage called a "sinus tract." To avoid this, misplaced stitches must be removed and replaced correctly.

Many practitioners wait until they are finished with the entire repair and check only once at the end. But why in the world would anyone want to risk having to break down an entire repair to correct the situation if a stitch is, indeed, misplaced? I recommend checking after each step that would be likely to leave a stitch that penetrates the anorectal wall: after each layer of rectal mucosa repair, after sphincter repair and after placing a deep layer of stitches in the posterior yoni wall. Of course, if you feel you have just misplaced a stitch during repair, it will be simplest to deal with it right then, before proceeding with the repair.

Examining for stitches

Put a cover glove over the gloved hand you will use for the rectal examination. Now insert a double-gloved finger into the anus and examine the upper rectal wall to feel for misplaced stitches. To be sure, palpate beneath each stitch, using the pad of your index finger and a finger of your other hand in the yoni for guidance and to assist by applying counterpressure, if necessary.

If in doubt, look. Have an assistant hold a good light. Use the finger in the rectum to guide your yoni finger to the stitch in question. Place the pad of your yoni finger against the suspect stitch and press down and forward very gently and carefully. Identify the area with your rectal finger, then remove the rectal finger and look. If the tear is not very long, this should allow you to visualize the area as the anal tissues will be very lax at this point. Get down below the level of the anus so you can look up, rather than severely distorting the sutured area in an attempt to make the stitch visible. This tissue is fragile, and you could easily poke a hole through your line of sutures if you are not careful. If you still cannot see, use your yoni finger to depress the yoni wall as described and use your rectal finger to open the lumen by applying pressure to the posterior rectal wall.

Removing a stitch that was accidently placed through the rectal wall

These suggestions are useful whether you are removing a stitch that has penetrated the rectal lumen from the yoni wall or from the rectal mucosa.

Interrupted stitches: When removing a single stitch, it is ideal to cut the knot off from above and pull the loop out of the tissue from below. First grasp the loop of suture from the rectal side with a small instrument. Cut the stitch from the yoni side of the tear. Grasp the knot with an instrument and, then snip the loop to either side of the knot. Lift the now-detached knot off the loop and place the instrument holding it to the side (this avoids releasing the knot and having it get lost in the tissue or bedclothes). Use the instrument attached to the anorectal side of the loop to pull it out from the anorectal side, thus avoiding dragging contaminated suture through the tear.

If grasping a loop from the rectal side proves impossible, lift the stitch from the yoni side with tissue forceps and cut *only one side* of the loop, near the knot. Then grasp the knot and pull the strand through from the yoni side. Be certain that all scraps of suture material are removed from the yoni and rectum before you proceed. (For details regarding replacing stitches, see the appropriate chapter for the layer you are suturing.)

Irrigate the wound, replace the stitches and reexamine rectally to be sure the new stitches do not penetrate the lumen.

Continuous stitches: If you must remove a continuous stitch, depending upon where in the line of stitches you find the error, you can either remove and replace the entire row or remove the one problematic stitch and then restitch over the area, starting from above the removed stitch and extending a couple of stitches below it. Because this is a continuous stitch, it is best to pull it from the yoni side so you can see what you are doing and disrupt as few of the adjacent stitches as possible, even though contamination of the wound is more likely when suture is removed from the yoni side. If the mistake occurred in the middle of the tear, assess whether overlapping the sutures seems feasible. If so, start a new anchor stitch, so that it overlaps the last two or three basting stitches adjacent to the area with the missing stitch and continue your repair. If neither method seems like it will provide adequate support, you will need to remove and replace the entire row of stitches. To do so, grasp the knot at the internal apex and use suture scissors to cut the looped end on either side of the knot and lift the knot away. Then use thumb forceps to gently lift the cut loop and work it up through the tissue. Continue to do this until the thread you are removing is unwieldy. Whenever that occurs, trim it and continue to remove stitches until you arrive at the last knot (if one is already in place). Trim one side of that knot and pull the knot to remove the last bit of suture. Irrigate the wound, replace the stitches and reexamine rectally to be sure the new stitches do not penetrate the lumen.

Visible fecal matter

If there is fecal matter in the lower bowel, it should be removed as completely as possible with a gloved finger and gauze pad. Irrigate the area with diluted povidone iodine mixed with water (about 2 oz in an 8 oz peri-bottle diluted with clean water) or normal saline (1 tsp salt to 1 quart water). To do so, place an absorbant towel under a large bowl or bed pan beneath the woman's bottom to catch the fluid. Open the tear from the yoni side to expose it to its depth, and forcefully squirt the solution into the area so that it flows from the yoni side, directing the stream above the location of the misplaced stitch and using the entire bottle of solution. Then irrigate again with normal saline. See the chapter entitled "Postpartum Care and Comfort Measures" regarding preventing infection.

Repairing the Anal Sphincters: General Considerations

NOTE: The repair of either anal sphincter is a serious responsibility. Do not attempt it unless you are sure of what you are doing and have the proper materials and equipment. If you have never observed a sphincter repair and have no experienced person to supervise you, I recommend hospital transport whenever possible. If the repair is done incorrectly or heals poorly, the woman could be partially or completely incontinent of feces for the rest of her life.

Third- and fourth-degree tears are collectively referred to as obstetric anal sphincter injuries (OASIS). Severe tears like this are primarily a product of clitorotomy extension, although they can certainly happen spontaneously as well.

When there is third-degree damage (rectal mucosa is intact), some practitioners start by repairing the yoni mucosa, then do any deep intrayoni repair that is needed, and then repair the sphincters. However, I recommend that you start with the sphincters and then do the rest of the repair. If there are cervical tears or upper yoni wall damage or both, repair the cervix first and then the upper yoni wall before beginning any other repairs.

Before you start, it is vitally important to be sure your third-degree tear isn't really a fourth-degree tear. If it is, the rectal mucosa must be repaired prior to the anal sphincters. See the preceding chapter, entitled "Repairing the Rectal Mucosa."

Obstetric recommendations intended to ensure an optimal repair

Doctors recommend that anal sphincter repairs take place on an operating table to provide optimal lighting and positioning of the mother. They also recommend that the repair be performed under general or at least regional anesthesia to allow relaxation of the sphincters, which they feel is essential to allow adequate retrieval of retracted ends and to allow sewing them while they are not under tension; getting the stitches properly placed is easier, and they are less likely to be pulled out as others are placed to complete the repair. You should explain these recommendations to the mother before you begin. You must also honestly assess whether you feel you can perform the repair at home. If the damage is extensive or you believe anesthesia will make for a better repair, advise the mother.

Suture materials and surgical equipment used for anal sphincter repair

The anal sphincters can be repaired with 2-0 or 3-0 absorbable synthetic monofilament suture. The advantage of a monofilament is that you do not have to worry about braided strands harboring infectious organisms. As of this writing, most sources specifically recommend the use of Polydioxanone (PDS II) by Ethicon (Maxon is Syneture's closest equivalent) on a CT-1 or T-12 taper point needle to repair either of the anal sphincters. These materials are preferred because of their very long half-life, which provides extended support, allowing plenty of time for the ends of the sphincter to scar together. Unfortunately, these sutures' longevity also means they are more likely to irritate and cause discomfort and may even result in knot migration to the skin surface, leading to pain and even infection at times.

Whatever you choose, do not use Vicryl Rapide as it dissolves too rapidly for use in these repairs. Historically chromic gut has been used, but the staying power and lack of inflammatory reaction associated with the use of synthetic suture is a big advantage.

You will also need two to four Allis clamps and four small hemostats. Because of the complex nature of these repairs, it is almost essential to have an assistant to help you.

Avoiding knot migration: Migration of suture material and surgical knots can occur as suture breaks down. Migration refers to the movement of suture material through the overlying tissue as remodeling occurs and as the body tries to reject the foreign material before it has dissolved. Migrated material may eventually extrude through to the skin surface. The risk for migration appears to be greater when longer lasting suture material is used. During sphincter repair, the risk of knot migration can be minimized by being sure to bury the knots beneath the superficial tissues of the perineal body, which is accomplished when you only include the sphincter and its capsule in each stitch (Fouda, 2009).

Prognosis for women who sustain anal sphincter injury

If you identify the sphincters correctly, sew the ends with stitches that don't come out, and the wound remains free of infection, it would seem reasonable to assume that the wound will heal fine. In reality, a good suture job and adequate healing, by themselves, do not necessarily ensure an optimal outcome as far as muscle tone and long-term anal continence are concerned. Immediate complications include infection, dehiscence and fistula formation. The incidence of problems after birth is high. After repair of the external sphincter some 20 to 40% of these women report some sort of anal continence issues at 12 months after the birth. Most describe problems such as incontinence of flatus or fecal urgency (Fernando et al., 2007). In other sources, the reported incidence of problems following repair were even more discouraging, with 25 to 59% of women reporting some type of anal incontinence (Sultan & Thaker, 2002). Problems are more common in women who have a complicated course of healing, and there is some debate regarding what type of repair heals best (discussed in the chapter entitled "Repairing the External Anal Sphincter"). Differences in outcome are also related to different repair techniques and the expertise and training of the practitioners involved. Education and training in sphincter repair has been notoriously inadequate in medical curriculums. Long-term complications may also plague these women, with symptoms developing with the onset of neurologic changes or muscle atrophy as they age (Rogers et al., 2002c).

Women who have sustained anal sphincter injury during a previous birth run a higher risk of developing anal incontinence or worsening symptoms with subsequent yoni birth. This is especially true for women who had transient fecal symptoms after the first birth that involved sphincter damage. Prophylactic clitorotomy does not reduce this risk. Those who are already symptomatic should be advised that surgical delivery is an option that may reduce their risk of further anal incontinence (Fernando et al., 2007). The woman must weigh this risk against the considerable risks of surgical delivery itself to herself and her baby.

Repairing the Internal Anal Sphincter

Historically, tears in the internal anal sphincter (IAS) have been largely ignored. Not so today, as urogynecologists have recognized the devastating effects of lax sphincter function on a woman's daily life. The IAS plays a role in fecal continence. Disruption of both the internal and external anal sphincters increases the risk of anal incontinence compared with women who have damage to the external sphincter alone (de Leeuw et al., 2001). Since the IAS is largely responsible for maintaining the resting tone of the anal sphincter complex, damage to it is associated with incontinence of flatus and passive soiling (Sultan & Thakar, 2007).

To understand some of the specific issues presented by midline anal sphincter disruption DeLancey and colleagues (1997) undertook a study involving 20 women who sustained fourth-degree lacerations. Visible defects in both the IAS and the EAS were found in all 20. Both the IAS and EAS were usually retracted posterolaterally. In a few, minimal dissection was required to expose the separated ends. Extension of the IAS laceration above that found in the EAS was noted, except in cases where the laceration was confined to the part of the IAS that directly underlies the EAS. In such cases, the IAS was found to be intact above the upper margin of EAS damage. Looking down into the tear where the two layers overlapped, the EAS lay on top of the IAS and the two muscles were often fused into a single mass. This did not occur above the upper margin of the EAS, where the two parts were separate. In those women who did not receive regional anesthesia, the constant muscular activity of the IAS caused it to retract into the surrounding tissue and it could only be found when specifically searched for and retrieved. The IAS was easier to identify after the mucosa and submucosa of the anorectum was reconstructed, as pulling those layers to the midline also helped pull the IAS medially into view.

Identifying parts of the tear

A tear that clearly divides the external sphincter and also reveals or divides more than the first bit of the anorectal muscosa is likely to include a tear into the IAS. Reidentify the IAS before you begin repair. The most distal border of the IAS is set back about 3.7 mm or a little more from the anal verge. Therefore, it is possible to have either external sphincter damage; a tear that extends down the perineal skin, over and around the external sphincter and into the most distal part of the rectal mucosa; or both, that does not involve the IAS.

It is also possible, though very rare, to have IAS damage while the rectal mucosa and the external sphincter remain intact; this type of tear is much more difficult to identify, especially if you do not have a high index of suspicion. If such an IAS tear is relatively short, you may be able to place a stitch or two to close it by using instruments to retract the overlying tissues and retrieve the IAS ends. If you suspect an extensive tear, however, the woman should be transported to the hospital, examined with an endoscopic ultrasound probe and repaired by a surgeon. This is because such tear is likely to require tissue dissection before repair can be performed. However, because such a circumstance is exceedingly rare, always assume that the EAS is damaged when IAS injury is detected.

Also recall that the IAS is about 3 cm wide (tall) but has no separate proximal (upper) border because it is continuous with the outer layer of the rectal wall. Thus, unlike tears in the external sphincter, which is a distinct band of muscle, tears of the IAS will have an internal apex. As is true for other tears, it is a good idea to identify this apex because you want to know the extent of the tear so that you can take that into consideration when you assess how many stitches are required to reunite the sides. Plus, it is always wise to identify the internal apex of any tear, because not doing so may leave a much more extensive tear undetected. If the IAS is not bleeding and it is hard to reach above the internal apex, not beginning the repair above the apex is acceptable in this case, however, because the IAS is sandwiched between two other layers of tissue that are also being repaired, thus it is unlikely that lochia will seep into the space above the first stitch. Even so, it is still important to begin your repair at the level of the internal apex.

It is now considered best practice to repair the internal sphincter as a separate structure. If connective tissues are still linking the internal and external sphincters and both are torn, you can gently separate the layers just enough to allow you to place stitches in the internal sphincter. The internal sphincter glistens and looks like a flatter, broader band of fresh raw fish meat as compared to the rounded, beefy red appearance of the external sphincter.

Repairing the internal anal sphincter

Both halves of the IAS should be identified and grasped with Allis clamps, and the edges brought to the midline. You may need an assistant to hold these clamps in place until you can insert the first stitch, as the muscle is likely to retract to either side otherwise. The need to apply gentle traction to retrieve the ends confirms that you have indeed grasped the muscle and not just the surrounding fascia (Rogers et al., 2002b, 2002c).

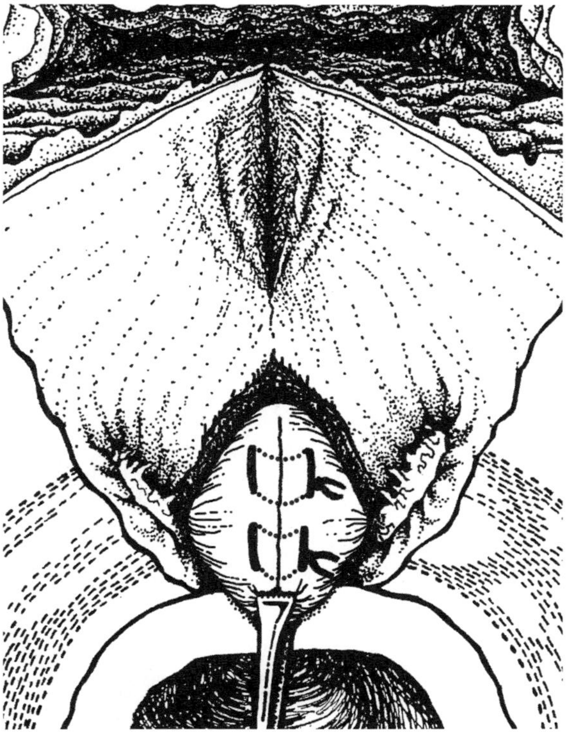

Two horizontal mattress stitches reunite the torn sides of the internal sphincter. (Allis clamp applied at 6 o'clock)

Once each half has been identified, repair is a simple matter of placing either interrupted stitches or horizontal mattress stitches to reunite the sides. I recommend using horizontal mattress stitches, as they will better distribute the stress that the elastic muscle places on the repair. Space whichever you choose about 0.5 cm apart and leave an 0.5 cm space between the two entry and exit points of each side of the horizontal mattress stitch. Be sure you are entering and exiting the tissue well back from the edge, in completely intact muscle (not frayed ends). Leave at least

0.5 cm between the needle entry and exit points and the edge of the muscle on either side. Bring the sides together, where they may evert slightly, which lets you know they are making adequate contact to heal, but do not exaggerate the eversion. Although overlap techniques have been considered for repair of the IAS, they probably are not suited to this repair since the IAS is composed of smooth muscle. Thus, stitches that are placed under tension in the IAS are more likely to rip out than those placed in the EAS (Sultan et al., 1999).

Once you have finished, proceed to the next chapter covering the repair of the external anal sphincter.

Repairing the External Anal Sphincter

The external anal sphincter (EAS) primarily controls voluntary fecal continence, including passage of solid stool. The EAS, along with the puborectalis muscle, provides the squeeze tone of the anal canal, but only 10 to 20% of its resting tone.

Approaches to the repair of the external anal sphincter

Repair of the capsule: In 1955, Fulsher and Fearl reported excellent results using a technique wherein the ends of the EAS were left unsutured and only the surrounding capsule was repaired. No doubt this technique is still used by some, although the original results have never been reproduced in a study. For a completely severed sphincter, you would place four stitches (as described) in the capsule, not the muscle itself. For this method to effect good healing, it is imperative that the capsule be fully restored (Kolder, 1990). Suturing the muscle itself is the current standard of practice and what I strongly recommend.

As of this writing, the literature describes and debates two basic approaches to EAS repair: the overlap technique and the end-to-end technique.

Overlap technique: Sultan and colleagues (1999) were the first to report the use of an overlap technique for the primary repair of birth-related EAS damage. (**Primary repair** refers to a repair performed in the first instance of the type of damage in question.) Prior to that, overlap repair was only used by colorectal surgeons in secondary repairs for women being treated for fecal incontinence. This works because, even though the torn ends are not reapproximated, this is muscle tissue, which heals by scarring. Thus, a substantial region of raw, overlapped tissue that is held in place by long-acting suture provides a broad base of contact so that the two halves can scar together. Although otherwise not advisable, overlapping the ends also tightens the muscle, which seems to work well to support continence.

There has been much discussion in the literature as to whether the overlap method offers superior results to the more classic end-to-end technique that is easier to perform and certainly the more reasonable choice for home repair. Currently, even though some studies have found more favorable results using the overlap technique, as of this writing, there is no reliable evidence to show that the overlap method is superior to the end-to-end method for reuniting the ends of the EAS during a primary repair.

Regardless of the method employed, the overlap technique is an extremely difficult type of repair because it is so easy to wind up with twists in the muscle ends. There are basically two approaches to this type of repair. Each begins with identification of the ends of the external anal sphincter and its surrounding capsule. These structures are dissected away from the surrounding tissue enough to allow mobilization of the ends so that they can be overlapped at least 2 cm. This is accomplished by dissecting the tissue with surgical scissors by making little snips around the muscle end, taking care to include the whitish capsule as you do. The separated ends are then grasped with Allis clamps, pulled, along with the surrounding capsule, to the midline and beyond so that they overlap. If 50% or more of the sphincter is torn, the remaining intact fibers are also divided so that the ends can be fully overlapped (Fernando et al., 2006). There are then two ways to approach the overlap technique:

Overlap style: Fernando and colleagues (2006) describe this approach. Two or three horizontal mattress stitches are placed across the top to draw together the torn halves. Each stitch is started in the torn muscle half on your dominant side. The needle enters the surface of the muscle about 1.5 cm from the torn end and exits in the center of torn end. The needle then enters the center of the other torn half and penetrates about 0.5 cm. At this point a U-shaped bite is created as the needle exits the tissue adjacent to the entry point. Finally, the needle reenters the center of the end on your dominant side and exits the surface of the muscle. The ends of the suture are then trimmed long and grasped with Allis clamps. Another two or three stitches are placed in the same manner. Once all the sutures are placed, they are tied off one by one, resulting in a small flap of tissue from the dominant side where the two halves overlap. This flap is then tacked to the surface of the nondominant half of the sphincter muscle with two or three small interrupted stitches. This method is still quite tricky but is easier to accomplish than Method 2 described below because of the positioning of the stitches.

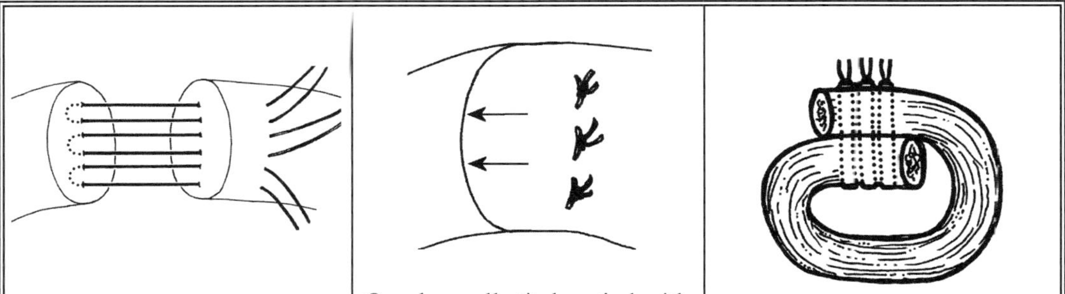

Overlap: horizontal stitches untied

Overlap: all stitches tied with loose flap to be tacked down where arrows are pointing

Stacking: three stitches in place

Stacking style: The other description of the overlap repair shows stacking the muscle ends in a "double-breasted" fashion (Power et al., 2006). This produces a more truly "stacked" configuration, but involves considerably more challenging needle work and dexterity to maintain the muscle ends in the desired position while executing the stitch. The needle is held at a 90° angle in the holder (as usual) and passed through both halves using a forehand motion, starting at the top of the upper half of the muscle through the bottom half and out of the tissue (the forehand motion assumes that the upper part of the EAS is the "far side" of the wound–see page 363 for an explanation). Then the needle is repositioned in the holder to make the second half of the stitch, which is accomplished by passing the needle through the bottom half and then the top half of the EAS using a backhand motion. The ends of the suture are now both sticking out of the top of the stacked ends. Grasp them with Allis clamps. Then place two or three more stitches. Then each suture is tied off.

Overlap repair requires regional anesthesia to relax the muscles sufficiently to allow for this much overlap as well as considerable tissue dissection and manipulation. If a woman desires this type of overlap repair, she should be transported to the hospital to have it done.

End-to-end repair: The end-to-end technique has been used for decades. It effectiveness has only been called into question since the 1990s. One of the reasons for the failure of any approach to repair of the EAS is that sutures are placed too close to the torn ends. Because the muscle fibers run side to side, it is imperative that you enter and exit the tissue well back from the torn or frayed ends, in intact muscle. Since end-to-end repair is the more practical and reasonable technique to use at home, I will describe it in more detail.

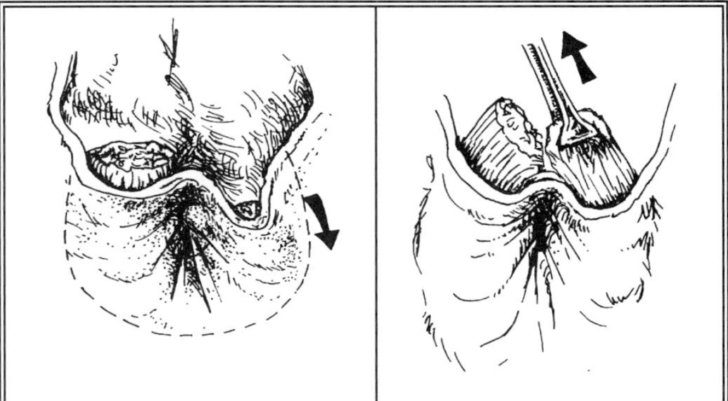

Torn and retracted sphincter end on your right	Retrieving the retracted end

Retrieving a retracted portion of the external sphincter: To understand what I am about to describe, imagine a doughnut-shaped object with a large, round piece of elastic inside that fills in the circular shape. The tube shaped "skin" of the doughnut represents the sphincter capsule, and the round elastic, the EAS itself. When the EAS is torn, sometimes the torn half of the EAS remains flush with the torn end of the tube skin. In other cases, the muscle is retracted down inside the capsule. If this is the case, you will need to retrieve it with an Allis clamp before you begin repair. In the typical situation during which retraction has occurred, one or both ends of the sphincter have completely detached from the capsule and retracted down inside a palpable hole. To retrieve the retracted end, simply open the clamp about 0.5 cm wide and reach directly down into the hole formed by the capsule. Feel around with the open clamp in the bottom of the hole until you meet resistance. Open the clamp slightly more to fit it around the muscle end, lock it and pull up gently. You will note an elastic resistance when you have, indeed, grasped the sphincter.

Much less commonly, one side of the torn EAS is only partially detached from its' capsule. It can be found retracted against the side, but not drawn down into the capsule (which will present as an opening immediately next to it). This can be confusing when you first encounter it. However, you must look carefully and identify both ends of the sphincter before proceeding or you run the risk of not sewing the ends together properly.

If you reach down into the capsule pocket with an Allis clamp and cannot find the sphincter (you are likely to pull and feel strong resistance and come up with a very small scrap of tissue instead), examine the side walls of the pocket for the stringy, latitudinal fibers of the external sphincter. Once located, grab the sphincter by holding the opened clamp at a slight angle (to allow for gathering a substantial portion of the muscle), clamp it and pull it out toward the center of the capsule, then up toward the midline.

Once all retracted portions have been retrieved, arrange each clamp so that it grips the muscle beyond any frayed ends to ensure that you place your stitches through an undamaged diameter of muscle. To accomplish this, you may have to use a second Allis clamp to hold one end while you reposition the other clamp. You may have to rearrange the clamps to allow the placement of different stitches. As you sew, it is okay to include the adjacent sphincter capsule; this will strengthen the repair.

If no ends are retracted, you may place the same type of stitches, but need not use your Allis clamps to do so. (This is unlikely. At least one end usually retracts, even when the other remains unretracted and visible on the opposite side.)

Repairing a partially torn (< 75%) EAS: If 75% or more of the EAS is torn, repair as for a fully severed sphincter.

While a portion of intact EAS provides some residual rectal continence, this doesn't mean it is okay to guess about what you are doing with the part that is torn. If in doubt, transport to the hospital!

What you will repair depends upon the degree of damage. If the surface of the mostly intact EAS is merely frayed, you can repair the capsule of the muscle and need not use Allis clamps. Recall that the capsule is composed of fascia and will not hold a stitch well, so be sure to take a bite well back from the edge to increase the likelihood that the stitch will stay.

If the tear is extensive enough that part of the severed muscle is retracted into the capsule, pull that side out with an Allis clamp and place one or two interrupted stitches or horizontal mattress stitches through the fattest part of the muscle well back from the frayed ends to reunite the retracted end with its other half. Any stringy ends can be tucked into the capsule of the sphincter.

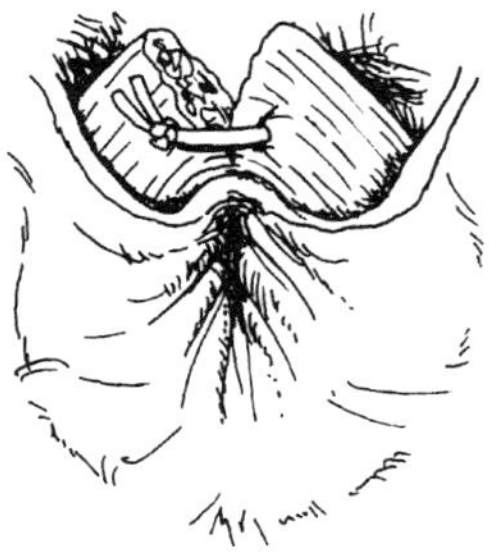

Take a stitch and tie it off. Assess its integrity by doing a rectal exam.

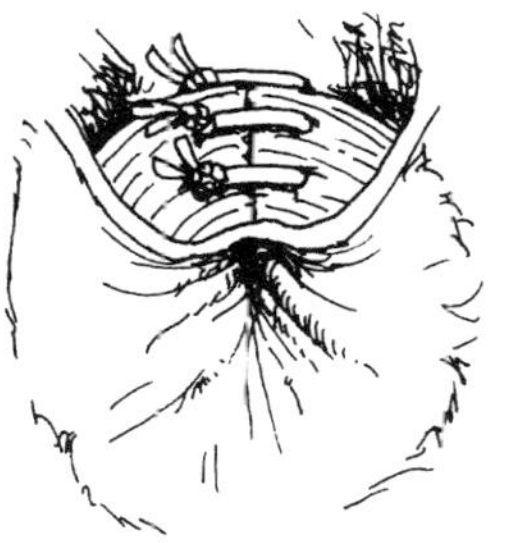

Place as many stitches as necessary to hold the ends together, spacing them evenly to unite the torn portion (usually 2 or 3).

The type of stitch to use depends entirely upon how well it will hold the capsule or sphincter together. Part of ensuring integrity is to take your bites far enough back into the intact part of the muscle so they won't pull out. Once it is in place, test the integrity of the first stitch by inserting a double-gloved finger in the anus and pressing up against the sphincter gently. If the stitch threatens to rip out, remove it and begin again. If you put in an interrupted stitch and find it to be inadequate, you should replace it with a figure-eight horizontal mattress stitch. Of course, you could just start with figure-eights in the first place. Space the stitches evenly over the torn portion (usually 2 or 3 are needed if less than 75% is torn). Interrupted stitches are illustrated here.

Be sure to check rectally for any misplaced stitches. Remove them, irrigate the area, and replace them as necessary.

Repairing a fully severed (>75%) EAS: After having assured yourself that there is no rectal mucosa or IAS damage or after repairing such damage, proceed with the repair. Because of the maneuvering space you will need, always repair the cervix, upper yoni wall, anorectal muscosa and IAS before suturing the EAS or anything else.

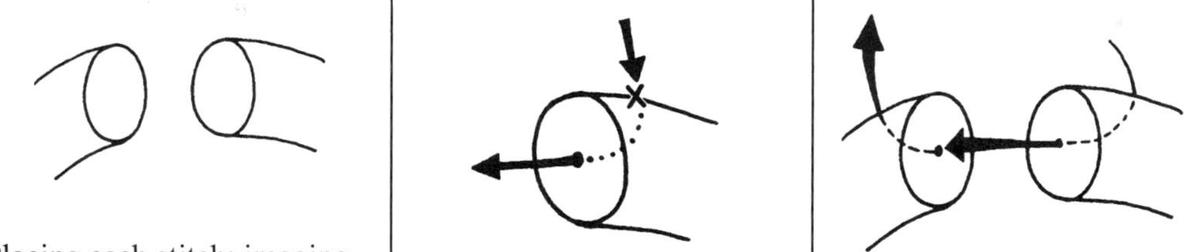

Placing each stitch: imagine the ends of the sphincter as shown.	Insertion of the needle for the first half of the stitch	Finishing a stitch

To visualize what you will be doing, imagine each round end of the sphincter facing the other (the left side mirrors the right). You will be placing interrupted stitches starting well back from the torn end in the intact part of the muscle. The needle is inserted from the outer surface of the muscle through the center of the ends at four points: A, B, C and D (9, 6, 3 and 12 o'clock). Again, including the sphincter capsule is fine, as this will help to strengthen the repair. Please note that the traction and length of the sphincter ends is *greatly* exaggerated in the drawings that follow to emphasize where each insertion point is located and that the needle is to be inserted well back from the muscle ends. During an actual repair, this much access would require dissecting the external sphincter away from the surrounding tissue, which is entirely unnecessary. Sufficient access can be achieved without doing so, but we are attempting to illustrate the locations of each stitch by elongating the muscle ends and to emphasize the importance of starting each stitch well away from the end of each muscle half.

The symbols in these drawings show where you will be entering and exiting the tissue to place each stitch (A=●, 9 o'clock; B=○, 6 o'clock; C=×, 3 o'clock; D=▲, 12 o'clock).

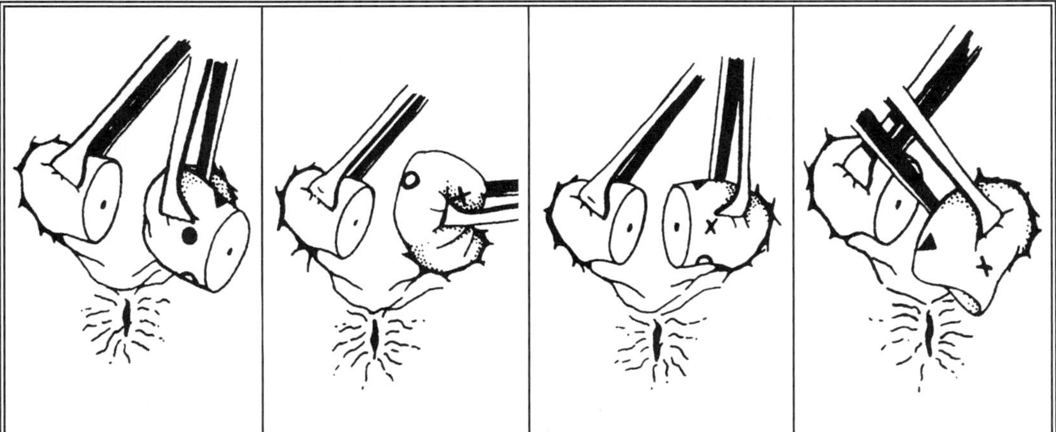

A	B	C	D

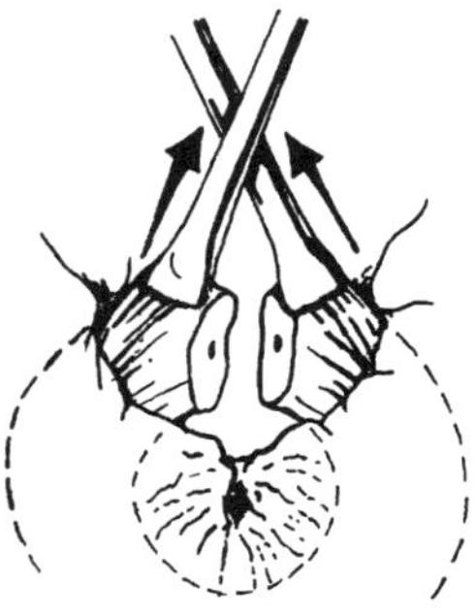	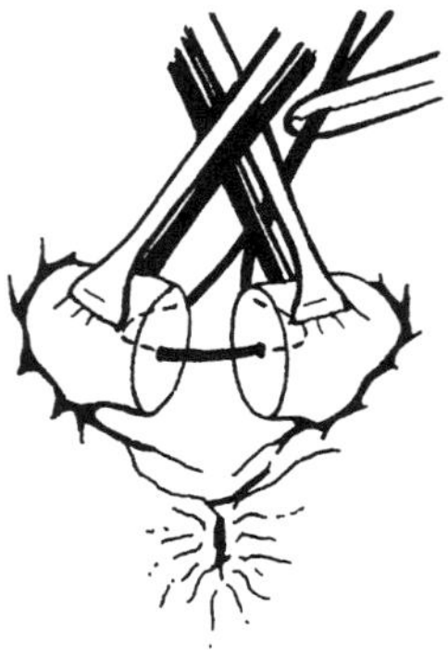	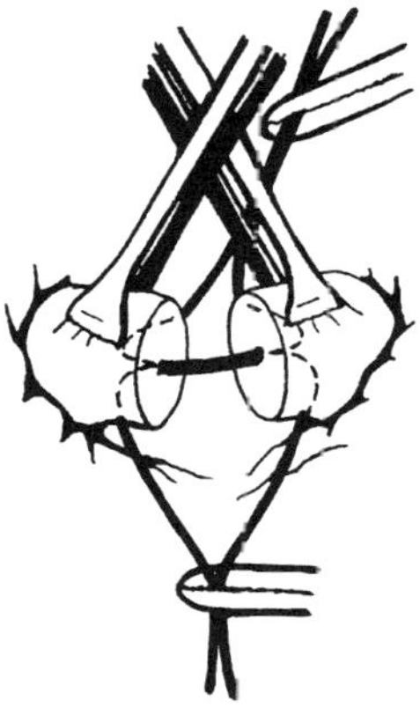
To begin repair, grasp both ends of the sphincter with Allis clamps. Pull them up to the midline. Have your assistant hold them in place.	Start an interrupted stitch at A (●). Cut the ends 4" long and grip them in a hemostat; have your assistant hold them up. Do not tie the ends yet.	Place a stitch in the same fashion through B (○). Do not tie it off. Hold ends as before in another clamp.

- Place two more stitches: one at C (✕) (hold ends but do not tie them yet) and one at D (▲) (hold untied ends).
- Be sure all sutures are correctly placed and that the EAS ends are not twisted.
- If the muscle is twisted, carefully check each stitch until you find the one that was misplaced, remove and replace it.
- Tie off all sutures using two square knots (4 throws), starting with A (●); then B (○), then C (✕), and finally D (▲).
- Double-glove and check rectally to be sure the sutures are secure. To do so insert your finger into the rectum, press up and toward you while looking down into the yoni.

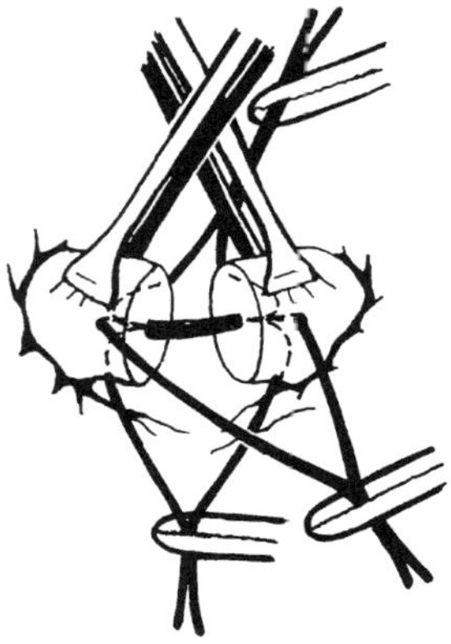	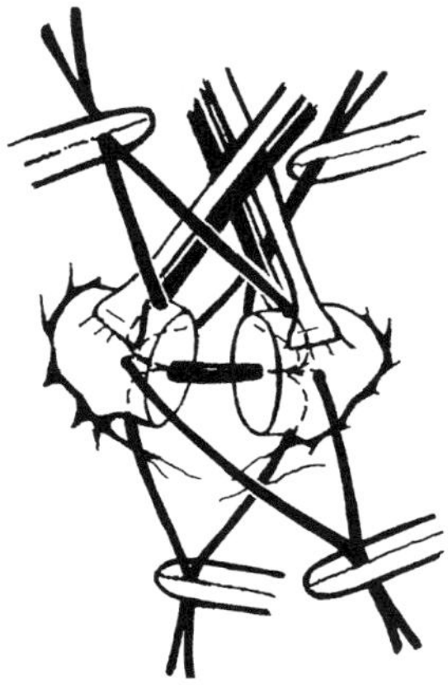
Placing a stitch at C (✕)	Putting in the final stitch at D (▲)

- Before you remove your rectal finger, be sure no stitches have been misplaced through the rectal wall. If so, remove them, irrigate the area, replace them and then check again.

At this point in the repair, continue as for a first- or second-degree tear. To proceed from here, refer to the chapter entitled “Repairing the Posterior Yoni Wall.”

References and Further Reading on Third- and Fourth-Degree Repair

References Used for Multiple Chapters

Briel JW, et al. "Clinical outcome of anterior overlapping external anal sphincter repair with internal anal sphincter imbrication," Dis Colon Rectum, 41(2):209-214, Feb, 1998. (Comment in Dis Colon Rectum, 42(5):688-689, May, 1999.)

de Leeuw J, et al. "Risk factors for third-degree perineal rupture during delivery," BJOG, 108(4): 383-387, Apr, 2001.

Evans J, MD. Clinical observation and discussion of 4th degree repair, Sep 7, 1989.

Fernando R, et al. "Repair techniques for obstetric anal sphincter injuries: a randomized controlled trial," Obstet Gynecol, 107(6):1261-1268, Jun, 2006.

Fitzpatrick M, et al. "A randomized controlled trial comparing primary overlap with approximation repair of third-degree obstetric tears," Am J Obstet Gynecol, 183(5):1220-1224, Nov, 2000.

Fornell EU, et al. "Obstetric anal sphincter injury ten years after: subjective and objective long term effects," BJOG, 112(3):312-316, Mar, 2005.

Hakelius L. "Reconstruction of the perineal body as treatment for anal incontinence," Br J Plas Surg, 32(3):245-252, Jul, 1979.

Mahony R, et al. "Internal anal sphincter defect influences continence outcome following obstetric anal sphincter injury," Am J Obstet Gynecol, www.ajog.org, 217.el-217.e5, Mar, 2007, accessed Mar, 2007.

Power D, et al. "Obstetric anal sphincter injury: how to avoid, how to repair: a literature review," J Fam Prac, 55(3):193-200, Mar, 2006.

Rogers R, et al. "Obstetric anal sphincter lacerations: an evidenced-based review, Part 2: Repair techniques," Female Patient, 27(3):31-36, May, 2002a.

Rogers R, et al. "Obstetric anal sphincter lacerations: an evidenced-based review, Part 1: Anatomy and risk factors," Female Patient, 27(4):21-24, Apr, 2002b.

Rogers R, et al. "Repair of a fourth-degree obstetrical laceration," 25 minute DVD, ACOG Audiovideo Library. American College of Obstetrics and Gynecology, Washington DC, 2002c.

Sparks R. "The 'sponge perineum': an innovative method of teaching fourth-degree obstetric perineal laceration repair to family medicine residents," Fam Med, 38(8):542-544, Sep, 2006.

Sparks R, et al. Repair of Fourth-degree Lacerations: Instructor's Guide, www.fmdrl.org/index.cfm?event=c.getAttachment&riid=800, accessed Aug 31, 2007a.

Sparks R, et al. Repair of Fourth-degree Lacerations: Resident's Guide, www.fmdrl.org/index.cfm?event=c.getAttachment, accessed Aug 31, 2007b.

Sultan A, Thakar R. Chapter 4: "Third- and fourth-degree Tears," in Sultan A, et al., eds. Perineal and Anal Sphincter Trauma. Springer-Verlag, London UK, 2007.

Sultan A, Thaker R. "Lower genital tract and anal sphincter trauma," Best Pract & Res Clin Obstet Gynaecol, 16(1):99-115, Feb, 2002.

Sultan A, et al. "Primary repair of obstetric anal sphincter rupture using the overlap technique," Br J Obstet Gynecol, 106(4):318-323, Apr, 1999.

Williams A, et al. "How to repair an anal sphincter injury after vaginal delivery: results of a randomized controlled trial," BJOG, 113(2):201-207, Feb, 2006.

World Health Org. "Essential surgical care: a clinical procedures e-learning tool kit," www.steinergraphics.

com/surgical/001_02.2.html, accessed Feb 15, 2008.

Repairing the Rectal Mucosa

Lawrence L. Personal correspondence, Win, 1992.

Ethicon, Inc. Wound Closure Manual. Johnson & Johnson, Somerville, NJ, 1994.

Repairing the Anal Sphincters: General Considerations

Fouda A. "The management of obstetric anal sphincter injury (evidence based)," slide presentation. http://tiny.cc/291Yn. Accessed Aug 20, 2009.

Fernando R, et al. Green-top Guideline No. 29: "The management of third- and fourth-degree perineal tears," Royal College of Obstetricans and Gynaecologists (RCOG), Mar, 2007.

Repairing the Internal Anal Sphincter

DeLancey J, et al. "Internal and external anal sphincter anatomy as it relates to midline obstetric lacerations," Obstet Gynecol, 90(6):924-927, Dec, 1997.

Repairing the External Anal Sphincter

Fulsher R, Fearl C. "The third-degree laceration in modern obstetrics," Am J Obstet Gynecol, 69(4):786-793, Apr, 1955.

Kolder V, MD. Editing comments, Aug, 1990.

NOTES:

UNUSUAL REPAIRS AND OTHER PROBLEMS

PERIURETHRAL AND LABIAL REPAIRS

Periurethral and labial tears will usually heal very well on their own. This area is so sensitive and receives so much abrasion from clothing that healing is frequently better when no attempt is made at repair. Attempts to repair too-shallow areas may end up causing more discomfort than if left alone.

To decide whether labial repair is indicated, you must judge how deep the tear is and how likely it is to heal together on its own. Is it bleeding heavily? If so, a few stitches may be essential. Otherwise, my criteria for repair is as follows:

1. If the tissue is torn completely through its width (i.e., across its narrow part or latitudinally), is hanging away from its opposite side in a chunk or is sagging down from its original location leaving a big raw gap, it may need repair. The likelihood of this kind of damage healing properly without assistance is remote. Also, leaving such a tear unrepaired encourages it to adhere to another area of damage, rather than to heal back to its original location.
2. If the damage is longitudinal, I usually leave it to heal on its own. However, if it is so deep that it forms a flap large enough to be folded backward during normal activity or be rubbed apart with walking, I repair it. If left unrepaired, tears of this type produce excessive stinging and burning during the first days postpartum. If no repair is done and tissue must regranulate over large raw areas, tenderness will be prolonged postpartum.

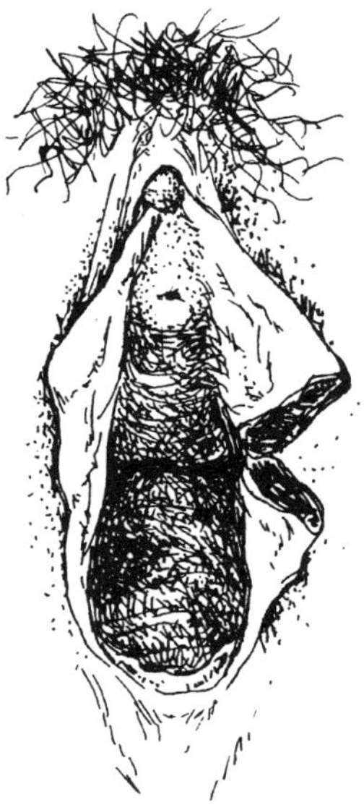

Tear across the width of the labia (lateral tear)

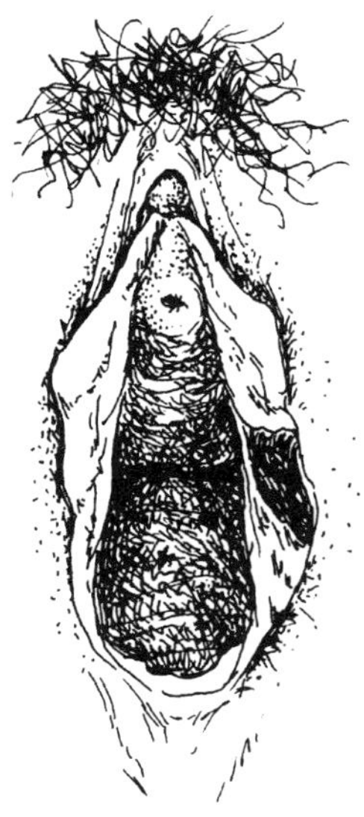

Torn lower half sags

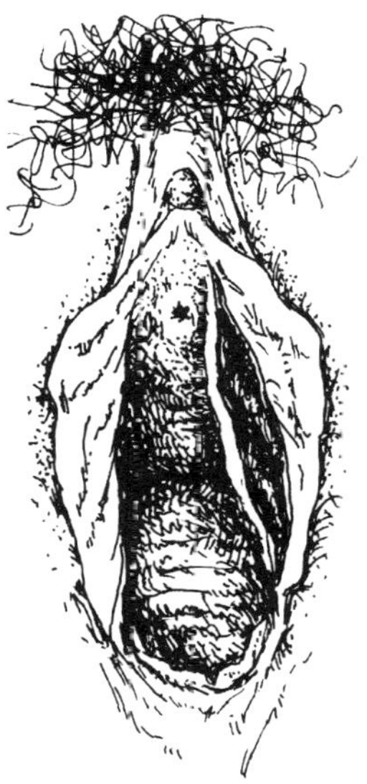

Deep longitudinal tear

When repair is necessary, you may have some very odd-looking pieces to put back together. The stitches you use and the number you take will depend entirely upon the size and location of the tear. If you are having difficulty deciding how to proceed, place an **alignment stitch** with long threads above the upper apex of the tear. Exert gentle upward traction on the strands, which will cause the tear edges to come together (in most cases); this will help reveal what goes where (Sorger, 1991).

Suture materials for labial and periurethral repair

The labia should be repaired with 4-0 absorbable synthetic on a small or very fine (PS-4, RB-1, PR-4, or T-31) cutting or taper point needle. Though this tissue is delicate, it is still tougher than mucosa. A cutting edge works well, but should not be used if the tissue is friable, as it may be in a woman who has been poorly nourished or who has a connective tissue disorder. Synthetic suture's slower breakdown time greatly increases the likelihood that the repair will remain intact for as long as needed. For this reason, both chromic gut and Vicryl Rapide are unsuited for labial or periurethral repair.

Special considerations when working in the periurethral area

Most periurethral tears need not be repaired since they typically stop bleeding when pressure is applied. Repairing near the superficial clitoral parts or the urethral meatus needs to be carefully considered. You are much more likely to put a stitch through nerves in this area. To avoid this, stitches should be as shallow as possible. When repairing near the urethra, it is necessary to insert a catheter so that you do not accidently suture the orifice closed. (Don't put a stitch through the catheter!)

Some form of anesthetic is necessary due to the sensitivity of the area. The rare times I have needed to do this type of repair, I have used very little anesthetic, leaving enough sensation so that the mother could let me know if I was getting too close to nerves. Topical spray or gel anesthetic is an excellent choice.

General considerations when repairing the labia

Anesthetic is also important in the labial area because it is so sensitive. Since this tissue distorts dramatically with swelling, use as little as possible (although very slight edema may help with identifying edges). Misalignment of such soft tissue is easy. Be sure it lines up correctly before you begin (not always obvious at first). Realign the tissue before each stitch.

If you are having real problems seeing how to align the tissues, place an alignment stitch (see above) and have an assistant hold the threads with gentle traction as you place the first few stitches to get a better idea of how to proceed. Be careful, though, because too much traction could really distort this delicate tissue.

I use running mattress stitches as much as possible for labial repair because they subject to less irritation and subsequent early breakdown. My second choice is a basting stitch. I often use a combination of the two. Other practitioners feel they get good results with interrupted stitches; however, it is difficult to gauge the appropriate tightness of stitches in this delicate tissue (tension along a continuous line of stitches can be adjusted as you proceed) and it is a good idea to use as few knots as possible.

In any case, be sure stitches are shallow; they should unite the edges and a little of the underlying tissue but not encompass the depth of the tear. This will avoid puncturing blood vessels and penetrating into nerves. Remember, this tissue does not contribute to pelvic support and is normally very mobile, so restoration of function requires preserving mobility as well as vascular and neurological tissues in as undamaged a state as possible. Be especially careful when you tie your knots. It will be easy to drag on the tissue with the final knot; better for a knot to be a bit loose than too tight. To repair tears across the labia begin where the labia joins the vestibule on one side. If the area of the labia minora is plump enough to permit it, both sides of the tear should be repaired, leaving the raw central parts in contact so they can heal well.

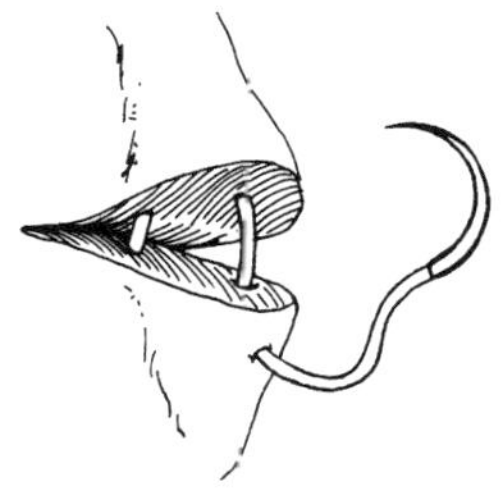

Placing stitches in the center of the torn tissue

To repair a lateral tear

Lateral tears can be reunited as illustrated next. If the labial tissue is not thick enough to allow a more internal stitch, sew the outside of the tissue (you may have to sew both sides of the labia in some cases).

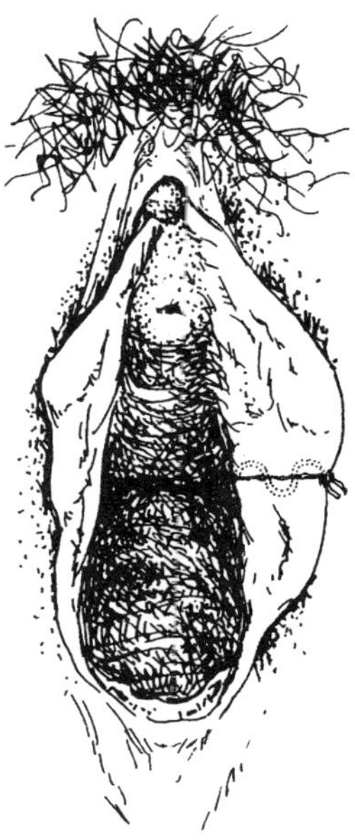

Lateral tear closed with running mattress sutures

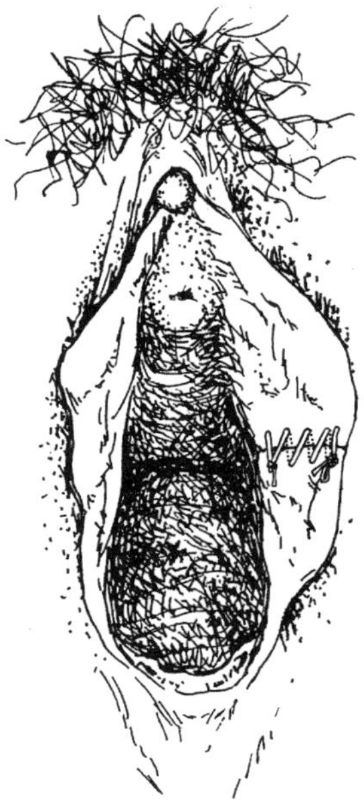

Lateral tear closed with basting stitches

To repair a longitudinal labial tear

Longitudinal repair is illustrated on the next page.

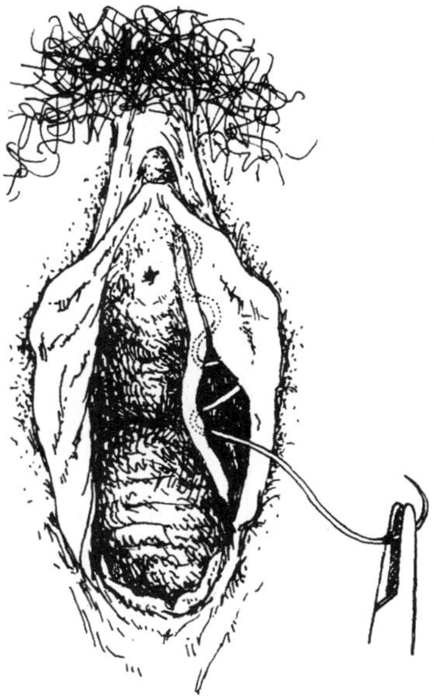

Closing a longitudinal tear with a running mattress stitch

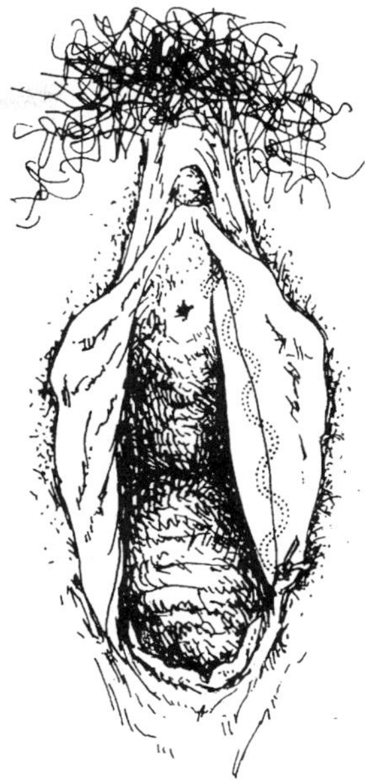

When you use a running mattress or another continuous stitch, you only wind up with two knots.

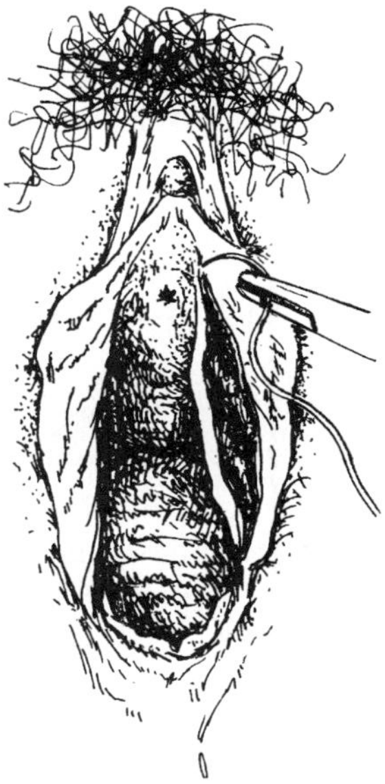

Beginning a repair with a basting stitch, which will leave more suture outside the tear

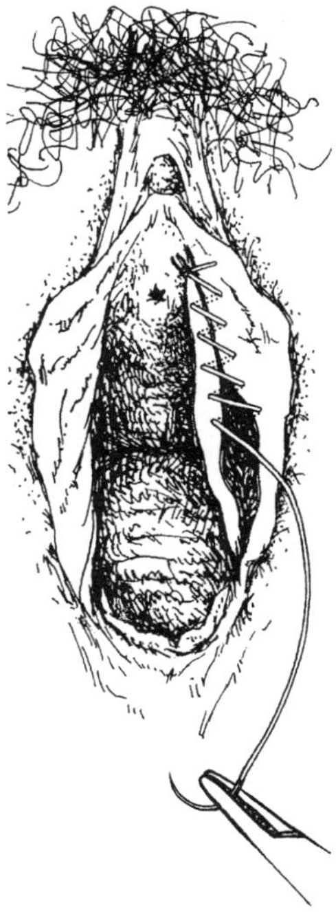

Carry the stitch to the posterior apex

SKIN TAGS

Rather than routinely and indiscriminately trimming off all skin tags that may occur, it is always best to reconstruct the tissue, leaving as much of the original tissue intact as possible because the tissue must regranulate across the surface of the wound and removing skin tags may make the wound wider. A deeper scar will result if too much tissue is removed. However, tags that are too small to suture or those dangling by a thin pedicle should be detached, as they will become irritated during normal activities and may become necrotic, which can lead to infection. When you take all this into account, the need to remove skin tags is a relatively rare occurrence.

Removal of skin tags

Before you begin your repair, carefully remove any *very* small skin tags that may get in your way. For example, small ragged tags along the perineal skin edge can be trimmed to provide a cleaner edge to repair. A skin tag is small enough to warrant removal if it is very thin or small with a tiny base. If it appears thick enough to allow blood flow, it should probably be repaired or left to heal on its own.

Sometimes a skin tag is borderline; too small to sew and seemingly too large to remove. Talk over options with the mother. You can always remove it later if you leave it alone or try to repair it and it doesn't work. At other times the question will be how the original location of the tag will heal. If a tag has left a big raw area on the other side, not reattaching it will leave that area to regranulate, creating a tender spot for weeks or even months. As an alternative to stitching the tag back in place, it may be possible to stitch that raw area so that the edges are held together (discussed later in this chapter).

To remove a skin tag, pick it up with an Allis clamp. (An Allis clamp allows you to grasp the tag across the base and helps ensure a clean cut.) Be sure the tissue is not bunched up in the clamp, as this will interfere with removal. You don't want to cut it off and simply create a shorter tag in its place. On the other hand, if you grasp it too close to its base, you will not leave room for your scissors blades and may cut off a bigger, deeper piece than you intended. Proceed as follows:

- •Hold a gauze soaked with anesthetic around the tag, especially at the base, use a spray anesthetic, or inject a tiny bit of numbing agent, especially if removal is not being done immediately postpartum.
- •Clamp the tag with your instrument and lift it away from the underlying tissue at an angle that allows good visibility and a clean cut. It may help to lift the tag with another instrument prior to clamping it with the Allis clamp. Leave it clamped a minute or two to encourage hemostasis and deaden the tissue.
- •You may want an assistant to hold the tag up while you cut.
- •When ready to cut, put slight traction on the clamp to afford maximum visuability of the base of the tag. This increases the chance of a clean, smooth cut.
- •Using sharp surgical scissors, trim the tag as close to the base as you possibly can. Try to do this in one, clean snip by opening the scissor blades just enough to extend the tips past the edge of the tag by about 3 mm. Place the joint of the blades against the nearest edge of the tag, then cut.

- There may be minor bleeding once the tag is removed. Have a gauze soaked with witch hazel, shepherd's purse infusion or calendula extract ready to help arrest bleeding. (You can also use alcohol-based tincture that has been placed in a small amount of boiling water for a few minutes to burn off the alcohol.)
- If tags need removal during the weeks after birth, the same techniques apply.

Repair of skin tags

The decision to repair a skin tag is made when it has a large enough base that trimming it off will leave a long, wide, raw area to heal. Repair of skin tags takes artistry and skill; it's an iffy business at best, even for those with a great deal of experience. Sometimes problems occur such as sensitive places where the tag has been tacked up or it does not heal as you intend. Using 4-0 absorbable synthetic (not chromic gut and not Vicryl Rapide) with a very fine cutting or taper point needle vastly improves your chances of a successful repair. Use topical anesthetic or inject very little. It is very hard to judge how to sew a swollen skin tag.

In the majority of cases, tag repair is the last thing you do before final closure behind the hymenal ring. This is because you can't always tell how to put a tag back together without first repairing the surrounding tissue and because the majority of tags you will repair will occur near the introitus.

Start your anchor stitch in the yoni mucosa or beneath the surface of the perineal skin depending upon where the tag is. Now run the suture beneath the tissue, exiting at the base of the tag. Begin tiny subcuticular running mattress stitches or tiny basting stitches to unite the edges of the tag to the underlying tissue. Go all the way around the tag, being careful to match the edges together as much as possible. Don't pull so tightly that the edges roll or pucker. Don't use interrupted stitches; they expose much of the suture, and several knots make irritation more likely. In addition, knots are difficult to tighten appropriately, due to the delicacy of the tissue. The fewer knots, the better. If the tag is narrow, you may be able to take small bites down the center of the underside, attaching one raw side to the other with a row of running mattress stitches. Here are some examples of different repair techniques:

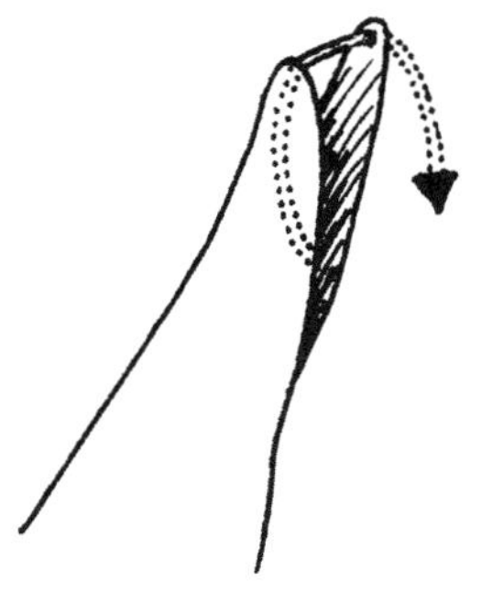

Tacking the tip of a tag in place

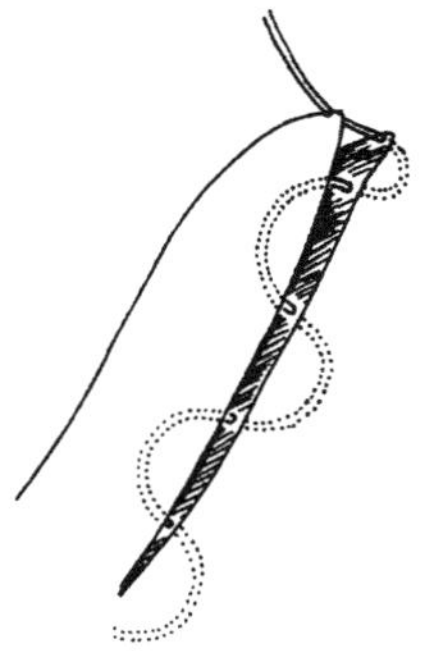

Repairing the edge of a tag with running mattress stitches

Iatrogenic skin tags at the introitus

Skin tags may have been created because a previous repair was unanatomically tight either unintentionally (due to poor technique or a tricky repair), or quite intentionally, via the use of a "husband's stitch" or "lover's knot." Typically, a tag is formed when the mouth of the yoni is opened to its original, larger size during a subsequent birth (see the illustrations on page 557). The resulting tag naturally lies where it was before the first repair (below where it was previously attached), leaving a raw place above it where the tight area has torn away. Raw areas may also be left when you remove a skin tag; the same repair techniques (given in the next subsection) apply.

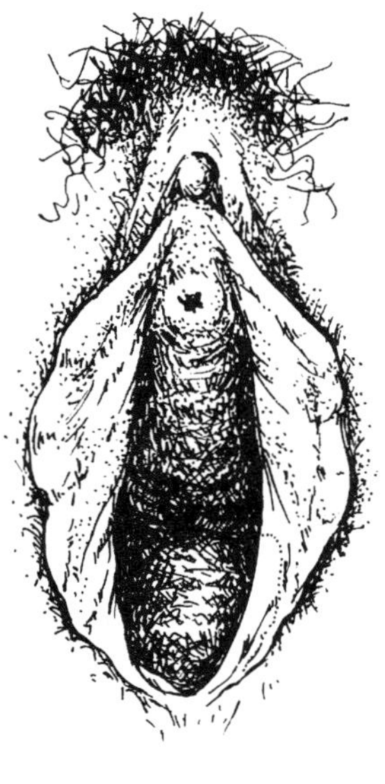	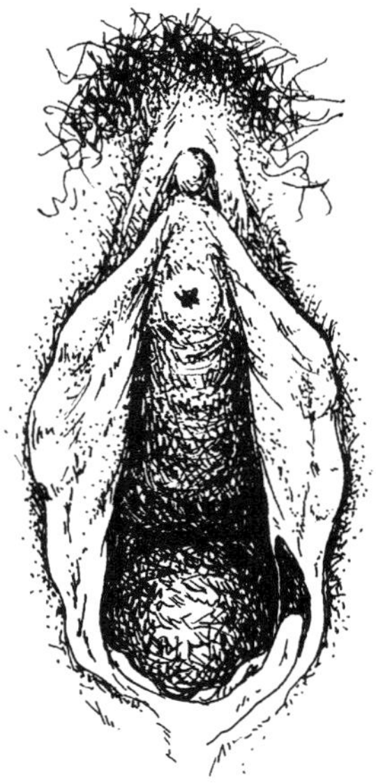	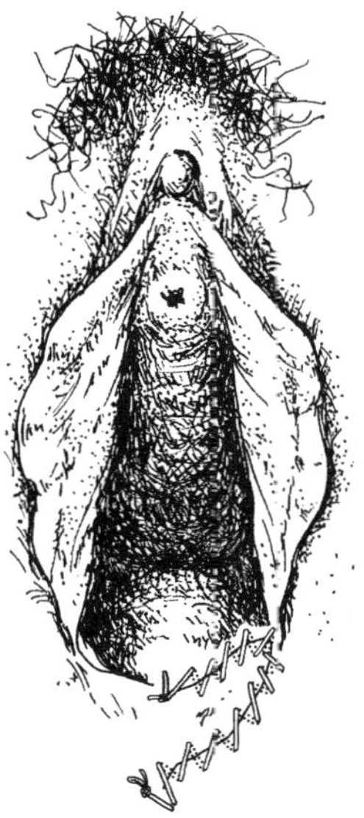
Tight, shiny area on (your) right of introitus	The tear leaves a raw area where it was sewn too tightly.	Main part of tag repaired with basting stitches

Since you don't want to (again) sew the introitus too tightly, the only solution is to do the best you can to recreate the original mouth of the yoni. Do this by attaching the tag to the underlying area where it naturally rests. At this point there will be a variably long, narrow raw area above the tip of the tag, where it was improperly attached previously.

Repairing a raw area left by a skin tag

Frequently, you can stitch the raw area by bringing the two edges together, which causes the middle of the area to fold inward and results in a clean, closed surface. However, if the area is very wide (> 0.75 cm or so), this technique may leave the adjoining tissue puckered. If the area is very narrow, a stitch will not close it very well, as there isn't enough raw surface to fold in with the tension of the suture. This is a judgment call. Hold the edges together to gauge how the area will accept being sutured.

Running mattress stitches are best used for a wide, deeper area, and basting stitches for one more narrow or shallow. If neither seems appropriate, try a few interrupted stitches. For a shorter raw area, you might try a single interrupted stitch from side to side, across the center. In the following illustrations, only the repair of the raw area itself is illustrated for clarity. (See the chapter entitled "Special Tricks and Techniques" for details on the interrupted running mattress stitch.)

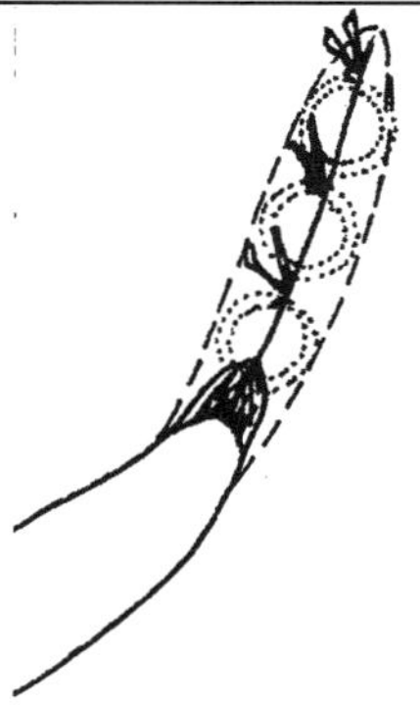

Interrupted running mattress stitches

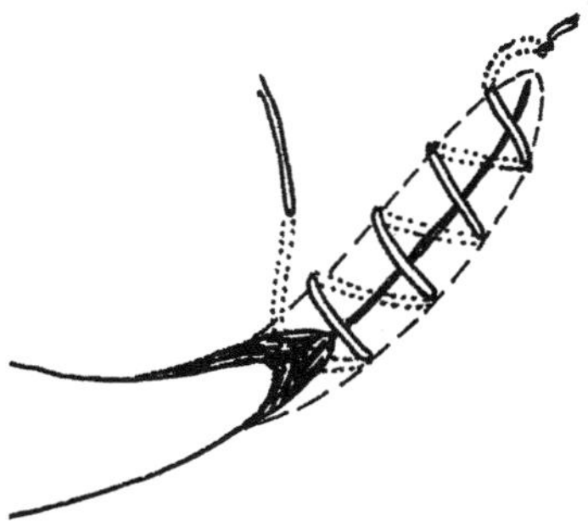

Basting stitches

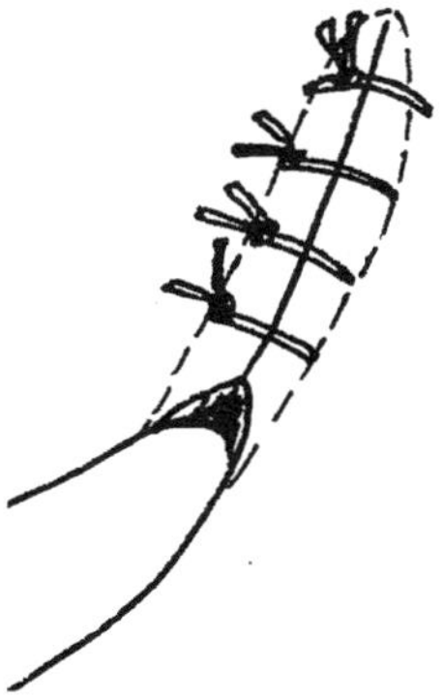

Interrupted stitches

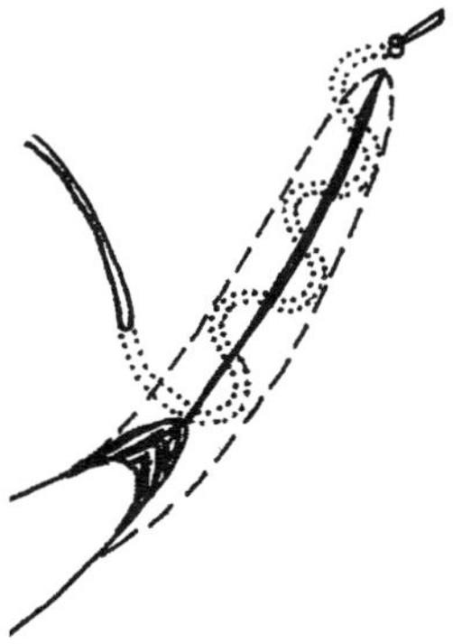

Running mattress stitches

If a woman has previously been infibulated, one of these techniques can be used on the raw edges of the incised scar to reestablish a more anatomical introitus if the scar tissue will allow it (buried sutures are harder to place in thick scar tissue). (See the chapter entitled "Traditional Female Genital Modifications" for more details on this practice.)

When a raw area or skin tag must heal on its own

If a raw area or a larger tag at the introitus is impossible to repair, you must leave it to heal on its own. Wait for 5 to 6 days and then have the mother apply vitamin E straight from capsules to the area several times daily. I was astonished to see a large tag reduce in size and disappear completely by the six week postpartum visit after it had been left hanging by the doctor who performed the repair.

PUERPERAL HEMATOMAS

A hematoma (HE-ma-TOE-ma) is a blood blister that results from a broken blood vessel seeping underneath the skin. The incidence of puerperal hematomas ranges from 1 in 300 to 1 in 1000 births. Women at increased risk of developing hematomas include nulliparas; those whose infant weighs more than 8 lbs 13.5 oz (4000 g); and those with preeclampsia, a prolonged pushing phase, multiple pregnancy, vulvar varicosities, or a clotting or connective tissue disorder. Nonetheless, the most frequently associated risks are clitorotomy and forceps delivery. Hematomas develop following injury to a blood vessel within the tissues; this may occur spontaneously but is more likely to happen during an instrumental delivery or during disruptive care such as overzealous manipulation of the uterus after the birth (i.e., uterine massage).

Apart from birth trauma, hematomas may develop secondary to such accidents as nicking a vessel with the needle during repair, failing to catch a small lacerated vessel with your anchor stitch or failing to adequately close an area that has been bleeding diffusely. The stretching of deep tissue during pushing can also result in hematomas, even with no external tears.

Very rarely, a hematoma may form during pregnancy and may even obstruct labor. Prolonged pressure in one location from the presenting part may cause a vessel to necrose (neck-ROS), leading to the gradual development of a hematoma over the next several days. Small cervical hematomas may also occur in the anterior lip, but these will usually not enlarge.

Birth-related hematomas are classified by location (e.g., vulvar, vulvovaginal, paravaginal, or in the broad ligament with extension into the retroperitoneal space). **Vulvar hematomas** usually occur when branches of the pudendal artery, including the inferior rectal, transverse perineal or posterior labial branches, are injured as a result of clitorotomy or laceration. The damaged vessels are usually located in the superficial fascia of the pelvis. The superficial compartment of the urogenital triangle communicates with the subfascial space of the lower abdomen below the inguinal ligament. Extension of bleeding in the urogenital triangle is limited by Colles fascia and the urogenital diaphragm, while the anal fascia limits extension of bleeding in the anal triangle. As a result, bleeding spreads toward the skin where the loose subcutaneous tissues expand more easily, allowing a visible swelling to develop. Hematomas can extend from the posterior margin of the urogenital triangle (at the level of the superficial transverse perineal muscle) anteriorly over the mons to where the fascia is fused at the inguinal ligament. Necrosis caused by pressure against tissues surrounding the hematoma may lead to rupture with external hemorrhage.

Hematomas of the yoni and paravaginal regions are usually associated with injury to the uterine artery, most often its descending branch. These hematomas are commonly associated with forceps delivery but may also occur spontaneously. In contrast to the vulva, vessels in the yoni are surrounded by soft tissue but are not surrounded by superficial fascia; therefore, vessel trauma may result in a large accumulation of blood in the paravaginal space or ischiorectal fossa.

Uncommonly, a **broad-ligament hematoma** develops when a torn vessel lies above the pelvic fascia and a hematoma develops above the fascial layer in the broad ligament. As the hematoma enlarges, extension and dissection into the retroperitoneum may occur and form a palpable tumor above the inguinal ligament. Dissection may also extend cephalad and reach the lower margin of the diaphragm.

Early on, a yoni or paravaginal hematoma produces a rounded swelling that projects into the upper portion of the yoni canal and may almost occlude the lumen. If bleeding persists, the hematoma starts to enlarge in a retroperitoneal direction, presenting a palpable mass that can be felt above the edge of the inguinal (Poupart) ligament (which extends from the anterior, superior ilial spine to the pubic tubercle). Alternatively, the hematoma may dissect tissues in an upward direction, eventually reaching the lower edge of the thoracic diaphragm. Branches of the uterine artery may be injured when this type of expansion occurs.

Signs and symptoms

Most hematomas start to develop at the time of the injury, although, on occasion the onset of bleeding is delayed. Visible hematomas typically develop gradually, eventually presenting as fluctuant, purplish swellings. Depending upon its exact location and direction of expansion, a vulval or yoni hematoma may cause perineal, yoni, urethral, bladder or rectal pressure and often produces severe pain. A vulvar hematoma is easily identified when severe perineal pain is accompanied by a rapidly developing, tense, fluctuating and sensitive mass of varying size covered by discolored skin. When such a mass presents next to the yoni, it may not be recognized immediately. However, when a woman reports increasing pressure, if not pain, and an inability to void you should visually inspect to rule out a round, fluctuant mass that is starting to fill the yoni's lumen. The more rapidly the swelling occurs, generally the more severe the pain, which can be excruciating. If the mass develops higher up in the pelvis, it can produce rectal pressure that may mimic a full bowel, but straining to pass stool will be unproductive and result in more pain. Small yoni or cervical hematomas may not present any of these symptoms. A coagulation disorder can lead to large hematomas that will not stop bleeding (Kolder, 1990).

Broad-ligament hematomas present with lateral uterine pain that is worse with palpation, extension of pain into the flank (side of the torso), a painful swelling in the rectum that can be felt during a high rectal examination, a ridge of tissue that can be palpated just above the pelvic brim that extends to the side (the edge of the distended broad ligament) and abdominal distension (Varney, et al., 2004). Hematomas that reach up between the folds of the broad ligament may escape detection unless part of the mass can be felt on abdominal palpation or unless hypovolemia develops. If there is a hematoma deep in the pelvis behind the yoni fornices, there may be uterine pain on either side above the pubic bone that becomes more severe during palpation. Other symptoms include extension of the pain up between the ribs and the thigh, a painful bulge high in the rectum, a palpable ridge of tissue just above and along the top edge of the pelvic brim, nausea and abdominal distention. Hematomas of the broad ligament can rupture into the peritoneal cavity and cause sudden, severe shock (Oxorn, 1986; Varney et al., 2004).

Ruptured or not, hematomas can provide a breeding ground for infection and, if sufficiently large, can lead to anemia or even death.

Treatment for a hematoma

Small to moderately sized hematomas that stop enlarging can often be left to absorb on their own. If enlargement proceeds, however, the tissues that overlie the swelling may rupture as a result of pressure-induced necrosis and profuse hemorrhage may follow. At other times a discharge of large clots is extruded from the rupture. Subperitoneal hematomas may release a large quantity of blood under the peritoneum that can even prove fatal; some subperitoneal hematomas dissect behind the ascending colon up to the level of the hepatic (right colic) flexure (the sharp bend where the ascending colon meets the transverse colon).

If you have discovered a hematoma somewhere in or next to the yoni wall or vulva that you can see, watch to see if it is enlarging. Periodically check it by palpating very gently. Too vigorous palpation may dislodge the clot trying to form and cause more bleeding. Ask the mother to report any sensations of increasing pain or pressure, which could also indicate enlargement.

Whether a hematoma is actively bleeding or not, a cold pack can help arrest bleeding and reduce pain. If a hematoma seems to be forming, apply a cold pack immediately after your repair. Take an exam glove and tie off all but one or two fingers (depending on the size of the hematoma). A condom can also be used. Fill with water, tie the end, and put it in the freezer. While that one is freezing, take another glove and tie off the fingers in the same way. Place crushed ice in the other fingers and palm. Tie off the end and place the fingers in the yoni next to the hematoma. Gently slide a gauze pad or two beside the fingers (opposite the hematoma) to hold them in place. Change the ice pack frequently, very carefully removing the gauze and glove so as not to disturb the clot (Lowe, 1989).

Give homeopathic Arnica (30 C or 200C) three to four times hourly during the first 8 hours to help alleviate swelling and bruising. Do not leave the mother until you are satisfied that the hematoma is not enlarging and that she is stable. Analgesics should not be given to ease the discomfort, as this may mask symptoms of enlargement.

If there is a hematoma deep within the pelvis, you can still apply a cold pack inside the yoni. You must watch the mother carefully for signs of concealed blood loss, such as shock and she should not be left unattended until you are convinced that the hematoma has stabilized. Plan to spend the night or have an assistant do so. She should immediately report increasing pain or pressure. (For information on caring for a hematoma associated with an infection, see the chapter entitled "Perineal Infections.") Transport to the hospital if the hematoma is invisible (i.e., it cannot be visually monitored), is very large or continues to enlarge.

Bio-technical medical management

More interventive medical management of vulvar hematomas should be sought when the mass continues to enlarge, when pain is severe or when rupture occurs or appears to be threatening. In most cases, the mass is promptly lanced over the area of maximum distention. After that blood and clots are evacuated, and any bleeding vessels that can be identified are tied off. The cavity may then be closed with mattress sutures.

Often, however, no bleeding points can be found. In that case, the yoni is packed with gauze for 12 to 24 hours (note this applies counterpressure to the outer wall of the evacuated hematoma cavity; the cavity itself is not packed). Hypovolemia and anemia are prevented with adequate transfusions, a necessary component of care in about 50% of cases.

Subperitoneal and supravaginal hematomas are more difficult to treat. They can be drained by cutting into the area via the perineum and emptied, but it is difficult to stop the bleeding by this route. In most cases, laparotomy in a hospital is required (Cunningham et al., 2005).

When the bleeding is otherwise uncontrollable, angiographic embolization has been successfully used to stop it. This procedure involves introducing a catheter into an artery. Under X-ray visualization, the catheter as it is guided to a specific location along the vessel. Once the catheter is in position, the blood supply to the area is slowly tamponed off by injecting particles that end up in the small vessels that feed the target area, thus bringing the bleeding to a stop (Malak, 2009).

Also see the postpartum care recommendations for women who have had a hematoma in the chapter entitled "Postpartum Care and Comfort Measures."

Cervical Lacerations

The cervix typically sustains a small degree of trauma during dilation, especially with the first baby. This accounts for the bloody show of labor. Women who have cervical scars are more prone to cervical tears, but if precautions are heeded (see the chapter entitled "Preparing the Perineal Tissues for Birth"), even these women are unlikely to sustain cervical trauma that requires repair.

The cervix is constructed so that the sides are less fibrous and less muscular than the front and back lips. While tears can occur at any point around the os, they are often on the sides. Typical cervical lacerations present as longitudinal (vertical) splits, at 3 or 9 o'clock, which extend up from the edge of the cervical lip toward the uterus. Previous scar tissue may also predispose a specific area to weakness.

Suture materials and equipment

Use 2-0 chromic on a small (SH, T-5) taper point needle for repair. You will also need two ring forceps and tissue forceps.

Types of cervical trauma

Typical cervical trauma involves the breaking of tiny surface blood vessels, bruising and swelling with an occasional hematoma on the anterior lip. These types of damage usually present no problem. Homeopathic Arnica given orally (30C or 200C) several times during the hours right after the birth will help reduce swelling and relieve trauma.

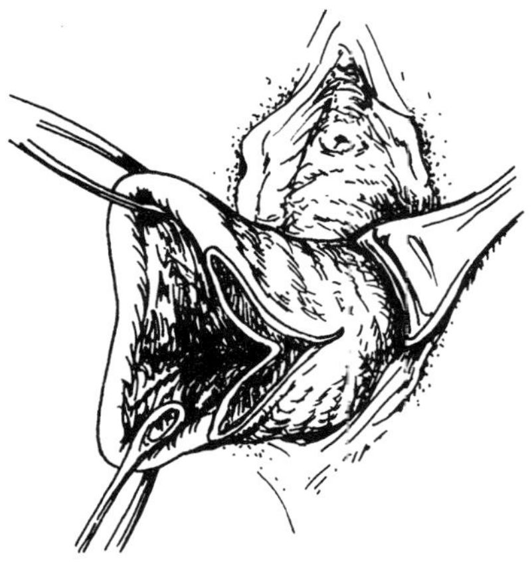

Deep cervical tear

Cervical tears less than 1 cm in length can be left to heal on their own. Any cervical laceration may bleed profusely (particularly those longer than 1 cm). If you discover a longer tear or cannot find the apex (even if the tear isn't bleeding), transport. Tears may also occur where the base of the cervix meets the lower segment of the uterine cavity; these types of tears are probably more likely to occur with instrumental delivery (forceps, vacuum extraction). Rarely, cervical tears extend into the lower uterine segment. If not adequately repaired, deep cervical tears will provide an avenue for uterine contamination and increase the possibility of postpartum infection.

Very rarely, the muscle within the cervical body tears and retracts, leaving the mucosal surface tissue intact. A thin bridge of mucosal tissue is left uniting the anterior and posterior cervical lips (Greenhill & Friedman, 1974). Such tears might occur if an anterior lip has been strained excessively and dragged down to the introitus for a length of time before birth. To assess for cervical body damage, see "Inspecting for cervical damage" in the chapter entitled "Examining the Perineum after Birth."

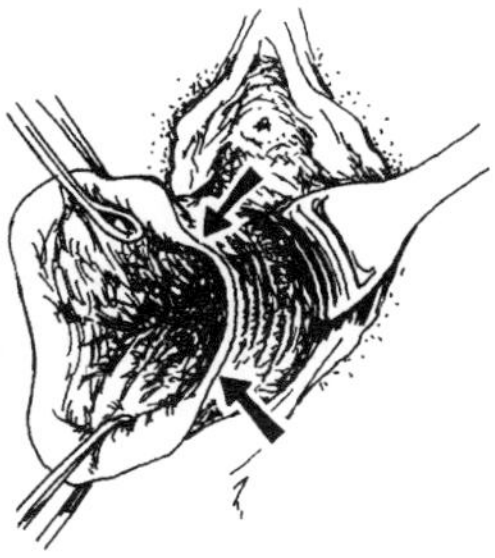	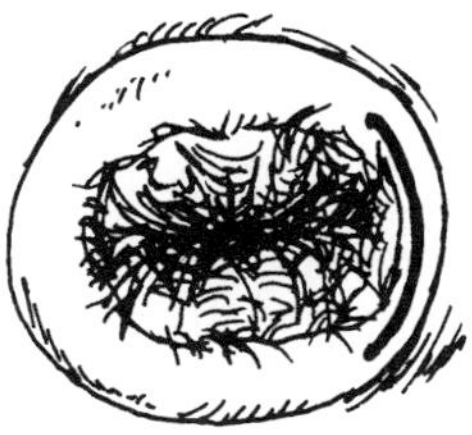	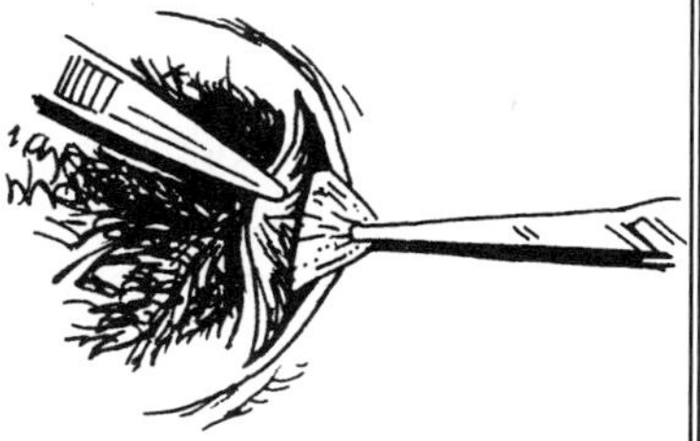
Occult tear in the layer underlying the surface (arrows show where this defect is located)	Dissection along this line . . .	. . . reveals the underlying re-tracted tissue.

Cervical repair

The first step is to achieve adequate view of the cervix. This is accomplished by using a yoni retractor and having an assistant hold the tissue steady while you do the suturing. Once the retractor is in place, grasp the cervical lip with two ring forceps on either side of the tear. This stabilizes the cervix and holds the edges of the tear straight. The forceps must be placed close to the tear edges, but not so close that they cause you to include the rings as you sew. To avoid this, place the rings on the lower edge of the cervix so they are at least halfway over the lip (to afford good traction) but as close to the edge as possible. If good traction cannot be maintained without excessive pressure, move the rings a bit higher up on the cervix (Varney et al., 2004). Once the forceps are placed correctly, give the handles to an assistant to hold in place while you sew.

Profuse bleeding or a deep tear may hinder identification of the internal apex. For many tears, tightening the ratchet tension on the ring forceps may help reduce bleeding. If not, place one or two interrupted sutures as close to the tear's internal apex as possible and leave the ends long. Then put gentle traction on these strands to pull the internal apex of the tear down into view. These sutures may also help arrest bleeding until you can get the repair started. If this technique does not reveal the apex, the tear may extend into the lower uterine segment, in which case I strongly urge you to transport to the hospital.

If all is going smoothly, the next step is to place an anchor stitch above the internal apex of the tear to catch any retracted blood vessels. Interrupted stitches can be used, but if the tear is bleeding, a locked mattress stitch or figure-eight is a better choice. The stitch can be placed from the outer to the inner surface of one edge of the tear and finished by bringing the needle from the inner to the outer surfaces of the os to the other side. Don't pull the stitches so tightly that the edges wind up rolling in on themselves. You may also take stitches that do not go completely through the cervical wall as long as bleeding is controlled.

Take special care not to sew the mouth of the cervix closed by accidently stitching through to the other lip (i.e., do not attach one lip to the other). This is where tissue forceps to help identify entry and exit points can come in very handy.

If the tear extends high into the cervix, there is danger of entering a ureter as you sew. (Remember, the ureters run high up along each lateral fornix.) To avoid this, care must be taken not to puncture the yoni fornix as you maneuver the needle. Try to point the needle more up (toward the uterus) than out (toward the upper yoni walls) when you enter and exit the tissue. Using a small needle helps, but the danger of puncturing a ureter is increased by not having adequate retraction to see what you are doing.

Repairing an occult tear requires splitting the cervical mucosa along the lower edge, retrieving the retracted muscle and holding it in place while it is rejoined to its original location under the mucosal tissue. Do so by passing the needle through the muscle layer as the mucosal surfaces are sutured along the edges (Greenhill & Friedman, 1974).

To repair the cervix properly, the yoni must be retracted sufficiently for visualization. This is hard to manage at home. Hospitals will have all the necessary equipment to do this correctly. If the tear is bleeding profusely, use ring forceps to clamp it as close to the internal apex as possible (preferably over the crotch of the apex, where bleeding is most likely to originate), administer homeopathic Arnica every 5 to 15 minutes and transport to hospital.

Detachment of the cervix

A combination of edema, lack of circulation and poor oxygenation may lead to tissue necrosis and cause some or all of the cervix to be sloughed off. The separation of the entire cervical ring is called annular detachment. Detachment usually occurs from the intense pressure of a persistent anterior lip or an excessively rigid os. This may also occur when a cerclage has been placed to close a loose (medically referred to as an "incompetent") cervix and labor begins before it has been removed. However, it happens most commonly in first-time mothers who have had prolonged labor with ruptured membranes and a low baby, in combination with a thin, rigid cervix and strong uterine contractions.

Even though this is rare, if the labor history is positive (extremely thin, rigid cervix followed by sudden advancement for no apparent reason) and a piece of unidentifiable tissue is passed (either a portion or a ring) before or after the birth, you need to examine the cervix with this in mind. If detachment has occurred, be sure to check carefully for bleeding and for tears which extend into the lower uterine segment. Because the tissue has been pinched off due to pressure, bleeding is unlikely, and repair rarely necessary. If bleeding does occur, it needs to be controlled with figure-eight stitches along the edge of the stump.

Prognosis for future pregnancies: Subsequent contraction of the uterine opening (stenosis) from scar tissue may occur, resulting in a backup of menstrual blood (hematometra). Severe stenosis may prevent normal dilation in subsequent labors. Otherwise, the prospects for normal yoni birth in the future are mixed. There are cases of normal gestation followed by yoni birth, as well as spontaneous abortion from a loose (incompetent) os (Oxorn, 1986). During future pregnancies affected women may benefit from taking oral evening primrose oil as well as local applications of vitamin E and evening primrose oils to the scarred cervix prenatally to help soften the scars and ease the birth. Taking 1 drop of gelsemium (Carolina yellow jasmine) tincture daily mixed in ½ cup of water and sipped during the day for the last four weeks of pregnancy may help as well (see precautions in the "Preventing Cervical Damage" section in the chapter entitled "Protecting the Perineum during Labor and Birth").

This event happens very rarely and hopefully will never happen to your clients because you will deal with swollen or rigid cervices in a timely fashion. Using oral herbal therapies and homeopathics, position changes, and, if need be, pushing a stubborn lip out of the way or breaking up rigidity with massage are certainly better than this!

Repairing the Anterior Yoni Wall

Damage to the anterior yoni wall (ceiling) is fortunately very rare. This is a difficult area to see, much less repair. The same dangers and precautions apply here as with the rectal mucosa, because the urethra or bladder wall could be penetrated during suturing. In addition, these tears frequently require retractors for adequate visualization. Stitches must be small, close together, and encompass both apexes of the laceration. Unfortunately, you cannot stick your finger into the urethra or bladder to discover a misplaced stitch. Unless the tear is very shallow and requires no stitches, it is wise to transport or call for backup.

When there is blood in the urine

Blood in the urine means a hole exists somewhere along the urinary tract. If possible, two layers of stitches are placed in the same manner as for double-layer repair of the rectal mucosa. The first can be small, closely-spaced interrupted stitches, for ease of removal should one be misplaced. Immediately below that layer (when looking up at the ceiling of the yoni), a second layer of basting stitches can be placed, if it seems necessary and if the tissue depth will allow it. You must examine the tissue and weigh the need for a repair that completely seals the lumen of the urethra without placing too many stitches that may impair healing. An indwelling catheter should remain in place for 10 days in the hope that the wall will heal intact. If the tear is located so that repair is impossible, an indwelling catheter is placed anyway so that, with luck, spontaneous closure of the fistula will result. If a fistula forms despite these precautions, further repair is usually delayed for 2 to 3 months to allow the area to recover from the birth (Oxorn, 1986).

Catheterizing to check for bladder damage

Whenever there is deep upper vault damage, you should catheterize to rule out bladder damage before you begin your repair. Remember that you are trying to find out if there is blood in the urine, so pay attention to keeping the flow of urine free of other fluids. If the urine is clear of blood, you will want the catheter to remain in place for the duration of the repair. For this reason, place a Foley catheter if you have one.

- Clean up as much blood as possible from the area.
- Insert a gauze tampon to minimize bloody contamination of the urine from lochial flow, if necessary.
- Put on fresh, sterile gloves.
- Open the labia minora widely with your nondominant fingers.
- Provided the mother is not allergic to iodine, soak three sterile cotton balls in povidone iodine solution (not scrub solution, as it is sudsy)
- Wipe the urethral region with the cotton swabs. Wipe downward three times, using a fresh cotton ball for each pass. First wipe one either side, then directly over the urethral meatus.
- Have your assistant peel back the wrapper at the drainage end of the catheter so that you can remove it, taking care that the tip does not touch anything.
- Lubricate the tip with sterile lubricant gel or povidone iodine gel (or solution).
- Put the flared drainage end of the catheter in a clean pan.

- •Hold the catheter so that the tip is extended about two inches beyond your fingertips. Carefully open the labia minora with your nondominant hand. Gently insert the catheter into the urinary meatus. This sounds hard, but it is easy. The meatus is 0.5 to 2.5 cm below the clitoral glans and looks like a little pucker in the tissue. If you cannot find it due to swelling, use your finger to put traction upward, just below the clitoral glans, to the side of the urethra. This should expose the meatus.
- •Gently feed the catheter into the urethra, allowing it to find its own way until urine starts to flow from the other end. If this proves difficult, insert a finger into the yoni to guide the catheter tip along the upper yoni wall. If a tear causes the tip to protrude into the yoni, very carefully withdraw the catheter and transport.
- •As the flow tapers off, assist drainage by gently pressing along the top of the pubic bone. Start from the edges of the abdomen (just above the pelvic crests) and move in toward the center. Having the mother bear down may help as well.
- •Watch carefully for bloody urine.
- •If you plan to proceed with repair, leave the catheter in place to help you identify the urethra as you stitch. A straight catheter can be used for this purpose, but you must be careful not to pull it out as you work. You can also use a Foley (balloon) catheter if you have one. Use a syringe to inflate the little balloon on the tip of the catheter to help hold it above the bladder neck. If you only have a straight catheter, clamp the tubing off with a hemostat, attach the hemostat to an upper drape (this will minimize the chance that you will accidently remove the catheter during the repair). Remove the clamp to drain the bladder periodically during the repair. More details about the use of a catheter can be found in my HOLISTIC MIDWIFERY, VOL. II.

See the chapter entitled "Postpartum Care and Comfort Measures" for tips to reduce the chances of infection after catheterization.

Positioning the mother for repair

Position the mother so that you can see well. Achieving this at home will be challenging, at best, and is another good reason to transport whenever it is feasible. Placing her on her belly with her pelvis just off the end of a table and her lower legs flexed at the knees and supported from below may afford better visualization of the upper yoni wall. Two people could support her legs at the appropriate angle, or her knees could be propped on chairs; this might be a time when a sturdy kitchen or dining room table is the best place to suture. Likewise, leaning her over a soft couch back with her upper body supported somehow might work if you have the furniture and enough assistants available to support her. Some such position will afford you the best view, but it will be uncomfortable for the mother, to say the least. Have good light and enlist your assistant to hold the tissue open; use a retractor if you have one. Alternatively, you can use a blade from a disassembled speculum to retract the tissue (the assistant can hold this in place as you work), but it will be far easier and less tiring to insert a retractor before you begin. Transporting the mother to a hospital that has a surgery table that can be adjusted to accommodate the necessary position is reason enough to transport to the hospital whenever possible.

Suture materials

Use only 4-0 absorbable synthetic (not Vicryl Rapide) on a small or very fine taper point needle.

General considerations for repair

Lacerations of the upper yoni wall may require two layers of small, closely spaced sutures. When a second layer is used, the stitches can be spaced slightly wider apart than the first layer. The object is to create a urine-tight closure. If the wound is not deep enough to require two layers, a single row of locked mattress (especially useful with bleeding) or basting stitches may be used. If bleeding is profuse, several figure-eight stitches can be placed.

Leave a catheter tip in place during repair to ensure that the urethra is not stitched closed. Not only is the catheter itself easier to palpate than the urethra, but you will be able to tell if your needle is trying to penetrate the catheter, which will help prevent sewing the urethral lumen closed.

Even when no large vessels are torn, bleeding sometimes continues after the repair is completed. When this occurs, the yoni should be packed with sterile gauze to reduce the flow. The gauze can be soaked in astringent and hemostatic herbs. Give homeopathic remedies orally.

If you begin the repair and find that it is more complicated than you anticipated, stop and reconsider transport or calling for backup. If bleeding is profuse, pack the yoni with gauze prior to transport. Mistakes in this area are serious because of the proximity of the bladder and urethra. IF IN DOUBT, TRANSPORT TO THE HOSPITAL FOR REPAIR!

INCLUSION CYSTS

Epithelial inclusion (dermoid) cysts may develop in the skin or in the yoni mucosa as the result of a previous improper repair and are particularly common among women who have undergone traditional female genital surgery. Cysts can appear either before or during pregnancy. They may form when surface tissue has been submerged because of poor suturing technique, commonly occurring when tissue edges are either inverted or overlapped; suture has passed through the skin surface, or stitches have been sewn too tightly. As a result, the repair heals with secretory tissue beneath the mucosal surface (there are no glands in the yoni mucosa). Cysts that occur along the perineal scar are created when glands have been submerged during a previous repair.

Hormonal activity and yoni secretions stimulate the submerged tissue causing a discharge-filled cyst. The woman may note cyst formation along the old scar after the previous birth or as the current pregnancy advances. Examination reveals a fluctuant mass along the line of a scar. If it is located somewhere other than along an old scar, you may be dealing with a different type of cyst; have it checked out. An inclusion cyst occasionally causes discomfort before birth. If so, it can be drained by puncturing it with a sterile needle and pressing out the milky contents. It is likely to refill. During pushing, palpate to remind yourself where the cyst is located. After the birth it may be difficult to distinguish, especially if it ruptures during pushing.

Removing an intact cyst from the yoni mucosa

Small, uninfected cysts may be left alone or removed under local anesthesia. The most important consideration regarding removal is whether doing so could result in further damage and scarring of existing sensitive tissue. Removal of small cysts can sometimes be accomplished without the need for transport. If a small cyst is still intact, use a pair of sharp/sharp tipped operating scissors to detach the entire cyst immediately below its base in the yoni tissue, being careful not to puncture it as you do. Use smooth tissue forceps to stabilize the cyst and then gently lift it out of the tissue still intact. If the cyst does not release fairly easily, call a more experienced colleague for consultation or transport to the hospital for more expert care. Once removed, place the tissue in a container provided by the lab for tissue examination or, failing the availability of such a tube, place it in a new, chemical free blood collection tube and send it to the lab for a pathology study (check with the lab regarding the color of the tube's top because, as of this printing, these colors were being changed) . Prior to sending it to the lab, place the tube in the refrigerator to prevent the tissue from drying out. Then proceed with the repair, as necessary.

Removing a ruptured cyst in the yoni mucosa

Cysts sometimes rupture during pushing or may require lancing prior to removal. If the cyst is small and filled with material, it can be lanced over the most distended part. Then locate one edge of the cyst and grasp it securely across as much of the edge as possible with an Allis clamp. Gently and slowly peel it away from its attachment point, using firm, even tension. A plane of cleavage should form easily and the cyst should peel away with little trouble. Try to pull at an angle; otherwise you may tear a piece off without removing the entire capsule. Examine the capsule to see if it appears complete (as you would with amniotic membranes). Then proceed with the repair as usual (Kolder, 1990). If removal proves difficult, abandon your attempts and transport for the repair.

Lancing and removing a large cyst, however, is trickier and I strongly recommend that you avoid doing so yourself without first getting some supervised hands-on training.

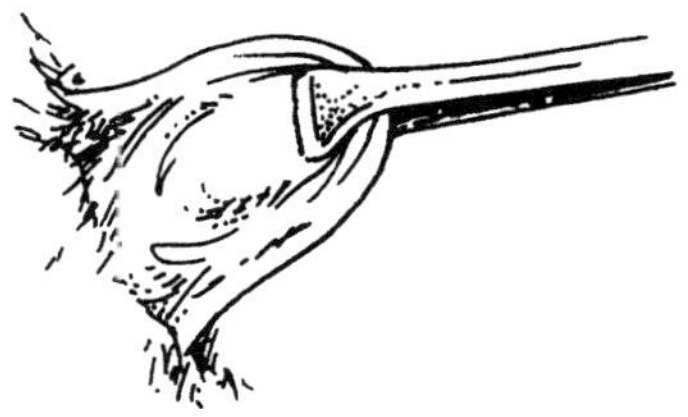

Removing a small cyst capsule

Dealing with a cyst in the skin

External cysts that underlie the vulval skin also present in a wide variety of sizes. These cysts may be lanced and drained if they are infected, obstructive or otherwise problematic. Whether doing so would further damage surrounding tissues, especially nerves or blood vessels, must be considered. During pregnancy, attempting to remove a cyst can result in a severe hemorrhage (Chalmers & Omer-Hashi, 2003).

If the midwife must deal with a small cyst, the best option is to open it by puncturing it over the fullest part of the surface of the cyst. A full-length incision is then created and the cyst drained. After that the edges of the cyst are sutured separately, leaving an area that used to be enclosed by the cyst in the center that must epithelize to heal. This procedure is known as marsupialization. Some cysts can also be excised entirely. Either process may be extremely painful and runs the risk of damaging tissues. Surgery on cysts is best performed in a hospital under general anesthesia.

DEALING WITH BLEEDING VESSELS

Fortunately bleeding vessels are an uncommon complication, especially with tears. Be alert for torn vessels if you have excessive bleeding and the uterus is low and firm, if there are varicosities in the yoni or vulva, or if you have done a clitorotomy. Keep in mind that continuous oozing or the formation of a large and expanding hematoma may point to a coagulation disorder.

Distinguishing a vein from an artery

A bleeding vessel may be either a torn vein or artery. Venous bleeding produces a continuous flow of blood, while an artery produces a pumping or pulsating flow. This is because venous blood flow is passive while arterial blood is under pulse pressure from the beating heart. Even so, arterial blood pressure is only about 3 pounds per square inch (psi). The flow from an ordinary garden hose is about 45 pounds psi. and can be stopped with pressure from your thumb. Therefore, relatively light pressure is required to control arterial or venous bleeding, especially from small vessels. Excessive pressure may further traumatize the vessel and surrounding tissue (Anderson & Romfh, 1980).

Sometimes the uterus will produce what may sometimes be construed as a slightly pumping blood flow. You must systematically rule out all uterine bleeding as well as bleeding from all other sources such as the cervix and upper yoni wall before you conclude that you have damage to a vessel in the injured tissues.

Checking for a bleeding vessel

To check for a bleeder, mop up the area with a gauze pad. Try to increase visibility by holding a gauze pad soaked with witch hazel bark or calendula extract firmly over the bleeding area. This alone will often stop the bleeding (but not if a large vessel is torn). You may have to expose the vessel by stretching the tissue slightly and pressing down, especially if it is concealed beneath a fold of tissue (Hobbs, 1990).

Tears sometimes bleed a lot with no vessel in particular being damaged. In this case, getting the repair done as quickly as possible is the best solution. Use figure-eight stitches, as necessary, to control bleeding. Watch carefully for a developing hematoma due to bleeding behind the sutures from a vessel you may have missed.

If there is a torn, bleeding vessel, you need to stop the bleeding before beginning closure. This is easier said than done. Once you locate the vessel, have your assistant maintain pressure on the area while you quickly set up your equipment (or vice versa). Homeopathic remedies can help arrest bleeding as well.

Cauterizing a bleeding vessel

Vessels or areas that are bleeding diffusely can sometimes be cauterized with a 75% silver nitrate/25% potassium nitrate swab. Barely moisten the swab and apply it directly to the bleeding vessel or area, twist it a bit to rub in the solution, and then hold it against the vessel for a minute or so. This will usually stop the bleeding if the vessel is small. However, if a large vein or an artery seems to be damaged, ligate it whenever possible (Leonard, 1991; Sorger, 1990).

To ligate a bleeding vessel

When you are ready to proceed, expose the vessel as previously described. Clamp the end with the tip of a hemostat so that it is in a straight line with the natural angle of the vessel (as shown). In some cases, this alone with allow a vein to clot off and arrest bleeding. Leave the clamp in place for a few minutes and then carefully remove it, if it was easy to find in the first place; if it was not, do not run the risk of removing the clamp, but ligate it just to be sure. If you do release the clamp and the vessel starts to bleed again, go ahead and ligate it. If an artery is torn, ligate it without waiting.

Have your assistant hold the hemostat and apply slight traction on the vessel. You should use 4-0 absorbable synthetic to tie it off. Encircle the hemostat and start the first throw of the knot over its tip. Then, slide the loop down around the vessel and tighten it by extending one or both index fingers to either side of the hemostat's tip to ensure that each segment is parallel the tissue surface as the knot is tightened. Tie it tightly with 2 or 3 complete square knots (i.e., 4 to 6 throws). Make sure to tie the vessel securely; if it comes loose after you have done the rest of your repair, you may have a hematoma on your hands.

Special Tricks and Techniques

Here are some uncommonly needed techniques. Studying them now may prevent an unnecessary transport in the future.

Repairing a pocket tear in the yoni mucosa

A pocket is a hole that is deeper and more narrow than the rest of the tear but that does not go through the bowel wall or into the urinary tract. It forms a place for lochia to pool, which invites infection. Be sure a pocket isn't really the retracted side of a torn sphincter (which is likely if it is right behind the lower perineal skin surface). When you get to the pocket, recheck with your finger to find the bottom of the hole. Assess whether to close the pocket as you close the rest of the tear. If you feel this will not work, run your suture beneath the tissue and bring the needle up beside the hole. Take a deep stitch from one side of the hole to the other to close it. Usually one stitch will do it. If not, take another stitch above the first one to close the top. If the pocket seems deep enough to involve muscle, open a new pack of 2-0 suture. Take a deep interrupted stitch at the bottom of the hole, then do a rectal exam to be sure it hasn't penetrated the bowel wall. Close the top with your continuous suture from the mucosa. These holes are hard to make look right. However, do not put in lots of stitches; the tissue will begin to pucker, which will distort the rest of the repair and may cause it to heal poorly.

Pocket tears will sometimes bleed profusely although you cannot identify a torn vessel. Figure-eight stitches, pressure, herbs and homeopathic remedies can be used to help stop the bleeding. If it will not stop, you need to transport to the hospital.

Very rarely, the surface of the perineum will separate from the underlying tissue, creating a wide (from side to side), deep (from top to bottom), and shallow (from front to back) pocket behind the perineum. There may be little or no damage to the fourchette or perineal surface. Check the bottom of the pocket to rule out sphincter damage. If none is found, you can take basting stitches along the pocket following to the path of the tear (i.e., from side to side). Be sure to close the bottom of the pocket as you do so. Do not pull the stitches too tightly.

Dissecting the perineum to gain access for deep repair

If a deep perineal pocket tear has resulted in a damaged or severed sphincter or the baby has been born through a rupture in the perineum, leaving the introitus of the yoni intact, the perineum will have to be dissected in order to gain access for repair. This must be done carefully with very sharp surgical scissors. Open the scissor blades about half-way and place the joint against the edge of the tissue. Be sure to keep them at a right angle to the perineal surface as you cut. One clean cut is ideal, but if the area that needs to be dissected is long, several clips may be necessary to avoid chewing the tissue (which results from opening the scissors too widely). Make every effort to start each clip in line with the previous one so you don't create a jagged incision. Take care not to cut any further down the perineal surface than is absolutely necessary to gain access to the sphincter. Unless there is no alternative, I recommend hospital transport when such dissection is necessary.

Finding an invisible internal apex of a tear

If you can't see the internal apex of a tear, but are pretty sure you can feel it, proceed as follows:

- •Take an appropriately spaced interrupted stitch or two as close to the internal apex as possible. Tie these off and leave the ends long.
- •Now pull down on these sutures just enough to bring the apex of the tear into view.
- •Have an assistant maintain traction on the strands while you place a stitch above the internal apex of the tear. Place any other necessary stitches between the anchor stitch and the locating stitches.
- •Cut the long ends on your locating stitches and continue your repair (Oxorn, 1986).

Removing misplaced stitches

Even the most experienced clinician can occasionally make a mistake in suture placement. This might occur when tears are very ragged or when a tear at the opening of the yoni is very uneven. The mistake will usually be discovered after only one stitch has been misplaced. In some cases it is possible to slowly and carefully work the suture and needle back through the tissue in order to avoid cutting the strand. Of course, this causes tissue trauma, and you should only opt to do this if you felt placing a knot or interrupting the line of continuous sutures would result in even more tissue trauma. Do not attempt this with stitches in the rectal mucosa or upper yoni wall. If you are near the beginning of the repair, you might also opt to remove the suture and begin again. You could also cut the strand near the needle and tie it off as described below, and then open a new packet of suture.

If you have made an even more unfortunate error and are confronted with several misplaced stitches, I recommend cutting the strand near the needle and carefully removing all the poorly placed stitches by pulling the thread back through the tissue. When you get to the last stitch which needs removal, create a loop as you pull the strand out of the tissue on one side and, using your loop as one thread, tie it to your single strand (i.e., the one to which the needle was attached). (This is a modified form of the closure technique previously described in the chapter entitled "Repairing the Perineum.")

Sulcus tears

Sulcus tears occur in the grooves to either side of the yoni floor or ceiling (where the floor or ceiling meets the wall of the yoni). Tears may extend up one or more of these grooves, usually along the lower ones. If only one groove is involved, repair is exactly the same as for centrally located tears. The grooves of the just-stretched yoni can be deep. Be sure to hold the tissue open widely, so you are sewing the edges of the tear together and not suturing the sides of the yoni wall adjacent to the torn groove. This is facilitated by using a retractor.

If the tear forks at the perineum and extends up both grooves of the yoni floor, there will be two internal apexes. Repair the longest tear first. When you get to the hymenal ring, put that suture aside (pin it to your drape over the mother's pubic bone) and use a separate pack of suture to repair the other fork. Start at the second internal apex and work your way down to the base where it meets the first tear. Using the longest strand of suture, continue as you normally would. You can tie and cut the shortest of the two sutures, or use the technique of closure at the end of the chapter entitled "Repairing the Perineum."

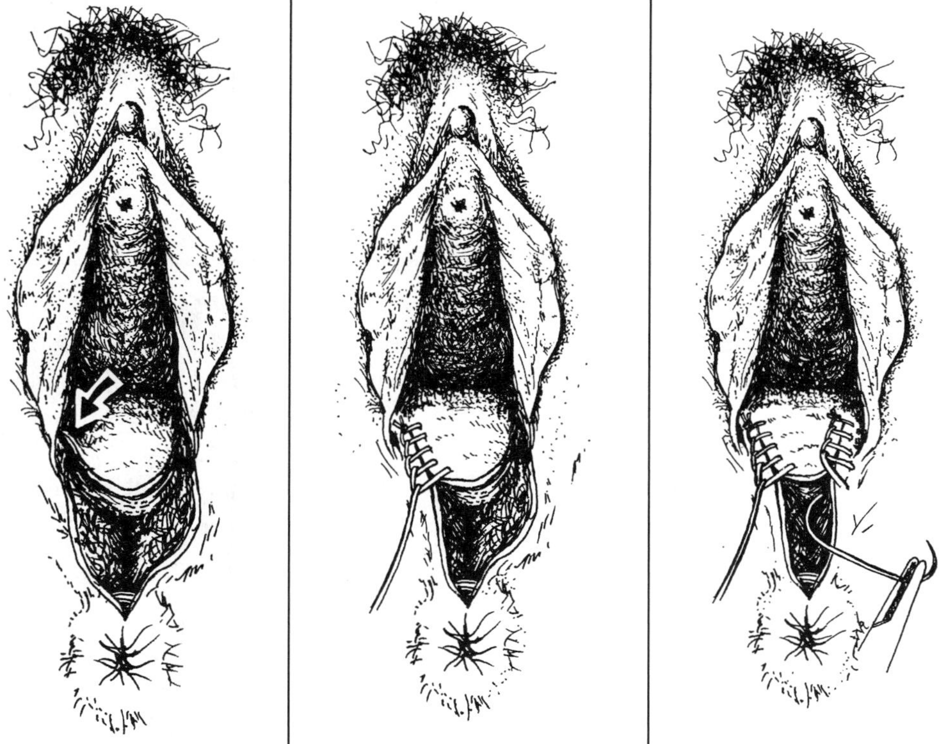

Start with the longest side of the tear first.	Stop here, and close the other side with a new packet of suture.	When finished, continue the repair as usual.

In the examples above, a locking stitch has been used. However, a basting stitch can be used with equally good results.

Repairing a mediolateral tear or cut

Mediolateral tears divide all tissue on an angle as they extend down the perineum. These tears are very rare and usually occur along an old mediolateral clitorotomy scar.

If you have a cut or tear that goes off at an angle, the inner side (the edge nearest the midline of the yoni) will tend to retract more than the outer edge. There is likely to be more muscle damage at a more superficial depth than is usually the case. This is because the puborectalis muscle is shallow along the sides of the yoni, where it is unprotected by the anal sphincter and the perineal body.

To compensate for the angle, sew parallel with the line of the tear by holding the needle holder in line with the edges of the tear, not straight in front of you. There is more tissue on the lateral side of the tear than on the medial side. Thus, more tissue should be included in the lateral side of the stitch than in the medial side of the same stitch. Stitches along the lateral side are placed more deeply than those on the medial side more shallowly, in part, to avoid entering the rectum. The stitches along the lateral side are also spaced at a normal width, while those on the medial side are placed a little closer together than is usual. These modifications should not be too exaggerated. If done correctly, they will bring the inside edge to the outer edge, which is what you want. It is a good idea to practice on foam rubber and then some sort of meat before attempting this kind of repair for real.

Be sure to do a rectal exam to check for misplaced sutures; remove them, irrigate the area (if necessary), and replace them as needed (Varney et al., 2004).

Tears that have side deviations (forked tears)

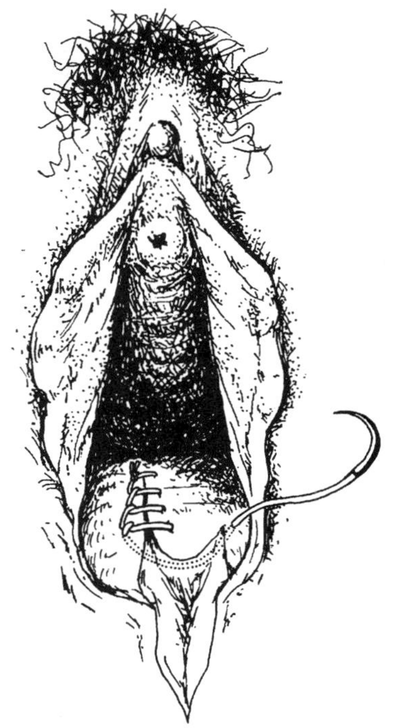 Here, the longest fork has been closed with a locking stitch. The needle is then passed through the tissue to bring it up at the internal apex of the shorter fork.	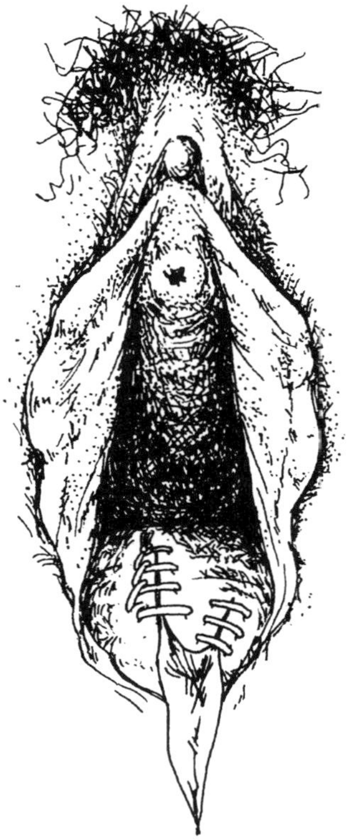 The short side has been closed with a basting stitch. From here, continue the repair as usual.

Occasionally a tear in the yoni mucosa has a short detour off to one side of the main tear. (Compare with a sulcus tear; they are not the same.) Start your repair at the deepest internal yoni apex, as usual. To repair the fork, use either locked stitches (if alignment of the tissue is a problem) or basting sutures.

If you repaired the long side of the fork with a locked stitch, use the Hobbs maneuver to secure the last lock. Take a stitch underneath the yoni mucosa, directing the needle so that you exit at the internal apex of the short fork. Take care not to pull the suture tight (you are merely moving to another point, not holding anything together). Now sew down to where the fork meets the main tear. When you arrive at the point where you left off in the main tear, continue your repair as usual.

When one longitudinal edge of a tear protrudes more than the other

When two edges of a tear present a "stair-step" effect, you must avoid leaving one raw edge exposed as you suture. Use the same size stitches that you normally would, but place your stitch deeper (i.e., further below the tissue surface) on the side that is low and more superficially (closer to normal depth or more shallow) on the side that is too high in the subcutaneous layer. Accomplish this by either bringing your needle out in the center of the tear before inserting it at a different depth on the other side or by pressing against the high side of the tissue in order to alter the depth of your needle insertion point as you make your stitch on the high side (using pressure is less precise and I recommend removing the needle whenever practical). When you exert traction on a running stitch, this technique will bring your elevated edge down to meet the other side. The edges for subcuticular repair should then match perfectly (Sorger, 1991).

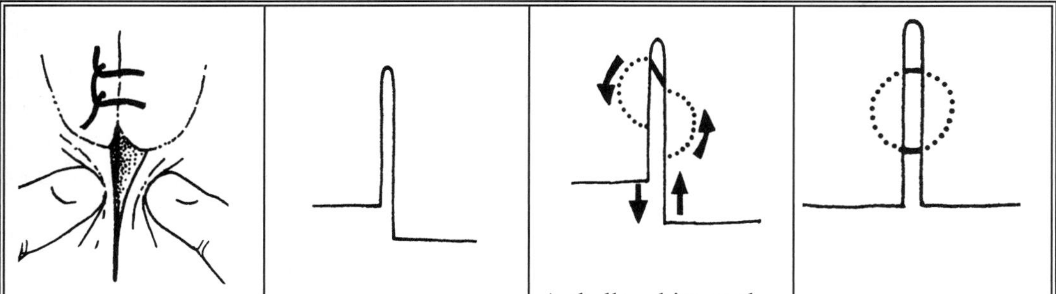

Exposed edge of tissue (shaded area) where edges meet	Looking down on the tear, the edges are mismatched.	A shallow bite on the high side and a deeper bite on the low side . . .	. . . evens out the edges when the stitch is pulled together.

The "U" (interrupted running mattress) stitch

This special stitch constitutes an interrupted running mattress–style suture; the concept is similar to the buried circle stitch, but like a usual running mattress stitch, it is placed parallel with the tissue edge (not deep to it). It can be used to join cervical or labial tears. It may also be used in the lateral walls of the yoni, as well as anywhere else a single, hidden stitch is desired. It must be at least as long as it is wide to prevent rolling and puckering of the tissue. It may be placed slightly deeper from the tissue surface than a normal running mattress suture. Depth of placement depends upon what is being repaired (Reese, 1992).

Fig. 1: Enter the tissue as shown, under and parallel with the tissue edge.

Fig. 2: Exit the tissue, coming out at a depth parallel with your entry point. Bring the needle completely out of the tissue before beginning the second half of the stitch. Enter the tissue directly across from your exit point and complete the stitch.

Fig. 3: Tie the stitch; note that the knot will be buried when you finish. Place your next stitch immediately above your knot (you will exit the first half of the next stitch where the arrow is pointing).

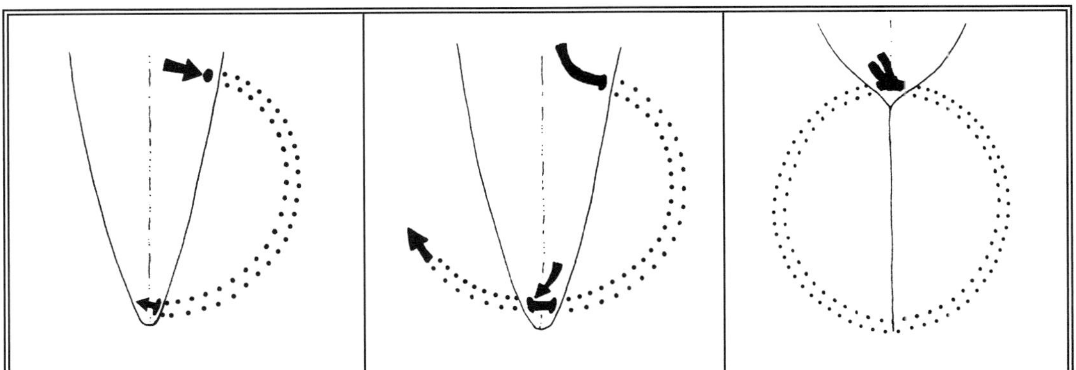

Fig. 1	Fig. 2	Fig. 3

(These stitches should be small; these drawings are greatly enlarged to show detail.)

If the free end of the suture strand is quite short and you must tie a knot

Leave the needle attached to the suture and use it to help tie your knot. Using a needle holder–type tie, use the needle as a handle to wrap the strand around to make your loops and hold the loops in place. Then use your needle holder to help pull the free end through the loop. This will often allow you to complete a knot that would otherwise be impossible to accomplish with short ends. You must be very careful not to puncture yourself as you do this: be sure to use your thumb forceps rather than your fingers to manipulate the needle.

ALTERNATIVE CLOSURE TECHNIQUES

Using tissue adhesive

Although not recommended for perineal repair, synthetic tissue adhesive has been successfully used by some midwives. It might be a good alternative to offer when women refuse conventional sutures. Tissue adhesive works best when the wound is moderately shallow, has no pockets to collect lochia and does not require other sutures. It has also been used instead of subcuticular sutures after placing basting stitches in the perineum. Adoni and Anteby (1991) and Bowen and Seligner (2002) studied the use of tissue adhesive for clitorotomy repair but all the women in the adhesive group were conventionally sutured first to close the deeper parts of their perineums and tissue adhesive was only used to close the skin layer. They experienced significantly less postpartum discomfort than those whose skin was conventionally sutured. It must be emphasized that this is *not* how midwives are typically using tissue adhesives, as most midwives are seeking to forgo suturing altogether. Therefore, it must be reiterated that a deep, serious laceration can be hiding behind skin edges that meet nicely, mimicking a superficial tear. Only the most superficial tears are suited to repair with tissue adhesive: tears that are this shallow can be left to heal on their own.

Tissue adhesives are only used to bridge and seal across the surface of a wound. Care must be taken to avoid penetration of the adhesive into the depth of the wound. Cyanoacrylates that enter the wound can cause acute inflammatory reactions, giant cell reactions, inclusion body formation (in which the body encapsulates the foreign material) and seroma (a specific type of mass resulting from the localized accumulation of tissue serum). When the adhesive enters damaged tissues, it can remain there for over a year. In large amounts, these glues can produce painful exothermic heat.

Wounds that are candidates for closure using tissue adhesive have edges that are straight and that lie together naturally. Insert a tampon, then clean and dry the wound. For this a hair dryer set on warm can be used to dry the skin thoroughly. Insert your extended, gloved finger between the edges of the wound and lift it out from the tear; this will bring the wound edges forward slightly. Have your assistant stabilize the wound edges by placing their fingers on either side of the wound to hold the edges together, taking care to match them correctly. Have her also hold a gauze pad against the area immediately below the apex.

Crush the plastic Dermabond applicator and squeeze it until adhesive covers the applicator tip. Apply a 5 to 10 mm wide layer of adhesive centered over the wound edges. Several strokes of the tip are applied until an obvious layer is formed. Continue wound support for 60 seconds to allow the glue to dry. After another 15 to 20 seconds, more glue can be applied. Two or three separate layers are applied to complete closure.

Glue removal: Liquid adhesives can drip and run into areas adjacent to the wound. Any drips should be removed immediately before they dry. If they do dry, Lansinoh cream can be applied to the drip to speed breakdown and peeling. Forceps can also be used to gently flake off adhesive after it is completely dry. Do not use acetone-based glue removers, which are toxic and should never be the used in the genital area.

Aftercare: Women whose tears are repaired with tissue adhesive should observe the same precautions as those who have refused sutures entirely. The area should be kept as dry as possible for the first 24 hours. After that, showering is not contraindicated but prolonged soaking should be avoided. Expect the adhesive to flake off in 3 to 7 days. Allergic reactions are very rare, but may include inflammation and swelling (Quinn & Kissick, 1994). If the wound does come apart, it can be left to heal on its own. Alternatively, sutures can be placed. Which you will choose will depend on the mother's preference, the extent of the laceration, the condition of the wound and the timing of the breakdown.

Using sea vegetables as tissue adhesive

Gilpin-Blake and Elliott (2001) learned about the use of seaweeds for healing wounds from a native American shaman who used this method to treat burns and lacerations. This method flies in the face of what is known about wound healing because it calls for lining the raw wound with seaweed, which, according to the current understanding of how wounds heal, should interfere with first intention healing (see the chapter entitled "How Wounds Heal" to review this information). There is very little in the literature on the use of seaweed to close wounds, and I have never used it myself. However, these authors have used it extensively and report good results. It offers an option for women who refuse all other types of repair.

You will need flat sheets of seaweed, either unseasoned kelp leaves or nori will work. Cut a piece of seaweed that is twice the length and width of the tear and fold it in half. Moisten it with sterile water (bottled sterile saline is a suitable liquid, but boiled water will do as well). Once it is soft, place the piece of seaweed down the trough of the tear, covering both walls of the tear with smoothed, wrinkle-free plant material, then align the sides of the wound and gently press them together. Once the tissues are approximated in this manner, moisten another patch of seaweed and "tape" it over the center of the tear down the perineum. Each time the woman uses the toilet, she should replace the external patch. The authors report miraculous results with this method of closure, with wounds healing and becoming nearly invisible by the 24 hour mark. Midwives that I talked to directly report great difficulty in getting the seaweed to stay put, and I could find no midwives in Portland who are using this method of repair as of this writing.

REFERENCES AND FURTHER READING ON UNUSUAL REPAIRS AND OTHER PROBLEMS

REFERENCES USED IN MULTIPLE CHAPTERS

Cunningham F, et al. Chapter 35: "Obstetrical Hemorrhage," in Cunningham F, et al. WILLIAMS OBSTETRICS, 22nd ed. McGraw-Hill, New York NY, 2005.

Kolder V, MD. Editing comments, Aug, 1990.

Oxorn, H. Chapter 34L "Episiotomy, lacerations, uterine rupture, inversion," HUMAN LABOR & BIRTH. 5th ed. Appleton-Century-Crofts, Norwalk CT, 1986.

Peyton V. Chapter 20: "Episiotomy and obstetrics tears," in Lynge C, et al., eds. 20 COMMON PROBLEMS: SURGICAL PROBLEMS AND PROCEDURES IN PRIMARY CARE. McGraw-Hill Pro., New York, NY, 2001.

Sorger L., MD. Editing comments, 1991.

Varney H, et al. Chapter 79: "Cutting an episiotomy and repairing episiotomies and lacerations," VARNEY'S MIDWIFERY, 4th ed. Jones & Bartlett, Sudbury MA, 2004.

PUERPERAL HEMATOMAS

Kiefer D, et al. "Management of hematomas incurred as a result of obstetrical delivery," www.uptodateonline.com/patients/content/topic.do?topicKey=~BNCPyXh9VXvxVI#subscribeMessage, updated Jul 31, 2008, accessed May 4, 2009.

Lowe C, CNM. Conversation regarding hematoma care. Win, 1989.

Malak J. "Angiographic embolization," www.noblood.org/ask-professional/5507-angiographic-embolization. html, Accessed May 4, 2009.

Sorger L, MD. Editing comments, Feb, 1991.

Varney H, et al. Chapter 44: "Screening for and midwifery management of puerperal abnormality," in their VARNEY'S MIDWIFERY, 4th ed. Jones & Bartlett, Sudbury MA, 2004.

CERVICAL LACERATIONS

Fahmy K, et al. "Postpartum colposcopy of the cervix: injury and healing." INT J GYNAECOL OBSTET, 34(2):133-137, Feb, 1991.

Greenhill J, Friedman E. Chapter 65: "Parturitional trauma" in their BIOLOGICAL PRINCIPLES AND MODERN PRACTICE OF OBSTETRICS. WB Saunders. Philadelphia PA, 1974.

INCLUSION CYSTS

Chalmers B, Omer-Hashi K. FEMALE GENITAL MUTILATION AND OBSTETRIC CARE. Trafford Pub., Victoria BC, Canada, 2003.

Mubiayi N, et al. "Epithelial inclusion cyst formation after buried vaginal mucosa. Diagnosis and management," GYNECOLOGY, OBSTETRIQUE & FERTILITE, 31(12):1013-1017, Dec, 2003.

Webster JC. A TEXTBOOK OF DISEASES OF WOMEN. WB Saunders. Philadelphia PA, 1907.

DEALING WITH BLEEDING VESSELS

Anderson R, Romfh R. TECHNIQUE IN THE USE OF SURGICAL TOOLS. Appleton-Century-Crofts, New York NY, 1980.

Hobbs V, Midwife. Editing comments, 1990.

Leonard C, CM. Discussion regarding use of silver nitrate swabs, Jan 12, 1991.

Sorger L, MD. Conversation regarding the use of silver nitrate postpartum, Dec 1990.

Special Tricks and Techniques

Reese K, MD. Conversation, Yale-New Haven Hospital, April 1992.

Alternative Closure Techniques

Adoni A, Anteby E. "The use of Histoacryl for episiotomy repair," Br J Obtet Gynaecol, 98(5):476-478, May, 1991.

Bowen M, Selinger M. "Episiotomy closure comparing enbucrilate tissue adhesive with conventional sutures," Int J Gynaecol Obstet, 78(3):201-205, Sep, 2002.

Coulthard P, et al. "Tissue adhesives for closure of surgical wounds," Cochrane Database Syst Rev, (2):CD004287, 2004.

Heimstetter, G. personal communication. Permabond Internat, Bridgewater NJ, 1995.

Jueneman F. "Stick it to um," Industrial Research Dev, 19, Aug, 1981.

Gilpin-Blake D, Elliott S. "A natural alternative to suturing," Midwifery Today, (60):32, Win, 2001.

Quinn J, Kissick J. "Tissue adhesives for laceration repair during sporting events," Clin J Sport Med, 4(4): 245-248, 1994.

POSTPARTUM CARE OF THE PERINEAL TISSUES

Postpartum Care and Comfort Measures

Many women you care for will have little to no broken tissue trauma. However, all will experience stretching and some degree of bruising; swelling is common too. Most of the suggestions in this chapter can be used for these women as well as those who have more extensive trauma.

Heat and the postpartum period

According to Chinese medicine, birth causes a rapid reduction of internal heat in the mother's system. Women are usually warm during pregnancy as a result of increased metabolism (i.e., internal heat). After birth, women frequently shake, as if they have chills. The Chinese explain that this is due to the Ming men (life gate fire) being opened by the birth.

The Chinese consider the Ming men to be the basis of all strength. This energy center is located between the kidneys; it extends down the lower back and the abdomen, and from two fingerbreadths below the navel to the pubic bone. The kidney energy governs sexuality, reproduction, growth and decline. The gate of life opens to allow passage of the baby and, with proper postpartum care, closes again, contributing to stronger lower back and kidney energy.

Postpartum shaking is symptomatic of the internal heat loss that has taken place. The Chinese feel that applying cold encourages this internal cold and may create long-term complications such as the weakening of the back or kidneys. Therefore, ice should be used only in the most extreme cases of swelling or hematoma formation. Otherwise, offer heat-producing fluids (such as ginger tea) and hot packs applied to the perineum, as well as ensuring that both mother and baby are warm, to help balance out the rapid heat loss that follows birth (Lang, 1987).

The herbal bath

Once the placenta is out, any necessary sutures are in place, and mother and baby are stable, both may get into an herbal bath. Whether a woman has torn or not, the bath helps to soothe, heal and cleanse the yoni area. It also helps dry and heal the baby's cord stump. Be sure to confirm that the mother is not allergic to the herbs you will be using.

The tub should be scrubbed with an abrasive cleanser, unless the material it is made of contraindicates it (then use a nonabrasive cleaner). Rinse thoroughly; check for dirt and grit; wipe, rinse or clean again. Be sure to get around the drain and the overflow drain. Squirt with povidone iodine and wipe, then rinse once more. Fill with temperate water, no more than 100° F [37.8° C] if you plan to put the baby in the bath. Water that is too hot will make the mother more prone to fainting as well.

Moonflower, a division of Cascade HealthCare Products, has a prepackaged herbal bath pack that is easy to include in your customized birth kit for parents to order. A bath may also be made from one or more of the following herbs (Leeds, 2005):

- Calendula flowers (healing, antiseptic and anti-inflammatory)
- Comfrey leaf (promotes cell growth and healing–current research has raised the concern that Comfrey may promote superficial healing of the skin, enclosing a deeper wound

that is not yet healed and thus increasing the risk of infection. I have never observed this myself and used comfrey extensively in herbal baths when I was in practice. It is something to keep in mind, however, especially if the wound is deep or involves rectal tissues.)

•Golden seal root (tonifies mucous membranes and is antimicrobial, but very expensive and endangered.)
•Lavender (promotes oxygenation [from deep breathing this fragrant herb], relaxation and calmness)
•Marshmallow root (demulcent herb that soothes tissues)
•Mullein leaf (soothing to raw mucous membranes)
•Oregon Grape root (can be substituted for Golden seal root)
•Plantain leaf (demulcent, astringent and mildly antiseptic, good for drawing out infection and healing old wounds)
•Rosemary leaf (antiseptic and reduces swelling)
•Sage leaf (astringent, antiseptic and warming)
•Uva ursi leaf (astringent, anti-inflammatory and healing to the urinary tract)
•Shepherd's purse (promotes clotting)
•White oak bark (astringent herb good for shrinking hemorrhoids)
•Witch hazel bark (astringent, good to shrink hemorrhoids or varicosities)
•Yarrow flowers (antiseptic and astringent)
•Yerba mansa (astringent, antibacterial, antifungal and tonifying to mucous membranes)
•A whole bulb of fresh garlic (antiseptic, stimulates circulation)
•Sea salt (½ cup in a normal-sized bathtub creates a mild saline solution)

From among these herbs, choose several that are readily available in your area and that have the qualities each woman may require. For example, comfrey or mullein, rosemary, uva ursi, shepherd's purse, garlic and salt might be chosen. Ideally, a ½ oz each of the loose herbs (or any combination of suitable healing herbs you concoct) should be prepared as an infusion; that is, steeped (not boiled or simmered) from the onset of labor until the mother and baby are ready for their bath. Choose a large glass, stainless steel or enamel pot. Fill it three-quarters full of water, remove the boiling water from the heat, and then add a half ounce of each herb. Cover the pot and let it sit for the duration of labor. This makes a medicinal strength infusion for use after birth.

The garlic should be peeled enough to remove the outer paper (no need to peel every single clove), then whizzed in a blender or food processor with enough water to process. It can be added now by tying it up in a bit of cheesecloth or it can be placed in the colander before the infusion is strained. (Occasionally, a friend or relative, overwhelmed with the birth experience, has attempted to steep prepackaged herbs without first removing them from the plastic bag. You might want to check to be sure all is going well with preparations.)

If prepackaged bath herbs are not available, check the kitchen. Some women may have rosemary or sage in their kitchen, but today many women do not cook, so you should be sure to carry these standbys in your bag. Either can be used alone, along with salt, for a bath.

When bath time is near, fill the tub and strain the herbal infusion through a colander lined with an clean, old T-shirt or a cloth diaper; the cloth can then be pulled together and tied to make a big tea ball and dropped into the tub as well. Add the salt directly to the water and use your hands to stir to dissolve. Do not make the mistake of dumping the herbs directly into the tub, as this will make a huge mess and clog the plumbing.

Even the most stable woman who has experienced minimal blood loss can feel faint on her feet after birth. A warm bath may accentuate this tendency. Be on hand when she first gets into the bath, until she is settled and stable, and once again when she is ready to get out. While she is in the bath, you should be waiting nearby in case she feels woozy.

During the first few days postpartum I have had frazzled fathers attempting to prepare baths in my absence. One mother found herself soaking in collard-green liquor (he inadvertently dumped the infusion). Another father carefully disposed of the infusion and saved the herbs! Be sure helpers know how to prepare the bath.

Baths once or twice daily for the first few days postpartum are soothing and healing. In most situations, soaking more frequently than twice a day can waterlog the repair and prolong healing.

Drying the perineum after a bath

Some women enjoy drying their stitches with a hair dryer or exposing them to a high-wattage light bulb for a few minutes after their bath; this helps to remove excess water form the area and avoids waterlogging the repair. However, since moist wounds heal best, it is not necessary for the perineum to be kept as dry as possible at all times. Infrared heat lamps should be used very carefully; a sunburned perineum will not feel better.

Hot packs

Hot moist herbal packs placed against the perineum help to stimulate circulation. This will carry away local anesthetic and edema, as well as promote oxygenation and enhance healing.

Ice packs

If swelling is very extreme the perineal area can benefit from the application of ice. (Homeopathic Arnica taken orally can be used instead of, or in addition to, ice. It does not expose the mother to the internal chilling that ice promotes.) Ice should not be applied for longer than 24 hours except in the event of a hematoma that is enlarging.

Ice packs can be made by liberally dribbling maternity sanitary napkins that have been cut in half with comfrey leaf infusion. Freeze several for use after birth. (Soaking rather than dribbling creates large ice chunks, which will be unpleasant for most women). A quick ice pack can be made by filling a sterile glove with crushed ice and tying off the end.

Hot ginger tea (1 tsp powdered or fresh grated ginger to a cup of water given orally) and warm blankets can be used to help offset the chilling effect of the ice.

Pelvic floor exercises

When the home is all on one level, normal activity should not pull out the stitches of most types of repairs when they are done properly and the knots are secure. Strenuous activity that puts pressure or strain on the perineal area or the climbing of stairs should be avoided for the first six weeks. Any exercise involving opening the legs widely or pressure down into the pelvis (such as sit-ups or jogging) should be postponed until the tissues have had a chance to knit together and restore their tone (preferably six weeks). Other exercises can stress the perineal area as well, such as biking or horseback riding, and should be avoided for at least four weeks for most repairs, and at least six weeks if labial or skin tag repair has been done or if a tear was left unrepaired.

While suturing can restore the structure of the perineum, only pelvic floor exercises will restore its proper function. Pelvic floor exercises will help orient healing muscle fibers and promote a stronger healed area (Montgomery, 1989). Women should keep up their prenatal schedule of daily pelvic floor exercises, starting immediately after birth. This will increase circulation in the area, reduce edema, disperse injected anesthetic and promote healing. Prenatal exercise makes identifying stretched muscles during postpartum exercise easier. Encourage women to do this vitally important exercise fifty times daily for the rest of their lives (Noble, 1995). Walking can be resumed shortly after birth (as long as the mother is not carrying anything heavy, even the baby) to help tone the pelvic floor as well, but she should build up her time and stamina gradually to avoid overdoing it (Rosenberg, 2005).

Relief of postpartum pain

After-birth pains and swollen perineums can cause discomfort and restless nights. Afterease tincture (by Wishgarden Herbs) can help take the edge off uterine cramping. This combination contains black haw root bark and cramp bark (both of which calm the uterus), motherwort (calms the uterus and the nerves) and yarrow (good for aches and slowing bleeding). It can be included in your custom birth kit from any one of the specialty midwifery supply houses such as In His Hands or Cascade HealthCare Products. External therapies, along with homeopathic Arnica, can help as well. One of the best positional therapies is for the mother to lie on her belly with a small pillow or rolled-up towel pressed against her uterus. This will help to contract the uterus and relieve severe cramping (Varney et al., 2004). The application of a heating pad across the lower abdomen may also help some women.

Herbal relaxants and sedatives include skullcap, St. John's wort and valerian tincture. Up to half a dropperful can be taken to help with sleeping. If no hematomas are suspected and other remedies are not helping, there is no point in women staying up all night being miserable. Acetaminophen (Tylenol) is the most suitable over-the-counter analgesic for the postpartum period, although it is hard on the liver. Salicylate (aspirin) agents are less desirable since they cause clotting dysfunction by disrupting normal platelet activity. Ibuprofen, another anti-inflammatory, is frequently given to women postpartum. Side effects may include nausea, gastrointestinal bleeding, diarrhea or constipation, headache, dizziness, fluid retention and hypertension as well as platelet dysfunction. It must be used with care and with attention to the heaviness of the lochial flow. It is not officially recommended for use during nursing.

If a woman seems to be in an unusual degree of discomfort, rule out serious problems before recommending analgesics. You don't want to mask the symptoms with drugs until you know what is happening. Homeopathic remedies are not contraindicated because they do not work by masking symptoms.

Hematoma care

If a hematoma has formed, do not leave after the birth until you are satisfied that it is not enlarging. It can take hours to be sure and you should probably plan on spending the night or having a well trained and experienced apprentice do so. Be sure the mother and family understand that if she is feeling increasing pressure or pain, or seems to be going into shock, someone should call you at once. To avoid masking increasing pain or pressure, the mother should not take any analgesics (herbal or otherwise) until you are satisfied that the hematoma has stabilized. (Homeopathic remedies are not contraindicated and may stop the bleeding.) Be sure the parents know what danger signs to look for: pallor, clammy skin, disorientation, visual or hearing disturbances, or excessive drowsiness (especially in the presence of other symptoms). If the mother does go into shock, the main thing is to keep her warm, lie her down (feet higher than head), keep her awake, and call an ambulance right away: family should not wait to hear from you or for you to arrive before going to the hospital in such a case.

If an existing hematoma is traumatized, clotting may be disrupted and the hematoma can begin to actively bleed. Women will need to stay quiet for the first several days after birth. However, if the mother has varicosities (which is likely), she should not stay in bed full time, as this encourages clot formation in her veins. (See the entry entitled "Hemorrhoids and varicose veins" later in this chapter.)

Homeopathic Arnica can be given to relieve the trauma. (Arnica is indicated for any kind of bruising and is generally a good remedy to give after the birth.) Shepherd's purse and astringent herbal tinctures (10 drops each, 3 times daily) can be given in combination to help stop the bleeding. Keep in mind that internal bleeding may lead to anemia (see the next entry in this chapter entitled "Postpartum nutrition and supplementation").

Pooled blood makes infection a possibility. Increase Vitamin C to 3000 mg daily and recommend echinacea root tincture (½ dropperful 4 times daily for the first 2 weeks postpartum). Watch for signs of fever, local tenderness, inflammation and expanding redness. (See the chapter entitled "Perineal Infections.")

Postpartum nutrition and supplementation

After birth, women need to continue to eat well (including more protein than when they were pregnant) to promote healing, general recovery and an adequate milk supply. If excessive blood loss has occurred, check the hemoglobin 32 hours after the bleeding stops and recommend supplementation as appropriate. A low hemoglobin predisposes a woman to slow recovery and poor healing as well as making her more prone to infection. (See my book UNDERSTANDING DIAGNOSTIC TESTS for anemia therapies.)

Five hundred mg vitamin C with bioflavonoids daily and vitamin E (1200 IU daily) can be taken to help slow the lochial discharge and encourage healing. Zinc (15 to 25 mg daily) can also be taken to promote healing, especially if the woman has a history of malnourishment. It should be taken after meals to avoid nausea. If women are taking JuicePlus+, they can continue. Homeopathic Arnica (30C twice daily) helps reduce swelling and bruising and relieves trauma.

Wearing sanitary pads, underwear and slacks postpartum

Wearing underclothing and sanitary pads over perineal tears is not a problem, although the more air that reaches the perineal area, the better.

If there are carefully repaired skin tags or labial tears, however, it is best that nothing be worn directly against the vulva for the first seven days postpartum. The woman should also sit in positions that keep her legs together for the first week to avoid stressing the area. This allows it to heal with as little abrasion and irritation as possible. The mother can place extra underpads or clean towels beneath her bottom when she is in bed. Pads and panties should be worn only when it is absolutely necessary.

Be sure to mention that the use of menstrual tampons, cups or sponges are not appropriate in the immediate postpartum period. Not only might one find its way through the open cervix, but they increase the likelihood of infection.

Toileting

Although women are often instructed in elaborate toileting rituals in hospitals, in most cases the actual risk of infection is very slight. The woman should sit very gently on the toilet, so as not to pull her stitches (or unrepaired tear) apart, and avoid straining her bowels. It may help to support the perineum with her fingers during bowel movements by reaching down between her legs from the front and using the flat of her fingers to apply counterpressure to the perineum (especially if rectal or muscle damage has been repaired) (Noble, 1995). She may also rinse herself off with plain water, saline solution (¼ tsp salt to 1 cup water), herbal infusion or water with a squirt of povidone iodine added. This is not mandatory to prevent infection, but squirting water on her genitals may help when burning during urination is a problem. The mother can also pat herself dry at the toilet, moving from front to back.

If burning with urination is severe (usually only during the first 24 hours), she can dilute the flow by urinating in the herbal bath before getting out, or while sitting in a sitz bath or a shallow tub of plain or mildly salinated water.

It is normal for a woman to go 24 to 36 hours after the birth before she has a bowel movement. This is because her bowels have been emptied very well from the stimulation of birth, and she has frequently missed at least one full meal. Remember that increasing rectal pressure from a hematoma may mimic a full bowel. If a woman is complaining of constipation with painful, nonproductive straining at the toilet, check it out. True constipation in the immediate postpartum period following a yoni birth is exceedingly rare.

Identifying a subluxated coccyx

Sometimes the coccyx is knocked out of joint by the baby's descent, causing severe postpartum pain. If so, it may confuse the picture when a woman is complaining of pelvic pain. If not corrected, the surrounding tissues will swell, making it difficult or impossible to reposition the coccyx correctly. Repositioning can be accomplished by having the mother lie flat on her stomach on a hard surface and applying firm pressure to the sacrococcygeal joint with the heel of your hand (Gaskin, 1978). If this doesn't work, you can try repositioning it by inserting your gloved index finger into the rectum and manipulating the coccyx into place, using your other hand externally to assist. If this doesn't work either or proves too difficult (do not force it, as you are not trained to adjust it; you are trying to encourage it to go back into place), a chiropractor or osteopath should reposition the coccyx as soon as possible. Waiting only encourages more inflammation. Homeopathic Arnica can be given to help relieve swelling.

Care after urinary catheterization

Catheterization makes a woman prone to the development of a urinary tract infection. Extra vitamin C with bioflavinoids (up to 3000 mg daily for one week) and uva ursi leaf or mullein infusion (1 to 2 cups daily for the first few days postpartum) can help reduce the chance of this.

Bedrest in the postpartum period

Bedrest during the days and weeks postpartum is a time honored practice that is found in many indigenous cultures. Honoring this time to allow the mother undisturbed contact with her baby and relief from her normal domestic duties is a given in many cultures. During a set period of time, often 40 days or 6 weeks, the mother is cared for so that she can care for her baby. There are often a variety of rules for this period, including recommendations for diet as well as other aspects of baby and mother care. In today's white western, rat race-paced societies it is easy to overlook this important time and simply attempt to resume like as usual; this tendency should be resisted and midwives should prepare their clients for this instruction to rest well ahead of the birth.

The rule of thumb is, unless there are varicose veins (discussed next): spend the first two weeks in the bed (of course she can get up to bathe, dress, use the toilet and eat meals, overall this means spending about 80% of her time in bed). The next two weeks should be spent "near the bed" and the final two weeks are spent "around the bed." More advice that is good for every mother to follow can be found below under "unsutured tears."

Hemorrhoids and varicose veins

Hemorrhoids commonly appear or become aggravated during pregnancy (review hemorrhoid anatomy on page 102). They arise from highly vascular submucosal cushions of the anal canal, which differ from the rest of the GI tract. Rather than forming a continuous ring, this mucosa is present in only three areas: 2 o'clock on the posterior anal canal, 5 o'clock on the anterior aspect and 9 o'clock on the left lateral anal wall. Hemorrhoids are the abnormal dilation of veins in one or more of these cushions.

Internal hemorrhoids, if large enough, may eventually be pulled down through the anal opening. Closure of the sphincter then strangulates the prolapsed hemorrhoid, occasionally leading to thrombosis. If hemorrhoids arise below the pectinate line, they present at the anal opening as external swellings where they more commonly undergo thrombosis. An external skin tag can form from an old skin fold that was once a thrombosed hemorrhoid. Trauma, irritation, sedentary jobs and straining during defecation increase the risk of thrombosis.

Hemorrhoids make many a woman's postpartum recovery miserable. Rutin, a bioflavonoid, is remarkably helpful for shrinking hemorrhoids in some cases (up to 50 mg daily). Women can also prepare a witch hazel or white oak bark infusion by pouring 1 pint of boiling water over 1 oz of the herb and steeping for 10 hours. Refrigerate the infusion (to preserve it). The woman should soak a gauze pad or square of old diaper in the infusion, and apply the pad to her sore hemorrhoids several times daily. She may use it hot or cold, as she prefers. It will shrink the hemorrhoids quickly, even if they are very enlarged. These herbs are very astringent, so she should avoid soaking her stitches. But if hemorrhoids are a problem and there are sutures near her rectum, two 15 minute soaks a day may help. Reducing the edema will also help the area heal.

Hemorrhoids may be gently replaced inside the anus with a gloved finger and a bit of vitamin E oil after each bowel movement. You can leave her some gloves so she can do this herself. This will also help to relieve venous congestion.

Varicose veins in the vulva will usually shrink remarkably once the pressure from the pregnancy is gone. If a woman has varicosities in her legs as well, she should not stay in bed full time, as this encourages clot formation in her veins; light, gentle activity is important. If support hose have been worn during the pregnancy, she can continue wearing them for 4 to 6 weeks postpartum (i.e., until the blood volume reduces and the vessels return to their nonpregnant size). If hot spots, whitish swelling, leg or foot pain, fever or malaise should develop in a woman with varicosed veins, do not massage the area because this could cause a clot to become dislodged and travel to the heart or lungs, which could be fatal. The woman should continue light activity; this will usually help these areas resolve. If not, she should consult an obstetrician without delay.

More about the care of varicose veins will be found in Vol III of HOLISTIC MIDWIFERY.

Unsutured tears

In addition to all of the other suggestions given above, advise the woman to keep her legs together and minimize abrasion from clothing for at least two weeks (because a wound is weakest at the 7 to 10 day mark). This means no tailor sitting; no pants, underwear, sanitary napkins, tampons, cups or sponges; no swinging her legs over and out of a waterbed or car; no running up and down stairs numerous times daily; no sexual activity that involves disturbing the stitches and no lifting anything heavier than her newborn. She should refrain from all activities that strain the perineal area.

Fresh comfrey or another soothing herbal poultice such as plantain leaf can be applied 3 to 4 times daily to promote cell regeneration. To prepare, whiz fresh, clean leaves in a blender or food processor with just enough water to process. (This concoction can be made in advance and frozen in an ice cube tray. The cubes can be thawed one at a time, as needed.) If no fresh comfrey is available, steep dry comfrey for an hour or more. Place some of the wet leaves in a gauze pad soaked in infusion. Carefully apply either preparation twice daily. The woman can also drink comfrey infusion freely throughout the day.

Anal sphincter or rectal mucosa repair

To minimize the chances of infection, a 15 minute hot rosemary sitz bath should be taken two or three times daily. In addition to the recommended supplements for all tears, one dropperful of echinacea root tincture may be taken 3 to 4 times daily.

It is important to maintain good bowel function. The mother should refrain from eating foods she knows cause her constipation and eat plenty of fruit. Prune or black cherry juice can be taken daily to promote soft stools. Although some babies get gas when their mothers drink prune juice, most have no adverse reaction to black cherry juice. If damage was extensive or the woman has a history of difficult bowel movements, consider suggesting a stool softener, available over-the-counter in drug stores, for the first couple weeks postpartum. Some women hold back their first bowel movement for fear of hurting themselves. Explain that resisting the urge to go will only cause more fluid to be absorbed from the stool and make passage more difficult. This will not help the stitches. The woman should relax and let go, supporting the perineum with her fingers if this is more comfortable for her (Noble, 1995).

When misplaced stitches have been removed from the anorectal wall

Follow the precautions to minimize infection given in the previous section. Increase the sitz baths to three or four daily. Have the mother call you at the first sign of infection.

Resuming sexual activity

Most first-time parents eagerly await the return to "normal life." It doesn't happen, and sexuality is no exception. Even when no tears have occurred, not only does the perineum need time to return to its nonpregnant state, but it will never be exactly the same. Nursing means a woman has someone touching and wanting something from her all the time. For many women, it does not help to have her partner wanting something from her, too. In addition, hormonal changes and fatigue influence a woman's desire for sex (or lack thereof). Many women feel the need for rest and personal space when baby is asleep. This is sometimes interpreted as rejection by the partner, who probably hasn't had a day filled with lots of close contact and touching. During this adjustment period, it is very important to encourage the couple to communicate their feelings to each other in a nondefensive manner.

Taking all of the above into consideration, women should feel they want to be sexual before relations resume. Physiologically, the cervix should be closed and the perineum healed. Closure of the cervix is usually signaled by the cessation of the lochia at about two to three weeks, but it is really best to wait six weeks if there has been a tear or a repair of a cervical or perineal laceration. There should be no discomfort or bleeding. Explain these things to partners and encourage them to think in terms of creative intimacy and giving rather than receiving.

Once a woman is ready to resume yoni penetration with her partner, advise her that postpartum hormones will tend to cause yoni dryness. Water-based lubricant can be used, along with positions which minimize pressure. If perineal damage has been extensive, or raw areas have been left to regranulate, the longer she waits to resume penetration, the better.

Examining Tears and Repairs in the Weeks Postpartum

Normal discomfort after a tear or repair

Any report of discomfort should be investigated. When anesthetic is used topically and you have repaired as I have recommended, most women will be almost pain free by 24 hours. Frequently, most of the pain is gone shortly after the suturing is finished. Even unrepaired labial tears are only sensitive the first day. (This is not the rule when large quantities of local anesthetic have been used, which can leave women quite uncomfortable for a week or more.)

Cases of excessive natural swelling are exceptions to this rule. The quality of some women's tissues seem to produce more swelling when traumatized. I've noticed this to be especially true for fair-skinned women, particularly redheads. In my experience, such swelling, either natural or induced, causes significant discomfort for several days, lasting until the edema resolves. This is true regardless of the extent of the tear or the type of repair that has been done. Homeopathic remedies, local applications of cold (for the first 24 hours) and then heat, and time are the only remedies.

However, women vary in their responses to suturing. Women with extensive repairs are usually sensitive for a few days (but invariably report that it is nothing like the discomfort they felt during a previous recovery from a lidocaine-loaded hospital repair). Slight itching is frequently reported a few days after birth. This is a normal by-product of suture breakdown and the healing process, not a concern. Severe itching may indicate an allergic reaction to the suture, to an anesthetic or even to an herb being used for healing.

Often, repaired skin tags are sensitive, especially at the point where they are tacked up at the tip. Once healing is well underway (past 10 days), vitamin E oil can be expressed from an punctured capsule directly onto the area. Areas left raw can be similarly sensitive, and vitamin E can help heal those as well. In very rare cases, if the tear has been excessively deep or difficult to repair, or if the mother is especially sensitive, it may take even longer for it to feel right again. Nonetheless, if all is going well with your repairs, you should hear about significant postpartum discomfort from only a small minority of your clients.

Examining tears and repairs

When you are learning, you should check all tears at every postpartum visit whether they have been repaired or not. Checking tears will help you learn what heals best with sutures and what without. Once you've become more sure of your skill, a simple inquiry regarding pain or tenderness may suffice. Unusual or complicated repairs, or those with which you have had little experience, should be checked at every visit, so that you can learn how they heal.

During your exam, remember that the tissue heals from the inside out. The skin will invariably separate slightly as healing takes place no matter how well you have put it together. When you are first learning, you may even conclude that the whole repair is threatening to break down. It probably isn't. Repairs look very different during the process of transforming into healed tissue.

Once healing commences, tissue edges and raw surfaces will at first appear mottled creamy pinkish white, as they begin to form a new layer. Do not mistake this healthy response for a sign of infection, which may cause the wound surface to have a yellow, greenish or beige discharge. Dead tissue will appear black. After a few days, the mottled light pink areas will become beefy red, signaling the appearance of healthy granulation tissue (Stotts, 1990). While the yoni mucosa is not subject to keloid scarring, some women form excessive granulation tissue in the yoni mucosa.

Therefore, you can't really judge how a tear will come together until the sixth week postpartum. This is especially true of skin tags, which often shrink remarkably. Give them a chance to heal before you decide to cut them off.

Removing partially dissolved synthetic stitches

If synthetic suture has been used, it may still be in the tissue for some time after it has served its purpose (due to its slower breakdown time), causing irritation and slight soreness. Localized tenderness or pain is more concerning. Pain accompanied by increased swelling or inflammation could be due to an allergic reaction or possibly an infection. Check further for what might be happening (see the following chapters).

Women may report that the sutures are falling out or causing irritation. Although I don't recommend removing partially dissolved sutures routinely, they can be taken out if the tear is healed and the mother is extremely uncomfortable. Do not do so before 15 days or so, depending on how the repaired area looks. Since synthetic is used for its staying power, removing it too soon will defeat its purpose.

To remove interrupted stitches when the knot is still intact (likely with synthetic), elevate the knot with tissue forceps or a hemostat and slip one scissor blade below the stitch. Cut one side of the strand below the knot as close to the tissue as possible. Hold the knot in a straight line with the thread's entry point and pull it in one continuous motion to remove the stitch. Try not to pull any suture that was left exposed above the skin surface during repair back through the tissue as it is being removed (Sherris & Kern, 2004).

Take care not to cut the exposed part of the loop in two places, which will leave a fragment of suture in the tissue. Be careful to note where knots are so you don't accidently drag one through the tissue. If continuous suture is still intact you may have to cut in several places before you remove it, but each loop should be cut and then removed one at a time to avoid confusion.

If you must remove continuous basting (over-and-over) stitches, begin by grasping one knotted end and using your stitch scissors with the C-shaped tip to cut the looped end. Then continue down one side, cutting each loop flush with the tissue surface. Then pull each stitch out as you would for an interrupted stitch.

To remove locked mattress stitches, again start at one end, grasp the knot and cut the loop. Continue down the length of the suture line, cutting each locking loop as you go. Then remove each stitch as for removing a simple interrupted stitch.

If intracuticular stitches must be removed, avoid unduly disrupting the wound by only cutting out those parts of the strand that can be reached easily. Since you are using dissolvable suture and since these stitches were buried, they will eventually disappear.

If the stitch does not come out easily, apply a saline-soaked gauze pad to the area for a few minutes and try again. (Make saline solution by adding ¼ tsp of table salt to 1 cup of water.) If it still won't come out after soaking, cut the bothersome end flush with the tissue and leave it alone.

Sometimes women note fragments of chromic suture coming out between 7 to 10 days postpartum. If there is no inflammation, this is due to the suture's normal breakdown process. In most cases this can be allowed to take place without stitch removal, since chromic will completely dissolve much more quickly than synthetic. If chromic suture requires removal, follow the same procedure as described for synthetic materials.

When suture or knot migration has occurred: If suture or a knot that was originally buried extrudes through the skin, use a hemostat to gently tug the end free and remove it; trim the loop if necessary. If pulling on the knot is painful, stop and apply topical local anesthetic and allow it to take effect before proceeding.

If suture has migrated up through the tissue so that it is visible but hasn't extruded through the skin, it is somewhat more difficult to remove. Cleanse the skin with povidone iodine or a similar product. Apply topical local anesthetic to the skin. Make a tiny stab incision using either a no. 11 surgical blade or the beveled tip of an 18-gauge syringe needle over the nonextruded suture. If using a needle, you may need to pick open the hole it makes a bit, which may require more local anesthetic once the skin is broken. Now insert a small, sterile, stainless steel crochet hook under the skin to hook under the suture and pull it out through the incision. You may then need to use a hemostat to grasp the end and pull gently to remove it. Do not pull too hard as the suture may still be attached to a loop, which may need to be cut with your stitch scissors. Then remove the knot by gently pulling on the end (Lam, 2007). It may help to use a gentle on-and-off tugging motion.

Identifying a fistula or sinus tract

Fistulas are holes that typically form between the yoni and rectal wall when a perineal tear extends into the rectum and is either unrecognized or improperly repaired or when the development of infection leads to the breakdown of a repair, leaving a hole. Depending upon its location, a healed hole or fistula may result in the involuntary discharge of urine or feces from the yoni or even the perineum if an anal fistula has formed.

Rectovaginal fistulas present with a yoni discharge that has a fecal odor, recurrent or chronic infection, and the passage of gas via the yoni. The passage of stool through the yoni is most often noted when the woman has diarrhea, unless the fistula is large. Associated sphincter incontinence may also be present resulting from disruption at the time of the original injury. If there is an underlying disease present, blood and mucus in the stool or diarrhea may be chronic. An anal fistula typically becomes infected, may present a bright red border around the skin opening and often drains a purulent discharge.

A small vesicovaginal fistula may mimic stress incontinence. Urine may also pool in the yoni at night, creating the impression that the woman is dry at night. Such damage must be surgically repaired.

The chapters entitled "Functional Disorders of the Urinary Tract" and "Anorectal Disorders and Incontinence" cover fistulas in more detail; if you suspect a fistula, refer to the appropriate chapter.

Cauterizing a sensitive area

Small sensitive areas that have not healed by the 6 week visit may be treated with a 75% silver nitrate/25% potassium nitrate swab. Barely moisten the swab and apply it directly to the sensitive area, being careful not to touch the surrounding tissue. Carefully paint the spot and then remove the swab, leaving the swab in contact with the tissue for just a second or two. Do not rinse.

This treatment will often result in a less sensitive area that heals well. Small pinholes along the line of the repair or any area that continues to feel sore may benefit. Still, application will cause intense burning for about 5 minutes and will lengthen the healing period somewhat. Most sensitive areas will feel better eventually without this treatment, but silver nitrate may speed the process (Leonard, 1991; Sorger, 1990). Vitamin E oil can be applied to the area starting the day after cauterization to help soothe and heal the tissue.

About 75% silver nitrate/25% potassium nitrate swabs: This combination of caustic chemicals has been called "toughened silver nitrate." It allows application to a specific area of tissue without the chemicals spreading to adjacent areas. Forming a dense surface film of coagulated albumin (protein) on contact, it seals the tissue and prevents deep penetration of the chemicals. It should not be washed off when used in the perineal area. These chemicals are recommended for application to wounds and weepy areas and for removal of small tags or overgrowths of scar tissue.

Effects and reactions: Silver nitrate blackens or grays on contact with skin, although this discoloration will gradually disappear. No such color change occurs when it is applied to an open wound. It has a marked germicidal effect and leaves the tissue free of bacteria to heal cleanly. Treatment commonly causes burning upon contact, but may also cause tingling, irritation, scaling and drying. Extreme reactions include excessive tenderness, inflammation and ring-shaped warts.

Storage: Exposure of the swabs to light may cause oxidation, which leads to darkening, but does not affect the therapeutic action of the swab. Humidity or moisture will often cause the tips to loosen and fall off, however. Therefore, swabs should be kept in a dry, dark place.

Mysterious lumps and bumps

A lump can be formed by a clogged vestibular gland, a hematoma, a cyst, a piece of suture that has migrated or an abscess. If you find a painless swelling that does not disappear by the 6 week exam, get a second opinion regarding what it may be. If it is painful, get another opinion immediately.

Scar or excessive granulation tissue often forms a very firm lump or ridge. If this occurs, massaging vitamin E and evening primrose oils into the area may help reduce it. (Also see the chapters entitled "Inclusion Cysts," "Puerperal Hematomas" and "Perineal Infections.")

If there are recurrent problems with your repairs

If you find many women complaining of discomfort, if repairs come apart or if pain persists for weeks and months postpartum, you need to reevaluate your technique. The reasons for any of the above problems could be:

- Sewing too tightly
- Putting too many stitches too close together
- Improper alignment of tissue
- Poor knot-tying technique
- Excessive use of anesthetic, rendering the tissue so swollen that accurate approxi-

mation of the tissue is impossible
•Attempting repairs that you are not yet skilled enough to tackle

If you are approximating tissues poorly, you probably need more help identifying structures that are damaged before you continue to suture without supervision. If poor technique seems to be the problem, go back and practice basic techniques. Women do not have to hurt after being sutured. Refine your technique and skills to minimize their postpartum discomfort and optimize the chance of a well-healed repair.

Allergic Reactions to Suture Materials

Identifying allergic reactions

Suture reactions are uncommon but tend to happen more with chromic than synthetic suture. A reaction may produce abscesses and a whitish discharge from the area. This does not necessarily indicate an infection, just excessive inflammation (white blood cell activity) due to the reaction. The sutures in the immediate area may come undone, or the whole repair may break down. When gut material has been used, an allergic reaction commonly presents with stitches falling out at about four days postpartum. Gut materials produce more inflammation in general, and the increased enzyme reaction from the allergy causes it to break down more rapidly.

To differentiate between a suture and an anesthetic reaction, rub a cotton swab soaked in anesthetic on the woman's inner cheek. If any reaction other than numbness (such as itching) occurs, she probably has an anesthetic reaction. Although the test is not 100% reliable, if it is negative, she may have a suture reaction or an infection. Reactions to either anesthetic or suture material may be accompanied by tenderness, swelling and irritation. Significant redness may also indicate an infection is present.

An allergic reaction to iodine-based antiseptic solutions may result in local redness, swelling and irritation. Some women may react to latex exam gloves. If a woman is highly allergic to latex, using vinyl gloves is the best alternative. If a woman knows she is extremely environmentally sensitive, have her order vinyl gloves to have on hand for you at the birth (if gloves are part of the birthing kits you have clients order; otherwise, order them yourself).

Treating allergic reactions

No matter what the underlying allergy, hot rosemary infusion sitz baths three times daily will help relieve the discomfort and resolve the problem (that is, if she is not allergic to rosemary). If allergies to herbs are suspected, use normal saline instead. When inflammation is apparent, freely irrigate the area with normal saline solution (1 tsp salt to 1 quart water) or Ringer's lactate twice daily before bathing for the first 24 hours. This will help carry away dead cells. Hydrogen peroxide could also be used the first time but should not be used repeatedly since it tends to cause minor tissue damage. However, it is good at removing surface debris from a wound. Otherwise, care for the area as suggested in the chapter entitled "Postpartum Care and Comfort Measures."

Be sure the woman understands that she had an allergic reaction and knows what she reacted to so that she can inform future care providers.

Perineal Infections

NOTE: Review the chapters in the part entitled "Basic Surgical Principles" before reading this chapter.

Luckily for mothers and midwives, the genital area is remarkably resistant to infection. This is partly due its rich vascular supply, resulting in well-oxygenated tissue from which toxins are promptly removed. The incidence of local abscess is about 1%, and superficial wound infections occur in 0.5 to 3% of hospital populations.

An undamaged perineum is at the least risk of infection. Infections are far less common among women who give birth at home and those who have not received clitorotomies, although any woman living in a hot, humid environment is at more risk because organisms tend to flourish in warm environments. Repairs are more likely to become infected in women who have had extensive tears or cuts repaired in the hospital (where there are more pathologic organisms) or who have rectal mucosa repairs. No data support the notion that an incision is less likely to become infected than a tear (Owen & Hauth, 1990).

In addition to the birth environment, many things can increase the likelihood of infection. These contributing factors include:

- Poor maternal diet, health or hygiene as well as anemia
- Smoking
- Diabetes
- Uterine infection (with infected lochia pouring over the sutured area)
- Inadequate asepsis during the repair
- An infected hematoma from which organisms may spread to surrounding areas
- Passage of the needle or leaving a stitch through the bowel wall during suturing (which carries contaminated matter into the repair) or leaving a stitch through the anorectal wall into the lumen of the bowel.
- A repair done in close proximity to the rectum, where stitches become contaminated
- Excessive edema or tight stitches (strangulates tissue, which reduces circulation and lymphatic flow)
- Poor hemostasis (leading to blood pooling and organism growth)
- Too many stitches, too close together, which impedes circulation
- An unrecognized or poorly repaired tear in the rectal mucosa
- A pocket tear that has been carelessly repaired or has been left open to collect lochia, thereby inviting infection
- Any type of immune suppressing condition

Identifying an infected laceration or incision

At each postpartum visit, evaluate the perineum for normal appearance and healing. An infected laceration or incision should be identified early so it does not become more serious. Signs and symptoms include the following:

- Localized pain
- Painful urination (dysuria)
- Low-grade temperature—usually below 101 °F (38.3 °C)

- •Edema
- •Heat, redness and inflamation along the edges of the laceration
- •Oozing of pus or gray-green exudate from the incision or tear
- •Wound separation or dehiscence (Varney et al., 2004).

Severities of perineal infection

Shy and Eschenbach (1979) described four degrees of severity of infection:

Simple, mild infection: Simple infections are limited to the skin and superficial fascia along the line of tissue damage presenting with swelling, redness and local tenderness; and, in some cases, a purulent yellow, beige or greenish discharge exuding from the suture line. Skin necrosis, systemic symptoms (such as changes in pulse rate or fever), and bullae (fluid-filled surface lesions) are not present. Mild infections are rarely life threatening but may cause significant discomfort for the mother.

Superficial fascial infection without necrosis: The two layers of superficial fascia that overlie the perineal region may be involved in an infection of intermediate depth. Two varieties of infection may occur: the most common is a superficial infection without necrosis. There is nothing strikingly different about these infections to distinguish them from the less common and more serious superficial infection with necrosis. The overlying skin is usually firm and may appear red. Severe systemic signs are not present. Thus, it is usually difficult to determine the actual extent of the infection without surgical exploration.

Oral antibiotics are called for, and the infection should begin to resolve 24 to 48 hours after antibiotics are begun. If there is no response or symptoms become worse during the first 24 to 48 hours of oral antibiotic treatment, prompt wound exploration in hospital is imperative: deaths have occurred when these types of infections were not followed up appropriately.

Superficial fascial infection with necrosis (necrotizing fasciitis [fah-SIGH-tis]): This life-threatening infection causes destruction of the superficial fascial layers that typically prevent deeper invasion by pathogenic organisms. There is a high fatality rate, ranging from 21 to 76%. It has an acute onset and a rapid course with prominent systemic signs and symptoms. The overlying skin may display marked edema and redness early on in this process. The circumference of the affected area often enlarges and becomes somewhat indistinct as the infection gets worse.

Signs of local infection rapidly progress to necrosis of both layers of the superficial perineal fascia as the infection spreads along facial planes. Along these facial "highways," the infection may travel from the fatty and membranous layers of the vulva to the abdomen, the lower abdominal wall, the buttocks or the thighs. The inferior fascia of the perineal membrane and levator ani muscles are usually spared, although deep muscle infections can occur as well.

Marked, localized tenderness with induration (firmness) is typically present, progressing to nerve damage; numbness may occur over time. Since the skin is not the primary site of infection, skin manifestations vary, and diagnosis cannot be made by visual inspection alone.

Nevertheless, swelling and redness with indistinct margins that fade into normal areas are characteristic, as is anemia, although anemia is frequently masked by fluid shifts that produce hemoconcentration as edema progresses.

As the infection advances, the blood vessels supplying the skin may become occluded, and the skin may start to breakdown, developing bullae, ulcers, coolness to the touch and a blue-violet to reddish-brown discoloration. Surgical exploration is required to discover the extent of the infection. Advanced tissue destruction (necrosis) and Fournier gangrene (necrotizing perineal infection) is demonstrated first by a wooden feel to the tissue. As necrosis becomes established, the tissue rots, revealed by a lack of tissue resistance to probing, either with the examining finger or an instrument (this means your probe punches almost effortlessly through the skin surface). Drainage of the area may result in a thin, bloody to cloudy gray discharge. If blisters form, the area may take on the appearance of a third-degree burn. **Crepitation** (kre-pee-TA-shun)—a dry, cracking sound or sensation elicited when finger pressure is applied to the affected tissue—may occur.

Aches, pain and fever progressing to restlessness, drowsiness and confusion present the picture of a woman who is extremely ill. In a significant number of cases, however, there is no fever and a general lack of severe overt symptoms, even though pain is typically out of proportion to these other signs in these women (Owen & Hauth, 1990).

Delayed recognition of necrosis often leads to death due to a combination of massive extracellular fluid accumulation and bacterial infection resulting in vascular and organ collapse.

Myofasciitis with or without necrosis/myonecrosis (MY-oh-knee-CROW-sis). Myofascitis involves the superficial fascia of the perineal membrane and surrounding musculature. It may develop as a progression of superficial fasciitis. Myonecrosis of the gluteal or psoas muscles can also occur when bacteria is introduced via the needle used to give a pudendal or paracervical block (something to consider if you are following a woman after birth who was transported and received either intervention). In these cases, the onset of pain begins soon after birth and is inconsistent with the normal appearance of the perineal area. This is because the infection is deep inside. Deep pelvic hematoma should be ruled out as it can mimic a hidden infection by causing internal pain and pressure. If infection is causing the symptoms, lab findings will be consistent with an infectious process. Immediate transport for surgical exploration and aggressive treatment is called for.

Infection-related microorganisms

Numerous organisms have been cultured from infected perineal tissues, including gram-positive cocci (typically group A hemolytic streptococci); gram-negative aerobes, which require oxygen to live; and various anaerobic strains, which require an oxygen-free environment in order to survive. It has been suggested that some organisms may act in concert to increase tissue damage. Although a variety of organisms may be involved in infections, it is often impossible to culture them without surgical débridement. This is particularly true of anaerobic organisms. In fact, the absence of a positive culture in a case of clinically evident infection strongly suggests an anaerobic infection. Antibiotic therapy should take this possibility into consideration (Owen & Hauth, 1990).

Whenever the mother manifests a serious infection, the baby should be watched carefully for signs of infection as well and be examined by a pediatrician as soon as possible if an infection is suspected. Be sure to observe scrupulous handwashing and barrier precautions so that a perineal infection is not inadvertently transmitted to the baby through careless technique.

Related organisms include *Beta*-hemolytic streptococci; in this case infection may develop early after birth but usually does not present until 3 to 5 days after birth. Methicillin-resistant *Staphylococcus aureus* and Strep-α is often found as well.

Although necrotizing soft tissue infections can be monomicrobial, they usually are synergistic polymicrobial infections. Elliott and associates (2000) found only 28 of 182 patients developed necrotizing skin infections from single pathogens; the rest had poly-microbial infections (average of 4.4 organisms in the original wound cultures). In this series, the majority of monomicrobial infections were caused by streptococcal isolates such as *Beta*-hemolytic strep (usually group A streptococci or *Strep. pyogenes*). Other frequently cited causes of monomicrobial necrotizing soft tissue infections include *Staph. aureus* and *Clostridium perfringens*.

In polymicrobial infections, the most frequently isolated organisms in necrotizing soft tissue infections are combinations of staphylococci (especially *Staph. epidermidis,* sometimes in combination with *Beta*-hemolytic streptococci, usually group A), enterococci, Enterobacteriaceae species (commonly *Escherichia coli*, *Proteus mirabilis*, *Klebsiella pneumoniae* and *Pseudomonas aeruginosa*), streptococci, Bacteroides/Prevotella species, anaerobic gram-positive cocci, and Clostridium species.

In a review of all types of necrotizing infections, Headley (2003) discovered that polymicrobial infections occurred in 59 to 71% of cases, while some 29% were caused by single pathogens. In 2% of infections, no organisms grew from intraoperative culture. Johnson and associates (1998) found that more than 90% of nonclostridial polymicrobial necrotizing soft tissue infections involved *Beta*-hemolytic streptococci or coagulase-positive staphylococci; the remaining 10% were attributed to gram-negative enteric bacteria. In some instances, fungi have also been cultured from polymicrobial infections.

Perhaps the only generalization that can be made about polymicrobial necrotizing soft tissue infections is that aerobic and anaerobic organisms are frequently found in combination. Because of culture results, necrotizing soft tissue infections have previously been categorized as type I or type II infections. Type I infections are mixed infections generated by anaerobic and facultative bacteria ("facultative" refers to organisms that can survive in more than one type of environment) whereas type II infections generally are caused by group A streptococci. Staphylococci also may be found in conjunction with group A streptococci.

Treating wound infections

Mild infections: Women with mild, localized infections that only present with heat, redness and inflammation can be treated expectantly with careful perianal hygiene and frequent herbal sitz baths. First, irrigate the tear or repair freely with normal saline (1 tsp salt to 1 quart water) or Ringer's lactate before each bath. Hydrogen peroxide could also be used the first time or two, but it should not be used repeatedly, because it tends to cause minor tissue damage and thus may impair healing over the long-term. If allergies are not an issue, the mother can begin to take three hot rosemary sitz baths daily. If the wound is quite deep or if the mother is allergic to rosemary, plain Epsom salts baths should be used instead; use ½ cup Epsom salts and mix thoroughly. Any of these rinses and soaks help clean the wound, promote healing and remove surface slough. The woman can also take a ½ dropperful of Echinacea root tincture 4 times daily and a total of 5000 mg of vitamin C with bioflavonoids spaced throughout the day. Follow the progress of healing with daily home visits until the infection is resolved. Unless it gets worse, a mild infection generally does not require antibiotics.

The area should be rechecked in 12 hours to be sure the condition of the wound is improving or sooner if the mother reports that symptoms are worsening. If the infection has not begun to resolve by 24 hours with the above therapies alone and the repair has not spontaneously broken down, the stitches should be removed (see chapter entitled "Examining Tears and Repairs in the Weeks Postpartum"). This will allow drainage, especially if the area is abscessed. If any symptom is worsening or if the woman seems to have an apparently unrelated systemic response of any kind in the presence of a perineal wound, transport immediately because either could be a sign of a deep and dangerous infectious process.

Moderate to severe infections: Treatment of more established infections—those that display perineal abscess or purulent drainage; systemic symptoms, such as fever; extensive repair breakdown or all of these—usually involves removing any stitches, opening the wound to allow drainage, biopsying and culturing the wound, débriding and cleaning the wound, and administering broad-spectrum antimicrobial drugs. Examination should include a recto-vaginal exam to rule out a missed rectovaginal injury that could be a source of wound contamination. After 6 days or so, if the wound is free of purulent discharge and covered with healthy, pink granulation tissue, it can be re-repaired. Ideally, it would be best to have all suspected wound infections evaluated by a hospital practitioner who has lots of experience treating perineal wounds (Tharpe, 2008).

Very serious infection: A serious infection may be present if ordinary treatment measures are not quickly resolving the symptoms. If redness persists or more generalized signs of infection appear (such as fever, aches and chills), antibiotics may be necessary. Whenever an infection seems serious, get an obstetrical consultation immediately.

Treatment of serious infections includes aggressive antibiotic therapy and surgical débridement of the infected tissue under general anesthesia by a physician. The removal of infected tissue should extend to clearly healthy tissue margins, after which temporary tissue grafts made from pigs, human cadavers or amniotic membrane may be applied in preparation for permanent tissue grafts. Grafts made from pig tissue are widely available and are less expensive but must be changed every two days. Cadaverous tissue is more expensive but may remain in place until the permanent grafts are established (Owen & Hauth, 1990).

If the surgeon recommends sitz baths as part of the postsurgery care plan, hot soaks in strong plantain leaf infusion (an excellent remedy for old, infected wounds) can be used for this purpose. The perineum should then be blotted dry with a clean towel and briefly exposed to a heat lamp.

<u>Débriding tissue at home</u>: If you are working where medical care is scarce, such as a resource-poor country, your only option may be to débride the tissue yourself. This can be done if the necrotic tissue is very superficial; otherwise hospital transport will be required, as débridement will require anesthesia and surgery. Do not attempt this yourself unless you have been trained.

If the necrotic tissue appears to be shallow (a crap shoot at best since you won't know until you begin débriding the wound), open the wound and use dry gauze pads and rub the surface of the wound until healthy bleeding tissue is exposed. To do so, first spray the area with topical 10% anesthetic; have normal sterile saline on hand to rinse the area as you proceed to débride the tissue. Do not repair the wound again at this time as this is likely to result in the formation of an abscess. Even if débridement is not necessary, the infected wound edges should be gently parted and allowed to drain. If the wound requires more than superficial débridement, which will be the case if there is significant necrosis, you will not be able to do this outside a hospital.

After débridement, the therapies already explained in this chapter should be continued as outlined. Antibiotic drugs are recommended if the area of involvement is extensive or not resolving rapidly. The wound can be allowed to heal by secondary intention or re-repaired once the entire wound is covered with a layer of healthy granulation tissue. If a third- or fourth-degree tear is involved, it is best to attempt repair when all signs of infection have resolved. Serious superficial infection (cellulitis [SELL-you-LIE-tis]) is indicated by an enlarging red area. Surgery is recommended whenever significant skin changes, including edema, appear outside the local wound area (Owen & Hauth, 1990).

<u>Hematomas and perineal infections</u>

Unrecognized hematomas can become infected and may abscess. If a hematoma appears to be involved in an infection and the line of sutures has not already spontaneously parted, it should be opened by removing the stitches, and the hematoma should then be drained. This is best done in a hospital setting by someone familiar with this type of treatment. See the chapter entitled "Puerperal Hematomas" for more information.

<u>The effect of an infection on suture materials</u>

Polyfilament synthetics, such as Dexon and Vicryl, are associated with a minimal inflammatory response except in the presence of infection, when they actually promote inflammation. This is attributed to the ability of bacteria to penetrate and colonize the spaces between the braided fibers in the strand. White blood cells, such as granulocytes and macrophages, are too large to enter between the fibers and therefore cannot destroy the bacteria. The result is a marked inflammatory response as the system tries to overcome the persistent presence of pathological bacteria in the strands of suture. Infection may slow the breakdown of synthetic materials somewhat (but does not prolong retention of its tensile strength). Thus, the suture remains in the tissue harboring bacteria and encouraging inflammation. If signs of infection are not resolving, remove synthetic suture promptly.

In contrast, infection has the opposite effect on gut material. Increased inflammation, with its accompanying enzyme response, causes it to break down rapidly. Loose strands of suture should be gently removed from the perineal area, with attention to knot location (i.e., don't pull the knot through the tissue). Then proceed with therapies as outlined above (Sanz, 1987).

I now include a very funny story involving a former client and a very supportive back-up doctor. This, the only perineal infection I have seen, involved a case of a very bad tear in an extremely swollen perineum. This labor had resulted in a hospital transport prior to birth, so the doctor sewed her up (after using a large amount of local anesthetic). I remarked that it looked as though he was sewing awfully tight. "No," he assured me, "this will heal fine." Well, a week or so later she had a perineal infection for which she needed antibiotics. When it came time to resume intercourse, she said her yoni would barely admit a finger.

Determined to solve the problem, she sent her husband to the local "marital aid" emporium to purchase a variety of differently sized dildoes, the only thing she could think of to uniformly stretch the tissues. Her husband had a hard time explaining to the clerk why he needed them (and in such variety), but his wife felt it only fair that he, as a primary stakeholder, participate in resolving the situation.

After a month or so of gradual stretching, she took her collection of dildoes to her doctor, deposited them on his office desk and informed him that these were what she had to use to overcome his suturing job. He was quite embarrassed, but the point was made!

If a Repair Breaks Down

NOTE: Review the part entitled "Basic Surgical Principles" before reading this chapter.

The incidence of repair breakdown, or simple dehiscence (de-HISS-ens), in the absence of infection, is not known for certain, but it appears to be an infrequent occurrence. Repairs are more prone to break down in the presence of:

- Unhealthy tissue
- Inadequate rest postpartum (moving around too vigorously)
- Stitches tied too tightly
- Stitches placed with poor technique (a rare cause)
- Allergic reaction to suture material or anesthetic
- Infection (especially in the presence of chromic gut stitches)
- Cigarette smoking, diabetes or other immune-compromising condition
- Clinically evident venereal warts
- Suture material that is too thick or too thin for the task
- Hematoma
- Trauma

Poor nutrition, anemia, avascular scar tissue from previous repairs, devitalization of tissue from the use of crushing instruments, or using suture material that is inappropriately sized can all contribute to poor healing, although the repair may not actually break down.

However, even when good surgical technique has been used and bleeding is well controlled, dehiscence sometimes occurs.

Recognizing dehiscence

Obvious dehiscence involves the coming loose of all, or nearly all, of the stitches and will be apparent on inspection. It may be harder to tell what is going on if there is only partial breakdown of a repair due to infection. Here, you must look for signs or symptoms of infection as well such as pain, fever, induration (firm feel to the tissue) and purulent discharge.

Superficial dehiscence

Breakdown of a repair in the absence of infection is uncommon. When stitches do come apart, mechanical trauma (for example, from beginning intercourse too soon) or an allergic reaction to suture materials may play a part.

If a minor repair totally disintegrates, herbal baths and compresses and the use of a heat lamp two to three times daily will usually result in a well-healed perineum. In most cases, any attempt to redo the repair is unnecessary.

Dehiscence of deeper tears

If the tear is more extensive, it will probably heal better if it is repaired. The procedure is as follows:

1. Inspect the area to establish the extent of breakdown and look for clinical signs of

infection or wound contamination.

2. Clean and débride the wound. First administer local anesthetic (such as a gel) several minutes prior to treatment. Remove suture fragments with a needle holder and a pair of tissue forceps. Then remove all inflamed, necrotic or partially healed tissue by scrubbing the wound with sterile gauze pads. Irrigate the wound with sterile saline, diluted hydrogen peroxide (just once) or diluted povidone-iodine solution (do not use scrub). If you cannot get down to clean tissue with gauze pads, the wound needs to be débrided more thoroughly in a hospital.
3. Administer broad-spectrum antibiotics if infection is present or there is significant cellulitis.
4. Cleansing and healing of the tissues should take place for the next 1 to 4 days. Scrub and clean the wound at least twice daily using disposable surgical scrub brushes impregnated with povidone-iodine or use gauze pads (which is the gentler option).
5. Between scrubs, use sitz baths frequently to keep the wound clean. At least three daily sitz baths of rosemary infusion (1 qt water to 1 oz rosemary steeped overnight) can help cleanse the area. On the contrary, if the wound is deep, use only normal saline solution as excessive absorption of an herb solution could be toxic to some individuals. Once infection is eliminated and healing is underway, comfrey sitz baths can be used to promote cell growth.
6. Rule out clotting and CBC (complete blood count) abnormalities via laboratory blood tests. This is done to determine if clotting abnormalities have developed secondary to infection or a hidden hematoma. A CBC would also determine if a marked reduction in red cells or hemoglobin is occurring or has occurred, and it would show the status of the white blood cell count, a barometer of the body's response to infection.
7. Wait for granulation tissue to develop. Once the wound is free of exudate and is covered with healthy, pink granulation tissue, which typically has occurred by 4 to 6 days after the repair broke down, it is ready to be re-repaired. Well-vascularized tissue will bleed superficially from the newly formed venule buds when wiped with a gauze pad. This waiting period greatly minimizes the possibility of forming a rectovaginal fistula. More prolonged delay in secondary closure leaves time for the tissues to contract as they heal and makes successful repair less likely. A somewhat longer time may be needed when the area is infected, but as soon as healthy tissue appears, it is time to do the repair.
8. If there is bowel involvement, give the woman an enema along with an oral electrolyte solution prior to repair. For the enema, lay her on her left side and administer it yourself (see the chapter entitled "Cleansing and Retention Enemas" in HOLISTIC MIDWIFERY, VOL. II for more details on how to give an enema.)
9. Débride the wound again immediately prior to repair and dissect the tissue as necessary to ensure good tissue mobility. When muscles are severed, they tend to retract. This is especially true of the anal sphincter. It is thus important to identify the ends of the muscle and its surrounding capsule and free them from the surrounding tissue to facilitate repair. This also occurs more extensively when the laceration or cut is mediolaterally oriented. This is best accomplished in a hospital setting with the mother under regional anesthesia.
10. Close the wound using a minimally layered technique following the recommendations found in the relevant chapters.

11. Allow ten days of rest and perineal care. Women can eat a regular diet if the rectal mucosa is not involved. If it is involved, bowel rest can be achieved with a 72 hour liquid fast followed by a low residue or a commercial nonresidue diet. Perineal care consists of sitz baths, each followed by drying the area with a warm lamp (excessive drying of the area is not necessary). Pelvic rest can be accomplished by avoiding undue strain on the area and letting family do the necessary housework. Most women will be hospitalized during this initial ten-day period.

Of eight women so managed in the initial study of this protocol, all experienced complete healing, normal external sphincter and muscle function and no pain on urination. Follow-up intervals for seven of the eight took place six months postpartum or later (Owen & Hauth, 1990; Parker & Brunner, 2003).

Future births

A good diet, attention to adequate healing (see chapter entitled "Postpartum Care and Comfort Measures") and perineal stretching for the next baby should bring women who have experienced such damage to birth with no significantly increased risk of problems.

References and Further Reading on Postpartum Care

Texts Used in Multiple Chapters

Leonard C. CM. Discussion regarding use of silver nitrate swabs, Jan 12, 1991.

Owen J, Hauth J. "Episiotomy infection and dehiscence," in Gilstrap L, Faro S., eds. INFECTIONS IN PREGNANCY. Alan R. Liss, New York NY, 1990.

Parker L, Brunner J. Chapter 32: "Gynecologic surgery for obstetric patients," in Rock J, Jones H, eds. TE LINDE'S OPERATIVE GYNECOLOGY, 9th ed. Lippincott, Williams & Wilkins, Philadelphia PA, 2003.

Sorger L, MD. Editing comments, Feb, 1991.

Stotts N. "Seeing RED and YELLOW and BLACK: the three-color concept of wound care," NURSING90, 20(2):59-61, Feb, 1990.

Varney H, et al. Chapter 42: "The normal puerperium," in their VARNEY'S MIDWIFERY, 4th ed. Jones & Bartlett, Sudbury MA, 2004.

Postpartum Care and Comfort Measures

Gaskin IM. SPIRITUAL MIDWIFERY. Farm Pub. Co., Summertown TN, 1978.

Glazener C, et al. "New postnatal urinary incontinence: obstetric and other risk factors in primiparae," BJOG, 113(2):208-217, Feb, 2006.

Lang R. "Mother roasting and postpartum care," SPECIAL DELIVERY, 1-3, 11, Win, 1987.

Lang R. MOTHER ROASTING: THE USE OF TRADITIONAL CHINESE MEDICINE IN POSTPARTUM CARE. Privately published by the author, Sep 16, 1985.

Leeds A. "The art of the sitz bath," in Midwifery Today Holistic Clinical Series. TEAR PREVENTION AND TREATMENT HANDBOOK. Midwifery Today, Inc., Eugene OR, 2005.

Lowe C, CNM. Conversation regarding hematoma care. Win, 1989.

Montgomery RD. "Healing of muscle, ligaments, and tendons," SEMIN VET MED SURG (SMALL ANIM), 4(4):304-311, Nov, 1989.

Noble E. ESSENTIAL EXERCISES FOR THE CHILDBEARING YEAR: A GUIDE TO HEALTH AND COMFORT BEFORE AND AFTER YOUR BABY IS BORN, 4th ed. New Life Images, Harwich MA, 1995.

Rosenberg J. "What if? tearing, stitching and pelvic floor healing," in Midwifery Today Holistic Clinical Series. TEAR PREVENTION AND TREATMENT HANDBOOK. Midwifery Today, Inc., Eugene OR, 2005.

Steen M., Cooper K. "Cold therapy and perineal wounds: too cool or not too cool?" BR J MIDWIFERY, 6(9): 572-579, Sep, 1998.

Wilma J, et al. "Anatomical and functional changes in the lower urinary tract following spontaneous vaginal delivery," BR J OBSTET GYNAECOL, 110(7):658-663, Jul, 2003.

Examining Tears and Repairs in the Weeks Postpartum

Lam S. Chapter 34: "Bidirectional, non-anchored suture lifts," in Shiffman M, et al., eds. SIMPLIFIED FACIAL REJUVENATION. Springer, New York NY, 2007.

Sherris D, Kern E. ESSENTIAL SURGICAL SKILLS, 2nd ed. Saunders, Philadelphia PA, 2004.

Snyder R, et.al. "Human papillomavirus associated with poor healing of episiotomy repairs," OBSTET GYNECOL, 76(4):664-665, Oct, 1990.

Sorger L, MD. Conversation regarding the use of silver nitrate postpartum, Dec 1990.

Perineal Infections

Ash S. Chapter 22: "Deep soft-tissue infections: necrotizing fasciitis and gas gangrene," in Schlossberg D, ed. Clinical Infectious Disease. Cambridge U Press, Boston MA, 2008.

Cunningham F, et al. Chapter 31: "Postpartum infection," in Cunningham F, et al. Williams Obstetrics, 22nd ed. McGraw-Hill, New York NY, 2005.

Elliott D, et al. "The microbiology of necrotizing soft tissue infections," Am J Surg, 179(5):361-366, May, 2000.

Hauth J, et al. "Early repair of an external sphincter ani muscle and rectal mucosal dehiscence," Obstet Gynecol, 67(6):806-809, Jun, 1986.

Headley A. "Necrotizing soft tissue infections: a primary care review," Am Fam Physician, 68:323-328, 2003.

Johnson M, et al. "Aspergillus: a rare primary organism in soft-tissue infections," Am Surg, 64(2):122-126, Feb, 1998.

McHenry C, et al. "Determinants of mortality for necrotizing soft-tissue infections," Ann Surg, 221(5): 558-565, May, 1995.

Sanz L. "Wound management: Matching materials and methods for best results," Contemp OB/GYN, 30(5):86-114, Nov, 1987.

Schneider G. "A postpartum emergency–necrotizing fasciitis," Contemp OB/GYN, 31(2):109-114, Feb, 1988.

Shy K, Eschenbach D. "Fatal perineal cellulitis from an episiotomy site," Obstet Gynecol, 52(3):293-298, Sep, 1979.

Tharpe N. "Postpregnancy genital tract and wound infections," J Midwifery Womens Health, 53(3):236-246, May-Jun, 2008.

APPENDICES

RECORD KEEPING

Good records are always important. Recording lacerations and repairs can help you monitor healing. If clients return to you for another birth, you have a detailed record of any previous damage. They also help you keep accurate statistics.

I suggest making up a form that does not require much thought to complete (so it gets filled out even when you are exhausted). Include a drawing of the external genitals (to draw in any tears or other damage) and a place to list details of your exam and any repairs. Be sure to include the dimensions of any tears, especially if you are not going to repair them. After birth, information can be recorded on your postpartum visit sheet. See the following page for a sample exam form.

PERINEAL EXAM & REPAIR RECORD

Mother's name__________________ Date_________
Time______

Clitorotomy performed:___ Type: 1st 2nd 3rdabc 4th
Tear past incision____ Reason for clitorotomy_____________
____

Periurethral/labial lacerations:__rents/no sutures req._____

___Sutures required? Description of damage:______________
____

External laceration/incision:_____ shallow/no sutures req.__
Sutures required?___ Length of tear down perineal body____
Description of damage:________________________________
____

Internal yoni laceration/incision:____ shallow/no sutures req.____ Sutures required?___ Depth of tear_____
Length of tear in posterior yoni wall
Description of damage:________________________________
____

Anal sphincter examined:____ Findings:________________
Rectal mucosa examined:____ Findings:__________________

Catheterization performed: positive/negative for blood.

Cervix examined:____ Findings:_______________________

Reason for lacerations:______________________________

Anesthetic administered:___ Type_______ Topical Inj.

Suture material used: Labia__________ Yoni__________
Perineum_________ IAS___________ EAS________________
Rectal mucosa_________
Tissue adhesive used: Synthetic__ Seaweed (type)_______
Location used:______________________________________
Repair done by_____________________

Mother refused repair________________________________

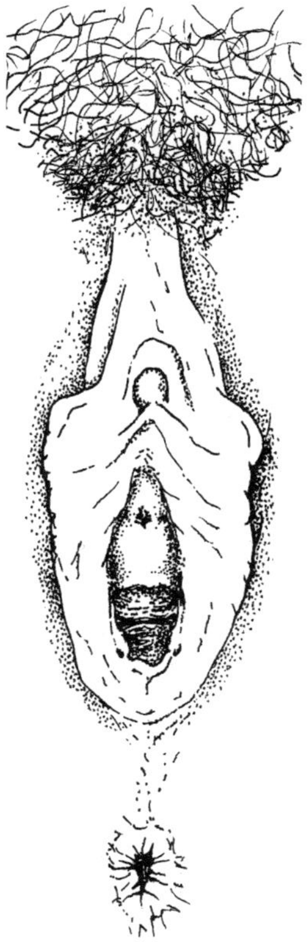

Mark the drawing to show where the tears are located. Make additional notes below:

Homeopathic Medicine

Since homeopathic remedies are mentioned in several places in the text, a brief introduction to the concept seems appropriate for those without experience with this form of medicine. Bio-technical (i.e., Western) medicine is based on the principle that opposites cure. If you have a bacterial infection, you take something to kill the bacteria. Homeopathy is based on the principle of "like cures like," also referred to as the Law of Similars.

Basic principles

In homeopathic prescribing, minute doses of every conceivable substance are carefully prepared in various dilutions for use as remedies. Homeopathy views the body as constantly trying to achieve a state of balance. Sometimes the best it can do is manifest a physical state that produces illness. When this occurs, a homeopathic remedy that in large (material) dose would produce the same symptoms is given in a highly potent, but physically dilute, therapeutic dose. The remedy selected would be the mineral, plant or animal substance that would most closely produce those symptoms in a healthy individual. Remedy pictures are discovered by giving healthy individuals the substance and having them keep a diary of any symptoms that arise. This process is known as proving a remedy.

How remedies are made

Remedies are prepared by using one of three dilution methods: decimal, centesimal and millennial. In decimal (X potency) dilutions, 1 part of the remedial substance is combined with 9 parts of inert solution. It is then successed (shaken) by firmly pounding the vial (as against the palm) for a time, and then diluted again. One part of that solution is then added to 9 parts of inert solution; and so it goes, each dilution being one X of potency. When 26X is reached, a chemist cannot find any of the original substance in the preparation. Even so, the more dilute the remedy, the more potent it is considered to be. This is because dilution and succussion release and raise the vibratory quality of the remedial substance on a molecular level. The centesimal (C potency) scale is prepared the same way except dilutions are 1 to 99, making each numerical potency higher than the equivalent number in the X scale. The millennial (M potency) scale is prepared using dilutions of 1 to 999 parts inert solution.

Finding the correct remedy

There are well over 2000 different remedies. To find the right remedy, questions are asked of the client regarding every aspect of her acute or chronic condition. In addition, personal preferences, habits, moods, etc., are recorded so that a total "symptom picture" emerges.

For example, if a person is jittery, hyper, can't sleep well at night and has loose stools, these symptoms would be noted down along with the details regarding the presenting complaint, such as a cold. In addition, other information (such as what makes the symptoms better or worse, times of day the symptoms are most apparent, food preferences and a host of other details) would be elicited as well. The most important symptoms are underlined three times and secondary symptoms are underlined twice. A good symptom picture has at least three symptoms that strongly indicate a certain remedy.

The homeopathic practitioner then goes to a resource known as a repertory and looks up the symptoms described (called rubrics), noting down what remedies are associated with each. As research proceeds, some remedies may be repeated from symptom to symptom. Repeated remedies are noted and the choice narrows down. Finally, a symptom picture emerges, and the remedy is chosen. In classic homeopathy, one remedy is taken at a time to determine its effectiveness, and it is changed as necessary.

When the remedy matches the symptoms precisely enough, it fits the energy pattern of the body at that moment, like a key in a lock, adding a burst of energy that strengthens the body's defenses and creates an avenue for the body to manifest balance in a more harmonious way. When a remedy is chosen perfectly, this can be a truly miraculous transformation. If the remedy does not match, usually nothing changes.

A few remedies, such as Arnica, have such a strong affinity for certain acute symptoms that they can be used confidently with a very basic symptom picture.

Using a homeopathic repertory

Because homeopathic prescribing is entirely dependent upon symptoms, various catalogues of symptoms have been developed. One of the most complete and well laid out is KENT'S REPERTORY. In this reference, thousands of symptoms are categorized according to their location in the body, as well as by general symptoms and the mental condition. Once you get your feet wet with a basic book (see the book list), I recommend getting a copy of KENT'S and the MATERIA MEDICA by Boericki (which is a catalogue of most of the remedies and their symptom pictures).

KENT'S classifies remedies using a three-point scale. Those in boldface are 3 points and have the strongest affinity for the symptoms described. Those in italics get 2 points and have more than an average affinity for the symptom. Those in plain type get a 1 and have some affinity for the symptoms; they can be thought of as supporting indications for other correlations. (This vital information is not written anywhere in the text!)

Since most books were written by Victorian physicians, the language is very outdated, which can make looking things up more difficult. Also, KENT'S can seem very overwhelming at times, in some cases listing hundreds of remedies for a particular symptom. But such a complete reference will really help track down the right remedy. Read the information in the beginning regarding how to take a case and study the examples given there as well. Robin Murphy, a naturopath, has updated KENT'S into modern medical language and has added a large number of new rubrics. His repertory can be obtained from Homeopathic Educational Services (see address below).

Prescribing

There is much controversy regarding dosage and potency. The higher the potency, the more precisely it must be prescribed to be effective. Very high potencies are used primarily for constitutional (deep-set) conditions, but if an acute condition is very serious, a high-potency remedy may be used at frequent intervals.

Potencies from 3X and 6C up to 200X or 200C are often prescribed for acute conditions. The lower the potency, the more frequently it must be taken for maximum effectiveness. Most homeopaths recommend beginning with 200C potencies when working with women during birth. A kit that contains each remedy in 12C, 30C, 200C and 1M potencies offers a well-rounded array to choose from, but it will also be quite expensive. Start out with a 30C kit of commonly used remedies (see the book list for sources regarding what remedies to include in your first kit), adding a few 200C potencies for those used most often at births.

Bach flower remedies

Bach flower remedies constitute a form of homeopathic medicine that balances different emotional states. They are 38 remedies that are prepared from the essences of 38 different flowers. Rescue Remedy is a combination of five of these and is intended to be used in all kinds of crisis situations. It contains star of Bethlehem (for shock), rock rose (for terror and panic), impatiens (for mental stress and tension), cherry plum (for desperation) and clematis (for semi-consciousness). It can be safely used for mother or baby in any situation regardless of whether other remedies or drugs are being administered simultaneously. It is also a good idea to give Rescue remedy to yourself and other helpers and bystanders whenever it is used.

Books on homeopathy

For more information on homeopathic medicine, refer to the following books and suppliers:

Beginner and intermediate texts on homeopathy (in alphabetical order)

EVERYBODY'S GUIDE TO HOMEOPATHIC MEDICINE by Stephen Cummings, MD, and Dana Ullman (This text serves as a basic primer.)
THE FAMILY GUIDE TO HOMEOPATHY by Dr. Andrew Lockie
FIRST AID AND ACUTE CARE: THE NCH STUDY GUIDE
A FIRST MATERIA MEDICA FOR HOMOEOPATHY by Margaret Roy (Step-by-step lessons for the beginner and offers a good foundation of knowledge)
HEALING WITH HOMEOPATHY by Wayne Jonas, MD, and Jennifer Jacobs, MD
HOMEOPATHIC MEDICINE AT HOME by Maesimund Panos and Jane Heimlich
HOMEOPATHIC MEDICINE FOR WOMEN by Dr. Trevor Smith
HOMEOPATHIC PHARMACY by Stephen Kayne
HOMEOPATHIC TREATMENT OF SMALL ANIMALS by Christopher Day
HOMEOPATHY FOR THE MODERN PREGNANT WOMAN AND HER INFANT by Dr. Sandra Perko. Benchmark Homeopathic Pub., 13526 Professional Building, Ste. 101, San Antonio, TX 78230-3002. (This hard-to-find book is perhaps the best repertory for midwives.)
HOMEOPATHY FOR PREGNANCY, BIRTH AND FIRST YEAR by Miranda Castro

Intermediate and advanced reference books (in order of recommendation)

MATERIA MEDICA WITH REPERTORY by Dr. William Boericke
HOMEOPATHIC REMEDY GUIDE by Robin Murphy, ND
MEDICAL REPERTORY by Robin Murphy, ND
HAHNEMANN REVISITED by Luc de Schepper, MD
HOMEOPATHIC CARE FOR DOGS AND CATS: A COMPREHENSIVE GUIDE by Donald Hamilton
THE ORGANON OF MEDICINE BY HAHNEMANN, translated by Wenda Brewster O'Reilly and based on Steven Decker's translation of the 6th ed.
THE SCIENCE OF HOMEOPATHY by George Vitoulkas (This work offers in-depth discussion

of the philosophy and methodology of classical homeopathy.)

Dictionaries

INTERNATIONAL DICTIONARY OF HOMEOPATHY by Dr. Jeremy Swain

YASGUR'S HOMEOPATHIC DICTIONARY AND HOLISTIC HEALTH REFERENCE by Jay Yasgur

Sources of remedies, books and education

Homeopathic Educational Services, 2124 Kittredge St., Berkeley, CA 94704, 800-359-9051, 9:00 AM to 6:00 PM Pacific time, M-F, www.homeopathic.com (books, tapes, computer programs and remedies)

National Center for Homeopathy, 801 N. Fairfax St., Suite 306, Alexandria, VA 22314, 877-624-0613, www.homeopathic.org (magazine, conferences, books, summer courses)

Foundation for Homeopathic Education and Research, 2124 Kittredge St., Berkeley, CA 94704, 510-649-8930 (research)

Rocky Mountain Homeopathic Press, P.O. Box 10265, Sedona, AZ 86336

Homeopathic pharmacies and related products

Boiron, 6 Campus Boulevard, Newtown Square, PA 19073, 610-325-7464, Fax: 610-325-7480, www.boironusa.com

Hahnemann Laboratories, Inc., 1940 4th St., San Rafael, CA 94901, 888-427-6422, Fax: 415-451-6981, www.hahnemannlabs.com (This pharmacy offers high-quality, high-potency remedies and home and professional kits.)

HomeoLab USA Inc, 3025 De L'Assomption, Montreal, Quebec, H1N 2H2, Canada, 800-404-4666, Fax: 514-252-8919, www.homeolab.com

Standard Homeopathic Company/Hyland's, Inc., 210 W 131st St., PO Box 61067, Los Angeles, CA 90061, 800-624-9659, Fax: 310-516-8579, www.hylands.com (This company welcomes midwives as wholesale customers.)

Weleda, Inc., 175 N. Route 9W, Congers, NY 10920, Contact: Finbarr Murphy, 914-268-0287 or 914-268-2764, Fax: 914-268-8574, www.weleda.com.

Apothecary Products, Inc., Burnsville, MN 55337, 800-328-2742 (Order screw-cap vials for your remedies; the one-dram size is easy to carry.)

Herbal Medicine

Herbs offer a powerful alternative to bio-technical drug therapy. They are nourishing and healing while helping to restore the body and its organs. They can, in turn, balance the system and overcome disease. Here is a summary of the basics. For more detailed information, books by both Susun Weed and Billie Potts are accurate and specific regarding the preparation and use of herbs for health and healing.

Even though researchers are always trying to equate herbs and drugs, they are not the same. Herbs are whole preparations, with all the associated vitamins and minerals, as well as active and passive ingredients (which balance the effect of the herb). Drugs are synthetically derived active principals, without any of the accompaniments nature intended to go along with them. Therefore, even though herbs should be used knowledgeably and with care, they are fundamentally different than drugs. Also remember that herbs have been time tested for hundreds of thousands of years, while most drugs haven't been in use even fifty.

Latin names for herbs mentioned in this text

Herbs may be referred to by both common and scientific names. Because one herb may be known by many common names (and one common name may refer to more than one plant), it is helpful to learn the scientific names of medicinal herbs.

Bayberry bark (*Myrica cerifera*)
Black currant (*Ribes nigrum*)
Black haw root bark (*Viburnum prunifolium*)
Borage seed oil (*Borago officinalis*)
Calendula flowers or marigold (*Calendula officinalis*)
Comfrey leaf or root (*Symphytum officinalis*)
Cramp bark or high cranberry (*Viburnum opulus*)
Echinacea root (*Echinacea augustifolium*)
Evening primrose oil (*Oenothera biennis*)
Garlic root (*Allium sativum*)
Ginger root (*Zingiber officinalis*)
Goldenseal root (*Hydrastis canadensis*)
Lavender flowers (*Lavandula officinalis*)
Marshmallow root (*Althea officinalis*)
Motherwort leaf and flower (*Leonurus cardiaca*)
Mullein leaf (*Verbascum thapsus*)
Oregon grape root (*Mahonia aquifolia*)
Plantain leaf (*Plantago major* or *P. minor*)
Rosemary leaf (*Rosmarinus officinalis*)
Sage leaf (*Salvia officinalis*)
Shepherd's purse leaf and flower (*Capsella bursa pastoris*)
Skullcap leaf and flower (*Scutellaria lateriflora*)
Saint John's wort flower (*Hypericum perforatum*)
Uva ursi leaf (*Arctostaphylos uva ursi*)

Valerian root (*Valeriana officinalis*)
White oak bark (*Quercus alba*)
Witch hazel bark (*Hamamelis virginiana*)
Yarrow flowers (*Achillea millefolium*)
Yellow jasmine (jessamine) (wild woodbine) root (*Gelsemium sempervirens*)
Yerba mansa root (*Anemopsis californica*)

Using herbs in your practice

Herbs are living beings, whereas drugs are lifeless. Therefore, in order to use herbs most effectively, it helps to develop a relationship with the energy of the plants and how they work. Believing they will work helps them to function most effectively. Whitney Pinger, CNM, has observed that herbs work well for her clients prenatally, but she does not observe that herbs work as well when they enter the hospital in labor. She feels the hospital environment interferes with the subtle action of the herbal medicine. This flies in the face of scientific theory with its double-blind studies. In fact, physicists are coming to the conclusion that everything is affected by everything else, derailing the double-blind study as the be-all-and-end-all of proof (helpful but not absolute).

As midwives skilled in the use of herbs have grown in numbers, we have observed that we have "herbal allies." That is, some herbs work great for some midwives and not for others (just as some tear prevention techniques work better for some than others). I get consistent results with my "ally herbs," sporadic results with others and seemingly little or no response with a few. Just because another midwife tells you that an herb works for her does not necessarily mean it will be as effective for you.

Start out with using harmless, nutritive herbs. Use some on yourself for minor complaints. Get an herbal guide and prepare some medicines. As you get used to using herbs yourself, you will become familiar with them and overcome any fears you may have about their danger or lack of effectiveness. As you begin to see good results in yourself, you can confidently recommend them to your clients. Most women I see are delighted with my knowledge of herbal use in pregnancy. However, if a client does not trust herbal medicine, she should not take it.

To prepare herbs for medicinal purposes

Gathering plant materials: Fresh plant materials should be gathered when the energy of the plant is in the part to be used: gather leaves before the plant flowers, flowers when the plant is in bloom, roots in the spring or fall before or after it puts out leaves (when the energy is in the root), barks in early spring when the sap is rising and seeds in the late fall.

Never completely clear out a patch of herbs. Always leave the largest and strongest as well as the weakest-looking plants. It is especially important to remember that if we take them all, there may be none the next time we need them.

Tinctures made with dry herbs: Use 1 weight oz of herb to 5 liquid oz of 100 proof vodka. Place both in a jar with a well-fitting lid. Label and date each jar and let the solution sit in a dark place for 6 weeks or more. This method is suitable for preparing dried roots, barks and seeds only.

Tinctures of fresh herbs: You may wash the herbs, if necessary, and dry with a towel. Pack a jar with cleaned herbs and cover with 100 proof vodka. Cap, label and date each jar and let sit for at least 6 weeks. Fresh flowers, leaves and stems, as well as all other fresh plant parts may be tinctured in this manner.

Tinctures may be drawn off for use and the plant materials left in the remaining solution if you like. A glass baster is ideal for this purpose and can be purchased in a cookware store.

Medicinal strength water-based infusions: Use only dried herbs for infusions. The rehydration process ruptures the dried cell walls and releases the medicinal properties into the water. Always boil the water, remove it from the heat and wait a minute or two. Pour it over the herb and let it steep, covered, for the designated amount of time. Refrigerate what is not used immediately. Prepare and steep various plant materials as follows:

Roots and barks: 1 pt water to 1 oz herb, steep 10 hours.

Light-textured leaves (nettles): 1 qt water to 1 oz herb, steep 6 hours or more.

Leathery leaves (uva ursi or rosemary): 1 qt water to 1 oz herb, steep 10 hours.

Flowers and oily leaves (peppermint): 1 qt water to 1 oz herb, steep for ½ to 1 hour, depending upon the potency of the herb being prepared.

Seeds: 1 pt water to 1 oz seeds, steep for ½ hour.

Decoctions: These are prepared from roots or barks only (not from leaves, flowers, or seeds, since the volatile essences tend to evaporate off). Start by making an infusion. Strain off the liquid and measure it. Heat the liquid until it begins to steam. Immediately turn the heat down very low. Continue steaming until the liquid is reduced by one-half to one-quarter of its original volume. If it is for external use, preserve it with a few drops of tincture of benzoin (which you can obtain at your local drugstore). Refrigerate the decoction.

Medicinal oils: These are tricky to make because they mold easily. To minimize mold formation, all fresh plant materials should be as moisture free as possible. Use only fresh plant materials gathered after the dew has been burned off by the sun. Do not wash plant materials. Carefully brush or scrub off dirt with a dry brush. Chop the plant material and pack firmly into an absolutely clean, dry jar, leaving a little space at the top. (If you need to wash a jar, scrub it thoroughly and dry with a towel. Then finish drying it with a hair dryer.) Cover plant material with olive oil, leaving no air space at the top. (Olive oil is preferred because it will not go rancid as quickly as other oils when stored at room temperature, and it is good for the skin.) Use a clean, dry chopstick to work the oil down into the plant material, leaving no air pockets. Leave in a cool, dry, dark place, putting something absorbent beneath the jar, as oil frequently comes over the top as the plant's gases are released. Decant after 6 weeks. Do not leave plant material in oil past six weeks, because it may mold or go rancid.

To make a salve, shave a little beeswax into the oil and heat in a glass or enamel pot only enough to melt it. Let it cool and check the consistency; add more wax if necessary.

Sources of herbs and related information

It is very important to obtain high-quality herbs and herbal preparations. Here are some sources and references you can count on:

Earth's Botanical Harvest, 36350 SE Industrial Way, Sandy, OR 97055, 800-428-3308 (Call to get a catalogue. This source offers prepared yoni remedies as well as other remedies.)

Eclectic Institute, 36350 SE Industrial Way, Sandy, OR 97055, 800-332-4372, Fax: 800-655-4372, www.eclecticherb.com (It provides high-quality, freeze-dried herbs.)

Emerson Ecologics, 800-654-4432, 8:30 AM to 7:30 PM Eastern Time, www.emerson ecologics.com (A source for many different lines of supplements and other natural healing products. Happy to open accounts for licensed midwives.)

Equinox Botanicals, 33446 McCumber Rd., Rutland, OH 45775, 740-742-1144, www.equinoxbotanicals.net (This is the source for an excellent Prenatal Uterine Tonic, echinacea tincture, Golden Healing Salve and a few other products.)

Frontier Natural Products Co-op, PO Box 299, 3021 78th St., Norway, IA 52318, 800-669-3275, Fax: 800-717-4372, 7:00 AM–6:00 PM Central Time M-F, www.frontierherb.com (Frontier offers high-quality bulk herbs.)

Herb Pharm, 20260 Williams Hwy, Williams, OR 97544, 541-846-6262, www.herb-pharm.com (Herb Pharm offers a variety of single-herb tinctures and loose dry herbs.)

Mountain Rose Herbs, Eugene, OR, www.mountainroseherbs.com (This group produces high-quality products.)

San Francisco Herb and Natural Food Co., 47444 Kato Rd., Fremont, CA 94538, 800-227-2030, www.herbspicetea.com (This company has a huge selection of herbs.)

Wish Garden Herbs, 3100 Carbon Place, Unit 103, Boulder, CO 80301, 888-301-2926, 303-516-1803, Fax: 303-561-1804, 9:00 AM–5:00 PM, M-F, www.wishgarden herbs.com (This midwife-run business has high-quality herbal products for use in midwifery-related care.)

Also check local woods, fields and your own backyard. Plants should be growing at least 8 feet from the road to cut down on pollutants. Many commonly used medicinal herbs and flowers, such as yellow dock, dandelion and plantain, and numerous others, grow almost everywhere in the United States.

Suggested reading (in alphabetical order)

HEALING WISE by Susun Weed, Ash Tree Pub., Box 64, Woodstock, NY 12498 (This book offers an overview of different healing modalities and an introduction to 5 common medicinal plants.)

HERBAL REMEDIES FOR WOMEN, by Amanda McQuade Crawford

THE NATURAL PREGNANCY BOOK: HERBS, NUTRITION, AND OTHER HOLISTIC CHOICES by Aviva Jill Romm & Ina May Gaskin

PEDERSON'S FIELD GUIDE TO WILD FLOWERS. (It can be found in local book stores.)

WISE WOMAN HERBAL FOR THE CHILDBEARING YEAR, by Susun Weed, Ash Tree Pub., Box 64, Woodstock, NY 12498 (This is the best book on herbs in pregnancy. Most of the preparations in HEALING PASSAGE have been derived from my personal experience or Susun's book. It is excellent on theory, how to prepare herbs and exact details of usage.)

WITCHES HEAL by Billie Potts. (This serves as a complete first-aid guide for women that covers general problems as well as gynecological concerns.)

WOMEN'S ENCYCLOPEDIA OF NATURAL MEDICINE, revised ed., by Tori Hudson

THREE-DIMENSIONAL MODEL OF THE LEVATOR ANI COMPLEX

Now here is a really fun project which should cinch your understanding of the pelvic musculature. Even with my own experience of writing this book, I really didn't fully understand how all the muscles work together until I ordered a model of the pelvic floor and started to work with it in three dimensions. However, that model, upon which the previous paper model was based, was shaped like a bowl. The new model of the levator ani complex included here has been modified to show the muscles toned and uplifted, as they are in life. It can be constructed with materials that are readily available from a craft store.

The model is roughly life size and includes its own, modified representation of the pelvis into which the soft parts fit. The sides of the pelvis have been left off so that you can more easily see the muscles from all angles. The use of modeling mesh and felt made it easy to show the shape of the muscles, but also made it much more difficult to include numerous additional very small, intermingled parts. For a 3-D understanding of the more superficial parts, refer to my FEMALE PELVIC ANATOMY lessons on the anatomy DVD. As this book goes to press, the anatomy DVD is about three-quarters finished.

Assembly Instructions

NOTE: Before you begin assembly, read through the all of these instructions, referring to the pages of figures that follow as you go.

Tools and equipment

Small ruler with cm increments

2 Pairs of scissors: one to use on the metal screen and another pair for cutting felt and paper. Both pairs need to be suitable for cutting small pieces accurately

Permanent black-ink marking pen with a small tip to use in mesh and a quilter's disappearing ink marker (available in the needlework section of any craft store) for use on felt

Small, sharp, long-blade Sharpie-type razor knife or new single-edged razor blades for cutting Styrofoam (Be sure that the blade is longer than the round of Styrofoam is thick, or you will not be able to cut out the space in the Styrofoam very easily).

Rolling pin, the largest, heaviest one you have

Needle and thread (If you want to get fancy, have colors to match your felt)

Thimble

Supplies

You will need ten standard 9 × 11" sheets of craft felt of the designated color for each of the following parts. The colors suggested here loosely match those demonstrated in the pelvic anatomy DVD. Use of similar colors will help you identify each part.

1) Medium (cadet) blue: puboanalis muscle
2) Lighter blue than (1) for fibers that run from the pubic bone to the coccyx that form the tendinous plate of the pubococcygeus
3) Aqua or turquoise: puboperinealis muscle

4) Green: iliococcygeus muscle
5) Light yellow (lighter than [8]): coccygeus muscles
6) Deep rose: puborectalis muscle
7) Light pink: yoni canal
8) Gold (darker than [5]): urethral canal
9) 2 squares of off-white, cream or ivory felt for the sacrum and pubic bone

1 package Activ-Wire Mesh 12 × 24" sheet (Small, 1/8 × 1/16" mesh) (This is a very fine sculptural and modeling wire mesh and may be the hardest item to find. Jo Ann Fabric stores carry it in the States. If you cannot find it, here is the source info: Item #166 made by Activa Products, Inc., Marshall, TX 75671, 800-883-3899/903-938-2224, www.activaproducts.com. If you are a student, talk to your class about ordering enough for all of you. They also sell this mesh in a large roll, which a school or group of students could buy and then sell by the piece.)

1 Styrofoam disc, 1" thick × 8" in diameter (This size can also be hard to find, call around. One inch 1" × 8" discs can be ordered from LACrafts.com.)

1 small package of strips of nonadhesive white or cream colored hook-and-loop tape (Velcro-type), a length of this tape can also be purchased from a roll in most fabric stores. Hook -and-loop tape is used to create the vaginolevator attachments (shown in red-purple on the DVD).

Straight pins with flat heads

A small amount of synthetic pillow stuffing material to stuff into the sacrum to help it hold its shape.

General notes on making the model

Figures: An extensive series of figures is included to help you assemble the model. They are grouped on the 3 pages that follow the instructions. It will help to make single-sided photocopies of these pages so you can refer to them more easily.

Patterns: The patterns have been printed double sided to save space in the text so you MUST MAKE SINGLE-SIDED PHOTOCOPIES OF THEM BEFORE YOU BEGIN. There are both FRAME mesh patterns and FELT patterns in this model. Make sure you are read each piece carefully and use the correct pattern for each type of material. Each piece is numbered and otherwise detailed like a dressmaker's pattern (thanks to Rhonda, an accomplished seamstress).

Working with the wire mesh: Open the package and unfold the mesh. Lay it on a clean, smooth surface and gently stretch and flatten it with your hands (do not stretch it so much that you distort the screen). Use the rolling pin to roll it out and flatten it as much as possible, avoiding creating creases.

There is no need to cut out the paper patterns for making the mesh parts. Lay the mesh over the paper pattern and use the permanent marker to outline the pattern onto the mesh. Use your "metal" scissors to cut the screen. Holding the screen over a piece of white paper may help you see the lines better. Remove wire mesh scraps from your work area to avoid entanglement with the felt.

Notes on working with felt: Be sure to refer to the supplies list as to which color you will use for each part. Felt stretches easily, so if you make a piece a little too short, you can gently stretch the felt to make it fit. If you stretch the felt a little too much, you can trim it to make it fit. Felt also snags easily on the screen mesh, tape and anything else, so it helps to clear your work space and then work with one piece of felt at a time. Remove felt scraps when you have finished cutting out your pieces (store them in a bag, in case you need them).

To make felt pattern pieces, cut out each paper pattern making sure to cut along the outside edge of the bold lines. Then lay the pattern pieces over the felt as close to one edge or corner of the fabric as possible (this ensures that you have enough of that color left for any other pieces you may need to cut out).

Hold the felt and pattern steady with one hand while you trace the outline of the pattern onto the felt with your marker, or use straight pins to pin the pattern to the felt. If you want a pristine model with no marker lines that show, use the straight–pin method for cutting out your pieces or cut just inside your marker lines; make your marker lines on the "inside" face of the felt (the face that will not show), or use a quilter's disappearing ink marker, the marks will last 48 to 72 hours. Cut along the bold lines with your best scissors.

Carefully copy all designated marks and dotted lines onto the felt (note that some marks do not need to be transferred, so follow the instructions carefully). One way to transfer the marks is to hold the marker on the marks for a moment to allow the ink to soak through the paper and onto the felt. Which side of the felt the marks need to be transferred to varies, so follow directions carefully.

Because felt is difficult to cut compared to some other fabrics and because these pieces are relatively small, do not attempt to stack the felt to cut multiple pieces of the same shape.

Tacking, whipstitching and overlapping: In these instructions, "tacking" refers to using needle and thread to sew basting stitches (Fig 1a) through the specified layer to attach parts together. These stitches may need to be large or small, as appropriate. Long dashed marks on the patterns or on the figure illustrations indicate stitching lines where tacking stitches should be placed.

Whip or overcast stitches (Fig 1b) can also be used when joining two pieces, usually along the edges. Short dashes indicate where a fold should be placed. Dotted lines indicate where edges should be overlapped and sewn together. Please refer to the accompanying illustrations for further clarification.

Fasteners: If you wish, you can put small snaps or hook-and-loop tape at many of the places where the pieces would otherwise be tacked to each other. Such fasteners would allow you to take the model apart and put it back together easily. This is particularly helpful if you will be using the model as a teaching aide. Do not attempt to use "dual lock" fasteners because they are difficult to sew and so thick that they distort the model. Use either black or beige hook and loop tape as a fastener so that you can easily distinguish the anatomical structures represented by white hook-and-loop tape (e.g., the vaginolevator attachments) from the fastenings that merely hold the model together. The instructions below for creating a model that disassembles will include both snaps and hook-and-loop tape. Note that the instructions pertaining to making a detachable model are bracketed by double asterisks (**). If you do not want to make detachable model, simply skip over these sections.

Creating a model that disassembles takes much longer than creating the model as one piece. It helps to make the model that does not disassemble first, to get a better sense of how the parts go together, before trying to make one that can be taken apart.

Making the model

NOTE: Numbers in parentheses refer to the number on each pattern piece.

Assemble the puboanalis muscle (part of the pubovisceral complex):

1. Trace onto mesh and cut out the **puboanalis muscle, frame (1)**.
2. Cut out the paper pattern for the **puboanalis muscle, felt (2)**. Using the medium blue felt, trace or pin the pattern onto the felt and cut the felt piece out. Be sure to cut along the bold lines, including those extending into the center.
3. Carefully transfer the marks for the vaginolevator attachment, the dots, the center ✚, and the alignment marks for the tendinous plate. There is no need to transfer the fold lines or stitching lines.
4. Place the felt piece (2) right side (the side with the marks) down, and lay the mesh frame (1) on the wrong side of the felt piece, aligning it as illustrated in Fig. 2.
5. Fold the top edge of the felt down toward the center, and the bottom edge of the felt up toward the center, encasing the mesh in the felt. Stitch through all thicknesses with a medium-sized basting stitch along the dashed lines as shown in Fig. 3, approximately 1/8" from the edges.
6. With the transferred marks on the inside, fold the strip in half by bringing the short ends together, creating a sharp crease at the fold line. Create a ridge by whipstitching along this crease, taking a ¼" bite, through all thicknesses. Stitch only the top half of the structure, leaving the bottom part ridge free, as shown in Fig. 4.
7. Trace onto mesh and cut out the **tendinous plate of the pubococcygeus, frame (3)**.
8. Cut out the paper pattern for the **tendinous plate of the pubococcygeus, felt (4)**. Using the light blue felt, trace the pattern or pin it to the felt and cut the felt piece out. There is no need to transfer the dashed line.
9. Lay the tendinous plate frame (3) onto the tendinous plate felt piece (4). Tack them together using medium-sized basting stitches (or a whipstitch if you prefer), approximately 1/8" from the edge, as illustrated in Fig 5.

If you are creating a detachable model, sew one side of a snap on the tip of the mesh side of the tendinous plate. Leave the other side snapped to it so it will not be lost. You will later sew it to the coccyx. Then sew one side of a piece of hook-and-loop tape on the mesh side below the snap. Stick the other side to its mate: you will later sew it to the iliococcygeus. Whipstitch around all edges of the hook-and-loop pieces, as if you were sewing a patch.

10. Open the puboanalis muscle part out flat, with the ridge side down. Align the tendinous plate at the center top, mesh side down, using the alignment marks, and stitch into place along the stitching lines, as shown in Fig 6.

Even if you are constructing a detachable model, permanently affix the tendinous plate to the puboanalis, as these fibers are continuous with those of the rest of this muscle; they are different colors only to emphasize that these are the only fibers that reach from the pubic bone all the way to the coccyx.

11. Create the puboanalis cuff by wrapping the flaps of the lower segment of the puboanalis muscle toward you, overlapping the edges slightly. Sew the overlapped edges together using a whipstitch, creating a cylinder, as in Fig 7.
12. Cut out the paper pattern for the **pubococcygeus fibers, felt (5)**. Using the light blue felt (the same color as for felt pattern piece [4]), trace or pin the pattern onto the felt, and cut one piece. Carefully transfer the bold slit line, and cut a slit along that mark.
13. Insert the tendinous plate of the pubococcygeus piece through the slit (Fig 8). Fold the edges of the felt pubococcygeus fibers over the edges of the puboanalis muscle and tack into place using basting stitches through all thicknesses, or whipstitching over the top of all thicknesses (Fig 9). Be sure the inside lower edge of the felt that is below the slit is flush with the lower edge of the tendinous plate of the pubococcygeus felt piece so that it covers the base of the tendinous plate completely. You will notice that the tips of the pubococcygeus piece extend beyond the edges of the puboanalis muscle: this is correct. These **pubovisceral complex attachment tabs** are used later to connect the pubovisceral complex to the pubic bone.

**Sew down the pubococcygeus fibers even if you want a model that disassembles. **

Assemble the vaginolevator attachments (parts of the pubovisceral muscle complex):

1. Cut out the paper pattern for the **vaginolevator attachments, hook & loop tape (6)**, or estimate the size and shape. Cut out two pairs of hook-and-loop pieces using pattern piece (6) as a guide. There will be four pieces in all; two hook and two loop.
2. Position one of the "hook" pieces (the bristly side) on the puboanalis muscle where indicated by the marks you transferred, and stitch into place. Whipstitch around all the edges of the hook-and-loop pieces, as if you were sewing on a patch. Do the same with the other hook piece on the opposite side of the model. Stick the loop sides of the pieces to their mates and leave them there for now, so as not to lose them (Fig. 10).

Assemble the puborectalis muscle:

1. Trace onto mesh and cut out the **puborectalis muscle, frame (7)**.
2. Cut out the paper pattern for the **puborectalis muscle, felt (8)**. Using the deep rose felt, trace or pin the pattern onto the felt and cut one felt piece. Transfer the marks for the puboperinealis attachments.
3. Lay the felt piece horizontally, wrong side up (puboperinealis marks down), and place the mesh frame along the lower edge, as in Fig. 11. Roll the mesh and felt as tightly as possible into a long, solid roll. If you can't get it started, stitch the lower edge of the felt to the lower edge of the mesh. Once it is rolled, use small whipstitches to sew the edge to the roll to hold it together (Fig. 12).

If making a detachable model, sew one side of hook and loop tape or one side of a small snap on each of the attachment marks for the puboperinealis muscle.

4. Sew this rolled piece, the puborectalis muscle, to the lower edge of the puboanalis muscle, passing around behind the cylindrical puboanalis cuff just below the ridge in back. Make sure the attachment marks for the puboperinealis muscle are on the inside (the same side

as the hook-and- loop tape for the vaginolevator attachments). An easy way to attach the roll is to first temporarily flatten the puboanalis cuff part and fold it upward, against the inside of the U-shaped part of the puboanalis muscle (Fig 13). Then hold the puborectalis roll alongside the resulting edge and whipstitch the pieces together, taking small bites on each side. Be sure to attach only the puborectalis muscle to the lower edge of the puboanalis so as not to accidentally sew the puboanalis cuff closed.

Even if you are making a detachable model, sew the puborectalis to the puboanalis muscle, as these parts are fused in life and because it is logistically difficult to attach them with fasteners.

5. Following the illustration in Fig. 14a, form the entire model into a U-shape, and curve the upper edges outward, like a flared collar on a shirt. The tendinous plate of the pubococcygeus should stick straight up, out and back from the rear of the puboanalis as shown in Fig. 14b.

Assemble the puboperinealis muscle (part of the pubovisceral complex):

1. Trace onto mesh and cut out the **puboperinealis muscle, frame (9)**.
2. Cut out the paper pattern for the **puboperinealis muscle, felt (10)**. Using the aqua or turquoise felt, trace or pin the pattern onto the felt, and cut the felt piece out. There is no need to transfer the fold line.
3. Place the puboperinealis frame lengthwise over the lower half of the felt piece and fold the felt along the fold line, enclosing the frame, similar to what you did in Fig. 2. Sew the three layers together using a medium basting stitch along the edges.
4. Line up the angled ends of the puboperinealis muscle with the ends of the puborectalis muscle, making sure the angled edges are in line with those of the puboanalis muscle edges, this should result in the puboperinealis muscle forming a loop that is angled down and back, as shown in Fig. 15. Tack the tips of this strip of muscle just inside the ends of the puborectalis muscle, with the upper edge of the puboperinealis muscle in line with the bottom edge of either side of the puboanalis muscle (Fig. 15).

If you have sewn hook-and-loop tape or a small snap at the attachment marks for the puboperinealis, now sew the other side of the fastener to the ends of the puboperinealis.

Fix the size of the anourogenital hiatus:

Set the size of the anourogenital hiatus by placing a spacer stitch to fix the side walls of the puboanalis muscle with a 2.5 cm space between them. To do this, have a threaded needle and a ruler ready.

1. Place your nondominant thumb and index finger on the outside of the U-shaped puboanalis muscle, near the open end (Fig. 16a).
2. Use your other hand and the ruler to measure a 2.5 cm gap between the sides of the open end of the U at the level of the dots on the puboanalis muscle and adjust your grip to maintain this gap (Fig. 16b).
3. As you assess where to place the stitch, keep in mind that both the yoni and urethral canals will eventually need to be inserted between this stitch and the puboperinealis muscle (see Fig. 42). Carefully tack the two sides of the puboanalis muscle together with thread so

that you span the 2.5 cm space. Insert the needle on the outside of one side of the U at the dot you marked earlier, and exit through the dot on the opposite site, so you have 2.5 cm of thread between your entry and exit points as in Fig. 17. Pass the thread through several times like this. This holds the gap at the open end apart at an appropriate width.

Assemble the wire mesh frame for the iliococcygeal muscle:

1. Trace onto mesh and cut out the **iliococcygeal muscle, frame (11)**. Be sure to trace the V-shaped solid and dotted lines. Cut along the solid line of the V on both sides.
2. Overlap the cut solid line of the V to the dotted line, so that the dotted lines meet. Refer to the paper pattern. This will give the frame piece two slight cone-shaped areas, similar to darts in fabric (Fig. 18). Tack the overlapped section together to hold it in place. The entire structure will resemble a bat with its wings spread. The side with the points of the darts (that is, the convex side) becomes the superior side of the muscle.

Assemble the felt pieces of the iliococcygeal muscle:

1. Cut out the paper pattern for the **iliococcygeus muscle, bottom layer, felt (12)**. Using the green felt, refer to the pattern piece layout shown on the same page to ensure you have enough felt. Trace or pin the paper pattern onto the felt, and cut the piece out.
2. Bring the sides of the Vs together so that they are just touching, and whipstitch together with small stitches, creating a dart on either side (Fig. 19).

If you are creating a model to be disassembled, cut four one-inch pieces of hook-and-loop tape. Sew one on each dot, running the tape from the dot toward the dart (may overlap the dart), and one by each side of the gap in the back of the muscle. Put the other sides of these pieces of tape on their mates to avoid losing them.

3. Lay the wire mesh frame piece over the felt piece with darts pointing up. Center the mesh so that the felt sticks out about 1/8" all around. Tack the mesh onto the felt using just a few stitches in the corners and in the center.
4. Fold the entire piece in half along the center fold line so that the mesh sides face each other. In the posterior center, stitch through all layers along the stitching lines, which will create a ridge (Fig. 20).
5. Fold each side down along the stitching line, creating a curved, winged piece with the darts (mesh side) pointing up and the ridge you just created along the bottom (Fig. 21).
6. Cut out the paper pattern for the **iliococcygeus muscle, upper layer, felt (13)**. Using the green felt, trace or pin the paper pattern onto the felt and cut the felt piece out. Transfer the dots and the small Xs to the side that will face up.
7. On each side of the felt piece you just cut out, bring the sides of the Vs together so that they are just touching. Whipstitch each V together, creating a dart on each "wing," like you did with the two pieces in steps 1 and 2. This piece should now resemble the mesh and felt form you finished in step 3.
8. Lay the felt for the ileococcygeus muscle, upper layer (13) over the mesh and felt form, sandwiching the mesh, darts pointing up. Baste or whipstitch around all edges and through all thicknesses.
9. Mold the iliococcygeus form to fit the curved upper U-shaped edge of the puboanalis form with the ridged part beneath the tendinous plate of the pubococcygeal muscle. Referring

to the paper pattern piece (13), align the tendinous plate with the dotted lines on top of the iliococcygeus and tack into place through all layers as in Fig. 22.

If you want to be able to detach the parts later, put a fastener at the two front inner corners (snaps work well here). Sew the other half of the hook-and-loop tape on the bottom of the tendinous plate to the upper surface of the iliococcygeus, at the middle of the gap.

10. Mold the upper edge of the puboanalis muscle into a gentle curve that will overlap the edge of the iliococcygeus muscle. Gently cup the sides of the iliococcygeal muscle up and out so that they act as an extension of the flared edges of the puboanalis muscle, like a wide shirt collar (Fig. 23).
11. Make sure the edges of the puboanalis part overlie the anterior edges of the iliococcygeal muscle at the Xs. Tack them together at this point, either using a stitch through all layers at the X, or a whipstitch over the edge of the puboanalis muscle, as shown in Fig. 24.

If making a detachable model, sew the other half of the fasteners that you sewed to the front, inner corners of the iliococcygeus to the puboanalis, just under the pubococcygeus fibers.

Assemble the coccygeus muscles:

1. Trace onto mesh and cut out the **coccygeus muscle, frame (14)**. Make two pieces.
2. Cut out the paper pattern for the **coccygeus muscle, felt (15)**. Using the light yellow felt, trace or pin the pattern onto the felt, and cut out two felt pieces. Flip the paper pattern piece over and cut out two more pieces, so that you wind up with two pairs of mirror-image pieces.
3. Sandwich one piece of mesh between one pair of felt pieces and tack together through all thicknesses with basting or whipstitches (Fig. 25). Repeat for the other side of the muscle. Lay the finished pieces in front of you as shown in Fig. 25 and mark the dots as shown. Set both completed pieces aside for now.

If you are attaching the muscles together with fasteners, remove the matching pieces of hook-and-loop tape from the dot ends of the iliococcygeus muscle and sew these onto the top felt layer of the coccygeus muscles. Two of them should go on the dot ends, with most of the tape hanging below the lower edge of the coccygeus muscle. The other two should go on the opposite end of the same edge, but entirely on the piece of felt. Cut two more one-inch pieces of hook-and-loop tape. Place one side of the tape along the inside short edge of each coccygeus muscle, and trim the edge of the tape so that it follows the curved edge. Sew the tapes to the undersides of the muscles, and place their mates on them. The mates will later be sewn to the back of the sacrum.

Assemble the sacrum and coccyx:

1. Trace onto mesh and cut out the **sacrum and coccyx, front, frame (16)** and the **sacrum and coccyx, back, frame (17)**.
2. Cut out the paper pattern for the **sacrum and coccyx, front, felt (18)**, and the **sacrum and coccyx, back, felt (19)**. Using the white felt, trace or pin the paper patterns onto the felt, and cut out both felt pieces. Transfer the dots to the wrong (inside) sides of the felt pieces. If you wish, transfer the details of the sacral anatomy onto the right (outside) side of the felt piece 18.

3. Lay the sacrum-coccyx front mesh (16) on the wrong side of the sacrum-coccyx front felt (18), and tack into place around the edges.
4. Lay the sacrum-coccyx back mesh (17) on the wrong side of the sacrum-coccyx back felt (19), and tack into place around the edges.
5. Lay the sacrum/coccyx back on top of the sacrum/coccyx front, mesh sides facing each other, matching the coccyx and dots (Fig. 26). Sew the pieces together from dot to dot along the stitching lines, with short basting or whipstitches.

If making a detachable model, sew the other side of the tendinous plate's snap onto the tip of the inside surface of the coccyx, being sure that it fits correctly into the gap in the ileococcygeus muscle.

Take the two unsewn mates on the coccygeus muscle and sew these along the edge of the sacrum and coccyx so that they correctly match the hook-and-loop tape on the inside edge of the coccygeus muscles. Most of the tape will stick out past the edge of the sacrum-coccyx back.

6. Cut out the paper pattern for the **sacrum side, felt (20)**. Using the white felt, trace or pin the paper pattern onto the felt and cut out a felt piece. Flip the paper pattern and repeat so you have two sacrum side pieces.
7. Curl the sacrum-coccyx form slightly into a parenthesis shape, with the shorter sacrum-coccyx front piece on the inside of the curve (Fig. 27). Now spread the front and back apart (Fig. 28). You will notice that this creates a curved V-shaped space between the two sides. This is where you will be attaching the sacrum side pieces. Get the left sacrum side piece positioned as shown in Fig. 29, and use a whipstitch over the edges to sew each side into place. Start at the point of the V and sew one side, then the other.
8. If you wish, now is the time to add a little fluffy pillow stuffing inside the sacrum to help it hold its shape. Be sure to do this carefully so as not to distort the shape.

Attach the posterior levator ani muscle complex edges to the sacrum and coccyx:

If you are making a model that disassembles, at this point you should be able to match the various hook-and-loop tape pairs and the snap to connect the posterior region of the levator ani muscle complex to the sacrum and coccyx.

1. With the concave curve of the sacrum toward the pelvic cavity, fit the tip of the coccyx into the V-shaped cut–out in the back edge of the green iliococcygeus muscle. Make sure the light blue tip of the tendinous plate of the pubococcygeus is on the top, as shown in Fig. 30. Tack the layers and edges together securely.

9. Refer to Fig. 31 to fit one half of the coccygeus muscles along the inside (pelvic) edge of the sacrum and coccyx. The lower edge of the coccygeus muscle should be level with the tip of the coccyx on the underside. Tack the scalloped edge to the sacrum-coccyx.
10. After both muscles are tacked to the bones, align (do not overlap) the dot at the narrow end of one coccygeus muscle with the dot on the iliococcygeus muscle. Using a whipstitch tack these muscles together at the dots (Fig. 32). The resulting V-shaped area created by the edges represents where the muscles would attach to the ischial spines on either side. Now your model should look like Fig. 33.

Assemble the section of the yoni canal:

NOTE: This model depicts only the portion of the yoni and urethral canals that span approximately from the distal mid-third to the distal upper third of the yoni. There is a little more of the lowermost end of both canals that project beyond the anterior edge of the yoni model to the introitus externally.

1. Trace onto mesh and cut out the **yoni canal, frame (21)**.
2. Cut out the paper pattern for the **yoni canal, felt (22)**. Using the pink felt, trace or pin the pattern onto the felt, and cut out one piece.
3. Lay the frame piece lengthwise in the center of the felt piece. Fold the sides of the felt piece toward the center so that they touch (but do not overlap), and sew the edges together using a whipstitch (Fig. 34).
4. Form the piece into a circle with the stitches on the inside. The edges of the circle should meet but not overlap. Sew the edges together with a whipstitch, using large, closely spaced stitches (Fig. 35).
5. Cut out the paper pattern for the **urethral canal attachment, hook & loop tape (23)**. Trace onto the hook-and-loop tape (or estimate the size and shape) and cut out. Sew the loop half of the hook-and-loop tape lengthwise to the top center of the yoni canal, over the stitches that close the circle, as shown in Fig. 36. Attach the remaining hook piece of the tape so as not to lose it.
6. Referring to Fig. 37, form the canal into a rectangle with the top and bottom about 3.5 cm wide. Now push in the sides of the tube to form four corners, creating the H-shape of the yoni canal at this level. Lay the canal on its side, then bend in the sides toward the center and flatten (Fig. 38).
7. Remove the loop pieces from the vaginolevator attachments you sewed onto the puboanalis muscle earlier, and sew these lengthwise along the upper, outer corners of the H at one end of the yoni canal on either side. The top edge of the tape should align with the dots shown on your left in Fig. 38 (the tape is attached along the sides of the top fold so you cannot see where this is on the other side in this oblique view). Affix the yoni canal into your model, by fastening the hook-and-loop tapes on either side, with the yoni inserted under the string spacer and resting on the puboperinealis muscle (Fig. 39). The yoni canal should be at a steep angle, which is best seen from overhead as shown in Fig. 48.

Assemble the section of the urethral canal:

1. Cut out the paper pattern for the **urethral canal, felt (24)**. Using the gold felt, trace or pin the paper pattern onto the felt and cut out one felt piece. Referring to the paper pattern, roll the felt tightly, starting with one short side. Use small whipstitches to sew the edge to the roll to hold it together (Fig. 40).
2. Remove the hook piece from the top of the yoni canal and sew it to the urethral canal lengthwise, over the previous stitching (Fig. 41).
3. Attach the urethral canal to the loop tab on the top of the yoni canal, tucking it under the spacer stitches (Fig. 42).

Make the Styrofoam pelvis:

NOTE: This model consists of only the pelvic brim, a pubic arch and a sacrum to allow you to better view the pelvic floor. If you are disoriented by the omission of the sides of the pelvis, please refer to the review of the bony pelvis that begins on page 31. If you are still confused, examine a complete 3-D female pelvic model, which every midwifery school should have on hand.

1. Cut out the paper pattern for the **pelvic brim (25)**. Please note that although the shaded areas are part of the pattern, they are merely to assist with alignment. DO NOT cut these shaded areas from the Styrofoam.
2. Use straight pins to attach the paper pattern to the Styrofoam round, positioning it so that both the shaded curve and the unshaded curve at the anterior edge follow the curved edge of the Styrofoam. Make sure that the pattern is centered from side-to-side as well, as shown in Fig. 43. Styrofoam discs are not perfectly circular, so move the pattern around the edge until you find a position that works. If the edges of the pattern do not meet both edges of the disc (that is, if the disc is larger than 8"), align the anterior shaded area along the edge and cut the **notch for the sacrum back** as deeply as the pattern will then indicate.
3. Transfer the dot in the center of the shaded area of the anterior edge to the "front" edge of the Styrofoam (on the 1" side), and place another dot above it on the top (flat surface) of the round, as shown in Fig. 44. Transfer the leveling indicator dot as well by marking it just outside the edge of the brim line.
3. Trace the two white bold-lined areas onto the Styrofoam with your marker, the **notch for the sacrum back** and the outline of the **pelvic brim**. Remove the paper pattern and use the razor knife to carve out the traced pattern all the way through the foam. Point the blade straight down and use a sawing motion to keep the walls of the cutout as straight as possible (Fig. 45). Try not to cut off the leveling indicator dot completely; make a new mark on the Styrofoam to replace it if you do. Gently remove the cut out pieces.

Attach the felt model to the back side of the Styrofoam pelvis:

1. Referring to Fig. 46, align the top edge of the felt/mesh sacrum back with the top outside edge of the notch in the sacral region of the Styrofoam pelvis. Attach it with straight pins pushed straight into the Styrofoam.
2. Align the felt/mesh sacrum front with the inside back edge of the pelvic brim and center it in place. Secure with straight pins (Fig. 47).

Assemble pubic bone and attach felt model to the anterior of the Styrofoam pelvis:

1. Trace onto mesh and cut out the **pubic bone, frame (26)**. To avoid distorting the mesh, cut along the solid line to reach and cut out the obturator foramina. Stitch the slit you created to reach the obturator foramina closed with small whip stitches. You can make this piece out of stiff but thin cardboard (posterboard will work well or a manila file folder) instead, if you want the pubic bone to retain its shape better.
2. Cut out the paper pattern for the **pubic bone, felt (27)**. Using the white or cream felt, trace or pin the pattern onto the felt and cut out a felt piece. Repeat so you have two felt

pieces. Transfer the "centering" dot to the outside surface of one felt piece.

3. Sandwich the mesh (or cardboard) between the two felt pieces and tack them together through all thicknesses with a couple of large basting stitches to hold the pieces together. Then sew around the edges with basting or whip stitches. Be sure to stitch around the obturator foramen holes as well. Once the edges are sewn, remove the tacking stitches. Set the pubic bone aside.
4. Using straight pins, attach the pubic bone to the front of the Styrofoam pelvis, lining up the center dots (Figs. 48 and 49). The top edge of the felt piece should be flush with the top edge of the foam (Fig. 49). Insert the pins at a sharp angle, so they do not stick out the other side.
5. Position the anterior portion of the puboanalis muscle so that it is centered to either side of the dot (Figs. 48 and 49). The urethra should be visible under the pubic arch from the front of the model (there can be a little gap between the bone and the urethra, but the puborectalis muscle should not be visible past the lower edge of the bone). Push the puboperinealis muscle back so that it is well underneath and slightly posterior to the front edge of the yoni. Hold the muscle complex in place.
6. Position the pubovisceral complex attachment tabs flat against the Styrofoam and insert pins through them at a sharp angle (so they don't stick through the other side) to attach the pubovisceral complex to the pubic bone. (The iliococcygeus will extend down, around and past the brim on either side.) Once the pubovisceral complex is in place, you can trim out the spacer stitches if you wish, although it is better to leave these in place.
7. Reshape the muscle parts as necessary to make sure that the top edge of the puboanalis muscle is uniformly flared, the inside edge of the iliococcygeus muscle is under (inferior to) the flared edges of the puboanalis muscle, and the sides of the iliococcygeus muscle are uniformly cupped upward (Fig. 50).
8. Bend the puboanalis cuff back so that it is angled toward the sacrum. You can tack it to the puborectalis muscle to keep it in place, if you wish, as it tends to bend out of position, even with the frame.

Attach the leveling indicator

1. The model is complete. To see how it looks in a woman who is standing, however, you will need a reference point. Cut out the **leveling indicator (28)**.
2. Starting at the leveling indicator dot you made at the "corner" of the pelvic brim, measure 5.5cm at an angle to the edge of the foam. Mark or place a locator pin at this spot on the edge of the foam (Fig. 51).
3. Pin the leveling indicator to the foam with the "top" of the leveling line meeting the mark or locator pin (remove the pin) (Fig. 52). When you hold the model up at eye level and position it so that the leveling line is horizontal, the pelvic brim is at a 58° angle, the average angle of the brim when a woman is standing (the range is typically 55 to 60°).

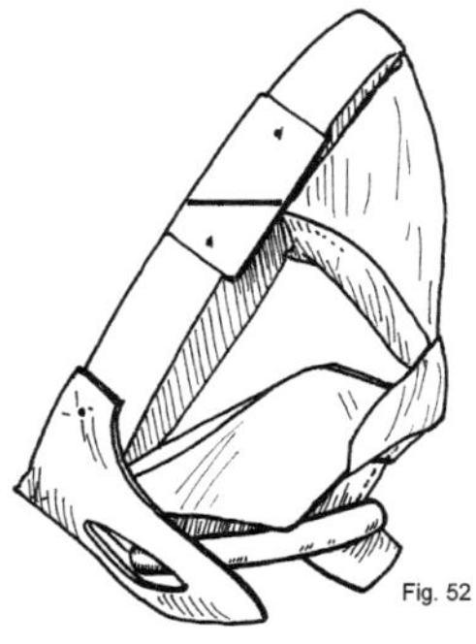
Fig. 52

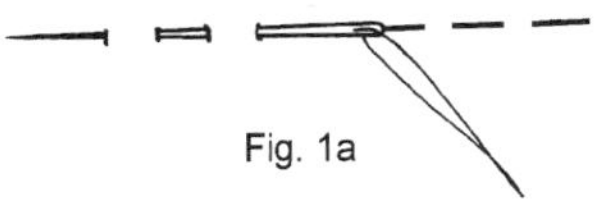
Fig. 1a

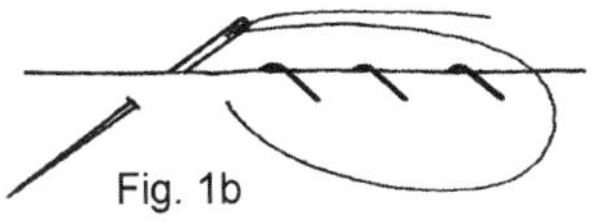
Fig. 1b

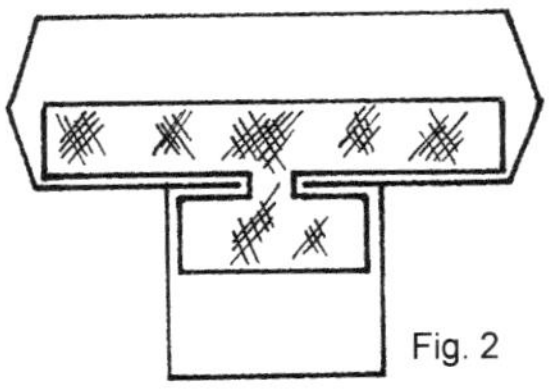
Fig. 2

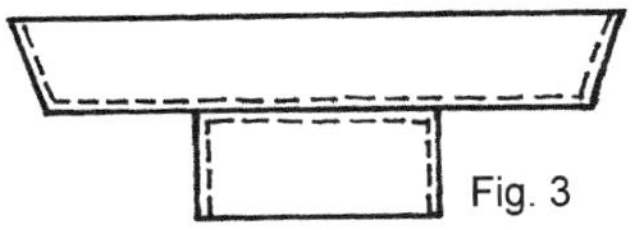
Fig. 3

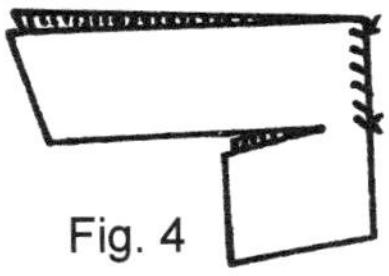
Fig. 4

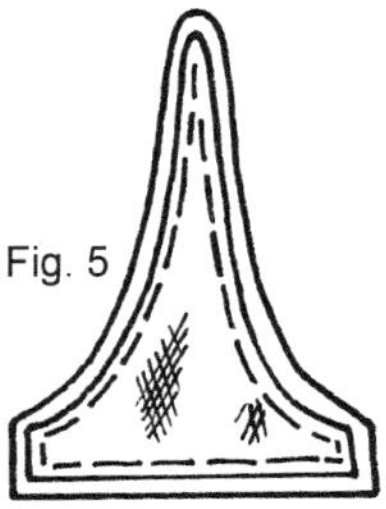
Fig. 5

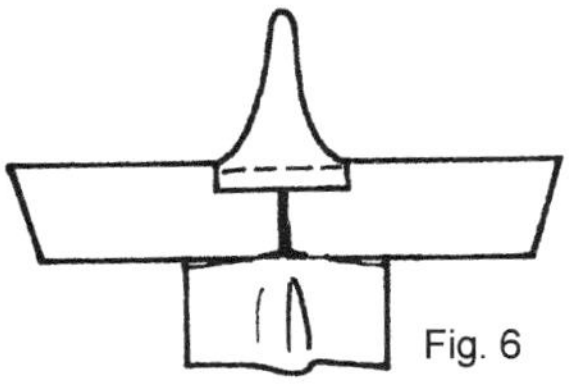
Fig. 6

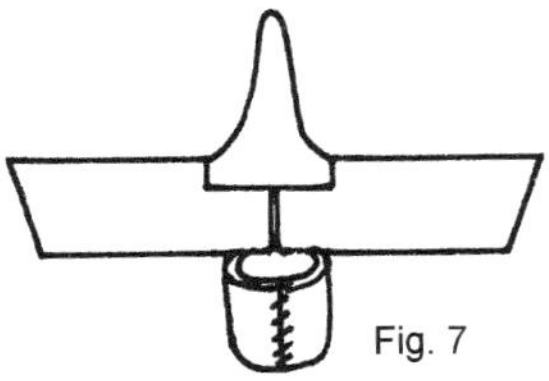
Fig. 7

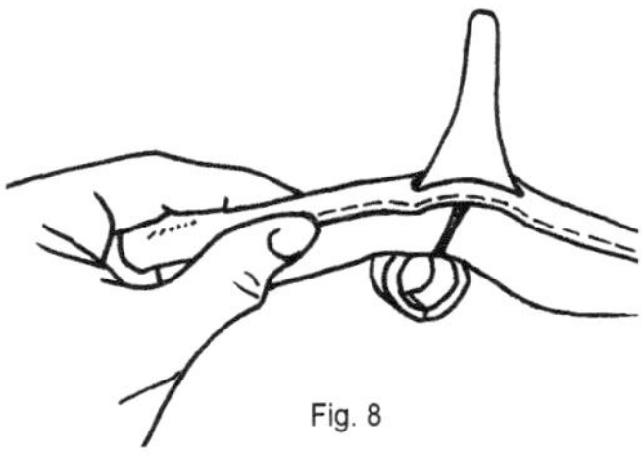
Fig. 8

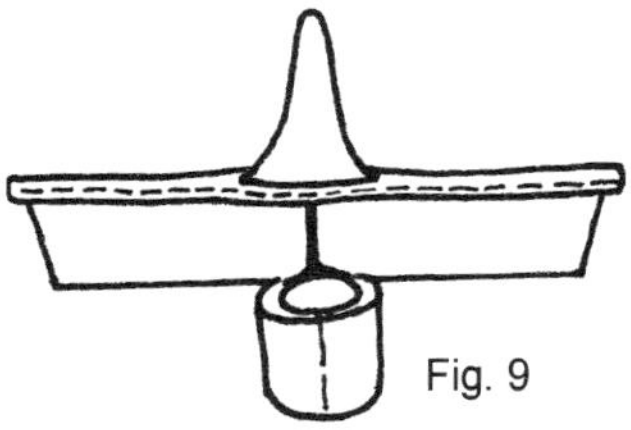
Fig. 9

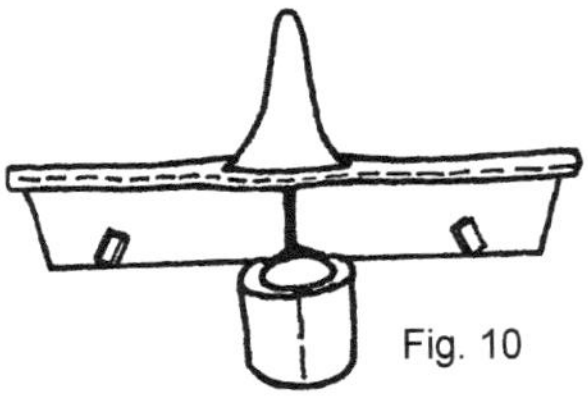
Fig. 10

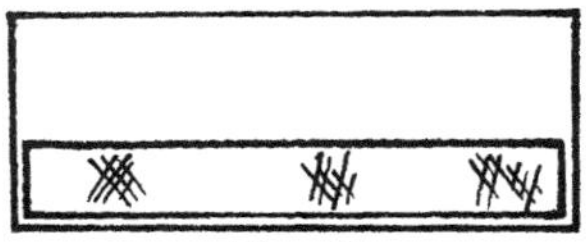
Fig. 11

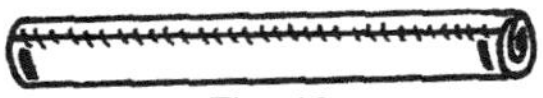
Fig. 12

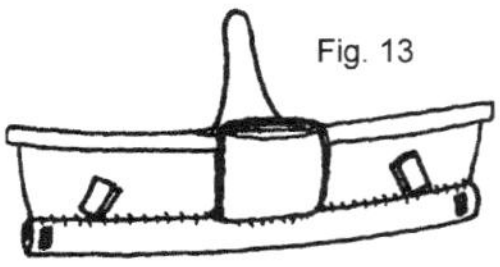
Fig. 13

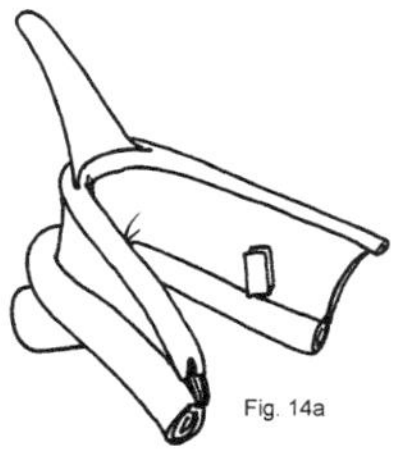
Fig. 14a

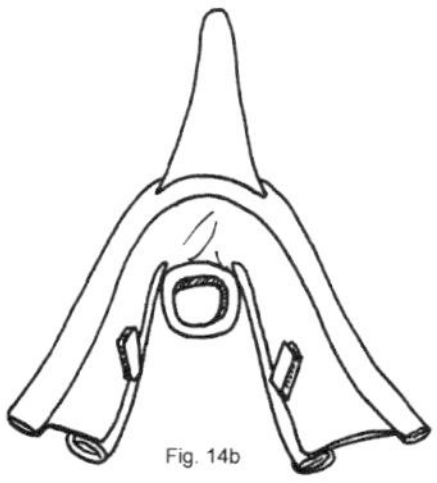
Fig. 14b

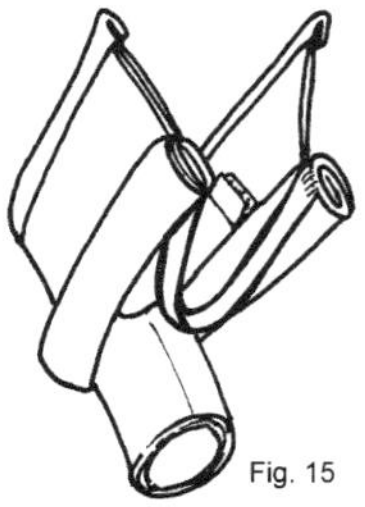
Fig. 15

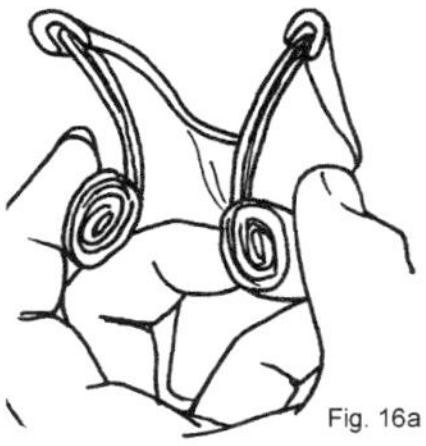
Fig. 16a

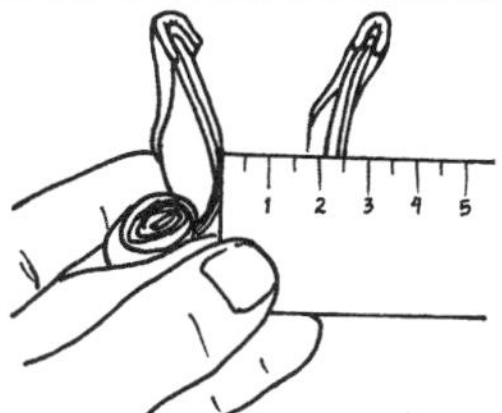

Fig. 16b

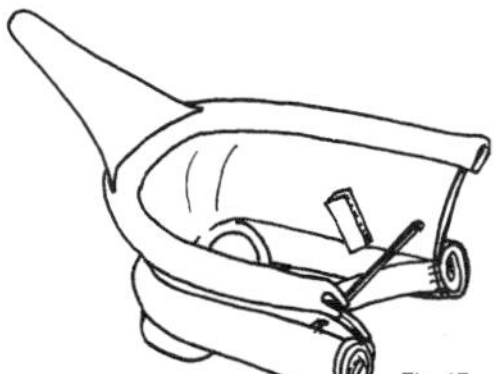
Fig. 17

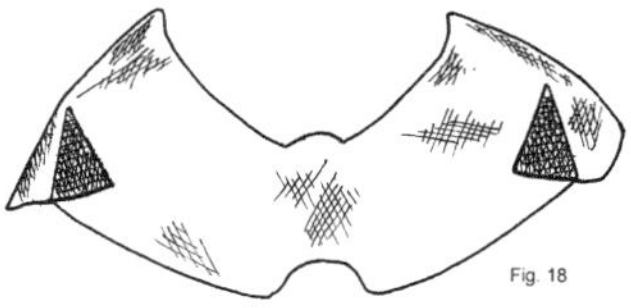
Fig. 18

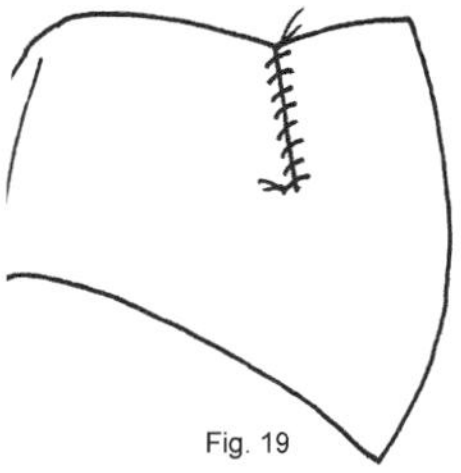
Fig. 19

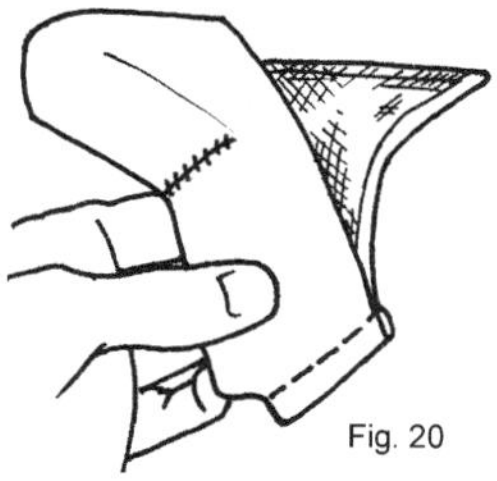
Fig. 20

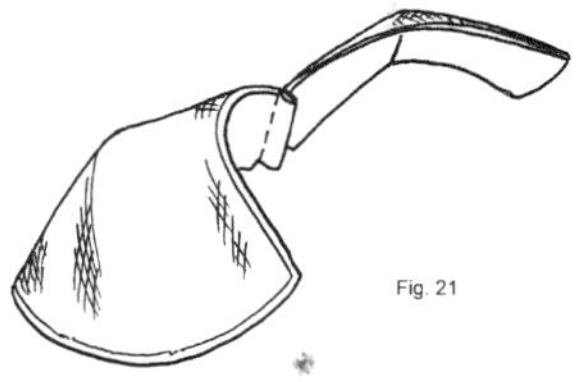
Fig. 21

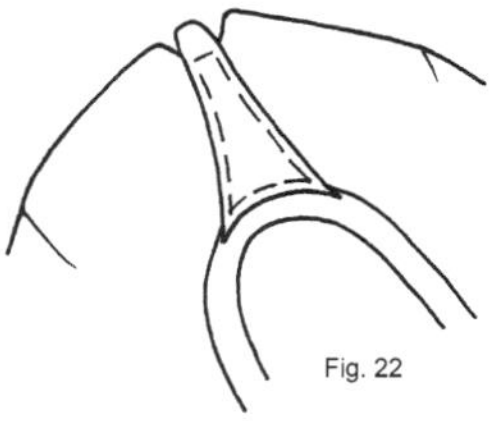
Fig. 22

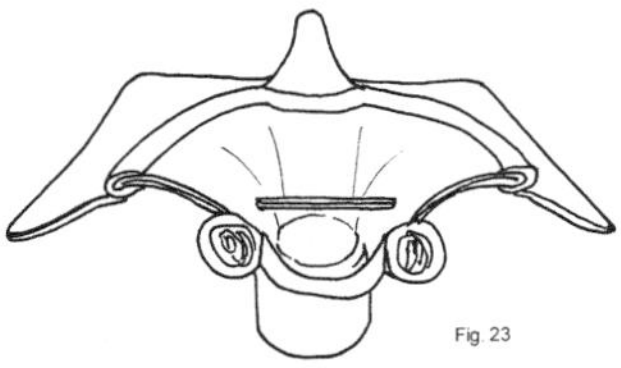
Fig 23

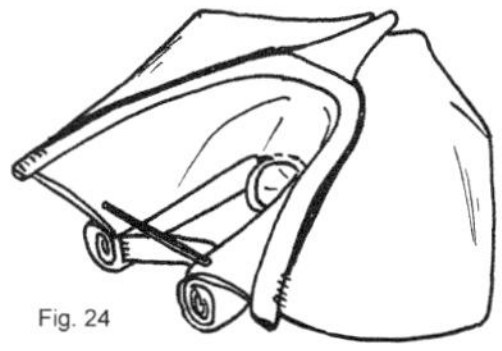
Fig. 24

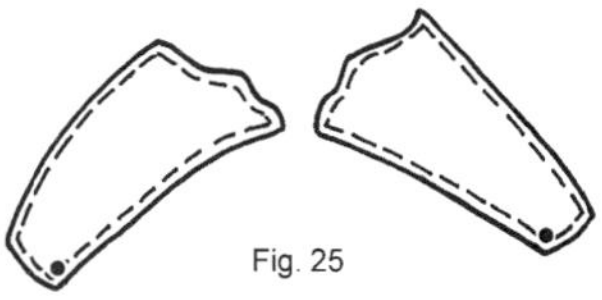
Fig. 25

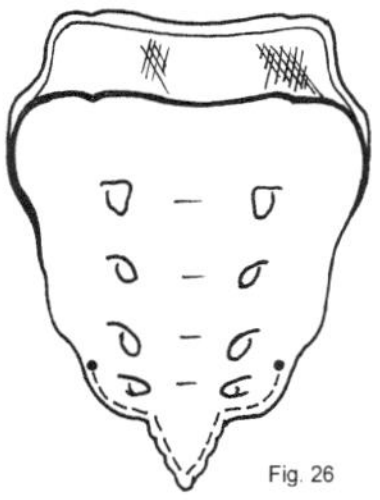
Fig. 26

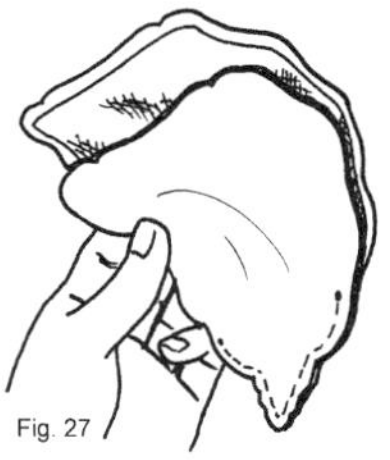
Fig. 27

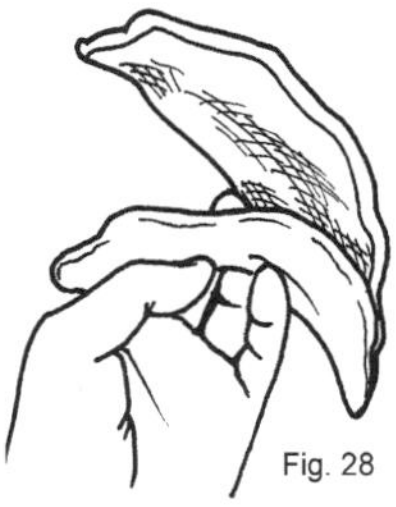
Fig. 28

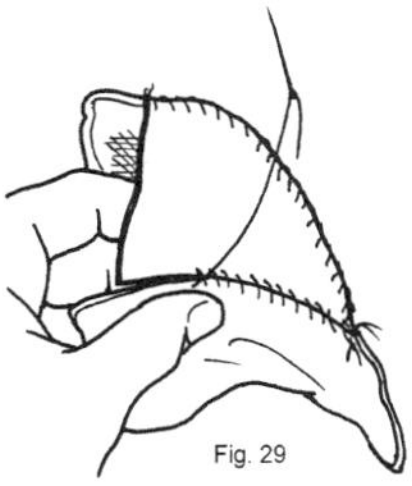
Fig. 29

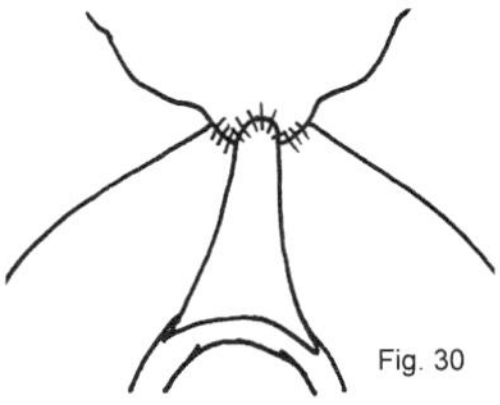
Fig. 30

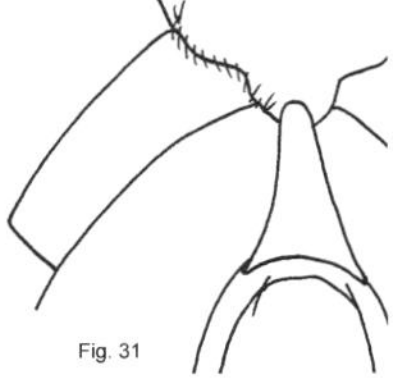
Fig. 31

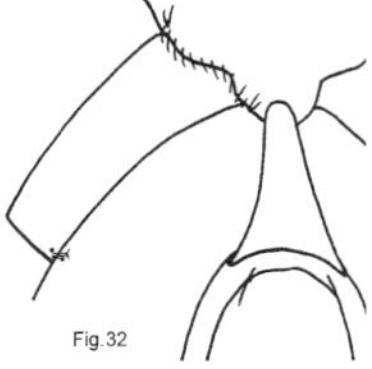
Fig.32

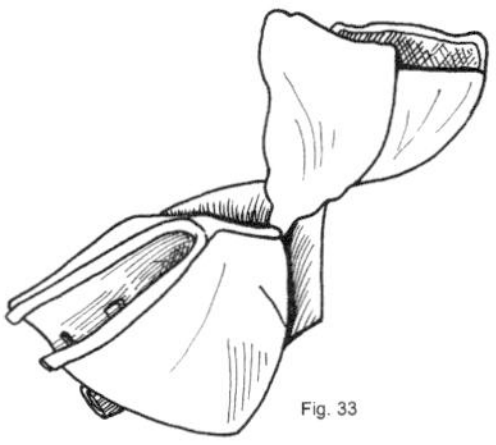
Fig. 33

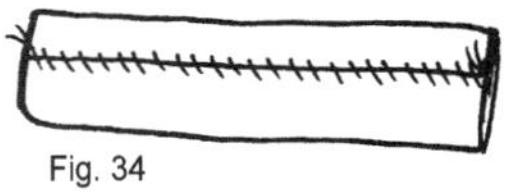
Fig. 34

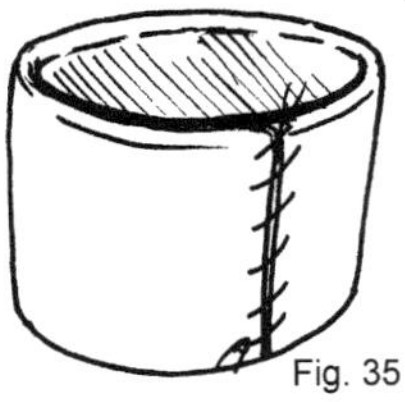
Fig. 35

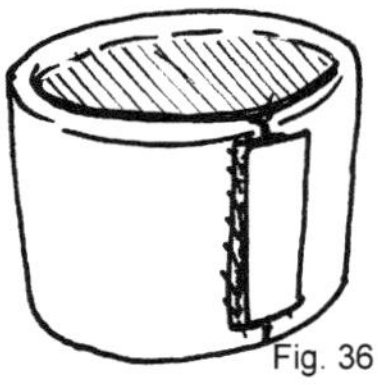
Fig. 36

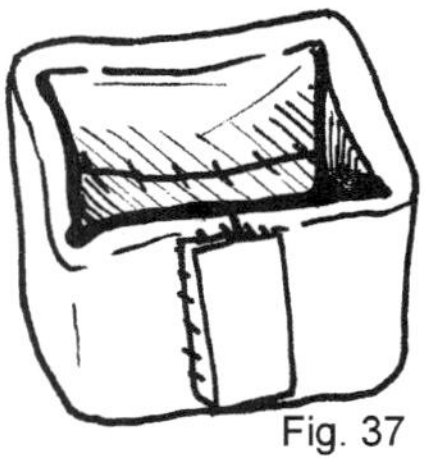
Fig. 37

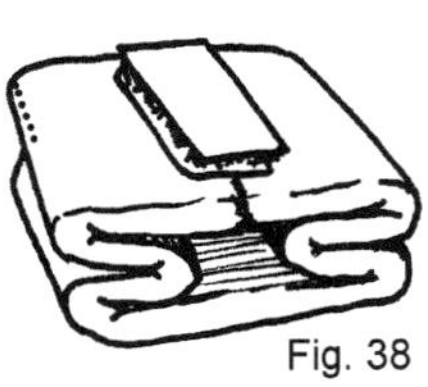
Fig. 38

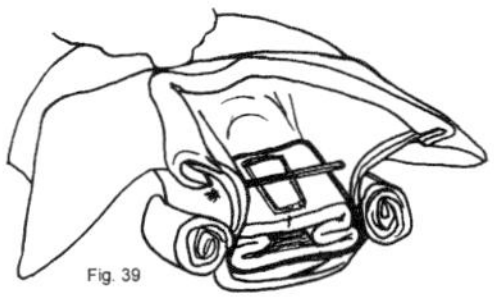
Fig. 39

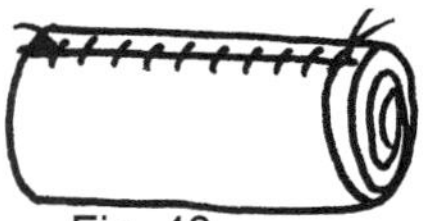
Fig. 40

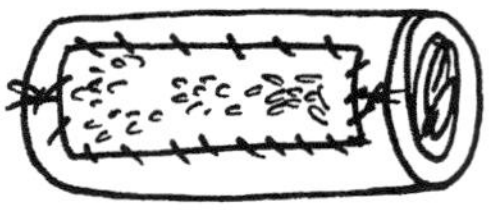
Fig. 41

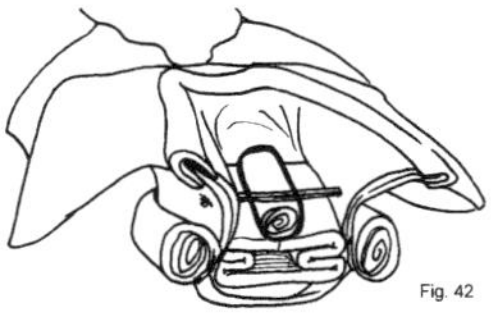
Fig. 42

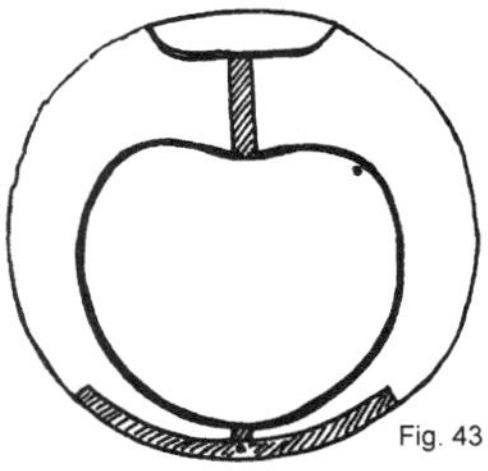
Fig. 43

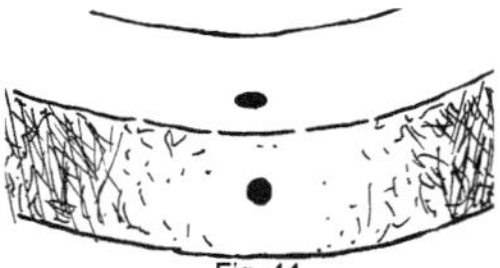
Fig. 44

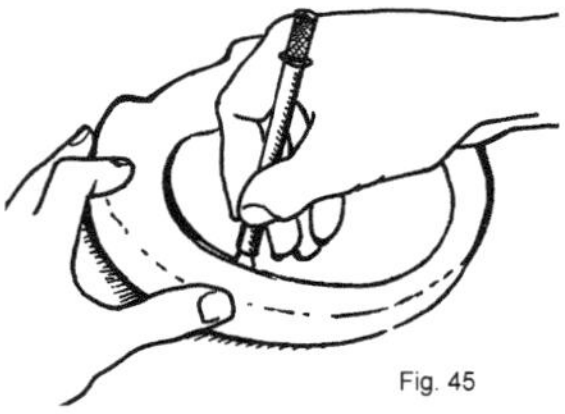
Fig. 45

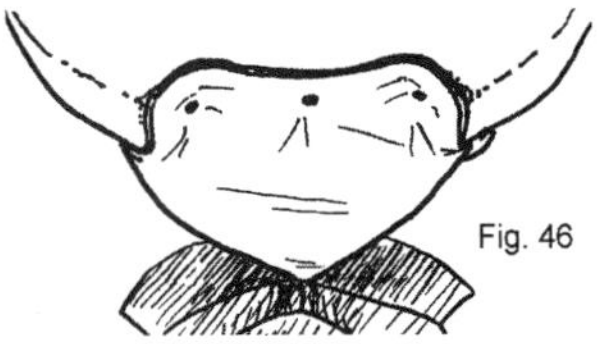
Fig. 46

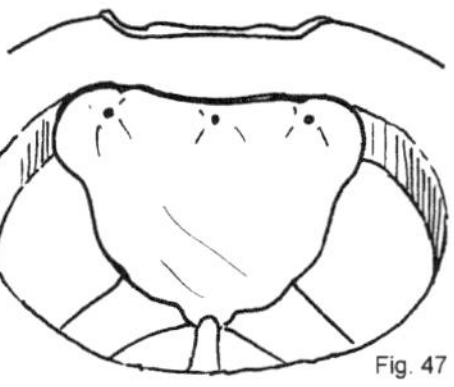
Fig. 47

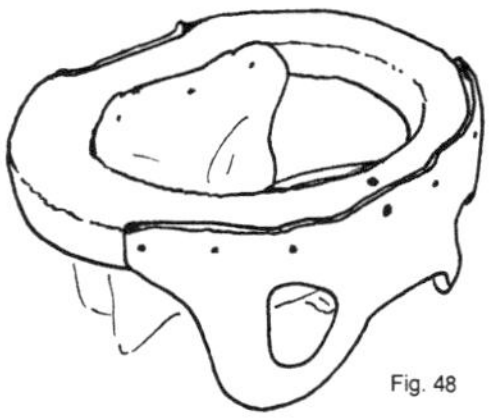
Fig. 48

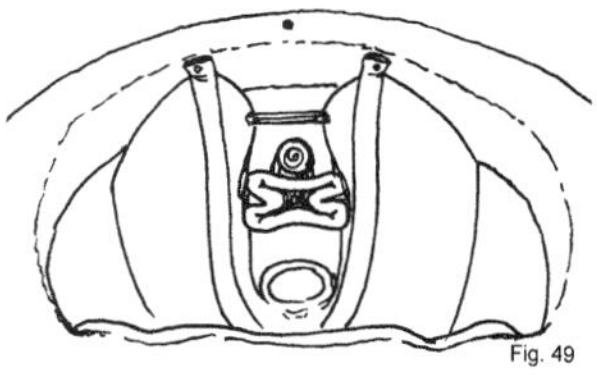
Fig. 49

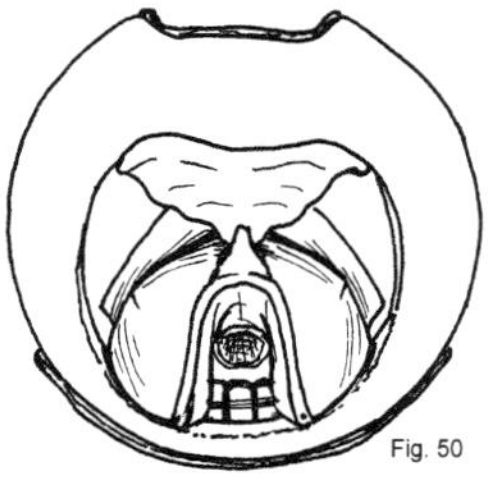
Fig. 50

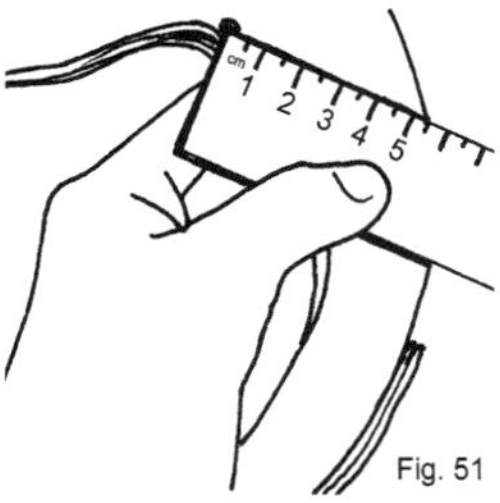

Fig. 51

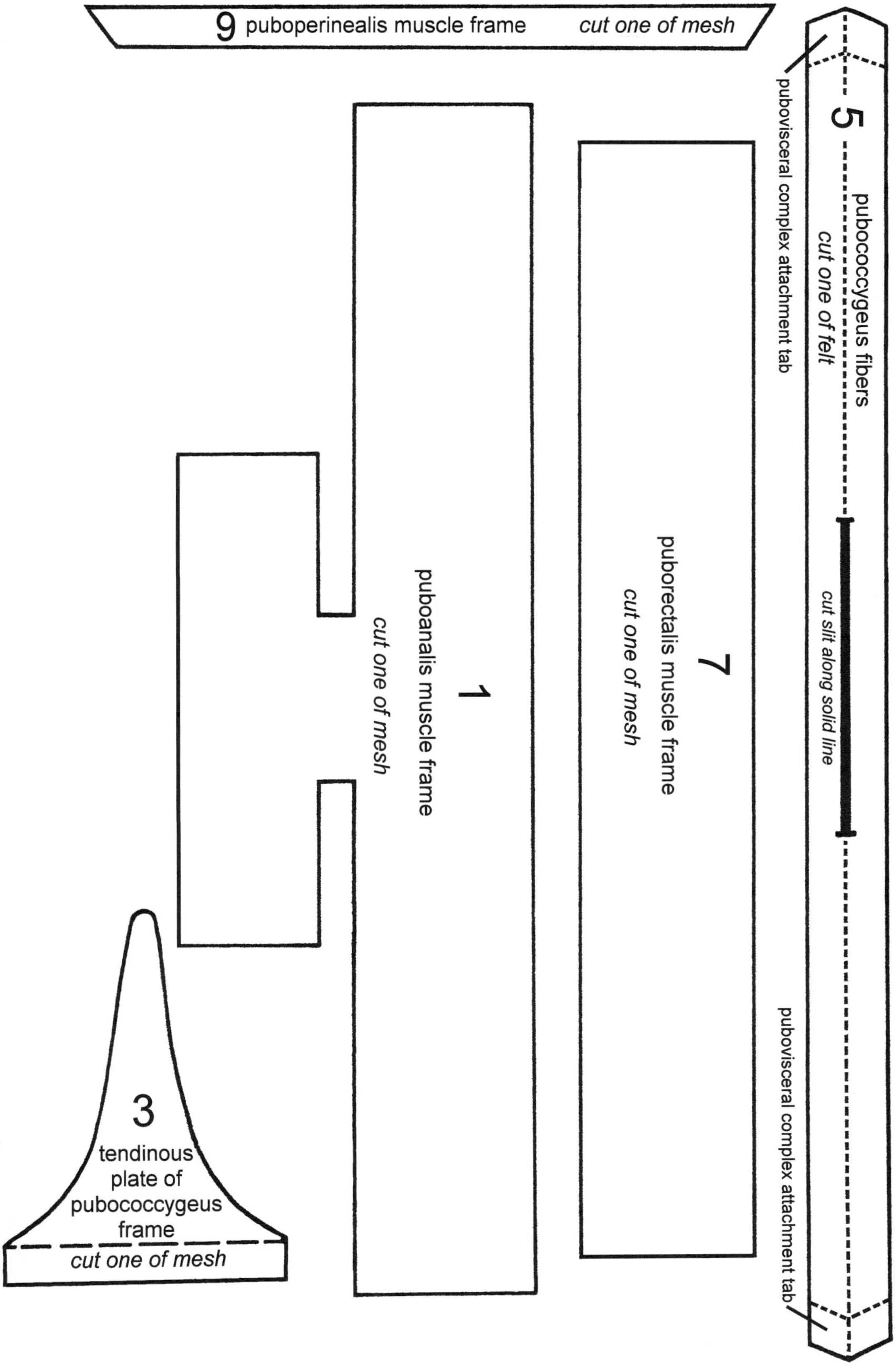
9 puboperinealis muscle frame
cut one of mesh
5 pubococcygeus fibers
cut one of felt
pubovisceral complex attachment tab
cut slit along solid line
pubovisceral complex attachment tab
7 puborectalis muscle frame
cut one of mesh
1 puboanalis muscle frame
cut one of mesh
3 tendinous plate of pubococcygeus frame
cut one of mesh

21

yoni canal frame

cut one of mesh

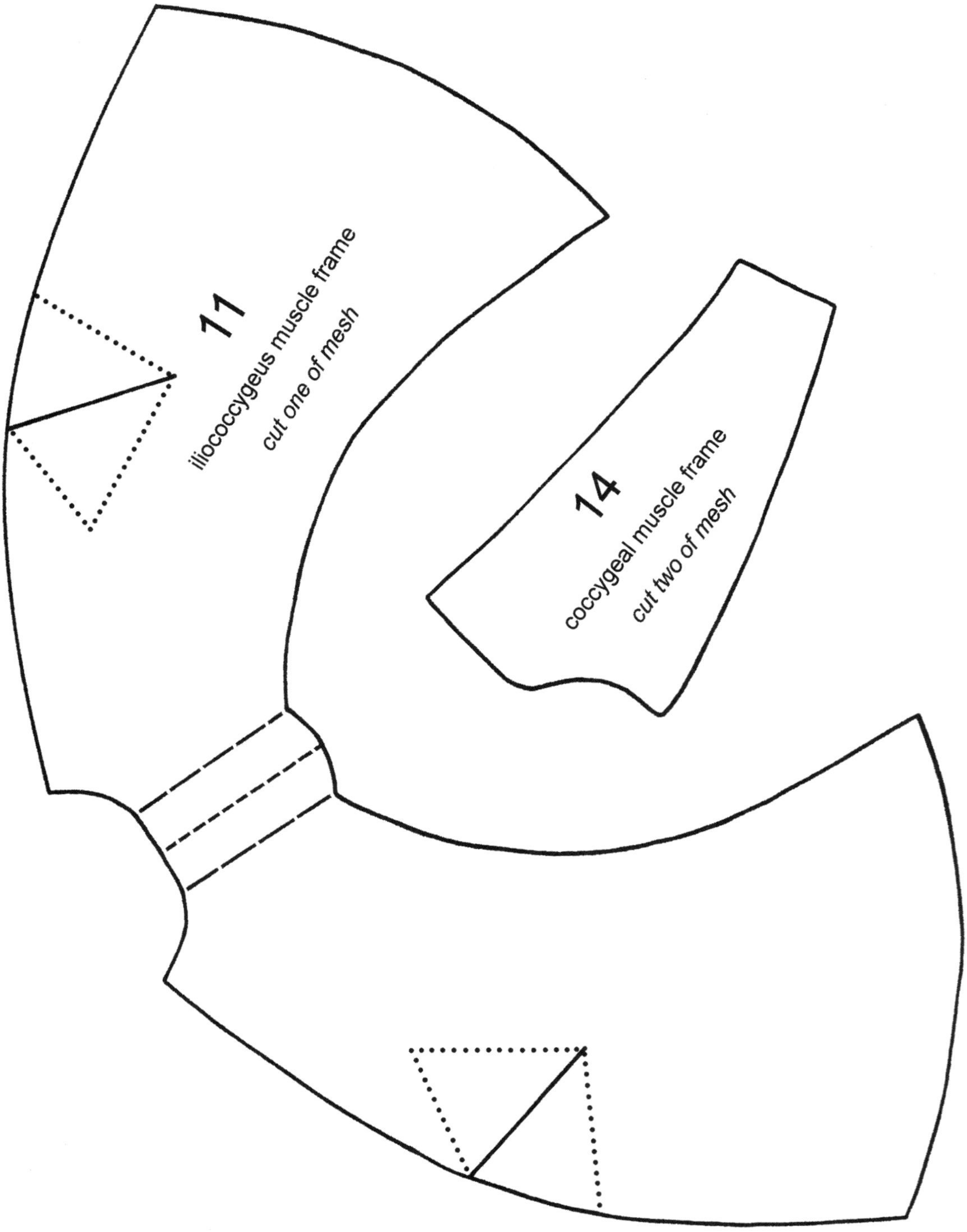

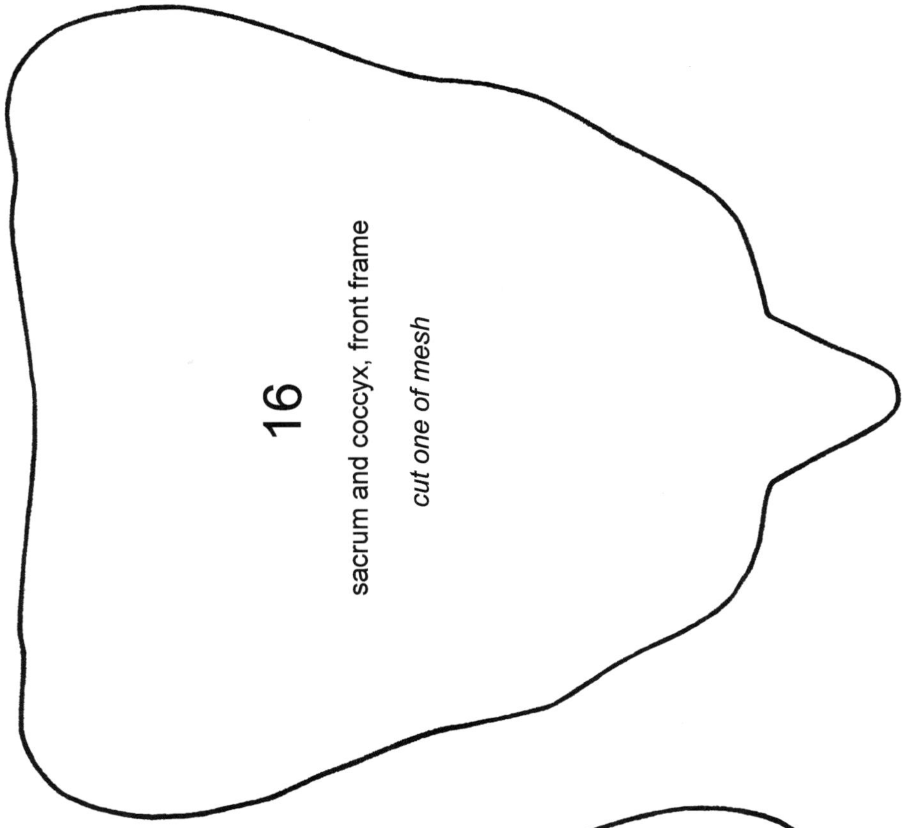
16
sacrum and coccyx, front frame
cut one of mesh

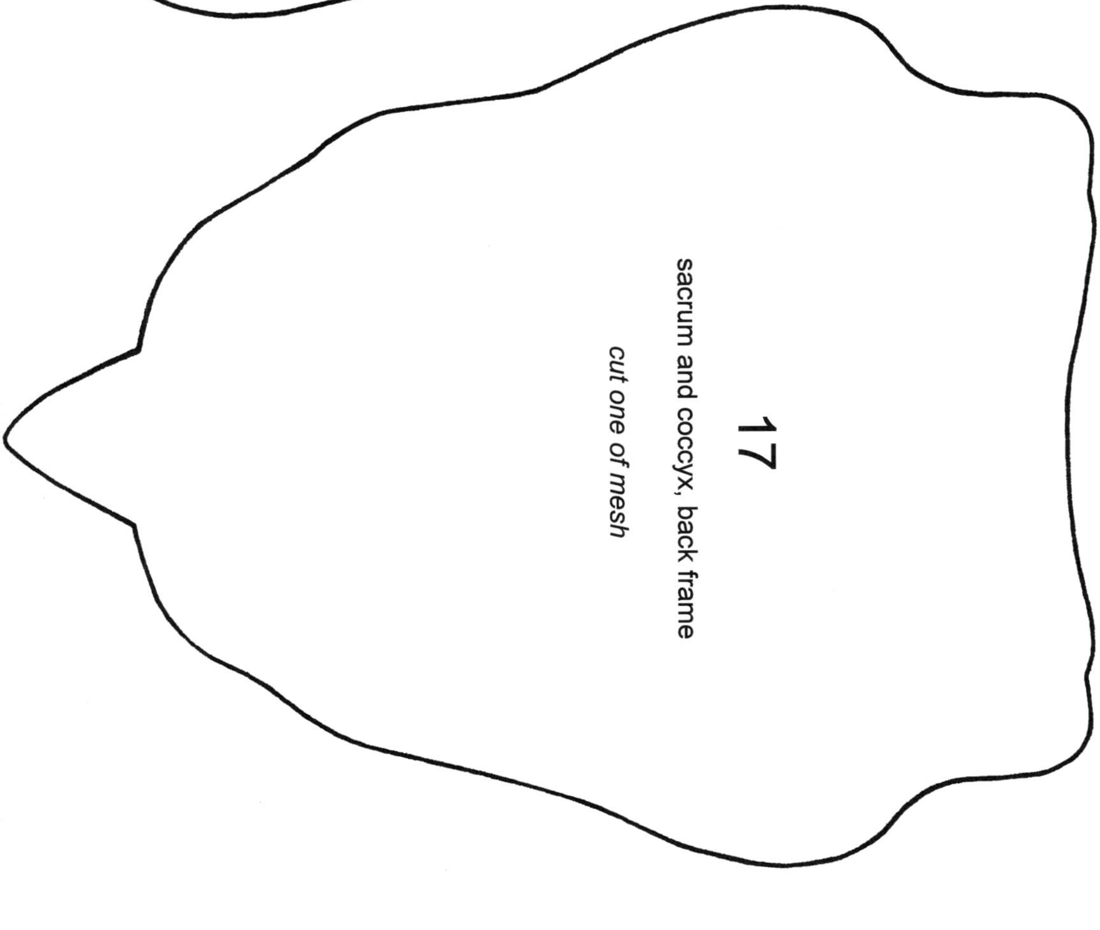
17
sacrum and coccyx, back frame
cut one of mesh

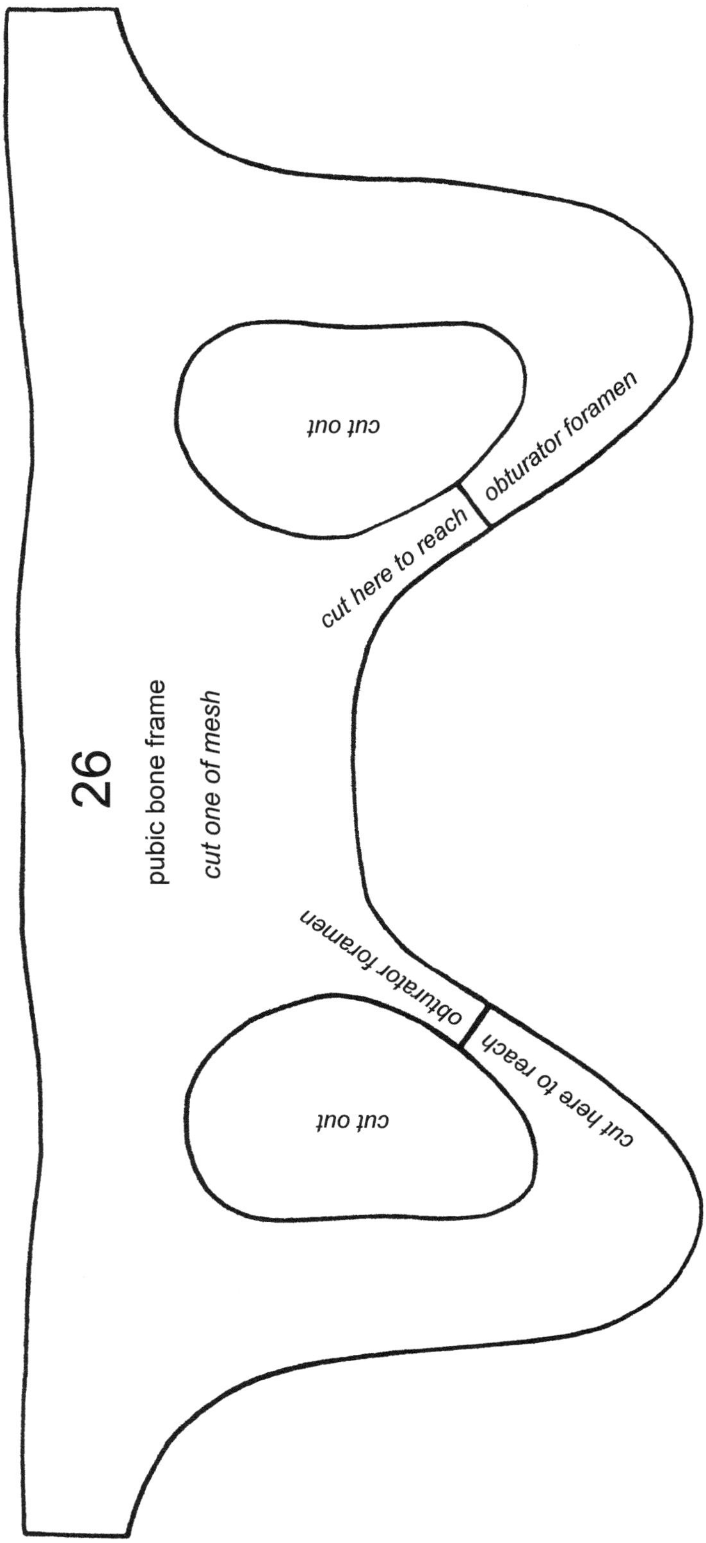
26
pubic bone frame
cut one of mesh
cut out
cut here to reach
obturator foramen
obturator foramen
cut here to reach
cut out

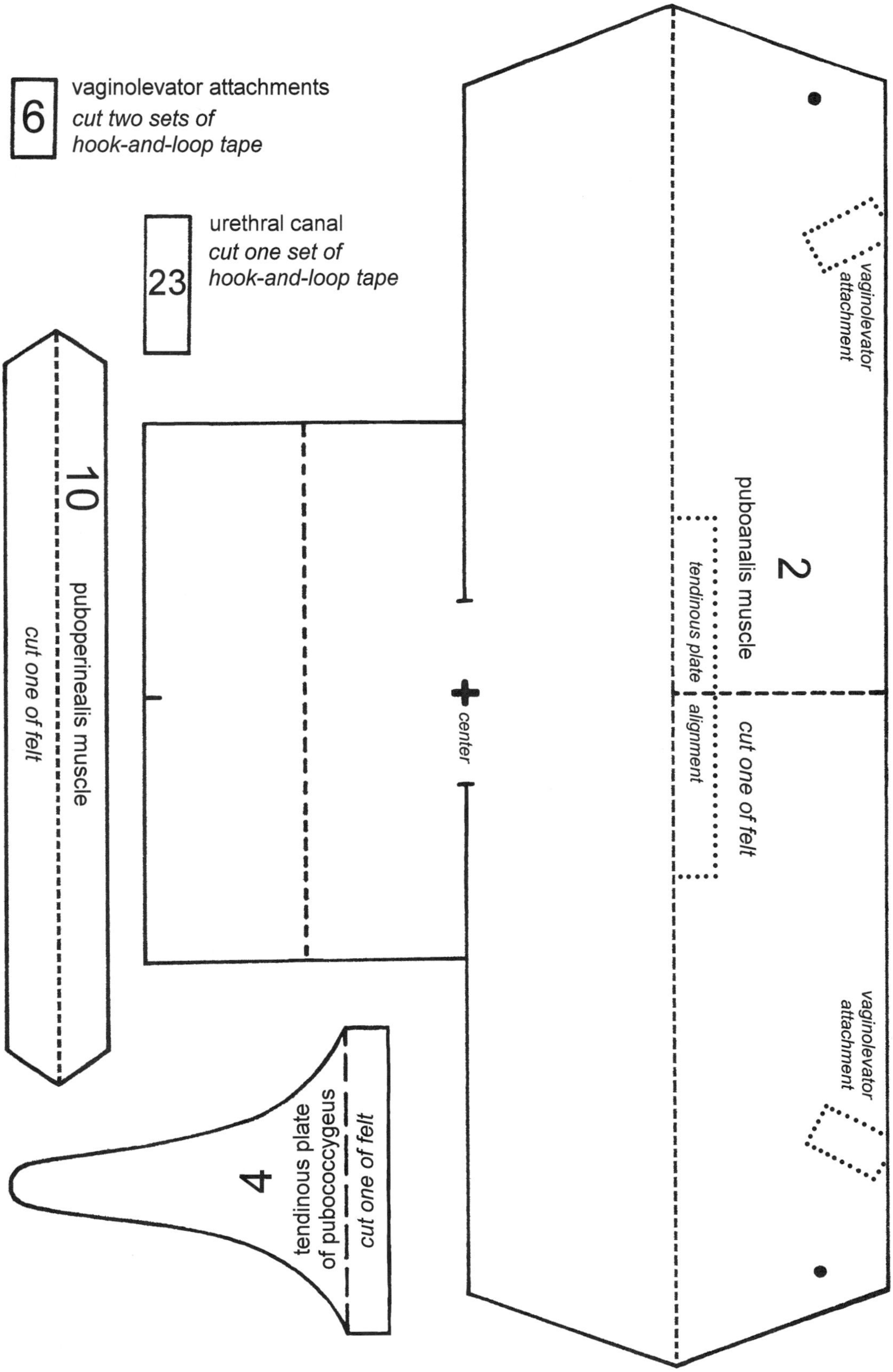
6
vaginolevator attachments
cut two sets of
hook-and-loop tape
23
urethral canal
cut one set of
hook-and-loop tape
10
puboperinealis muscle
cut one of felt
4
tendinous plate
of pubococcygeus
cut one of felt
center
2
puboanalis muscle
cut one of felt
tendinous plate
alignment
vaginolevator
attachment
vaginolevator
attachment

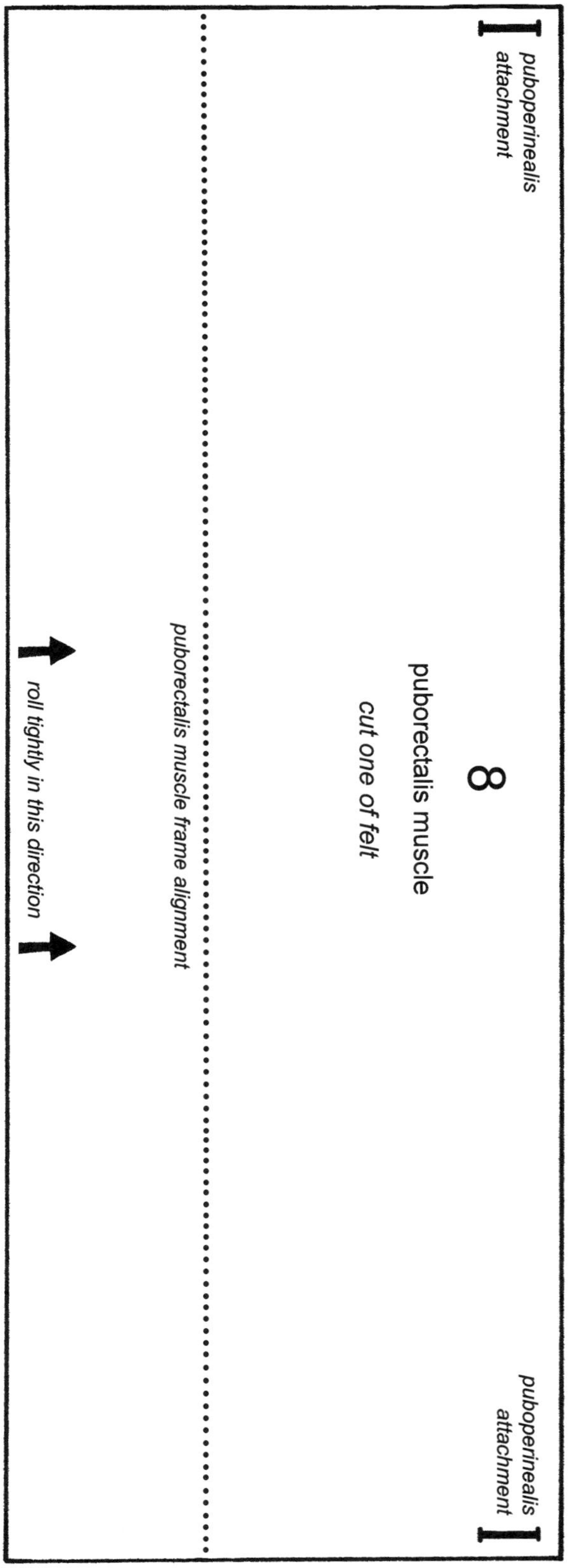
puboperinealis attachment
8
puborectalis muscle
cut one of felt
puborectalis muscle frame alignment
roll tightly in this direction
puboperinealis attachment

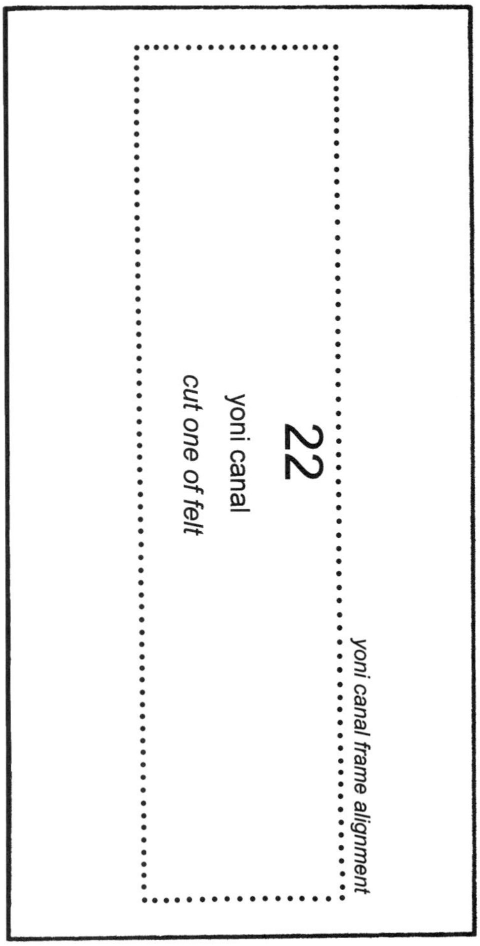
22
yoni canal
cut one of felt
yoni canal frame alignment

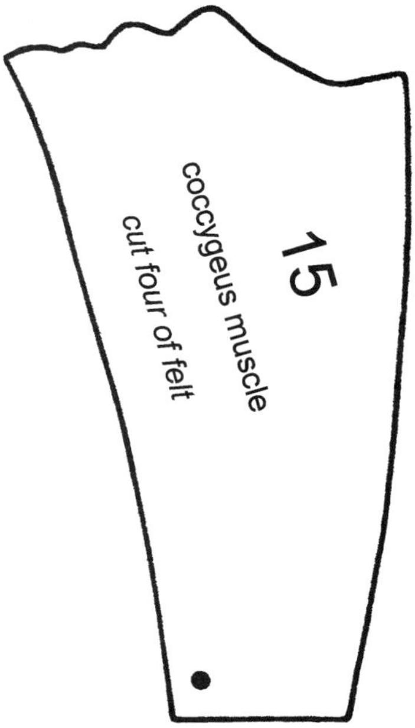
15
coccygeus muscle
cut four of felt

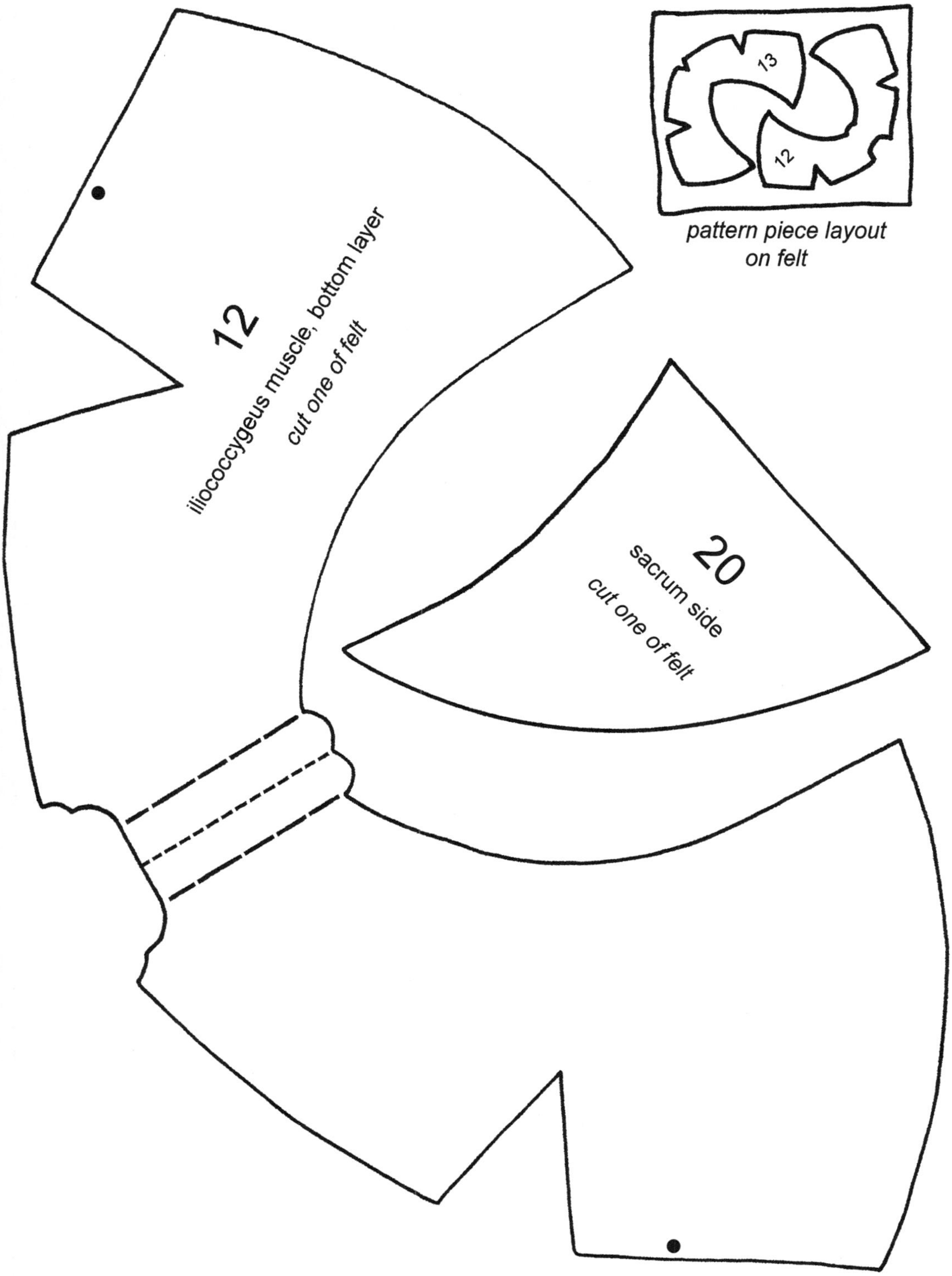

pattern piece layout on felt

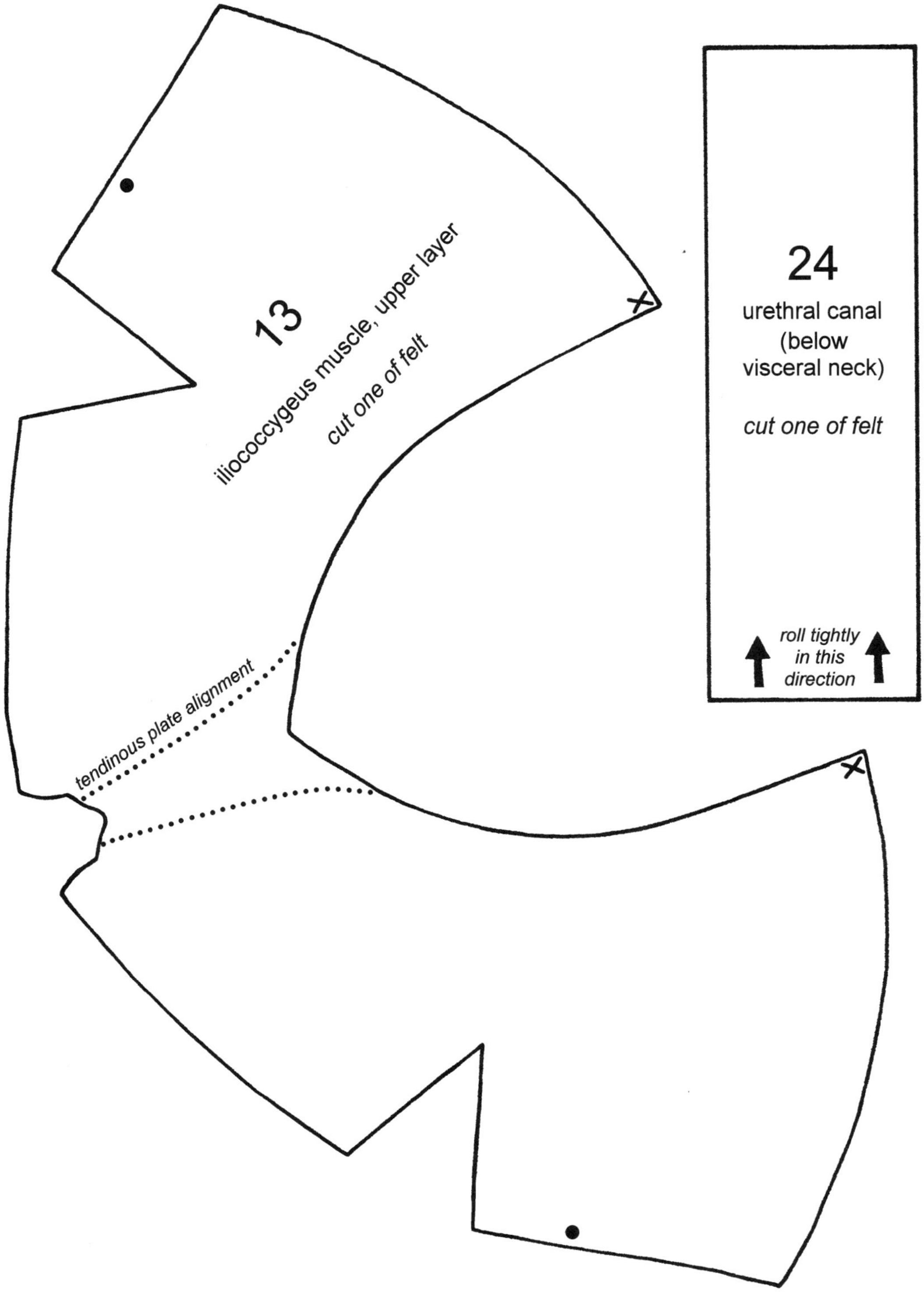
13
iliococcygeus muscle, upper layer
cut one of felt
tendinous plate alignment
24
urethral canal
(below
visceral neck)
cut one of felt
roll tightly
in this
direction

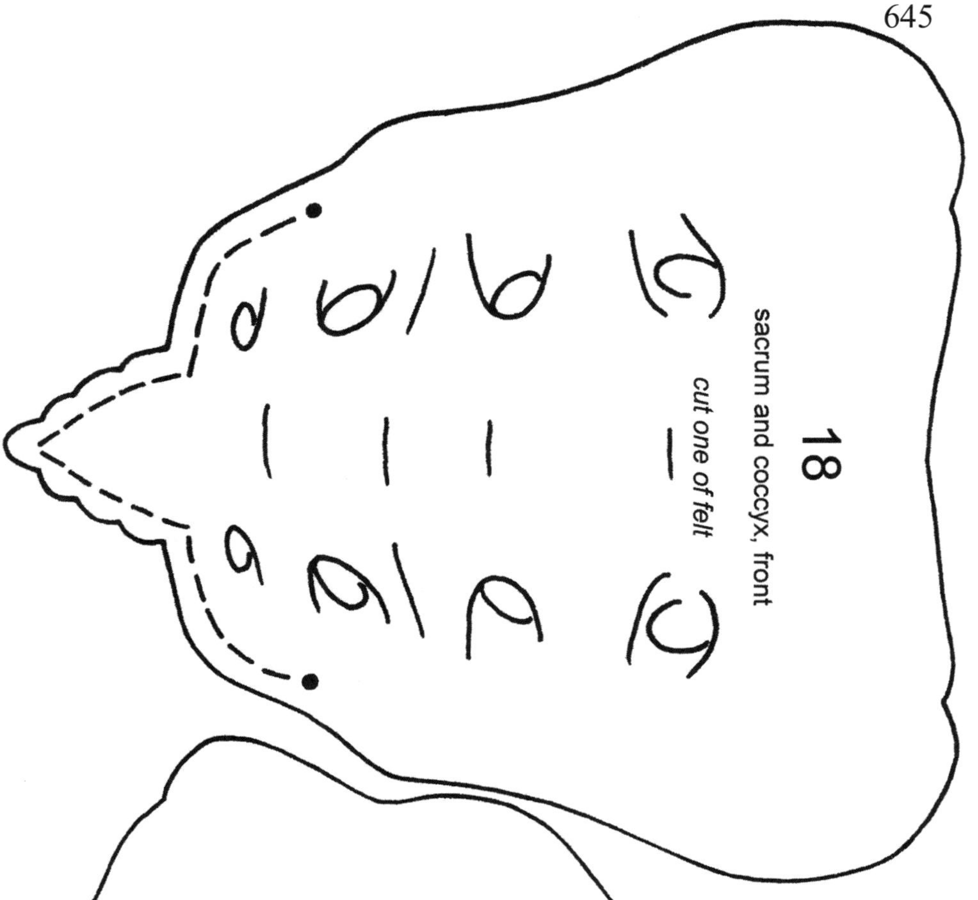
18
sacrum and coccyx, front
cut one of felt

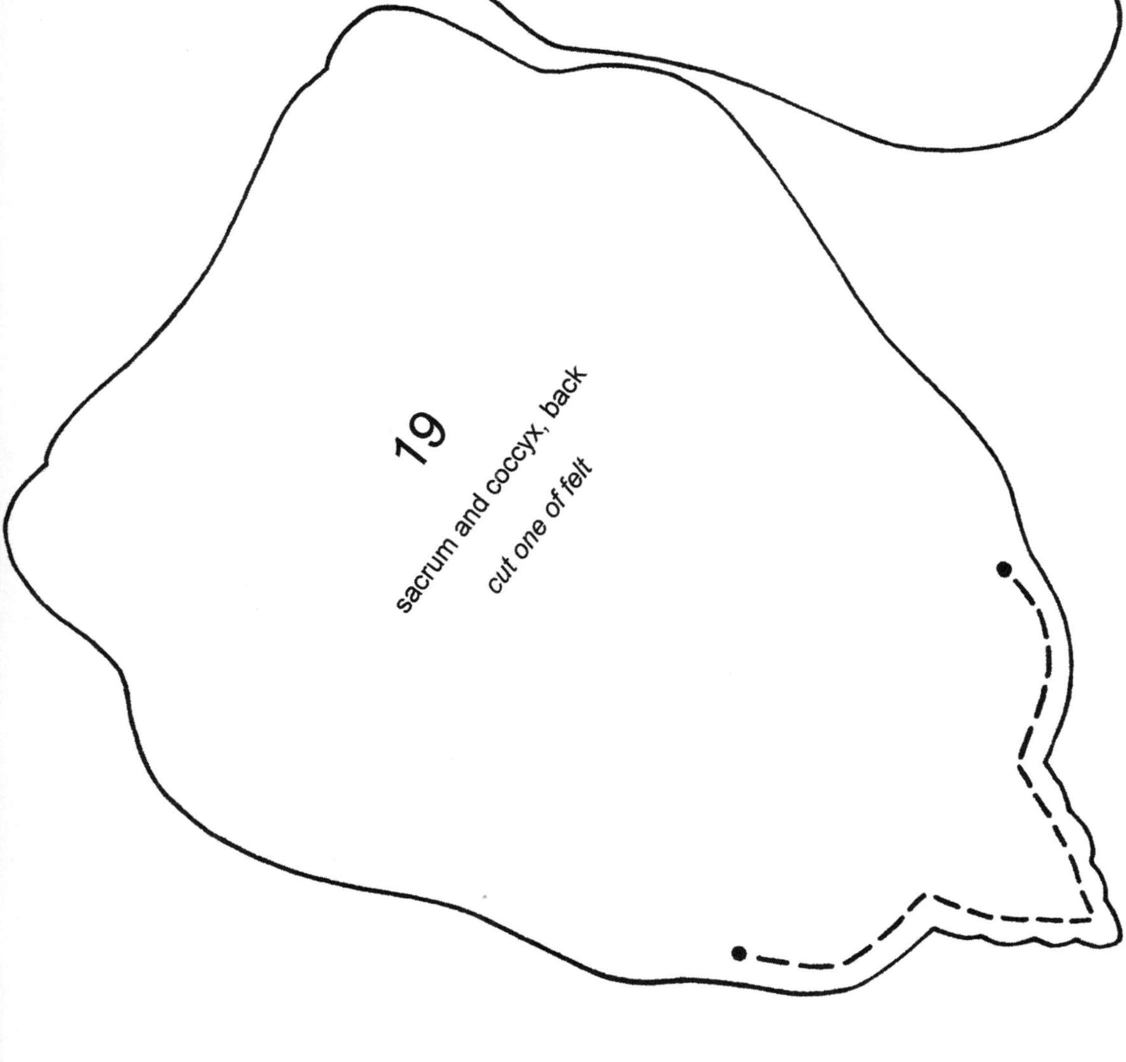
19
sacrum and coccyx, back
cut one of felt

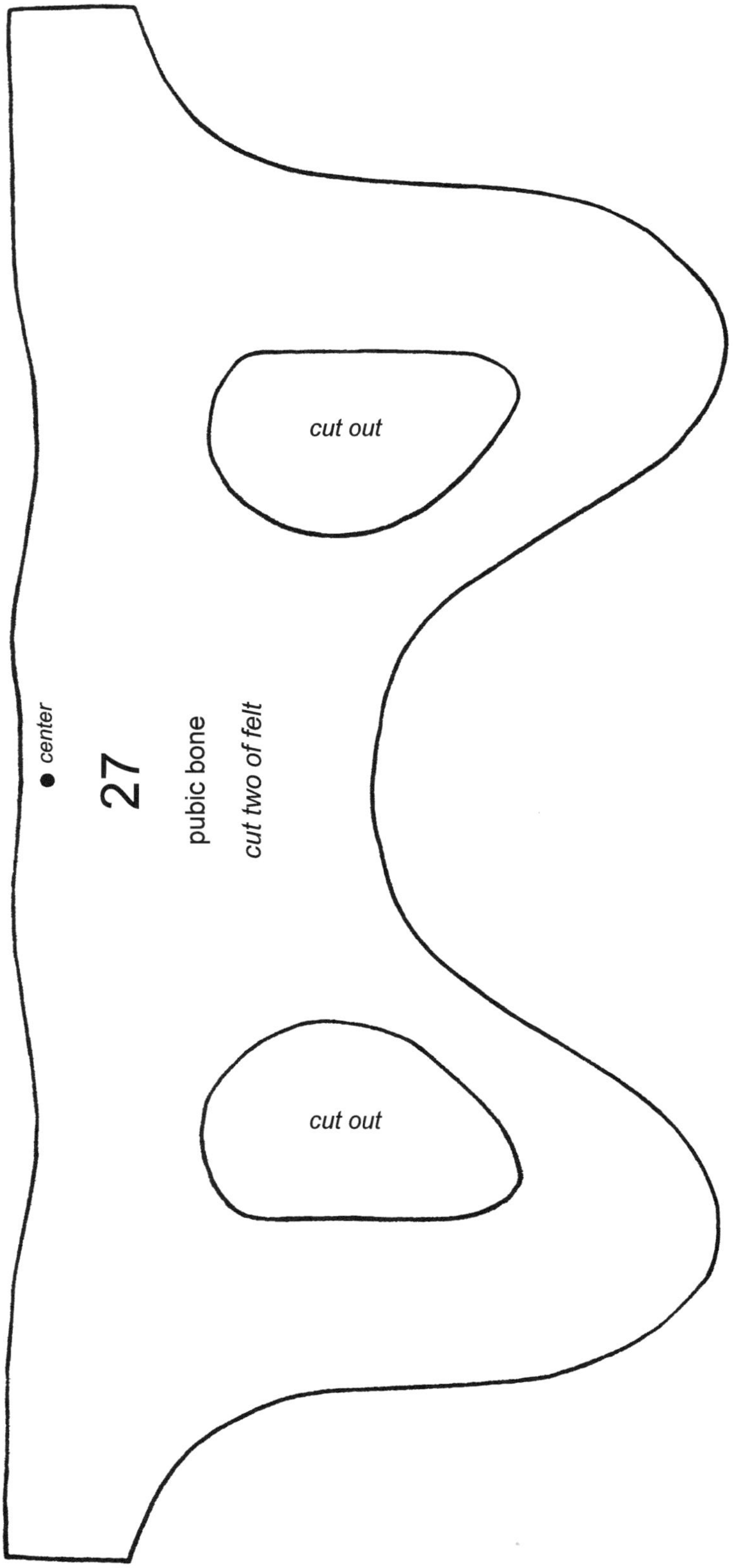
cut out
center
27
pubic bone
cut two of felt
cut out

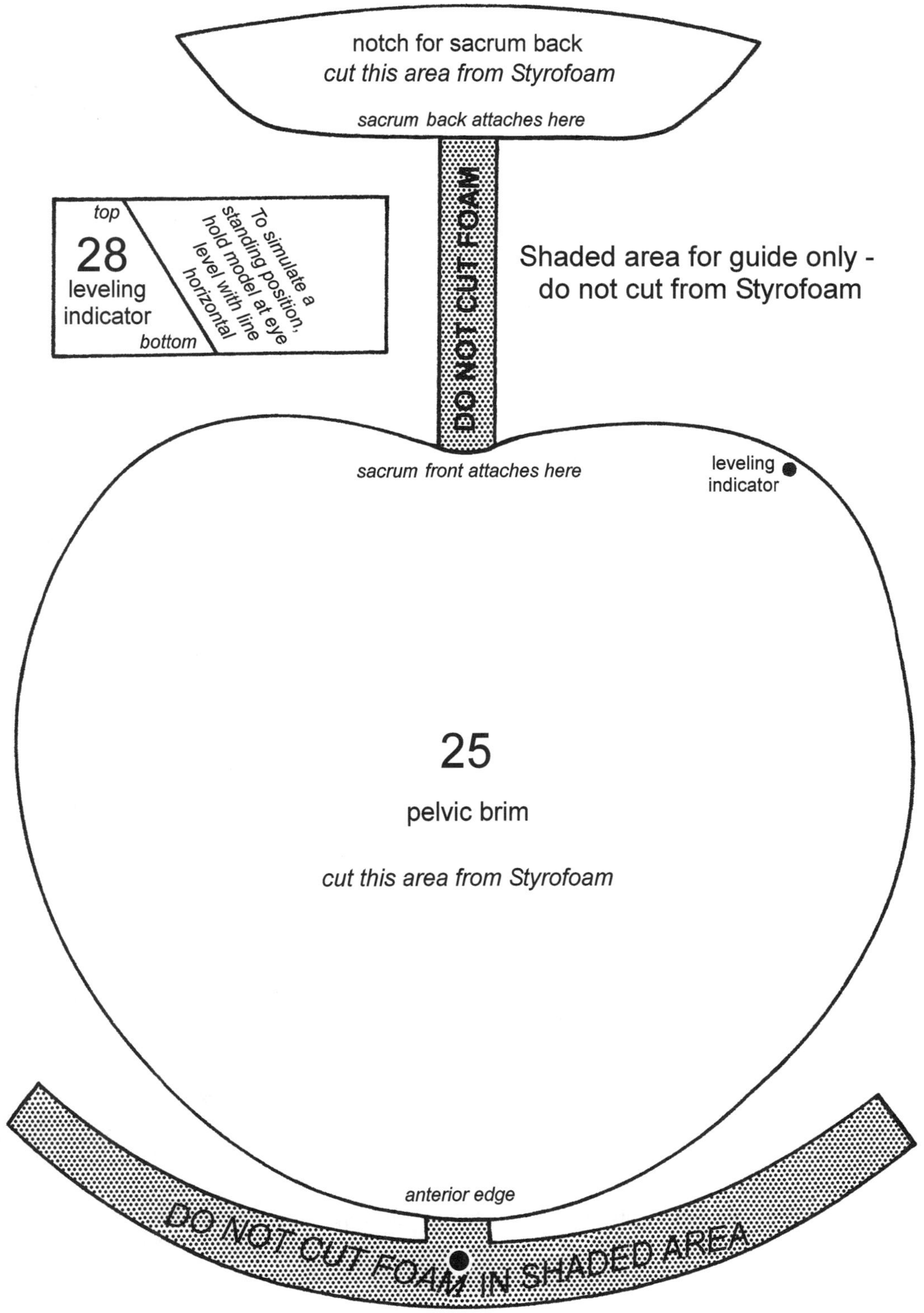
notch for sacrum back
cut this area from Styrofoam
sacrum back attaches here
DO NOT CUT FOAM
Shaded area for guide only - do not cut from Styrofoam
top
28
leveling indicator
bottom
To simulate a standing position, hold model at eye level with line horizontal
sacrum front attaches here
leveling indicator
25
pelvic brim
cut this area from Styrofoam
anterior edge
DO NOT CUT FOAM IN SHADED AREA

PRACTICE MATERIALS

As of this printing, the suturing video is still being reincarnated as an updated DVD. When it is published, an instruction manual will be included on the disc as a PDF file. In the meantime, if you want to practice suturing, you will need to gather together certain materials and equipment and follow along in the book. You will need:

- Indelible Magic markers in at least 2 colors--pink and red (to demarche tissue layers in foam)
- New single-edged razor blades (to cut foam and meat)
- Gloves (because you need to learn wearing gloves, and chicken may carry salmonella. Pigs may carry trichinosis.)
- Underpads (to use with raw meat)
- Cotton string to color or two colors of cording of some kind to use for knot tying practice (nylon string does not take color easily, and it tends to rub off)
- A 4" by 4" board with a small hook in the center for practicing knots
- Foam blocks to make 3-dimensional vaginal models. A wedge can be cut from the edge of the block that will approximate the shape of a tear the extends into the yoni floor and down the perineum. Study the cross section of a tear on page 470.
- Tape measure or small ruler (inches and centimeters) to space stitches
- Meat (optional): raw chicken skin can be used to practice labial and skin tag repair. Raw pigs feet can also be used, as pig skin is thin (for an animal), making it good for practice.
- Needle holder and small scissors
- ½ inch thick upholstery cording, paper surgical skin tape, and gauze can be used to make a sphincter model like the ones you see on the tape. Cover the end of the cording with one layer of gauze, then wrap a single layer of skin tape around (not over) the end and insert into a hole you have made in the foam. This was the best artificial sphincter I could devise that still allowed needle penetration. Even so, the sphincter is easier to pass a needle through than this model.
- Suturing needles and suture for practice. These can be either suture that you would ordinarily use for repair (nice for practice, but a very expensive proposition financially), or you can purchase 3-0 and 4-0 silk on spools and threadable needles of different sizes. This will give you a lot of practice material for relatively little money.

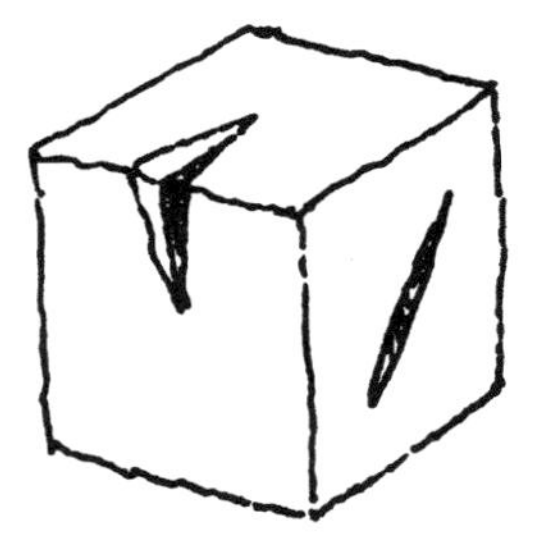

This block has a slit with a narrow wedge removed cut in the right side to practice basic stitches and a wedge cut from the edge to practice perineal repair.

Miami Medical carries threadable needles by Miltex but they do not carry silk suture on spools. You will need regular half-circle taper point surgeon's needles in sizes 6, 14 and 16 or17 (Miltex product code: MS-192A). Check www.miami-med.com, Miltex instruments, surgical needles. AliMed also carries these same Miltex needles, as well as spools of silk suture. Check their website at www.alimed.com. In the "Product finder" bar enter the code numbers given in the table below to locate these items on their website. They said they were happy to sell to midwives and their minimum order is only $25.00.

ITEM	SIZE/QUANTITY	ALIMED PRODUCT CODE
Silk suture	4-0, 100 yard spool	98SUT24-3
Silk suture	3-0, 100 yard spool	98SUT24-4
Silk suture	2-0, 100 yard spool	98SUT24-5
Regular surgeon's needle with eye (12 to a pack)	12 ½ circle, taper point–size 6 (equivalent to a CT-1)	98NES2-20
Regular surgeon's needle with eye (12 to a pack)	½ circle, taper point–size 14 (equivalent to a CT-3)	98NES2-24
Regular surgeon's needle with eye (12 to a pack)	12 ½ circle, taper point–size 16 (a little bigger than a PS-4)	98NES2-25

If you have connections with anyone who works in a hospital delivery or operating room, they may be able to bring you outdated or discarded non-sterile suture, which is great to use for practice, *if* you can get packets of suture with the proper sized needles. You need to be practicing with material similar to what you will actually be using. Obtaining the right sizes can be difficult if you are using leftovers from the operating room. This is why threadable needles are such a great alternative. If you are given partially opened packets of suture (that is, the sterile outer cover is removed but the foil is still intact) from an operating room, soak them in alcohol for 1 hour before storage.

With these materials and supplies, you can construct a variety of models and practice almost all the techniques presented.

I suggest trying to arrange some uninterrupted time for yourself or your study group. Have your materials at hand and something (a table, TV tray, cookie sheet, or breakfast-in-bed tray) on which to work. If you establish a time for your study group to get together and practice, you are more likely to get to it, and you will have each other's support and brain power to help you along.

I recommend breaking up your studies into several sessions, such as knot tying, internal exams on each other to learn anatomy, basic stitches, etc.. That way you will learn more and have more group practice before practicing on your own, as well as avoid being overwhelmed.

Sources of Suture and Other Materials

Anatomical Chart Co. Walters Flower Health, PO Box 1600, Hagerstown, MD, 21741-1600; 800-621-7500 (www.anatomical.com). Suppliers of the latex muscle models with plastic pelvis used for the anatomy lesson in the DVD, which is produced by Educational and Scientific Products, West Sussex, England.

Arista Surgical Supply, Alimed, Inc. 297 High St., Dedman, MA 02026. 800-223-1984. Arista has a full line of reasonably priced surgical instruments and other equipment.

Cascade Healthcare Products and **Moonflower Birthing and Herbal Supply**, 1826 NW 18th Ave., Portland, OR 97209. 800-443-9942; (www.1cascade.com). They carry suture, equipment, textbooks and numerous in vitro diagnostic tests.

To obtain a copy of **Caring for Women with Circumcision**, by Dr. Nahid Toubia, call the National Women's Health Information Center's toll-free referral service at 1-800-994-WOMAN or 1-888-220-5446, TDD. You may also contact RAINBO for this publication and as well as resources on community FGC education programs and materials.

deBy Birth Support, Seacoast Midwifery Services LLC, PO Box 381, Barrington, NH 03825. Cillia Bannenberg 603-332-7766; (www.birthchair.net). Cost $320.00 + $25.00 shipping and handling. See the web site for full details.

Eve's Garden, International, Ltd., 119 West 57th St., Suite 420, New York, NY 10019, (800) 848-3837. In New York (212) 757-8651. Carries battery operated aides and other devices that can be used to exercise the pelvic floor muscles.

Foam scraps can be found at many upholstery and fabric stores for little or no money. Inquire. Dense, fine grained foam is best.

Joy Chair, Artemis House, 7421 Meadowbrook Dr., Forth Worth, TX 76112.

A & A Medical/Rocket USA, Alpharetta, GA 800-424-1234. They stock a wide variety of ob/gyn instruments. They can also obtain left-handed surgical scissors in any style for about the same price as right-handed scissors, when ordered in quantities of four to six dozen.

The Sourcebook of Medical Illustrations, by Peter Cull, Parthenon Pub. Group, Park Ridge, NJ, 1990. This book is provides copyright-free illustrations which may be used and modified at the discretion of the user.

Snowden-Pencer Surgical Instruments Inc., 2058 Kilman Dr., Tucker, GA 30084, Customer Service in US and CA 800-843-8600. Source of excellent quality needle holders including all styles in left-handed (reverse ratchet) models.

Standard Process Labs., Inc., P.O. Box 652, Milwaukee, WI 53201, (800) 588-8740. Source for Collinsonia Root tablets. They sell only through practitioners that they authorize as distributors (usually chiropractors and naturopaths). They will consider independent midwives on an individual basis. Inquire about a service representative in your area.

(See chapters on Homeopathy and Herbal Medicine for relevant sources.)

INDEX